D1389760

# The
# Encyclopedia of
# Genetic Disorders and
# Birth Defects

## James Wynbrandt and
## Mark D. Ludman, M.D.

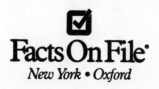

**Facts On File**
*New York • Oxford*

This book has been designed to be a valuable general information resource. However, it is not intended for use in diagnosis, treatment or for any other medical application. Questions regarding these aspects of genetic disorders and birth defects should be directed to appropriate medical authorities. Neither the authors, publisher nor any other party who has been involved in the preparation or publication of this work warrants that the information contained herein is in every respect accurate and complete.

**The Encyclopedia of Genetic Disorders and Birth Defects**

Copyright © 1991 by James Wynbrandt

Facts On File, Inc.          Facts On File Limited
460 Park Avenue South        Collins Street
New York NY 10016            Oxford OX4 1XJ
USA                          United Kingdom

**Library of Congress Cataloging-in-Publication Data**
Wynbrandt, James.
    The encyclopedia of genetic disorders and birth defects / by James
Wynbrandt & Mark D. Ludman.
        p. cm.
    Includes bibliographical references.
    ISBN 0-8160-1926-6
    1. Genetic disorders—Dictionaries. 2. Abnormalities, Human—
Dictionaries. I. Ludman, Mark D. II. Title.
RB155.5.W96 1990
616'.042'03—dc20 89-48278

British CIP data available on request from Facts On File.

Facts On File books are available at special discounts when purchased in bulk quantities for
businesses, associations, institutions or sales promotions. Please contact the Special Sales Department
of our New York office at 212/683-2244 (dial 800/322-8755 except in NY, AK, or HI).

Composition by Facts On File, Inc.
Manufactured by R. R. Donnelley
Printed in the United States of America

10 9 8 7 6 5 4 3 2 1

This book is printed on acid-free paper.

# Contents

# Preface

Genetic disorders and birth defects comprise a vast galaxy of anomalous conditions and exert an extraordinary impact on the human population. Attempting even a partial catalog of them is daunting, indeed. More than 4,300 "single gene" disorders have been reported, and are estimated to affect 1% of the population. The number of "multifactorial" disorders, those resulting from a combination of genes, is considered much greater. If late onset disorders are included, 60% of the population is thought to have a genetically influenced disease. Additionally, significant congenital anomalies, apparently unrelated to genetic influence, number in the thousands and are seen in approximately 2% to 3% of all live births.

We have included a little more than 600 entries in this encyclopedia, selected on the basis of the disorders' incidence and clinical and historical importance. We describe the condition, its prognosis, prevalence, mode of inheritance and the availability of carrier screening and prenatal diagnosis. For whom the condition is named and additional historical and anecdotal data are included where applicable and available. When known, the biochemical and molecular basis of the disorder is also given.

Entries for subjects and terminology important to genetic disorders and congenital anomalies are also included. Entry titles used within the text of other entries are in small capital letters the first time they appear, providing readers with numerous cross-references. However, we've attempted to make each entry stand alone, so that one can achieve a general understanding of a given topic without investigating additional entries. Resources to assist those seeking more information are also listed with many of the entries. These are mostly private organizations. The appendix contains an extensive listing of state, regional and federal government information resources. We urge readers to take advantage of these resources. Though entries were revised and updated through the final galley stage of this encyclopedia, rapid developments in the field of genetic and congenital anomalies add new knowledge to our understanding of this subject on an almost daily basis.

James Wynbrandt
Mark D. Ludman, M.D.

# Acknowledgments

We could not have created this encyclopedia without the help of many people and organizations. We wish to express our gratitude to them all, citing a few by name.

For their dedicated and tireless administrative assistance, we are deeply grateful to Gina Caimi and Deborah Hayes. For research and editorial assistance, heartfelt thanks to Don Sontup, Gayle Turim, Dina Stein, Gunnar Mengers, Betsy Hanson, Diann Peterson Trolle, Linda Smith, M.D., Michael Herring, Serena Chin, Leslie Brennan and Elizabeth Prata. For encouragement and guidance, Allan Schanske, M.D., Rena Petrella, M.D., Ram Verma, M.D., and Anita Lustenberger. Thanks also to Bob Markel and Kate Kelly for their support for this project. We would also like to thank Kurt Hirschhorn, M.D., who first interested Dr. Ludman in genetics, and who is responsible for the authors' collaboration on this encyclopedia. For their review and many helpful comments on the introductory essay, "A History of Human Genetics," very special thanks to Victor A. McKusick, M.D., and John M. Opitz, M.D.

Among the private and government organizations and their staffs that provided unfailing assistance, our gratitude to the March of Dimes Birth Defects Foundation, the Children's Defense Fund, the American College of Obstetricians and Gynecologists, the Centers for Disease Control, the American Academy of Pediatrics, the library and rare book collection of the New York Academy of Medicine, Johns Hopkins University, Mt. Sinai School of Medicine, the DuPont Institute, the National Institute of Health, the National Center for Health Statistics, the National Center for Education in Maternal and Child Health, the National Institute of Child Health and Human Development, the Administration on Developmental Disabilities, the Clearinghouse on the Handicapped and, of course, the many support groups, associations and other organizations and individuals that were so generous with their time, resources and expertise.

We also wish to acknowledge all those physicians and scientists who have contributed to the knowledge that we have endeavored to summarize and catalog here.

We dedicate this book to the individuals and their families who have been touched by a genetic disorder or birth defect.

Dr. Ludman would also like to thank all those who taught him what he knows about genetics: instructors throughout his training; students, who constantly challenge him to learn more; and colleagues at the Mount Sinai School of Medicine, in New York City, and in Halifax at the Izaak

Walton Killam Hospital for Children, Atlantic Research Centre for Mental Retardation and Dalhousie University. To his parents: Thanks for instilling the love of knowledge. And especially to his family for all the support they have given him throughout this project. Dr. Ludman's wife now understands all too well why books are often dedicated to authors' spouses!

James Wynbrandt
Mark D. Ludman, M.D.

# Introduction
# A History of Human Genetics

Less than a century ago, in 1906, English zoologist William Bateson suggested to the scientific community that the study of heredity be named "genetics." Millennia of misconception preceded this christening, and the explosion of knowledge that has occurred since continues at a remarkable pace. It is a science with a singular ability to influence life, both in the general and individual sense, at its most profound level, a field with a promising future and a rich history.

Interest in the subject is as old as mankind, and began with the realization that living things beget other living things in their own image, and the observation of unique differences among individuals. Conditions arising from genetic aberrations have also been observed throughout human history. For example, archaeologists have found remains of dwarfs dating to prehistoric times. No doubt various legends and myths were created to explain these variations, both normal and abnormal, explanations probably no more fanciful than many that existed, even in scientific circles, from the beginning of recorded history until the dawn of the 20th century.

In a void without scientific understanding, the public historically has grappled with the causes and consequences of these conditions and variations on its own, resulting in a long tradition of fables and fallacies.

Babylonians regarded the birth of deformed infants or stillborn fetuses as portents from the gods. Astrological records from Babylon and Nineveh dating to 2800 B.C. indicate a great familiarity with anomalous congenital conditions in humans. Specific deformities were linked to specific prophesies, heralding events from war to natural disasters such as an earthquake, as well as peace or the favorable reign of a monarch. The Greeks had their tales of cyclops and stories of hermaphrodites. In England in the Middle Ages, those who could not hear, and hence had not learned to speak, were thought to be stupid, and labeled "dumb." And in the relatively recent past, the curious have flocked to see "prodigies" (such as Tom Thumb and Chang and Eng, the "Siamese" twins), individuals whose physical abnormalities formed the basis of performing careers that often brought them great fortune and renown.

## *The Roots of Genetics*

What we now know as genetics has its roots in early history, with the development of agriculture. Animal and plant breeding were employed in Egyptian times; farmers crossed their best stock, surmising the offspring would also be superior. Babylonians are thought to have artificially cross-fertilized date palms. Stone carvings at least 4,000 years old from Chaldea (near the Persian Gulf) describe different pedigrees, showing the inheritance of specific traits of a horse's mane. Jews recognized a familial link in some diseases; according to the Tosafot, the commentary on the law of the Talmud, a boy need not undergo circumcision if his mother had previously given birth to two male infants who had bled to death at circumcision. This is obviously an allusion to hemophilia, a hereditary disorder seen almost exclusively in males, but whose pedigree pattern was not recognized by the scientific community until the 1800s.

It was likewise recognized that children often appeared to resemble their parents and that certain traits ran in families. Around 500 B.C., Pythagoras, the philosopher and mathematician, theorized that human life originated from a blend of male and female fluids, or semens, that came from within the body. Two centuries later, Aristotle, who believed males were primarily responsible for passing on hereditary characteristics, proposed that the semens were purified elements of blood, a belief that lingers today in phrases such as "blood relative" and "royal blood." Hippocrates, the father of medicine (ca. 460–377 B.C.), had his own ideas about these fluids: "The semen is produced by the whole body, healthy by healthy parts, sick by sick parts. Hence, when as a rule, baldheaded beget baldheaded, blue-eyed beget blue-eyed, and squinting, squinting." He had the mode of transmission wrong, but he clearly recognized the genetic nature of certain traits and disorders, as is further noted in his comments about epilepsy, the "divine" affliction (so called because those afflicted were said to have been blessed by the gods): "But this disease seems to me to be no more divine than others ... Its origin is hereditary like that of other diseases ... What is to hinder it from happening that where the father and mother were subject to this disease, certain of their offspring should be affected also?"

The Institutes of Manu in India during the first centuries of the Common Era proposed an agricultural model of heredity: Males provided the seed, while females provided the field in which the seed was planted and grew.

Despite these pioneering efforts, the nature of the connection between the parent and offspring, its method of transmission, how deformities arose, how hereditary patterns emerged or how they could remain hidden through generations, was completely unknown. For centuries it remained a riddle, referred to as "the mysterious force." Erroneous assumptions based on classical Greek concepts persisted through the Middle Ages. Among them: The sex of a child is determined by the dominator of the sexual act; characteristics of offspring arise from the heat of the womb, or which testis the sperm came from; sperm is secreted from all parts of the body during intercourse and responsible for reproducing that part of the body from which it was secreted. In the 1600s, the concept of the "manikin" was popular: each sperm contained a small but complete "manikin," which would simply grow larger in the womb, rather than develop as a plant from a seed. In the 1700s, a theory of heredity popularized by French naturalist George Louis Leclerc de Buffon postulated that the male determined bodily extremities (head, tail, limbs) while the female was responsible for internal constituents and overall size and shape. A belief that persisted beyond that century was that the "essence" from each vital organ of the parents' bodies somehow blended to create a new individual. However, foreshadowings of modern concepts of heredity began to appear. In the mid-1600s, Dutch scientist Regnier de Graaf advanced the idea of a new being arising from the union of sperm and egg. (The question of whether the primary component of heredity transmission was the sperm or the egg led to a lively dispute between the so-called "ovists" and "spermatists.")

During the 1700s, pedigrees, the patterns whereby traits are transmitted from generation to generation, were recognized for the first time. (Members of the Hapsburgs, the ruling family of the Austrian Empire, were known in the Middle Ages for a characteristic "Hapsburg nose" and jutting chin seen in portraits extending over several centuries.) In 1751, French naturalist Pierre Louis Moreau de Maupertuis invoked "elementary particles" as a transmission agent to explain a family in which several generations exhibited the trait of polydactyly (having more than the normal number of fingers and/or toes). In *Systeme de la Nature* he also suggested that mutations might account for the diversity of life.

Botanists became interested in plant breeding, leading to horticultural experiments that laid the groundwork for modern genetics. When new species of plants appeared, as they did periodically, efforts were made to explain their occurrence. In 1760, Joseph Gottlieb Kölreuter created the first experimentally-produced plant hybrid (the offspring of two different species), by mixing two species of the tobacco plant. This in turn helped generate extensive studies of the function of pollen. He also proposed, as had Maupertuis, that both parents contributed an equal hereditary element to their offspring. Yet, other than botanical studies, the scientific community showed little interest in questions of genetics and heredity, an attitude that changed remarkably in the 19th century, as a spirit of inquiry and innovative technologies spread.

In 1814, Joseph Adams published "A Treatise on the Supposed Hereditary Property of Disease," a remarkably prescient work in which he indicated an appreciation for many of the hallmarks of hereditary theory: He distinguished between recessive and dominant conditions, noted hereditary predisposition in some disorders and the role of environmental influence in their development, and surmised that higher rates of familial diseases found in isolated populations could be due to inbreeding. He even invoked the concept of new mutations, by stating that the reproductive ability of many patients with hereditary conditions would therefore eventually disappear were it not for their spontaneous appearance in healthy families.

## *Darwin and Mendel*

During the mid-19th century, attention shifted from different species to variations within a given species (population groups) and the question of why various populations of a species were not all alike. The major catalyst for the shift was Charles Darwin's (1809-82) monumental *The Origin of Species on the Basis of Natural Selection* (1859), which created an intense interest in the mechanics of evolution. Darwin was already well-respected for his first book, *The Zoology of the Voyage of the Beagle* (1840), an account of his five-year voyage on H.M.S. *Beagle*, on which he sailed as an unpaid naturalist. At one stop, the Galapagos Islands, 15 small rocky outcroppings straddling the equator some 700 miles west of South America, Darwin noted that species of birds that had migrated to different islands had evolved slight differences. He concluded the changes were the result of random variations. If the variation was beneficial, those possessing it were more likely to survive and multiply, a theory he called "natural selection." Darwin published his interpretation of these observations after his attention was brought to a manuscript by Alfred Russell Wallace, who was about to publish a paper with similar conclusions based on observations in the Malaysian islands. Darwin's theories, further delineated in *The Descent of Man* (1871), also addressed common ancestry among species, a concept often misinterpreted as man's having descended from apes. To this day, in the Western world, Darwin's theories of evolution are not universally accepted, primarily by those who find them incompatible with biblical accounts of the origin of life.

As science became more sophisticated in its outlook on genetics and heredity, so did the public. The hereditary nature of some disorders was now accepted. One of the characters in Nathaniel Hawthorne's *The House of the Seven Gables,* published in 1851, suffered from a disease (now speculated as being hereditary angioedema) that Hawthorne described as a fatal condition whose "mode of death has been an idiosyncrasy with this family, for generations past." Hemophilia was also known in New England to have a hereditary component. A familial link in color blindness had been recognized by the end of the 18th century.

It was also during this time that Gregor Johann Mendel (1822-1884) was conducting experiments with garden peas. Mendel, an Austrian, was a monk in Brünn (now Brno), Moravia (now a part of Czechoslovakia). Beginning his experiments in 1856, he noticed that pea plants had varying traits; some unripe pods were yellow, others green; some varieties were tall, while others were dwarfed. The position of the flowers, whether clustered at the top or distributed along the stem, also varied, as did the physical appearance of the peas themselves, being either smooth or wrinkled.

Using hybrid garden pea plants, Mendel's goal was to study the transmission of characteristics to their offspring, and the statistical relation of their subsequently-appearing traits. Mendel had studied physics and mathematics, and he carefully recorded and attempted to explain his observations. During this time, he was also in written communication with Karl von Näegeli, one of the most respected botanists of his day.

Prevailing theory of the time held that heredity was a blending process. According to this theory, if two pea plants, one producing wrinkled peas and one producing smooth peas, were crossed, the first generation of their offspring should produce peas halfway between smooth and wrinkled: a blending of the parental traits. This wasn't what Mendel found when he crossed two true-breeding strains (one always producing smooth, the other always producing wrinkled peas). The first ($F_1$, or first filial) generation produced plants that yielded only smooth peas. Cross-breeding these $F_1$ plants, he produced a second generation ($F_2$). Three-quarters of the $F_1$ plants produced peas that were smooth, and one-quarter produced wrinkled peas. Thus, the traits transmitted from parents didn't blend, but remained distinct, segregated, and had the ability to reappear in subsequent generations. This became the basis of his first law, the law of segregation. His hypothesis that the essence of heredity is particulate, that each trait is represented by only two alternate forms, one contributed by the male and one by the female, was a completely new idea, one that would eventually revolutionize genetics. (These alternative forms of traits are now known to reflect alternative forms of a gene, and are called "alleles.") He further proposed that these factors were either dominant or recessive: A dominant trait would override the influence of its complementary factor; the influence of recessive traits would recede when paired with a dominant complement.

Mendel presented his findings to the Natural History Society of Brünn in 1865, and they were published the following year in the society's proceedings, in a monograph entitled "Experiments in Plant-Hybridization." No one appreciated their importance. Näegeli was unimpressed, and suggested Mendel continue his experiments with another plant, the hawkweed. Mendel followed his advice, but the experiments proved frustrating, totally at odds with the results that would have been expected based on his experience with garden peas. This is not surprising, as it was later discovered that hawkweed reproduces asexually, and therefore inherits the genetic endowment of only one parent.

Eventually, Mendel was promoted to abbot of the monastery and no longer had the time to devote to his careful breeding experiments. He published only one other botanical paper, reporting his unsuccessful experience with hawkweed. However, he continued carefully to monitor and keep detailed records of meteorology. Upon his death, the succeeding abbot burned most of his papers.

## New Theories and Discoveries

In the absence of a unifying theory that Mendel's work would have provided, others struggled to explain hereditary transmission. Most theories incorporated the now-accepted notion that heredity was based on a system of self-replicating, living units, which had variously been called "physiological units," "gemmules," "idioplasm," "micellae" and "pangenes." These theories included Darwin's "provisional hypothesis on pangenesis," offered in *Variation of Animals and Plants Under Domestication* (1868), and English philosopher and naturalist Herbert Spencer's (1820-1903) "theory of physiological units," proposed in *The Principles of Biology* (1864), which somewhat approximated Mendel's much more refined theories. Dutch botanist Hugo De Vries weighed in with "intracellular pangenesis." Other plant geneticists came close to Mendel's idea of discrete hereditary units, hinting at ideas of dominance and segregation without managing to articulate an overall interpretation. Among the stumbling blocks was the still-accepted view that heredity was a blending of traits. There was also the insistence that theories explain the inheritance of acquired traits, a theory initially proposed by French naturalist Jean Baptiste de Lamarck (1744-1829) in 1809, and taken as an article of faith by many geneticists. According to this concept, a physical change in an individual can be passed on to offspring; for example, if enough mice in subsequent generations have their tails cut off, sooner or later, their offspring will be born without tails. (Despite his erroneous assumption, de Lamarck was perhaps the first to propose that species adapted to cope with changes in their environment, which would become a cornerstone in the theory of evolution.)

Francis Galton (1822-1911) contributed the idea of examining identical twins to study aspects of heredity. He deduced that twins must be genetically identical, and therefore were ideal to study the comparative influence of heredity and environment, which he referred to as "nature versus nurture." A proponent of the blending theory of genetics, he developed a method of statistical analysis he called "biometrics" that used complex mathematics to explain transmission of hereditary characteristics. In 1883 he formalized another idea that was to have a profound impact; he called it "eugenics," the improvement of a population by selective breeding of its best specimens. Though long practiced by farmers in plants and animals, Galton's concept of applying it to the human population was enthusiastically championed by many, initiating a eugenics movement that would hold sway for the next half century, until Nazi policies and atrocities committed in its name, as well as its ethical implications and practical problems, discredited it. In the United States and Canada, the movement was responsible for the passage of laws forbidding mentally deficient individuals from having children—statutes that were enforced through compulsory sterilization, and which remained on the books in some states and provinces until after World War II. The Cold Spring Harbor Laboratory, in Long Island, New York, one of the most respected genetics research centers in the world, began as the Eugenics Records Office, and became a center for the promulgation of many of these policies in North America.

Despite the continued prevalence of well-argued misconceptions, the 1800s was a century of scientific ferment, both literally and figuratively. Studies of the cell were well underway in the first half of the 19th century, with microscopy sufficiently advanced to be an invaluable research tool. (In the late 1600s, using a primitive microscope, Robert Hooke had seen structures in tissue he named "cells," giving birth to cytology, the science and study of cells.) In 1865, Louis Pasteur (1822-1895) proposed his "germ theory of disease," hypothesizing that disease could be spread by invisible microbes, or germs. Pasteur also described the concepts of inoculation, pasteurization and fermentation, the last of which led to the discovery of enzymes, organic catalysts involved in life-sustaining chemical reactions within the cells. (When first discovered, they were called "ferments.") Advances in chemistry also aided research into the secrets of heredity; by 1810 the distinction between organic and inorganic compounds had been established, and scientists set about trying to recreate the compounds in laboratories. In the mid-1850s, these efforts led to another discovery—synthetic dyes. The aniline dyes developed in England created several fortunes for the chemists involved in their discovery, and also proved to be invaluable genetic research tools. It was soon noted that various structures in the cell absorbed dyes in varying amounts, making them easier to view under a microscope. Soon, Scottish botanist Robert Brown identified a central area of the cell, which he named the "nucleus."

Further studies revealed that cells contained carbohydrates, lipids and proteins. In 1871, Swiss chemist Friedrich Miescher reported isolating a new substance from the nucleus of the cell, and named it "nuclein." When it was later discovered to have the properties of an acid, it was renamed "nucleic acid." However, the importance of his discovery would remain unrecognized for three-quarters of a century. Also in this decade, German biologist Walther Flemming discovered a staining technique that revealed tiny thread-like bodies within the nucleus. Due to their ready absorption of dye, they became known as "chromosomes," colored bodies. In 1882 Flemming published drawings of these structures based on his observations, showing them in a cycle of positions in which they regularly aligned themselves. He was observing, for the first time, the splitting and replication of genetic material during cell division. This process was soon formally dubbed "mitosis," from the Greek "formation of threads."

Pondering the doubling of genetic material that accompanied mitosis, German physician August Weismann theorized that there must be a mechanism for reducing the genetic material in sex cells, the sperm and egg that united to create one new being. Otherwise, the joining of cells with two complete complements of chromosomes would create offspring with double the normal number of chromosomes in the first generation and, if they continued doubling, an astronomical number of chromosomes several generations in the future. In the mid-1880s, the existence of this reduction mechanism, to be called "meiosis," was confirmed in observations made by Eduard von Beneden.

By the beginning of the new century it was known that nucleic acid and histone proteins were the basic components of chromosomes, and cytologists accepted chromosomes as the vehicle for hereditary transmission. But while some believed nucleic acid was the most important constituent of the chromosomes, many, particularly biologists, thought the proteins were more important. Nucleic acids were much simpler than the proteins. Far too simple, it was thought, to contain the information required to propagate a species. (A view that persisted in some scientific quarters until the 1950s.) But whatever the agents for hereditary transmission might be, as the 20th century dawned, the principles that governed their actions remained unknown.

## Mendelism

While working on papers attempting to explain the heredity riddle, and in the course of investigating previous work in the field, three botanists—Hugo De Vries, Carl Correns from the University of Tübingen, and Erich von Tschermak-Seysenegg, an agricultural assistant who worked near Vienna—independently and within months of each other came upon the work of Gregor Mendel. They immediately recognized its importance and incorporated his findings in their own published work, all in 1900. (The question has been raised whether all of them had at first planned to credit Mendel in their papers; but prior to publication, all became aware of their mutual knowledge of his theories, voiding any possibility of denying Mendel his due.) Once his work was rediscovered, "Mendelism," as it came to be called, was an overnight sensation. The major champion of Mendelism before the scientific community was English zoologist William Bateson (1861-1926). He had Mendel's paper translated into English and published in the *Journal of the Royal Horticultural Society* in 1900. Botanists and scientists across the Continent hurriedly duplicated Mendel's results, and hailed his theories' power and simplicity, which explained the results of many of their own experiments. Bateson also introduced the term "genetics" in 1906, formally proposing to the scientific community that the term be used for the study of heredity and variation. (It first appears in a 1905 letter of his; however, the term "cytogenetics" has been dated to 1903, used by American Walter S. Sutton in a paper, "The Chromosomes in Heredity," published in the *Biological Bulletin*.)

With Mendel's theories providing the framework, genetic research advanced quickly in the first decade of the 20th century. Physician and biochemist Archibald E. Garrod, conducting research aided by Bateson, established the idea of an "inborn error of metabolism," a block at some point in a metabolic reaction sequence that he postulated was due to the congenital deficiency of a specific enzyme. In 1902 he identified alkaptonuria (an essentially benign disorder whose most noticeable feature is that the urine of affected individuals turns black when left standing in light) as such an inborn error of metabolism. This is considered the first proof of Mendelian inheritance in man. Brachydactyly (having unusually short fingers or toes) and the human ABO blood groups were also held to be examples of Mendelian inheritance by 1910. Garrod's work is considered the beginning of both modern biochemical genetics and medical genetics. In the same year that Garrod identified alkaptonuria as an inborn error of metabolism, American W.E. Castle began a systematic study of heredity with laboratory rodents and, beginning in 1905, with the fly Drosophila melanogaster, studies that had large impacts on genetic research.

The term "gene" was introduced in 1909 by Wilhelm Ludwig Johannsen (1857-1927), a pharmacist's apprentice from Copenhagen who had gone on to become a respected geneticist and botanist, despite his lack of a university degree. He defined a gene as an accounting or calculating unit of heredity. He also introduced the term "genotype" (an individual's genetic make-up) and "phenotype" (an individual's physical appearance, which may or may not reflect his or her genotype).

By the middle of this first decade of the 20th century, assaults on Mendel's law of segregation of traits had proved futile, and it was now the foundation of hereditary theory. Variations that could not be explained according to his theories were now accepted as being caused by spontaneous changes. The Hardy-Weinberg equation of 1908 also helped bolster the case for Mendel. The equation demonstrated gene distribution in randomly-mating populations, and explained the unanswered question of why dominant characteristics do not increase at the expense of recessive characteristics, thereby eventually replacing them. Independently postulated by English mathematician G.H. Hardy and German physician W. Weinberg, it formed a cornerstone of population genetics, the study of factors involved in human evolution.

By the end of the decade, Mendel's laws were accepted as applying to humans and animals as well as to plants. (However, rearguard actions against Mendel's theories continued to be fought by Galton's disciples, the "biometricians," most notably Karl Pearson (1857-1936), who argued that Mendel's stark dominant and recessive approach failed to account for quantitative traits such as height, intelligence and body size. In an interesting coda to the battle, in 1918 English statistician and geneticist Sir Ronald Fisher (1890-1962) pointed out that there is no fundamental inconsistency between Mendelism and the blending concept of heredity; these quantitative traits involved the action of many genes, each behaving individually while blending with the action of others.) The concept of genes was also now accepted, as was their role in controlling the production of enzymes.

In 1910, American zoologist and geneticist Thomas Hunt Morgan (1866-1945) published his paper "Chromosomes and Heredity," ushering in the era of the "chromosome theory" of heredity. The foundations for this era had been laid in the previous decade. Sutton and Theodor Boveri of Germany independently suggested in 1903 that chromosomes were the carriers of genetic information and occurred in pairs, one inherited from the male and one from the female. Studies published in 1904 by A.B. Darbishire of two coat-color genes in the house mouse established the important concept of "linkage"; some individual traits tended to be inherited together. This was later demonstrated to be due to the genes for these traits being located on the same chromosome. (Mendel had been very fortunate; the genes for traits he chose to study were all located on different chromosomes of the pea plants, and thus were not linked. Had they been, it would have been virtually impossible to interpret the results of his experiments correctly.) Inheritance of sex-linked traits was demonstrated in plumage patterns on Plymouth Rock fowls in 1909. (Sex chromosomes had been observed almost 20 years previously, by H. Henking in 1891, and their function identified soon after the rediscovery of Mendel's laws.)

At Columbia University, Morgan established what became known as the "fly group." When he began his work, Morgan was not a committed Mendelist, but his work with Drosophila melanogaster soon changed his mind about Mendel, and made Drosophila the subject of choice for geneticists. Often called the fruit fly, but actually the pomace or vinegar fly, Drosophila could quickly and easily be cultivated for study of transmission of traits; one female could provide several hundred offspring in less than two weeks, and simple breeding methods allowed easy analysis of specific traits. (Years later, it would be discovered that Drosophila also has "giant" chromosomes in its salivary glands, greatly easing visual examination of this material.) In 1910 Morgan noted a variation in one of his flies: The eyes were white instead of red. Breeding it produced more white-eyed flies, and further experiments revealed they were always males, and eventually established the chromosomal basis of sex-linked inheritance. (In 1933, Morgan became the first geneticist to win the Nobel prize.)

In 1911, E.B. Wilson identified the X chromosome as the location of the gene for color blindness, the first time a gene had been assigned to a specific chromosome, a pioneering demonstration of gene mapping. Hemophilia was recognized as an X-linked disorder during this same period. Later in the decade sickle-cell anemia, a blood disorder found primarily in blacks, and whose characteristic "sickled," collapsed red blood cells had been first described in 1910, was identified as a recessive disorder.

During the period from 1910 to 1930, genetics slowly narrowed its focus from the chromosome to the gene. Research primarily involved experimental breeding, cytological observations, and direct chemical and physical study of chromosomes and the proteins and nucleic acids from which they were built. With the basic laws and principles elucidated, the dramatic breakthroughs of the first decade gave way to exploring the territory that had so recently been claimed. The discovery of the mutagenic properties of X rays was a major advance of this period. Previously, researchers had to wait for variations, which are useful for study and experimentation, to occur naturally, which rarely happened; genetic material appeared remarkably stable and impervious to alteration. But in 1927, Hermann J. Muller, who'd been a student of Morgan's, published "Artificial Transmutation of the Gene," a paper reporting that male flies exposed to heavy doses of X rays exhibited new variation rates 15,000 times above normal. He called these changes "mutations." (He received the Nobel prize for his work in 1946.) The following year, Lewis Stadler reported similar findings using maize, a corn plant, and barley.

Also during this period, unnoticed by most, an English microbiologist, Frederick Griffith, isolated a material from the cells that could influence heredity. Mixing the material with other cells, he found he could change hereditary characteristics of the bacterium he used in his research. His report of a "transformation" principle in 1928, overlooked at the time, represented the first isolation of DNA.

As improved health care conquered more infectious and nutritional diseases, the impact of genetically-influenced disorders became more apparent. Antibiotics prolonged the lives of those affected with some of these conditions, revealing their previously unrecognized hereditary nature. Cystic fibrosis, among the most widely distributed hereditary disorders in white populations, was first definitively described in 1937. In 1934, Ivar Asbjørn Følling, a Norwegian physician, identified phenylketonuria, a common metabolic disorder that had previously resulted in mental retardation, but was ultimately found (in 1954) to be relatively easy to treat. This would lead in the 1960s to the first large-scale screening program for early detection of an inherited disorder.

However, it was also during these years that the study of genetics was subjected to political and ideological assault, particularly in the Soviet Union and Germany. Nazi eugenic breeding experiments and Soviet "geneticist" Trofim Denisovich Lysenko (1898-1976) dealt devastating blows to the science. Nazi physician Josef Mengele conducted experiments using 1,500 pairs of twins. Lysenko, whose ideas held sway in the Soviet Union for a quarter of a century, preached a Socialist brand of Lamarckism, the theory of inheritance of acquired characteristics. He refused to acknowledge any hereditary property of chromosomes or genes, leading to the suppression of research and teaching of modern genetics in the Soviet Union from 1938 to 1963.

## The Building Blocks of Heredity

The 1940s marked the dawn of molecular genetics. The seminal development was Dr. Linus Pauling's work with the sickle-cell trait, in which he identified the flaw in the hemoglobin molecule that results in sickle-cell anemia. This change altered the molecule's electrical charge. Thus, it behaved differently in an electrical field, a fact Pauling used to detect the abnormal molecules themselves. (He won the 1954 Nobel prize in chemistry for his work.) This was also the era in which biochemical genetics flowered. George Beadle and Edward L. Tatum at California's Stanford University demonstrated the one-to-one correlation between genes and proteins. They began their experiments in the late 1930s with the mold Neurospora crassa. After inducing gene mutations with X rays, they proved that a subsequent nutritional deficiency in the mold resulted from the lack of an enzyme the mutated gene was responsible for producing. This confirmed and explained the "inborn errors of metabolism" whose existence had been hypothesized at the turn of the century by Garrod. (They shared the Nobel prize for their discovery in 1958.) By the end of the 1950s, a handful of the more than 250 recessive disorders then reported had been identified as enzyme deficiency diseases.

During this same period, DNA was established as the vehicle of hereditary transmission. In 1944, Dr. Oswald Avery at Rockefeller University in New York, building upon the earlier work of Griffith, demonstrated the transmission of characteristics from one strain of bacteria to another through DNA. By the end of the decade, the composition of nucleic acid was known, but its structure was not, setting the stage for one of genetics' major discoveries.

Drs. James D. Watson and Francis H.C. Crick of the Medical Research Council Laboratories in Cambridge, England, were among those trying to deduce the structure of DNA, basing their ideas on its behavior. They consulted extensively with Maurice Wilkins, a physicist who was attempting to make X-ray photographs of a DNA molecule. In 1953 Watson and Crick published their ground-breaking "Structural Implications of Deoxyribonucleic Acid," in which they proposed the double-helix model for DNA. Simultaneously, Wilkins published his X-ray photographs of the molecule, revealing a helical structure. (The three shared the Nobel prize in 1962 for their work.)

As described by Watson and Crick, DNA consists of two long, linked strands, resembling a tightly coiled spiral staircase. It is composed of smaller units called nucleotides, which in turn are made of a sugar molecule, a phosphate and any one of four nitrogen bases: adenine, thymine, guanine or cystosine. These nitrogen bases link up with complementary bases on the other strand, forming "base pairs." Adenine always joins with thymine, and guanine is always paired with cytosine. The model explained both how DNA was built, and how it functioned. It outlined how DNA replicated itself during mitosis, and how it orchestrated the production of enzymes and proteins. In effect, the two strands would "unzip," separating at the base pairs, and each strand would then form a template, attracting new bases to construct a mirror image, exactly like the other strand, which was now also building its complement. When mitosis was complete, there would be two sets of the DNA, both exactly like the original. For the production of proteins, only a portion of the DNA would unzip, attracting ribonucleic acid (RNA) to recreate portions of the DNA, which held the code to building proteins from amino acids. The RNA would then leave the cell nucleus, and itself become a template on which the proteins would be assembled. Watson and Crick's hypothesis was as simple and important in its own way as Mendel's postulations, providing a framework for all subsequent research in genetics.

There were other significant advances in the 1950s. After years of having to content themselves examining chromosomes from Drosophila, new techniques began to bring human chromosomes into better focus. In 1952, Dr. T.C. Hsu, at the University of Texas at Galveston, found that chromosomes exposed to a hypotonic solution, that is, one in which the concentration of sodium and chloride is less than in the cells, absorbed water and became more visible. By the middle of the decade the field of clinical genetics, the medical application of knowledge of genetics, was established, and a score of medical centers in the United States had medical genetics facilities. In 1956, Drs. Joe-Hin Tjio and Albert Levan, using improved staining techniques they'd developed, demonstrated that humans have 23 pairs of chromosomes, or a total of 46. (It had been thought since 1923 that humans had 48 chromosomes.) The technique led to the identification of conditions caused by chromosome abnormalities. In 1958, French pediatrician Jerome Lejeune announced at a conference at McGill University the finding of a chromosomal abnormality in Down syndrome, and his findings were published the following year. By the end of the decade, the chromosomal basis of Turner syndrome, Klinefelter syndrome and other chromosomal abnormalities had been identified. (Down syndrome had been identified by English physician J.L.H. Langdon-Down in 1866, and Dutch physician P.J. Waardenburg suggested as early as 1932 that it could be caused by a chromosomal abnormality.)

New methods to halt various stages of mitosis, using chemicals, such as colchicine, as well as hypotonic solutions, made study of the chromosomes easier by suspending them in more advantageous viewing positions. Another chemical, phytohemaglutinin, was found to stimulate the division of lymphocytes, white blood cells. This led the way to genetic testing using blood, rather than tissue samples, greatly easing investigation of human genetic anomalies.

With these growing chromosome visualization abilities, scientists were now making microphotographs of human chromosomes to allow for their study. They would cut the pictures apart, and arrange the individual chromosome pairs according to their size and the position of their centromere, the point at which the two chromosomes in a pair are joined. These blown up microphotos were called "karyotypes," and at a meeting of cytogeneticists in Denver in 1960, a standard method of arranging the human chromosomes in karyotypes was adopted, known as the

Denver classification. Though since amended, the Denver classification remains the accepted method of karyotype display.

During the 1960s, modern medical-scientific study of genetic and congenital anomalies came into its own, as did clinical genetics and genetic counseling. The first catalog of genetic disorders, composed of a survey of X-linked traits, was published in 1962, assembled by Dr. Victor McKusick of Johns Hopkins University. (McKusick's survey grew into "Mendelian Inheritance in Man," a catalog of known or suspected single gene disorders that, by the end of the 1980s, contained some 4,300 autosomal dominant, autosomal recessive and X-linked conditions.) Prenatal diagnosis became a reality with the development of amniocentesis. First used for an intrauterine transfusion in 1963, in 1966 M.W. Steele and W.R. Breg demonstrated how the procedure could be used to collect and cultivate fetal cells whose chromosomes could be then examined and tested for any number of genetic disorders. By the end of the 1960s, the procedure was perfected.

This was also the decade in which the actual "genetic code," the chemical instructions contained in the DNA, was cracked: The code consists of a triplet of adjacent nucleotides, on a strand of DNA, that form a single message. Each nucleotide triplet is called a "codon," and a gene was now defined as a series of codons that give the instructions for building a specific protein. Each codon may represent either a single one of the 20 amino acids found in humans, which make a protein, or it may be an instruction to stop or start production of a chain of amino acids.

But the size and complexity of DNA molecules continued to perplex researchers wishing to study individual genes, and slowed progress in determining their secrets.

The early 1970s brought developments that helped isolate segments of DNA, greatly assisting the study of individual genes and groups of genes. Swiss microbiologist Werner Arber, working with Escherichia coli (E. coli), common intestinal bacteria, and Drs. Hamilton O. Smith and Daniel Nathans of Johns Hopkins University, using the bacteria Hemophilus influenzae, announced the discovery of enzymes produced by the bacteria that could cut the DNA of some viruses and bacteria at specific points. These became the first "restriction enzymes," which would become a key tool for genetic researchers. Ultimately, it enabled the isolation of short segments of DNA, assisting the search for specific genes. All three shared the Nobel prize in 1979. (By the beginning of the 1990s, over 200 restriction enzymes had been isolated from bacteria, each of which can cut a DNA molecule at separate and specific points, based on the sequence of nucleotides on the DNA chain.) Once isolated, the function of some genes on these segments could be identified, or at least their location "mapped" to specific points on the chromosomes.

Modern gene mapping had its genesis in the 1960s with the creation of human-mouse "hybrid cells." Human cells were fused together with cultured tumor cells from mice, combining the genetic material of the two species. After several cell divisions, only a portion of the human DNA, identifiable fragments of human chromosomes, would remain. By examining the human protein products of the hybrid cells, the location of the gene that controlled its production could now be placed on the human chromosome. But the difficulty of obtaining specific chromosome fragments had hindered progress.

Once restriction enzymes were discovered, the ability to slice up DNA quickly and easily led to techniques to "re-combine" the resulting fragments of DNA. This allowed investigators to take specific fragments of DNA from one cell and graft them into the DNA of another. "Recombinant DNA," as the reconstituted genetic material was called, could be placed into the nucleus of bacteria to study the influence of the human genes, or to manufacture the enzyme the gene is responsible for producing. Using a combination of these techniques, by the early 1980s, human insulin and human growth hormone were being manufactured by genetically engineered E. coli.

Chromosome fragments created with restriction enzymes also proved vitally important in linkage studies, allowing the prenatal diagnosis of some genetic disorders even though the gene responsible had not been identified. This linkage was first used in 1978, to predict those at risk for developing sickle-cell anemia, demonstrated by Drs. Yuet Wai Kan and Andrees M. Dozy of the University of California at San Francisco. They found that some people have a benign variation in the DNA near the site of the gene for the production of hemoglobin. This was the first DNA polymorphism, an inherited variation in DNA sequence, ever found. These variations alter the points at which restriction enzymes would normally slice the DNA, creating DNA fragments of lengths not normally seen, called "restriction fragment length polymorphisms" (RFLP). By studying the DNA of many families of blacks, the researchers linked this natural variation to the mutant gene for hemoglobin production, which causes sickle-cell anemia. They found individuals exhibiting this DNA variation were much more likely to have sickle-cell anemia than those without it. Thus, using fetal cells collected via amniocentesis, linkage studies could indicate pregnancies at risk for sickle-cell infants, and pregnancies with greatly reduced risk. (Direct detection of the sickle-cell gene mutation became possible in 1981.)

DNA probes are another example of modern use of DNA fragments for diagnostic purposes. These are short, single-strand sections of DNA known to contain a specific group of genes, and irradiated so they can be radioactively tracked. The probe is exposed to selected fragments of DNA from an individual being tested for a specific genetic anomaly. If the probe binds with the DNA fragment from the individual, the two contain a complementary gene sequence. Thus, if a probe containing a mutation is used and binds with the individual's DNA fragment, then the individual's DNA must likewise be flawed.

New banding techniques allowing better visualization of chromosomes were another significant development of the 1970s. These bands are the individual chromosome's "fingerprints"; every section of each chromosome has a distinctive banding pattern when exposed to specific dyes. By 1976, high resolution banding techniques, which examined stretched out chromosomes, allowed the visualization of as many as 5,000 bands on the 23 pairs of human chromosomes. This enabled cytogeneticists to detect small chromosomal deletions in patients with a variety of disorders, ultimately assisting in the hunt for the genes that cause some of these genetic conditions. Concurrently, university centers and satellite clinics for study and treatment of genetic conditions proliferated. In 1979, the American Board of Medical Genetics was established. Also by the end of the decade, over 200 of the more than 700 recessive disorders then reported had been identified as enzyme deficiency diseases.

As the gene came closer into view, understanding of what exactly constituted a gene underwent further refinement. It was found that, rather than simply coding for an amino acid sequence of a polypeptide chain, almost every human and vertebrate gene analyzed has coding sequences, known as "exons," interspersed among intervening non-coding sequences, known as "introns," as well as "flanking regions," which are believed important in regulation of the gene's action. (Indeed, by the end of the 1980s, there were suggestions that even Mendel's laws might require modification, as new research found that, at least among mammals, genes inherited from the mother and father might not always be equal in their hereditary power; maternal and paternal genes appeared to differ in their ability to affect the development of some disorders in their offspring, through a process called "imprinting.")

During the 1980s, the number of identified genetic markers, normal genes often inherited along with or linked to an aberrant gene for a specific disorder, grew. Markers for cystic fibrosis, a number of cancers and Huntington's disease were identified. (However, in an example of certain limits of clinical genetics, only a small percentage of those at risk for developing Huntington's disease [that is, children and siblings of those with the disorder] indicated a desire to be tested; apparently a significant number of those at risk do not want to know if they will develop the disorder, or are fearful of learning that indeed they will.)

In what were probably the most important discoveries of the 1980s, by the end of the decade the genes for Duchenne muscular dystrophy, cystic fibrosis and chronic granulamatous disease, among others, were isolated and identified solely on the basis of their chromosomal location, without prior knowledge of these genes' products or an understanding of the basic biochemical mechanism of the diseases. This process has been termed "reverse genetics," as opposed to the more usual method of genetic research, whereby identification of a gene product and its function precedes its molecular characterization.

Efforts also began in earnest to create a complete map of the human genes. The Human Genome Project, as the federally-supported effort is called, hopes to identify every gene contained in the human genetic complement, or genome, a project estimated to require 15 to 20 years at a cost of $3 billion.

The discovery of oncogenes, another major advance of the 1980s, held the promise of one day revolutionizing the diagnosis and treatment of cancer. These are genes involved in the development of cancer. Anti-oncogenes have also been discovered, which appear to inhibit the development of cancer. It appears that several oncogenes need to be "activated" and several anti-oncogenes "deactivated" in order for the uncontrolled cell growth that characterizes cancer to occur. Oncogenes may be involved in regulating cell growth, perhaps triggering abnormal growth after exposure to virus or other environmental assaults causes a mutation. Drs. J. Michael Bishop and Harold E. Varmus of the University of California shared a 1989 Nobel prize for their pioneering work in developing the oncogene hypothesis.

If specific genes can be identified as promoting cancer, and the products they produce identified, it may be possible to identify at-risk individuals, and eventually develop methods to block the genes' destructive action. Treating disorders at this level is the goal of gene therapy. These therapies, though only at the research stage by the end of the decade, may one day enable mutant genes to be replaced by normal genes, rectifying whatever disorder is caused by faulty instructions given by a mutated gene.

But despite great strides, human genetics can still be maddeningly imprecise, particularly when applied clinically. Diagnosis of genetic disorders in a given case may be impossible. Exciting breakthroughs have not eliminated the heartbreak many families endure. The answers medical geneticists can provide are often far outnumbered by the questions they are asked. Advances that may one day reduce this impotence and uncertainty have brought us to the threshold of ethical, moral and legal dilemmas that are as challenging and imperative to address as are the technical and theoretical ones. These are issues that society as a whole, not just geneticists, will face in coming years.

Yet, given even its current limitations, genetics has improved the lives of many, and its benefits are certain to increase, providing help, hope and even life where before there was none.

# A

**Aarskog syndrome**    First described by Dr. Dagfinn A. Aarskog, professor of pediatrics at the University of Bergen, Norway, in 1970, this is a form of DWARFISM characterized by abnormalities of the hands, face and genitals. Inherited as an X-LINKED disorder, its full expression is seen only in males. (However, females who carry a single gene for the disorder tend to be below average height and may have minor facial or digital abnormalities.)

Infants appear normal at birth, and the slowing of growth generally does not become apparent until two to four years of age. Thereafter, height remains below the third percentile for age.

Facially, the forehead is prominent, with wide-set eyes (HYPERTELORISM), often mildly slanted downward and away from the nose (antimongoloid obliquity), with drooping eyelids (PTOSIS). Vision problems are frequent. The nose is short, stubby and upturned (anteverted nares). The ears are low-set and cupped. Mild mental retardation is common.

Hands are short and broad, and fingers may appear "double-jointed" (HYPERMOBILITY of joints). Other digital abnormalities may include short (BRACHYDACTYLY), incurving (CLINODACTYLY), permanently flexed (CAMPTODACTYLY) or webbed (SYNDACTYLY) fingers. The feet may exhibit a stubby appearance.

The penis exhibits characteristic folds of skin of the scrotum that surround it, in a manner that has been likened to a shawl worn around the neck, an abnormality that is called "shawl scrotum." The testis may be undescended (CRYPTORCHISM).

Puberty is often delayed, although life span is normal. Adult height is usually below 5 feet 3 inches (157.6 cm).

The basic defect that causes Aarskog syndrome is unknown. Considered relatively rare, approximately 50 cases have been reported worldwide. Prenatal diagnosis is not currently possible.

Diagnosis in individuals suspected of having the disorder is based on the presence of the characteristic symptoms.

**Aase syndrome**    See ANEMIA.

**abetalipoproteinemia**    (Bassen-Kornzweig syndrome)    First described in an 18-year-old Jewish female at New York's Mt. Sinai Hospital by Drs. F.A. Bassen and A.L. Kornzweig in 1950, this rare disease features intestinal fat malabsorption characterized by diarrhea and malnutrition. It may resemble celiac disease or CYSTIC FIBROSIS. Deterioration of the retina (pigmentary degeneration of the retina) leads to progressive loss of vision. Progressive loss of motor control with abnormalities of balance and gait (ataxic neuropathy), mental retardation (in one-third of cases) and abnormalities of the blood are also hallmarks.

Under microscopic examination, about 80% of red blood cells appear to have an abnormal shape, and are termed acanthocytes. These abnormal "burr-cells" are characteristic and appear to be covered by thorns. Other manifestations in the blood are very low levels of serum cholesterol and the absence of serum beta lipoprotein (which gives the disorder its name).

The disease usually begins prior to age one and the manifestations are progressive. While there is no cure, many of the manifestations of this disorder are the consequence of vitamin E deficiency, and treatment with vitamin E may alleviate some symptoms.

Inherited as an AUTOSOMAL RECESSIVE trait, of the approximately 40 published cases, 25% have been Ashkenazi Jews. The basic defect is thought to lie in the inability to produce the protein component of beta-lipoprotein, the apo B peptide.

**ablepharia**    See CRYPTOPHTHALMOS.

**abortion**    The termination of a pregnancy before fetal viability, that is, before the FETUS can survive outside the womb (usually consid-

1

considered to be between the 20th and the 28th week of pregnancy). Abortion may occur spontaneously, often referred to as a miscarriage. Alternatively, it may result from an induced procedure for terminating a pregnancy and thus preventing childbirth. Induced abortion is among the reproductive options available in conjunction with GENETIC COUNSELING.

## Induced Abortion

When induced abortion is performed for genetic concerns, it usually follows prenatal diagnosis of a specific condition, and is generally performed by the 20th week of pregnancy. Abortions may be induced with drugs, or performed by suction or surgical scraping of the embryo(s) from the uterus, or by injection of sterile hypertonic solutions into the womb. They may also be performed selectively in cases of multiple embryos, where continued development of all the fetuses threatens their collective health and that of their mother.

A small percentage of birth defects in infants born to young, unwed mothers may result from failed, self-induced abortions.

## Miscarriage

Miscarriages, spontaneous abortions, may be the result of many influences, though it is possible to determine the exact cause in only about half of the cases, often only after comprehensive examination of fetal remains. Among the causes are chromosomal or genetic abnormalities, maternal infections, exposure to toxins, substance abuse, nutrition and immunologic, endocrine and reproductive system abnormalities.

The rate of miscarriage is estimated to be approximately 10% to 20% of all recognized pregnancies among women who have never previously miscarried. However, due to the potential number of unrecognized pregnancies, the true rate may be significantly higher, with estimates ranging as high as 31% of all implanted embryos.

Approximately 85% of all miscarriages occur during the first trimester, or three months, of pregnancy, and half of these fetuses are estimated to be chromosomally abnormal. Half of these are thought to be the result of trisomies, the triplication of individual chromosomes (see CHROMOSOME ABNORMALITIES). Genetic factors may play a role in some of the remainder as well.

The rate of miscarriage increases with maternal age. Women who have had one previous miscarriage have a 25% risk of recurrence, rising to between 25% and 30% for those who've had two previous spontaneous abortions. Approximately one woman in 300 has had three or more miscarriages, referred to as habitual abortion. These women have a 30% to 40% chance of a miscarriage in any subsequent pregnancy. Their miscarriages are more apt to be the result of maternal factors, such as reproductive system abnormalities, rather than chromosomal abnormalities. However, there is a possibility that they or their spouses carry a chromosomal rearrangement.

Reproductive system abnormalities include abnormalities of the uterus, deficiencies of the ovaries' ability to produce the hormone progesterone, and deficiencies of the immune system.

Women with underactive immune systems appear to lack an antibody that normally blocks rejection of foreign tissue during pregnancy, possibly causing the rejection of the fetus. In perhaps half of the estimated two million American women who have repeated miscarriages of normal fetuses, the cause is thought to be due to underactive immune systems.

Women who miscarry are prone to the same hormonal imbalance that leads to postpartum depression following normal childbirth.

## Selective Termination

The selective aborting of some of the fetuses in a multiple pregnancy. Increased use of fertility drugs, taken by an estimated 20,000 women in the United States in 1990, has led to an increase in the number of multiple pregnancies, those in which more than one embryo develops; in some cases as many as nine embryos may develop. Continued growth of all the fetuses in some multiple pregnancies is incompatible with the survival of any of the offspring, and may endanger maternal health as well. Selective termination may be employed in these cases. It is accomplished by the administration of a toxic solution directly into the embryos that are to be aborted, guided by the use of fetal imaging equipment. This procedure has also been done to selectively abort one twin affected with a genetic disorder or birth defect, which has been prenatally diagnosed, while allowing the continued pregnancy of the unaffected twin. (See also GRIEF; MULTIPLE BIRTHS; QUININE.)

**absent nails**   See HEREDITARY ANONYCHIA.

**absent testes** (anorchia)   The absence of testes (anorchia) in individuals having otherwise well-differentiated male genitalia. It is not to be confused with agonadia, a more common condition in which not only are the testes absent, but the genital differentiation is abnormal as well.

Anorchia occurs in unilateral and bilateral forms, that is, either one or both testes may be absent. Unilateral is more common but at least 100 cases of bilateral anorchia have been reported.

Diagnosis cannot be made until puberty and should involve surgical verification that the testes are absent and not merely undescended.

The cause of this condition is uncertain, although familial tendencies exist. Cases have been observed in which only one of a pair of identical (monozygotic) twins was affected. It is theorized that the testicular tissue is present in all affected fetuses until about 14 to 20 weeks into embryonic development, after which they seem to have atrophied for some unexplained reason.

Treatment with male hormones can compensate for those hormones normally produced in the testes, but patients with bilateral anorchia remain infertile for life.

**acanthocytosis**   See ABETALIPOPROTEINEMIA.

**acanthosis nigracans**   A very rare hereditary skin disorder characterized by patches of gray or black, rough or velvety skin with a burned appearance, found around skin folds, most often about the armpits.

The lesions tend to be symmetrical (that is, a lesion on one side of the body will have a corresponding lesion on the other side), and may also appear on the neck, face, backs of hands, forearms, between the breasts, groin, genitals, inner thighs, buttocks and around the anus. These darkened areas are caused by the excessive accumulation of melanin in the skin. Small warts, freckles and other skin abnormalities may be associated with the lesions. Affected areas may become hairless, and fingernails may deteriorate.

The condition may be present at birth, but usually appears during childhood or early adolescence. It generally progresses during adolescence and regresses after puberty. In adults it is often associated with internal cancer.

Endocrine abnormalities are seen in approximately one-third of affected children. Those without hormonal abnormality are often obese.

A benign form known as Miescher's syndrome is believed to be inherited as an AUTOSOMAL DOMINANT TRAIT. A form that appears mostly in young adult females, Gougerot-Carteaud syndrome, may also be hereditary, though the mode of transmission has not been established.

For more information contact:

The National Arthritis and Musculoskeletal
   and Skin Disease Information
   Clearinghouse
Box AMS
Bethesda, MD 20892
(301) 468-3235

**acatalasemia**   See ACATALASIA.

**acatalasia** (also acatalasemia)   F i r s t discovered in Japan, this very rare disease of the oral tissue is most often seen in Orientals. The gum (gingival) and oral tissues are very susceptible to bacterial infection, and the condition may result in gangrene and destruction of the bones around the tooth sockets.

Inherited as an AUTOSOMAL RECESSIVE disorder, it is caused by the absence of the ENZYME catalase.

**Accutane**   The trade name for an acne medication (generic name isotretinoin), marketed since 1982, that has been shown to cause birth defects when used by women during pregnancy. Although only slightly more than 50 infants affected by Accutane had been reported to the Food and Drug Administration (FDA) by 1987, actual incidence was believed to be much greater. In one memorandum, the FDA estimated that from 900 to 1,300 infants were born with severe birth defects caused by maternal use of Accutane between 1982 and 1986. (Approximately 270,000 to 390,000 women between the ages of 15 and 44 took the medication during these years). They also estimated that from 700 to 1,000 spontaneous ABORTIONS could be attributed to the drug, and that 5,000 to 7,000 women had induced abortions due to concern of fetal exposure to Accutane. Officials compared the drug to THALIDOMIDE in its potential for causing fetal damage.

Major fetal anomalies related to Accutane that have been documented include brain anomalies, HYDROCEPHALUS, small head (MICROCEPHALY), small eyes (microphthalmia), abnormalities of the external ear, and cardiovascular anomalies. No dose, no matter how small, nor any exposure, no matter how short, can be considered safe; potentially all exposed fetuses could be affected.

Women using Accutane are advised to use a contraceptive, and, if planning to become pregnant, to discontinue use of the medication from one month before conception to one month after delivery.

**acetylator phenotype**   A genetic trait found in normal individuals that can help determine the likely outcome of some medical treatments and the impact of various doses of some commonly prescribed drugs. It refers to the speed with which the body breaks down the anti-tuberculosis drug, isoniazid. Those with a slow rate have an increase in adverse reactions to some drugs, such as isoniazid, hydralazine (a blood pressure medication) and some sulfa drugs. An individual is either a slow or fast acetylator. "Fast" is dominant to slow, thus an individual who is a "fast" acetylator has either one or two "fast" genes, while a "slow" acetylator has two "slow" genes.

**achondrogenesis**   A rare, lethal form of DWARFISM characterized by abnormal development of the skeleton, a large head (possibly exceeding 40% of body length) and severe shortening of the limbs and trunk. Total body length at birth is rarely more than one foot. Most affected infants are stillborn or survive only a few days after birth. More than 100 cases have been reported worldwide.

While the head size is actually normal, due to the dwarfing of the rest of the body it appears disproportionately large. The forehead is broad and the face and scalp are swollen (hydropic), with an extremely flattened nose and nasal bridge. The mouth is small, and the ears are low-set and blunted. The head appears attached directly to the trunk, as the neck is hidden by skin folds. The chest is extremely shortened, and the abdomen is disproportionately large. The limbs are extremely short, and are sometimes referred to as "flipper-like." There is almost a total absence of ossification (formation of bones) in the vertebral column. Heart defects and malformation of the respiratory system are also common.

Several types have been recognized, each inherited as an AUTOSOMAL RECESSIVE trait. They are differentiated by X-ray and microscopic examination of the cartilage. Types IA and IB (previously called Parenti-Fraccaro type) are believed to be caused by the failure of fetal cartilage to mature. Type II (Langer-Saldino type) is believed to be caused by the degeneration of fetal cartilage. (A disorder called Grebe disease has been referred to as "Brazilian achondrogenesis," but it is not actually a form of this condition.)

PRENATAL DIAGNOSIS is possible via ultrasound and X rays, which can detect the gross abnormalities of fetal development that characterize this condition.

**achondroplasia**  The most common and best-known form of short-limbed DWARFISM, characterized by relatively normal trunk size, disproportionately short arms and legs and disproportionately large head.

Achondroplasts have been noted throughout history. Skeletal remains of prehistoric achondroplasts have been unearthed by archaeologists. In Egypt, they appear to have occupied favored positions in royal courts of the pharaohs, and the deity Bes was depicted with achondroplastic features. A Roman statue of a gladiator with achondroplasia dates to the Emperor Domitian (A.D. 51-96). Don Sebastian de Morro, an achondroplast nobleman in the court of Philip V of Spain, can be seen in a portrait by Velasquez. There have even been suggestions that Attila the Hun had achondroplasia. (However, not all those so labeled have had true achondroplasia; many other forms of short-limbed dwarfism have similar features.)

Achondroplasia is a form of "rhizomelic dwarfism," so called because the limbs are shortened in a rhizomelic fashion: The bones closest (proximal) to the trunk display the greatest shortening. It is one of a group of congenital conditions called "chondrodystrophies," disorders affecting the development of bone from cartilage.

Facially, affected individuals have prominent foreheads, depressed nasal bridge and protruding jaw. The teeth are crowded, and upper and lower teeth often are poorly aligned (malocclusion). The skull may be somewhat squat (brachycephaly).

The upper spine tends to be straight, and the lower spine presents an exaggerated curve, giving a swayback appearance (lumbar lordosis). The shortness of the limbs is most pronounced in the thighs and upper arms. The legs are often bowed (genu varum). The feet may point inward (talipes varus). Additional limb abnormalities include inability to extend elbows fully, and hands with short, stubby fingers. The fingers are often abnormally positioned so that they appear to present three groups of digits (trident hand).

The basic cause of the chrondrodystrophy that characterizes this disorder is unknown. It appears to involve a disturbance in the production and formation of the cartilage at the end of the long bones (those of the arms and legs), which inhibits their elongation.

Achondroplasia is inherited as an AUTOSOMAL DOMINANT trait, though at least 80% of cases are believed to be the result of new mutations, often associated with increased paternal age. It is estimated to occur in one in 40,000 births, and accounts for approximately half of all cases of dwarfism. The total population of achondroplasts is thought to be approximately 5,000 in the United States and 65,000 worldwide. Yet while it is the most common form of short-limbed dwarfism, it is not as widespread as once believed; previously, virtually all infants with short-limbed dwarfism were routinely classified as achondroplastic.

While it can be diagnosed at birth, the disorder becomes more pronounced with age. Intelligence is normal, though developmental milestones may be retarded in infancy due to the physical problems associated with short limbs. Affected individuals are prone to middle ear infections in childhood, which, if not properly treated, can lead to significant hearing loss. Mean adult height for males is 52 inches (132 cm), for females 48 inches (123 cm). There is a tendency toward obesity and 50% of those under medical care exhibit some neurologic and spinal complications.

Prenatal diagnosis of achondroplasia is possible via ultrasonographic examination

(See ULTRASOUND) of the fetal bones of the limbs. Pregnancies of achondroplastic females must be carefully monitored, and delivery is always via CESAREAN SECTION. Should two achondroplastic parents each transmit the dominant gene for this condition to an offspring (that is, have a child who is HOMOZYGOUS for the trait), the result is a lethal form of achondroplasia.

For more information, contact:
The Human Growth Foundation
4720 Montgomery Lane, Suite 909
Bethesda, MD 20814
(301) 656-6904
(301) 656-7540

Little People of America
P.O. Box 633
San Bruno, CA 94066
(415) 589-0695

**ACHOO syndrome** (autosomal dominant compelling heliophthalmic outburst syndrome)    Benign hereditary condition characterized by nearly uncontrollable paroxysms of sneezing caused by exposure to intensely bright light, usually sunlight, after an individual's eyes have adjusted to a darkened environment. The number of successive sneezes is typically two or three, but has been reported as high as 43. It is also known as photic or solar sneeze reflex and Peroutka sneeze.

First described in medical literature in 1964, it was named by Dr. William R. Collie of Seattle, Washington, and three colleagues in 1978, all of whom described the condition in their own families. Limited surveys have found that the condition exists in as many as 23% to 33% of individuals, though many are unaware of possessing this reflex reaction. It is transmitted as an AUTOSOMAL DOMINANT trait.

**achromatopsia**    See COLOR BLINDNESS.

**acne** (acne vulgaris)    Common acne (an inflammation of the sebaceous glands most often seen on the face, with onset at puberty), has demonstrated a familial tendency, though the exact genetics are unclear. Medications taken to alleviate acne by pregnant or child-bearing-age women can have an adverse impact on fetal development. These medications include tetracycline and retenoic acids (see ACCUTANE). It is recommended that tetracycline not be used from the fourth month of pregnancy and not prior to age 12, because of its effects on tooth and bone development.

**acquired immunodeficiency syndrome**    See AIDS.

**acrocentric**    The two strands (chromatids) of most chromosomes are joined somewhere near their midpoint. This intersection is the centromere. However, the centromeres in the acrocentric chromosomes are located near one end. These are chromosomes 13, 14, 15, 21 and 22. These chromosomes are frequently involved in a form of translocation known as Robertsonian translocations, in which two chromosomes (e.g., a chromosome 14 and a chromosome 21) fuse at the centromere. This can have important genetic consequences. (See CHROMOSOME ABNORMALITIES.)

**acrocephalosyndactyly**    See APERT SYNDROME; CARPENTER SYNDROME; PFEIFFER SYNDROME.

**acrocephaly**    See CRANIOSYNOSTOSIS.

**acro-osteolysis**    A FAMILIAL DISEASE with onset in childhood in which the bones at the tips of the extremities dissolve. It is a severe type of an osteoporosis-like process. There is no history of trauma. Pain, swelling and deformity result. The cause is unknown, and most cases are autosomal dominantly inherited, although other inheritance patterns have been described. Only about 20 cases have been reported worldwide. The term acro-osteolysis has been used in a variety of syndromes in which the bones of the extremities of the limbs dissolve. These include

PYCNODYSOSTOSIS, RHEUMATOID ARTHRITIS, hyperparathryoidism and polyvinylchloride poisoning.

**acute intermittent porphyria**   See POR-PHYRIA.

**ADAM complex**   See AMNIOTIC BAND SYNDROME.

**adenosine deaminase deficiency (ADA)**   See SCID, under IMMUNE DEFI-CIENCY DISEASES.

**adrenogenital syndromes** (congenital adrenal hyperplasia; CAH)   A group of disorders characterized by genital abnormalities due to deficiencies of the enzymes of the adrenal glands, which result in disruptions at specific stages of the synthesis of the steroid hormone cortisol. Located above the kidneys, the adrenal glands produce hormones involved in the metabolism of sodium and potassium, and androgens, estrogens, and progestins, which are important in the development and functioning of the reproductive system.

Because of the failure to metabolize sodium properly, affected individuals also exhibit excessive sodium loss, which can be life-threatening, and, in some forms of adrenogenital syndrome, the individuals may be prone to hypertension.

The most common form (over 90% of cases brought to medical attention) is 21-hydroxylase deficiency. In females, this disorder causes the female genitalia to appear "masculinized." It is thus a cause of AMBIGU-OUS GENITALIA. The degree of masculinization of the genitals is variable, ranging from slight enlargement of the clitoris to development of a male phallus, and may lead the infant to be raised as a male. (Internally, there is development of the uterus and ovaries.) The nipples and genitals may exhibit excessive pigmentation. In the absence of treatment with hormones, no pubertal changes will occur.

Males appear normal at birth, but later may exhibit premature enlargement of the penis and precocious development of secondary sex characteristics.

In both males and females with 21-hydroxylase deficiency, bones develop at an accelerated rate. Though there is accelerated early growth, closure of the growing portion of bone prematurely results in ultimate short stature. Other associated features include excessive salt loss and dehydration.

Treatment is required and involves replacement of steroid hormones. Genital abnormalities may require corrective cosmetic surgery.

21-hydroxylase deficiency, an AUTOSOMAL RECESSIVE disorder, is estimated to occur in one in 12,000 live births in the United States, though incidence is increased among the Inuit or Eskimo Native Americans living in Alaska. The incidence among the Yupik Eskimos has been found to be one in 680. Newborn screening for the disorder is done in some places.

PRENATAL DIAGNOSIS is possible, using analysis of tissue obtained by CHORIONIC VIL-LUS SAMPLING or AMNIOCENTESIS. In females, treatment with steroids in utero may minimize the virilizing effects of the syndromes.

Another relatively common form of CAH is 11-hydroxylase deficiency (5% to 8% of cases of CAH), occurring in one in 100,000 births and appearing very much like 21-hydroxylase deficiency.

Another form, 3-beta hydroxysteroid dehydrogenase deficiency, results in genital ambiguity and incomplete virilization in males, characterized by a penis with a malplaced urethral opening, and defective development of the scrotum with undescended testes. These children also lose excessive salt in the urine.

Other rare forms are deficiencies of 12-hydroxylase, cholesterol desmolase, 17-, 20-lyase and corticosterone methyl oxidase, which together account for less than 1% of all cases of adrenogenital syndrome.

A final syndrome is nonclassic adrenal hyperplasia. This late onset disorder results from a deficiency of 21-hydroxylase and leads to excessive hair growth and infertility. It occurs in approximately three in 1,000 individuals in the general white population and about three in 100 Ashkenazi Jews and may be an important cause of infertility in this ethnic group.

**adrenoleukodystrophy (ALD)**  L i p i d storage disease and form of LEUKODYSTROPHY. Storage diseases take their name from the abnormal accumulation, or storage, of substances within cells. In this disorder, the accumulation of very-long-chain fatty acids in the white matter of the brain and in the adrenal gland interferes with the ability of cells to function. The disorder is believed to result from the absence of the enzyme that normally breaks down the very-long-chain fatty acid. ALD was first recognized in 1923, and was named by Dr. Michael Blaw in 1971. Several hundred cases have been reported around the world.

Inherited as an X-LINKED trait, adrenoleukodystrophy affects only males. In its classic and most severe form, affected infants develop normally until four to 10 years of age. Initial symptoms include attention deficit, memory lapses, vision problems and difficulty with walking and coordination. They are often described as walking into walls. The dysfunction of the adrenal gland may cause increased skin pigmentation, or "bronzing," as well as nausea, vomiting and weakness. Symptoms become progressively worse (though the rate of deterioration varies considerably), leading to inability to communicate (aphasia) or control motor functions (apraxia), dementia and blindness. Death usually occurs within one to 10 years of diagnosis. There is no treatment.

A milder, adolescent or adult onset form, adrenomyeloneuropathy, affects the spinal cord and results in stiffness and clumsiness in the legs, accompanied by general fatigue, weight loss, pigmentation and bouts of nausea and vomiting. Motor control of the legs deteriorates progressively over a period of five to 15 years, requiring the use of cane or wheelchair. Life expectancy is only moderately diminished.

There is also an AUTOSOMAL RECESSIVE neonatal form with features common to both X-linked ALD and ZELLWEGER SYNDROME. These children are neurologically abnormal at birth and die generally within the first five years of life. It shares the common features of leukodystrophy and adrenal dysfunction with X-linked ALD but has additional features of Zellweger syndrome, including characteristic dysmorphic facial appearance. This disorder is caused by more generalized abnormalities of the peroxisome, a subcellular organelle, a structure that is a component of the cell.

Diagnosis of ALD is made on the basis of high levels of very-long-chain fatty acids in plasma and/or cultured skin fibroblasts, and testing appears to be highly (close to 100%) accurate. Female carriers can be detected with approximately 90% accuracy by plasma and cultured skin fibroblast analysis. Prenatal diagnosis in at-risk pregnancies is also possible by examination of very-long-chain fatty acid levels in fetal cells obtained by AMNIOCENTESIS or CVS.

For more information, contact:

United Leukodystrophy Foundation, Inc.
2304 Highland Drive
Sycamore, IL 60178
(815) 895-3211

**adrenothyeloneuropathy**    See ADRENOLEUKODYSTROPHY.

**affective disorders**    See MANIC DEPRESSION.

**agammaglobulinemia**    See IMMUNE DEFICIENCY DISORDERS.

**agenesis**    The failure of a part of the body or an organ to develop.

**Agent Orange**    A chemical defoliant used extensively in the Vietnam War, and which many American servicemen were exposed to.

There has been considerable controversy concerning the impact of direct and indirect exposure to Agent Orange, including reports of increased incidence of CANCERS and other health problems in those directly exposed, and increased incidence of birth defects in their offspring. However, no conclusive link between paternal exposure to Agent Orange and birth defects in their offspring has been established. (See also TERATOGEN.)

**Aicardi syndrome**   Seen only in females, this severe developmental defect is named for French physician Jean Aicardi, who first observed it in 1965. It involves agenesis (lack of development) of the corpus callosum of the brain along with a degeneration of the retina.

The corpus callosum is the large bundle of nerve fibers normally found between and connected to the two cerebral hemispheres. This disorder is caused by the failure of the corpus callosum to form, or form completely. Most individuals show severe retardation. None can speak a complete thought or sentence, and some can speak only single words. They may be unable to hold their heads up, and all have seizures.

Skeletal abnormalities include severe vertebral and rib abnormalities.

The underlying cause for this disorder is unknown. It may be inherited as an X-LINKED dominant trait, with male fetuses dying *in utero*. Each case would represent a new mutation. However, no clear Mendelian inheritance pattern has been demonstrated.

It should also be noted that agenesis of the corpus callosum can occur as an isolated defect or as a part of a number of other syndromes. It can be seen in CHROMOSOME ABNORMALITIES (Trisomy 13 or 18, for example). When found in isolation, with no other associated brain anomalies, corpus callosum agenesis can be completely asymptomatic.

For more information, contact:

Aicardi Syndrome Newsletter
1502 Woodcliff Road
Baltimore, MD 21228
(301) 455-0317

**AIDS**  (acquired immunodeficiency syndrome)   Disorder characterized by a breakdown in the immune system, rendering affected individuals vulnerable to multiple infections (see IMMUNE DEFICIENCY DISEASE). It is caused by a virus termed "human immunodeficiency virus," or HIV. Definitive diagnosis of the condition is made by blood tests that reveal the presence of antibodies produced by the immune system in response to the virus. Those who have these antibodies are said to be HIV positive. Once manifestations of the disease occur, it has thus far proven invariably fatal. However, due to an incubation period that may range from several months to several years, not all HIV-positive individuals exhibit symptoms of AIDS.

While it has been predominantly associated with gays and intravenous drug users and their sexual partners, AIDS can also be passed from infected women to their offspring during pregnancy or delivery, resulting in infants who are born with AIDS. The first report of an infant with congenital AIDS was published in 1983. The mode of transmission is poorly understood, and estimates on the percentage of HIV-infected women who pass AIDS on to their offspring range from 30% to 70%. The U.S. government's Centers for Disease Control puts the figure at 50%. Additionally, the virus can be transmitted from infected women to infants by breast feeding.

The incubation period is shorter in infants than in adults, and symptoms may appear within three or four months of birth. Recurrent infections and fluid in the ears may be the first signs. Growth failure and craniofacial abnormalities may also be evident. Affected infants are prone to brain damage due to the effect of the disorder on the developing nervous system; as many of 75% exhibit some neurologic damage. Brain development may cease, and developmental abilities may regress. Infants become weak and apathetic. Other symptoms include failure to thrive, warts on the hands, a

### Table I
### Reported AIDS Cases[1] Among Children Under Age 13 by State

| State | Number | Percent of Total Cases Among Children |
|-------|--------|---------------------------------------|
| Arkansas | 1 | 0.1 |
| New Mexico | 1 | 0.1 |
| Wisconsin | 1 | 0.1 |
| Delaware | 2 | 0.2 |
| Hawaii | 2 | 0.2 |
| Idaho | 2 | 0.2 |
| Iowa | 2 | 0.2 |
| Kansas | 2 | 0.2 |
| Maine | 2 | 0.2 |
| Minnesota | 2 | 0.2 |
| Nevada | 2 | 0.2 |
| Oregon | 2 | 0.2 |
| West Virginia | 2 | 0.2 |
| Arizona | 3 | 0.3 |
| Indiana | 3 | 0.3 |
| Mississippi | 3 | 0.3 |
| New Hampshire | 3 | 0.3 |
| Rhode Island | 4 | 0.3 |
| Utah | 4 | 0.3 |
| Washington | 4 | 0.3 |
| Colorado | 5 | 0.4 |
| Oklahoma | 6 | 0.5 |
| Missouri | 7 | 0.6 |
| Tennessee | 7 | 0.6 |
| South Carolina | 8 | 0.7 |
| North Carolina | 10 | 0.8 |
| Alabama | 11 | 0.9 |
| Louisiana | 12 | 1.0 |
| Michigan | 13 | 1.1 |
| District of Columbia | 14 | 1.2 |
| Ohio | 15 | 1.3 |
| Virginia | 19 | 1.6 |
| Georgia | 25 | 2.1 |
| Pennsylvania | 26 | 2.2 |
| Massachusetts | 26 | 2.2 |
| Illinois | 28 | 2.4 |
| Maryland | 28 | 2.4 |
| Connecticut | 33 | 2.8 |
| Texas | 43 | 3.6 |
| California | 93 | 7.8 |
| Florida | 141 | 11.9 |
| New Jersey | 163 | 13.8 |
| New York | 364 | 30.7 |

[1]Cumulative total number of cases reported from June 1981 through September 1988 to the Centers for Disease Control.

Source: *The Health of America's Children, 1989.* Children's Defense Fund: Washington, D.C.

yeast infection known as "thrush" in the mouth, and swollen glands. Affected children are more susceptible to bacterial infections, rather than the viral and fungal infections more commonly seen in adult patients. These are similar to typical childhood bacterial disease, only much more severe and resistant to treatment. They are also susceptible, as are affected adults, to pneumocystis carinii pneumonia (PCP), which causes pneumonia, and, unlike adults, to lymphocytic interstitial penumonitis (LIP), a poorly-understood abnormality of the lung's immune response. Both cause severe breathing problems.

While exact statistics are difficult to ascertain, the incidence of those born with the virus has been rising dramatically, with a disproportionate number of cases occurring in urban minority communities. Of approximately 1,200 infants born with AIDS and identified by the Federal Centers for Disease Control (CDC) from 1983 to 1989, more than 80% were black or Hispanic (824 infant deaths had been attributed to the disorder by 1989).

There is no cure. Prognosis is poor, though it has been noted that infants born with AIDS may remain asymptomatic for several years, with some living beyond nine years of age. (One survived to age 13.) Among the experimental treatments that have been tried are AZT, an antiviral drug, and intravenous transfusions of gamma globulin, antibodies isolated from blood that help fight a variety of bacterial and viral agents.

It has also been estimated that more than 50% of the 20,000 hemophiliacs (see HEMOPHILIA) in the United States also harbor the AIDS virus, resulting from transfusions containing blood products from AIDS-infected blood donors. Prior to 1984, screening procedures for donated blood did not detect the presence of the virus. (By 1989, the CDC identified about 300 children under 13 infected by exposure to blood products.) Yet hemophiliacs who test positive for the virus seem to develop symptoms less frequently than affected members of other risk groups. Hemophiliacs with AIDS do not pose a greater threat of transmitting the disorder than do other affected individuals, despite their prolonged bleeding; the primary bleeding problem in hemophilia is an inability to staunch internal bleeding. Thus, fears of their spreading the disease by bouts of excessive bleeding are greatly exaggerated.

For more information, contact:

Mothers of A.I.D.S. Patients
P.O. Box 3132
San Diego, CA 92103
(619) 293-3985
(619) 576-6636

National Association of People with
  A.I.D.S.
2025 Eye Street, N.W., Suite 415
Washington, D.C. 20006
(202) 429-2856

T-4 Anon, First Things First
3917 Roanoke Rd.
Kansas City, MO 64111-4023
(816) 756-1895

**AIP**    See PORPHYRIA.

**Alagille syndrome** (also arteriohepatic dysplasia; Watson-Alagille syndrome)    A hereditary liver disease of infants and young children. It has many of the features of other childhood liver diseases (see ALPHA-1-ANTI-TRYPSIN DEFICIENCY, BILARY ATRESIA, GALACTOSEMIA), such as jaundice, failure to thrive within the first three months, itching, fatty deposits under the skin, and stunted growth and development during early childhood. However, this disorder also involves the cardiovascular system, spinal column, eyes, nervous system, kidneys and other organs.

Abnormalities in the cardiovascular system (peripheral pulmonary artery stenosis) and spinal column are usually benign and can help in diagnosing the condition. Abnormalities in the eyes and kidneys may lead to minor degenerative changes.

Though the first cases of this disorder were described by G.H. Watson and V. Miller in 1973, the eponymic designation of this disorder is for French pediatrician Daniel Alagille, who delineated more features of the disorder

in 1975 in the *Journal of Pediatrics*. This disorder is now recognized more frequently among children with chronic liver diseases. At birth, there is an insufficiency of bile ducts, causing bile to back up within the liver and damage liver cells. Scarring of the liver (fibrosis or cirrhosis) occurs in 30% to 50% of affected infants.

It has been suggested that individuals with this syndrome also present a typical facial appearance, with a prominent, broad forehead, deep-set eyes, bulbous nose and small, pointed chin.

Alagille syndrome is transmitted as an AUTOSOMAL DOMINANT trait. While many adults with the syndrome are leading normal lives, overall life expectancy for children is unknown. The severity of liver damage and complications caused by abnormalities in other organ systems is a factor in the long-term outlook. However, prognosis is generally better than for infants with other forms of childhood liver disease.

For more information, contact:

American Liver Foundation
998 Pompton Avenue
Cedar Grove, NJ 07009
(201) 857-2626
(800) 223-0179

The Children's Liver Foundation
7 Highland Place
Maplewood, NJ 07040
(201) 761-1111

**albinism**    One of the most widely recognized and striking of all genetic conditions, this describes a group of inherited metabolic disorders characterized by a reduction or absence of a pigment called melanin in the skin, hair and eyes. In addition to a lack of pigment, common features in all are visual abnormalities, including decreased visual acuity, rapid, involuntary back and forth darting of the eyes (nystagmus), increased sensitivity to light (photophobia), and crossed eyes, caused by a muscle imbalance of the eyes (STRABISMUS). They may be far-sighted (hyperopia) or nearsighted (myopia), and often have astigmatism, a condition wherein light focuses poorly on the retina due to abnormal curvature of the cornea. Some forms may be associated with other problems such as difficulties with blood clotting (see below) or hearing impairment.

(Albinism should be differentiated from hypopigmentation, in which there is a reduction of the normal amount of pigment, but vision is unaffected. Many forms of hypopigmentation are associated with deafness; see WAARDENBURG SYNDROME.)

Albinism occurs in plants, insects, fish, reptiles, amphibians, birds, marsupials and mammals. The Greeks referred to it as "leukoethiopes," from "leuko," the word for white. Pliny and Aulus Gellius described the condition in the first century. Historically, people with albinism have been singled out and occupied social positions ranging from outcasts to semigods.

Noah is thought to have been an albino, due to Midrashic accounts, which state "his hair was white as snow, and his eyes like the rays of the sun." However, there is a similar description of Christ, who has not historically been regarded as an albino, in Revelations 1:14: "His head and his hair were white like wool, as white as snow; and his eyes were like a flame of fire." The term albino was first used in about 1660 by a Portuguese explorer in describing white Negroes he had observed in Africa, and comes from the Latin "albus," meaning white. Early explorers to the New World found a high frequency of albinism in several Indian tribes. The English Rev. Dr. Spooner, a brilliant classicist whose amusing errors of speech became known as "spoonerisms," was an albino. His errors of speech are thought to be related to his nystagmus, which caused a jumbling of information from the printed page, leading to a verbal jumbling of speech.

Albinos are popularly thought to have red eyes, but actually most have blue or grayish eyes. In some types, the iris appears to have a violet or reddish hue, because light is reflected back from the reddish retina, similar to the effect seen in some flash photos where eyes appear red.

Visual problems are caused by pigmentary deficiency. The eye needs pigment to develop normal vision, though the reason for this requirement is unknown. The retina develops improperly during fetal life, and vision cannot be totally corrected, even with corrective lenses. Nerve signals from the retina to the brain do not travel along the proper nerve routes. Normally light enters the eye only through the pupil—the dark opening at the center of the iris. But in albinism, the iris doesn't have enough pigment to screen out excess light, and it passes through the iris, as well.

Treatment generally consists of attempts to alleviate ocular deficiencies. Surgery, though sometimes helpful for cosmetic reasons, does not seem to improve vision. Corrective and tinted lenses and specialized magnifiers and small telescopes may be of help in addressing vision problems. Albinism generally does not affect lifespan, though there is an increased incidence of skin cancer due to the lack of pigmentation, which serves to protect the skin from damage caused by ultraviolet radiation. Sunscreens are recommended for reducing exposure to the harmful ultraviolet rays.

There are two major forms of albinism: oculocutaneous albinism, in which pigment is reduced in the hair, skin and eyes; and ocular albinism, in which pigment is reduced only in the eyes. Overall, some type of albinism occurs in approximately one in 17,000 live births.

### Oculocutaneous Albinism

Researchers have described 10 types of oculocutaneous albinism. The most common types are termed either "ty-positive" or "ty-negative," based on whether or not there is any tyrosinase present. This is an enzyme that converts tyrosine, an amino acid, into melanin in the production of pigment. The determination is made by plucking a few hairs from the scalp of a person with albinism, and incubating the roots, or "bulbs," in a chemical solution of tyrosine. Hair bulbs that don't turn dark in this test are termed "ty-neg"—that is, they don't produce melanin from tyrosine. If the hair bulbs turn dark, they are termed "ty-pos"—melanin is present. A new test, the tyrosinase assay, measures the rate at which tyrosine in hair bulbs is converted to dopa, which is then made into pigment.

*Tyrosine-negative oculocutaneous albinism.* Without tyrosinase activity, the skin and hair stay white throughout life. There is a greater susceptibility to developing skin cancer than in ty-pos albinism.

Carriers can be identified through hair bulb analysis, measuring the rate at which they produce pigment, and prenatal diagnosis is possible through testing fetal hair bulbs obtained by fetoscopy. Visual problems are severe.

Ty-neg albinism occurs in about one in 28,000 blacks and one in 39,000 whites in the United States. A rare variant of this form, Hermansky-Pudlak-type albinism, exhibits a progressive and potentially life-threatening bleeding tendency.

*Tyrosine-positive oculocutaneous albinism.* At early ages, this form closely resembles ty-neg albinism. However, there is partial activity of tyrosinase, leading to the gradual accumulation of pigment with age. The hair becomes yellow or reddish and the skin may become freckled or have pigmented nevi. Ocular problems are less severe than in ty-neg, and tend to improve with age. This form is estimated to occur in one in 15,000 blacks and one in 37,000 whites in the United States. It is particularly common in some Indian tribes.

CHEDIAK-HIGASHI SYNDROME is a rare form of ty-pos albinism. While oculocutaneous symptoms are moderate, it is usually fatal in childhood due to leukocyte abnormalities that lead to repeated infections and a condition that mimics leukemia.

### Ocular Albinism

In these forms of albinism pigment is reduced only in the eyes. There are five recognized types. The most prevalent forms are X-LINKED and therefore affect primarily males. Female carriers can generally be identified through subtle abnormalities in the eye that are detectable through ophthalmologic examination. There is also an AUTOSOMAL RECESSIVE form of ocular albinism that affects males and females equally.

For more information, contact:
National Organization for Albinism and
  Hypopigmentation (NOAH)
1500 Locust Street, Suite 1816
Philadelphia, PA 19102
(215) 545-2322

American Foundation for the Blind
15 West 16th Street
New York, NY 10011
(212) 620-2155
(800) AFBLIND

National Association for the Visually
  Handicapped
305 East 24th St.
New York, NY 10010
(212) 889-3141

International Albinism Center
Box 485 UMHC
The University of Minnesota Hospital
  and Clinic
420 Delaware Street, S.E.
Minneapolis, MN 55455

### Albright hereditary osteodystrophy
(pseudohypoparathyroidism)   Syndrome marked by short stature, obesity and, in most cases, MENTAL RETARDATION. It is caused by errors of mineral metabolism, which frequently result in skeletal and dental abnormalities, including poorly formed teeth with delayed eruption and a proneness to develop cavities. Hand anomalies are common. The severity of expression of the disorder is variable. Life span is normal.

Affected individuals have elevated levels of serum parathyroid hormone (PTH), low levels of calcium and exhibit symptoms of hypoparathyroidism.

Affected infants frequently have seizures due to decreased concentration of calcium in the blood (hypocalcemia), muscle cramps and intermittent muscle spasms (tetany). These individuals don't respond normally to parathyroid hormone.

At birth, infants have prominent foreheads and a round face. The nasal bridge is low, and the neck is short. The most striking characteristic is shortening and malformation of fingers and toes, most commonly affecting the third and fourth digits.

This is an inherited condition, though its genetics are not entirely clear. The ratio of female to male reported cases is 2:1. Both sex-limited AUTOSOMAL DOMINANT and X-LINKED dominant inheritance have been suggested.

The basic defect that causes the disorder is unknown but is believed to involve deficient response to the secretion of parathyroid hormone. Treatment consists of cautious supplementation with vitamin D and calcium.

**alcoholism**    A chronic and progressive disorder characterized by the inability to control the consumption of alcohol. It may lead to death due to the internal consequences of long-term alcohol abuse, which include cirrhosis of the liver, cardiac arrest and cancers of the liver, pancreas, lung, colon and rectum.

Alcoholism is most likely a MULTIFACTORIAL disorder caused by the action of several GENES in concert with environmental influence. Inherited tendencies that may play a role include how an individual metabolizes alcohol, an individual's hormonal and behavioral response to alcohol, and his or her tolerance for levels of alcohol in the blood. Biochemically, those prone to alcoholism may experience more pleasurable effects than others. (A preference for alcohol can be selectively bred into experimental animals.)

A familial link has been recognized in alcoholism since ancient times, and numerous studies have found increased risks for the dis-

order among relatives of those affected. Estimates on the percentage of the general population that will develop alcoholism generally range from 3% to 10% of males and 1% to 3% of females. (Estimates of the number of alcoholics in the United States are generally put at approximately 10 million.) Sons and brothers of alcoholic males may have three to five times this risk, and daughters of female alcoholics three times. In identical (monozygotic) twins there is a concordance (both display the trait) of more than 50%, while the concordance is less than 30% for fraternal (dizygotic) twins of the same sex. Familial alcoholism tends to develop early in life.

Studies of adoptees indicate that heredity plays a stronger role than environment in producing alcoholics, with the rates among adopted children of male alcoholics more reflective of the risks associated with their biological than their adoptive fathers. Also, sons of alcoholics who are themselves not alcoholics have a higher tolerance for alcohol than sons of non-alcoholics. Researchers have also discovered biochemical differences between alcoholics in how white blood cells respond to alcohol. This may lead to a simple blood test for identifying those with a predisposition to developing the disorder.

Some ethnic groups show an increased incidence of alcoholism and some a markedly decreased tolerance for alcohol. Native Americans and individuals of Irish descent are among the former group, while Asians are among the latter. Many Asians lack an enzyme responsible for breaking down acetaldehyde, a toxic stimulant that is a byproduct of alcohol metabolism. Individuals with this enzyme deficiency become flushed, dizzy and experience headaches and nausea after ingestion of small amounts of alcohol. An estimated two-thirds of Asians exhibit ill effects from alcohol, while only about 5% of whites are similarly affected.

A small molecule, alcohol is easily absorbed throughout the body, and, in pregnant women, can enter the fetal blood via the placenta. The development anomalies that may

occur as a result are termed FETAL ALCOHOL
SYNDROME.

For more information, contact:

National Clearinghouse for Alcohol
Information (NCALI)
P.O. Box 2345
Rockville, MD 20852
(301) 468-2600

National Council on Alcoholism
12 West 21st St.
New York, NY 10010
(212) 206-6770

**Alexander disease**   A progressive and
fatal infant-onset disorder seen mostly in
males. A form of LEUKODYSTROPHY, it results
in defective formation or destruction of myelin, the protective sheath that covers nerve
tissue. Named for New Zealand pathologist
W.S. Alexander, who described it in 1949, it
is characterized by progressive enlargement
of the head, spasticity and dementia. Death
usually occurs one to two years after onset of
symptoms. The cause and mode of transmission are unknown, though AUTOSOMAL RE-
CESSIVE inheritance is suspected.

**alkaptonuria**   Inherited as an AUTOSO-
MAL RECESSIVE trait, this rare disorder results
from a lack of the ENZYME hepatic
homogentisic acid oxidase. Although this enzyme defect can be detected from birth by a
urine test, affected infants and young adults
are usually asymptomatic and fail to notice its
most characteristic manifestation—their
urine, if left to stand, turns brown or black.

This condition occupies an important place
in the history of genetics. It is one of the first
disorders in humans shown to be caused by
MENDELIAN inheritance; it was identified as a
recessive disorder by English physician
Archibald E. Garrod in 1902. It is also one of
the four disorders Garrod hypothesized were
due to an "inborn error of metabolism" (the
title of his 1909 monograph), an important
concept in human genetics whose value was
not appreciated until the 1940s. (The other

three of these metabolic disorders were ALBI-
NISM, CYSTINURIA and pentosuria.)

With age, dark spots may develop on the
whites (sclerae) of the eyes. Pigmentation also
develops in the cartilage, nails and skin, particularly on the cheeks, forehead, armpits (ax-
illae) and genitals. Ear wax (cerumen) is often
black or brown. A later symptom is arthritis,
especially in the spine. Joints often stiffen
completely (ankylosis).

Approximately 400 cases have been reported, with incidence described as unusually
high in the Dominican Republic and Czechoslovakia. Affected individuals have normal
intelligence and life span, although arthritis
may limit their mobility.

**allele**   One of two or more alternative
forms of any particular gene located on a GENE
pair. Gene pairs, found at corresponding positions (loci) on CHROMOSOME pairs, represent
two alleles.

Many genes have more than one allele, such
as those for blood type, with the alleles for
types A, B and O all found at the same gene
locus.

(Additionally, advances in molecular genetics have demonstrated that what were previously identified as simply either dominant
or recessive alleles may actually represent a
variety of forms of an allele.)

**allergy**   An acquired hypersensitivity to
normally benign substance. The word is taken
from the Greek "allos," meaning altered, and
"ergia," reactivity. Any substance that pro-
vokes an allergic reaction is known as an
allergen.

Allergic reactions are a unique form of autoimmune disease, possibly evolved from a
genetic mechanism that protected the body
against worms and parasites. The allergens
may in some way mimic these invading organisms. It appears that individuals inherit a genetic predisposition to develop a particular
allergy, though the mode of transmission is
unclear. It is likely to be POLYGENIC.

Common allergens include pollen, dust, hair, fur, feathers, scales, wool, chemicals, drugs, insect bites, and such foods as eggs, chocolate, milk, wheat, tomatoes, nuts, citrus fruits, shellfish, oatmeal, sulfite preservatives and potatoes. Evidence also indicates deer can make some hunters sneeze, cockroaches can prompt asthma attacks in asthmatics, and some individuals are literally allergic to exercise.

The prevalence of allergies is unknown, though it is thought potentially to represent the largest population of chronically diseased individuals in the United States. Common allergic conditions include hay fever (vasomotor or allergic rhinitis), bronchial asthma, eczema (a skin condition) and hives (urticaria). An estimated 40 million Americans have hay fever, 9 million asthma, from 10 million to 20 million have had occasional hives and an untold number have food allergies.

Symptoms of the reaction commonly involve the respiratory tract or the skin. In the respiratory tract this usually takes the form of congestion, runny nose, watery eyes, sneezing and breathing difficulty caused by swelling and constriction of the bronchial tubes. Cutaneous involvement includes itching, rashes and lesions.

Allergies usually develop following a number of exposures to a given substance, after enough antibodies are produced to trigger the response to the allergen. The antibodies are a class of immunoglobulins, IgE, with a specific form for each allergen. When allergens are present, the IgE antibodies attach themselves to cells in the lining of the nose and bronchial passages, where they bind to the allergens. This triggers the cells to eject histamine or histamine-like substances, causing an irritation accompanied by sneezing, itching and watery eyes. Severe reactions can cause death by blockage of air passages or a precipitous drop in blood pressure.

Atopic eczema, which is often associated with asthma and other allergic phenomena, is extremely common, affecting 0.7% of the population. Some believe that it may even be determined by an AUTOSOMAL DOMINANT gene with highly variable expression. The risk of developing some allergic problem where one parent is affected approaches 50%, and is slightly higher when both parents are affected.

For more information, contact:

American Academy of Allergy and
   Immunology
611 East Wells Street
Milwaukee, WI 53202
(414) 272-6071

American Allergy Association
Box 7273
Menlo Park, CA 94026
(415) 322-1663

National Institute of Allergy and
   Infectious Diseases
National Institutes of Health
Bethesda, MD 20205
(301) 496-4000

**alopecia**    A general term for any type of hair loss. There are specific forms of alopecia, with the most common being alopecia areata, a condition characterized by the loss of hair in distinct round or oval patches about the head, though hairless patches may appear anywhere. Onset is usually between the ages of 20 and 50, with the average about 30 years of age. In most cases, hair regrows after several months, though episodes may recur. Alopecia areata may progress, particularly in childhood cases, to alopecia totalis, resulting in total loss of hair of the head, or alopecia universalis, in which all body hair is lost, usually without regrowing. Between 5% and 30% of those with alopecia areata develop alopecia totalis.

It is estimated that 10% of alopecia areata and 20% of alopecia totalis demonstrate a familial aggregation. For those with a relative under medical treatment for alopecia, the chances of developing the condition are estimated at 100 times the general population's.

Familial forms of alopecia are thought to involve an abnormality of the immune system. Many cases go into spontaneous remission.

Treatments with the steroid cortisone and other drugs have been effective in some cases. (See also MALE PATTERN BALDNESS.)

For more information, contact:

H.A.I.R., Inc.
Help Alopecia International Research
P.O. Box 691487
Los Angeles, CA 90069
(213) 851-5138

National Alopecia Areata Foundation
P.O. Box 5027
Mill Valley, CA 94941
(415) 383-3444

**alpha-fetoprotein (AFP)**   A protein excreted by the FETUS into the AMNIOTIC FLUID and from there into the mother's bloodstream through the placenta. During the second trimester of pregnancy, usually the 16th week, a blood test to measure the level of maternal AFP can aid in assessing the presence of certain defects in the developing fetus.

Elevated levels of AFP are an indication of possible neural tube defects, which occur in about one to two of every 1,000 births. High levels can also indicate the possibility of multiple births, underestimation of the age of the fetus, other anomalies, low birth weight and fetal death. Low levels of AFP can indicate an overestimation of the age of the fetus or the more ominous possibility of genetic chromosomal disorders, such as DOWN SYNDROME.

The maternal blood test presents no risk to the fetus or to the mother, but it is not a positive indication of either neural tube defects or other disorders. However, an abnormal test result will allow the physician and patient to determine if further testing is necessary. Usually, a second AFP blood test will be performed as a confirmation of the first result. If the second test result is the same, a decision can be made to try ultrasonography (see ULTRASOUND), followed, if necessary, by a determination of the level of AFP in the amniotic fluid. Assaying the concentration of AFP in the amniotic fluid can be a more positive

confirmation of abnormalities, especially neural tube defects. Chromosome analysis can also be done on cells in the fluid to look for Down syndrome. However, this test requires AMNIOCENTESIS, which involves a small (less than 1%) risk of miscarriage, infection or fetal death.

**alpha-1-antitrypsin deficiency (AAT deficiency)**   An inherited disorder that can lead to hepatitis and cirrhosis in infants and, in its late onset form, emphysema in adults. It is a relatively common inborn error of metabolism. Transmitted as an AUTOSOMAL RECESSIVE trait, its incidence is estimated at between one in 700 and one in 2,500 live births.

The disorder gained attention in the medical community in 1963 when its link to the development of emphysema was demonstrated. Its association with juvenile cirrhosis was established a few years later.

The primary role of AAT is unclear, though it is known to be an enzyme-inhibitor that limits the action of enzymes active in the breakdown of protein. It may facilitate "safe handling" of these caustic enzymes, which are otherwise capable of digesting and destroying cells and proteins of the body.

There are over 75 genetic variants involved in the synthesis of AAT that may differ substantially in the levels of alpha-1 antitrypsin found in the body, leading to a wide variation in the manifestations and severity of this disorder. But what is inherited is the deficiency of AAT, not necessarily the disease. For unknown reasons, only 10% to 20% of babies born with the deficiency will develop liver disease. Individuals will either be asymptomatic, will develop a liver disease in the first weeks or months of life or will develop emphysema in middle age.

Symptoms of the disorder often appear in the newborn period. They include jaundice, swelling of the abdomen and poor feeding. If the onset is during childhood or adolescent years, symptoms include fatigue, poor appetite, swelling of the abdomen and legs or enlargement of the liver (hepatomegaly).

If they develop cirrhosis (scarring of the liver), the change in blood flow that results can cause significant complications. There may be nosebleeds, bruising, excess body fluid and enlarged veins in the inside of the stomach and esophagus (varices). Increases in pressure in these veins may make them leak, resulting in internal bleeding. Later complications include sleepiness after eating protein (due to increased blood ammonia levels) and increased risk of infection. Approximately 15% of those who come to medical attention develop cirrhosis.

Cirrhosis may be caused by abnormal forms of AAT, which are retained by the liver cells, where it may lead to liver damage. The alpha-1-AT deficiency's association with the development of emphysema may be due to the unchecked action of enzymes it is responsible for blocking. Released at the site of lung inflammation or irritation, the caustic action of the protein-digesting enzymes may eventually reduce elasticity in the underlying tissue, resulting in greatly reduced lung capacity.

It is estimated that 20,000 to 40,000 individuals in the United States have this disease. Two percent to 3% of the white population of the United States is thought to have a variety of alpha-1 trypsin deficiency that puts them at risk for developing emphysema, particularly if they smoke. This is because heterozygotes (carriers) of this variation are at risk of developing emphysema in later life.

CARRIER screening is available. PRENATAL DIAGNOSIS using RECOMBINANT DNA techniques is possible in a select number of laboratories. The gene is known to be on CHROMOSOME 14.

Research is currently underway on the treatment of this disorder by replacement therapy. AAT is given intravenously. Early results appear promising. Importantly, "treatment" includes avoidance of both cigarette smoke and environmental exposure to respiratory irritants.

For more information, contact:

The American Liver Foundation
998 Pompton Avenue

Cedar Grove, NJ 07009
(201) 857-2626
(800) 223-0179

The Children's Liver Foundation
155 Maplewood Avenue
Maplewood, NJ 07040
(201) 761-1111

**Alport syndrome**   See FAMILIAL NEPHRITIS.

**ALS**   See AMYOTROPHIC LATERAL SCLEROSIS.

**Alzheimer's disease (AD)**   An adult-onset degenerative brain disorder characterized by memory loss, deterioration of mental function and disturbances of speech and movement. It was first described in 1906 by German neurologist and psychiatrist Alois Alzheimer (1864-1915), who noted the "neurofibrillary tangles," damaged brain cells that are a hallmark of this disorder. (These distorted brain cells can only be seen upon autopsy; thus, definitive diagnosis of Alzheimer's disease cannot be made until after death.)

The disease was originally thought to be rare, but as knowledge of the disorder has grown, the extent of its impact on the population has been revised upward. By the latter 1980s the total number of those affected in the United States was thought to be 2.5 million. That number was revised upward again in 1989, when a major, federally financed study by Brigham and Women's Hospital in Boston found 10.3% of individuals over age 65 and 47.2% over age 85 had mental impairments most likely caused by Alzheimer's disease. If those figures are correct, 4 million Americans have Alzheimer's disease. It is considered the fourth leading cause of death among adults, responsible for more than 100,000 deaths a year. A 1986 study by Dr. D. Morrison Smith for Alzheimer's Society of Canada estimated that 300,000 Canadians had Alzheimer's, and that by 2020, 700,000 Canadians will have it. The National Institute on Aging expects that by the middle of the 21st century, 14 million Americans will be afflicted.

Most cases are sporadic, but familial forms of Alzheimer's disease are thought to account for 10% to 30% of those under medical attention. Most of these cases are thought to be MULTIFACTORIAL, precipitated by the action of several GENES in concert with environmental factors. But between 6% and 10% by some estimates of all those affected with Alzheimer's have inherited it as an AUTOSOMAL DOMINANT trait.

Onset may occur anywhere from the 30s to the 80s, though it rarely occurs before the age of 45; most cases occur after age 70. Early signs are forgetfulness and minor mood swings, leading to loss of memory, the ability for rational thinking and the ability to care for oneself. There is no cure, and affected individuals invariably succumb to infections, malnutrition or other complications within 10 years of onset.

This disorder is thought to involve the accumulation of large concentrations of amyloid, a protein, in abnormal brain structures of amyloid plaques and neurofibrillary tangles, as well as in the walls of the cerebral blood vessels. In 1989, researchers found the abnormal amyloid beta protein outside the brain for the first time, a development which may lead to a practical diagnostic test for the disease. Aluminum is present in increased concentrations in the brains of those affected as well, but this is thought to be a result rather than a cause of the disorder.

A gene believed to be responsible for a buildup of amyloid has been identified on the long arm of CHROMOSOME 21. Interestingly, this is the same chromosome that, when an extra copy is present, results in DOWN SYNDROME; individuals affected with Down syndrome frequently develop amyloid plaques and succumb to an Alzheimer's-like dementia in their forties.

A benign abnormality of platelets in the blood is observed in about half of those with Alzheimer's who are examined, and those who exhibit this abnormality tend to be more severely affected by the disorder. This suggests that the platelet abnormality is a genetic

marker for familial AD, and may itself be inherited as an autosomal dominant trait.

For more information, contact:
Alzheimer's Disease and Related
    Disorders Association, Inc. (ADRDA)
70 East Lake Street, Suite 600
Chicago, IL 60601
(312) 853-3060

**ambiguous genitalia**   A general term for maldevelopment of the genitals. These conditions have their genesis in the eighth week of fetal development, when the sexual organs begin to develop. At this time, in the female embryo, müllerian ducts develop into fallopian tubes and uterus, and in the male embryo, wolffian ducts develop into the epididymis, vas deferens and seminal vesicle. If there are errors in this process, the female reproductive organs may become overly masculinized, or the male organs may be inadequately masculinized.

Due to the psychological problems these conditions present for parents, a finding of ambiguous genitalia at birth has been described in medical texts as "a true genetic emergency." However, hormonal therapy and reconstructive surgery can often alleviate these conditions.

Among the disorders characterized by ambiguous genitalia are ADRENOGENITAL SYNDROMES, HERMAPHRODITISM and PSEUDOHERMAPHRODITISM.

**amelogenesis imperfecta**   Defective formation of the enamel of a child's teeth without any apparent accompanying disease or external cause characterizes this hereditary disorder. It occurs in AUTOSOMAL DOMINANT, AUTOSOMAL RECESSIVE and X-LINKED recessive forms.

Defects vary considerably with the genetic type. Dental abnormalities include thin, incompletely developed (hypoplastic) enamel; pitted, grooved and discolored enamel; lack of contact between adjacent teeth (malocclusion); teeth that do not grow through the gum (unerupted) due to partial absorption in their sockets; teeth sensitive to temperature changes; easily broken or pulverized (friable) enamel; enamel that is deficient in hardening (hypocalcification) or incompletely grown (hypomaturation) and soft enough to allow a metal probe to be pushed through; and teeth that turn brown or black from food stains.

Defects are apparent at the time of tooth eruption by visual examination and by X-ray examination, which may disclose a lack of contrast between the enamel and the basic bony tissue (dentin) of the teeth.

This disorder occurs in about one in 16,000 births among North American white children. It can lead to early loss of teeth, periodontal disease and psychosocial problems because of unsightly teeth. Orthodontics and special dental restoration procedures can be effective in correcting the problems.

The basic protein defect causing this disorder is unknown. Identification of carriers is possible in the case of the X-linked recessive type. Currently, there is no method for prenatal diagnosis.

**amino acid**    The building blocks of proteins, and members of a large group of organic compounds. While more than 80 amino acids are found in nature, only 20 are required for human life. Eight of these are only available from food, and these are called (essential) amino acids: isoleucine, leucine, lysine, methionine, phenylalanine, threonine, tryptophan and valine. During infancy, arginine and histidine are also essential; these amino acids are the end product of digestion.

A variety of inborn errors of metabolism in synthesis or breakdown of amino acids lead to inherited disorders of amino acid metabolism. These include PHENYLKETONURIA (PKU), HOMOCYSTINURIA and the UREA CYCLE DEFECTS. (See also AMINOACIDEMIA.)

**aminoacidemia**    (a m i n o a c i d u r i a; aminoacidopathies)    Any one of almost 100 inborn errors of AMINO ACID metabolism. They include ALKAPTONURIA, CYSTINURIA, HOMOCYSTINURIA and PHENYLKETONURIA.

**aminoaciduria**    See AMINOACIDEMIA.

**Amish**    A religious isolate population living primarily in Lancaster County, Pennsylvania. Intermarriage within the community has contributed to the documentation of a number of rare hereditary disorders in higher incidence than would be expected in a random population. The disorders include ELLIS-VAN CREVELD SYNDROME and cartilage-hair hypoplasia (METAPHYSEAL CHONDRODYSPLASIA).

**amniocentesis**    The most widely used invasive diagnostic procedure for prenatal detection of hereditary disorders and CONGENITAL defects.

During pregnancy, the fetus is surrounded by a sac of AMNIOTIC FLUID, which protects and cushions the developing embryo and into which fetal cells are released. In amniocentesis, these cells are collected, examined and analyzed, along with amniotic fluid itself, to provide information regarding the condition of the fetus and to detect possible genetic or metabolic defects. Normally, this procedure is performed at the 16th or 17th week of pregnancy to ensure that sufficient amniotic fluid is present to provide the amount of fluid required for proper analysis. It can take two to five weeks to culture and prepare the fetal cells in the laboratory for analysis, so the matter of the timing of this procedure is important in the event that amniocentesis discloses a defect or disorder that may indicate the option of terminating the pregnancy. Recently there has been much interest in the use of amniocentesis earlier in pregnancy (about 13 weeks); however, the safety and ultimate role of this procedure has not yet been determined.

Often the first step is injection of local anesthetic. A needle is then inserted through the mother's abdominal wall and GENETIC MARKERS the wall of the uterus, and into the amniotic sac. A syringe is used to withdraw a sample of the amniotic fluid.

ULTRASOUND is used in conjunction with amniocentesis to present an image of the fetus and its position in the uterus, and to aid the physician in guiding the needle into the amniotic sac. With the use of ultrasound and the image of the fetus projected on the screen, a skilled physician can guide the needle into and through a space as small as a quarter-inch in diameter.

A report published in 1963 described the technique, which was used in this account to give a blood transfusion to a fetus with maternal Rh blood factor incompatibility (see HEMOLYTIC DISEASE OF THE NEWBORN). In 1966, M.W. Steele and W.R. Bregg described how the technique could be used to collect and culture fetal cells for chromosomal analysis from the amniotic fluid. The technique was perfected for use in PRENATAL DIAGNOSIS by 1969.

Disorders that can be detected through amniocentesis include TAY-SACHS DISEASE, SICKLE-CELL ANEMIA, SPINA BIFIDA, NEURAL TUBE DEFECTS (NTD), ENZYME deficiencies, CHROMOSOME ABNORMALITIES and blood disorders. Using molecular diagnostic studies with linked GENETIC MARKERS, many other diseases, such as CYSTIC FIBROSIS and Duchenne MUSCULAR DYSTROPHY can now be diagnosed as well. Amniocentesis can also disclose the sex of the unborn child, although the procedure is not performed solely for this purpose.

Amniocentesis is an invasive procedure and involves risks, both to the mother and the fetus. Strict antiseptic procedures must be followed to prevent infection and extreme care must be taken to keep the needle from puncturing the fetus. Other potential adverse effects include hemorrhage of either the mother or the fetus, leakage of amniotic fluid, and spontaneous ABORTION. There is a one in 200 risk of miscarriage in addition to the normal risk of miscarriage at this point in pregnancy. The other potential complications are much less often encountered.

Despite its widespread use as a prenatal diagnostic procedure, the decision to use amniocentesis should be carefully considered by the physician and parents in consultation, with the risks weighed against potential benefits. However, it is commonly recommended for pregnancies of women over 35 years of age due to increased risk of DOWN SYNDROME and other chromosomal abnormalities, as well as in pregnancies involving a known and detectable risk of birth defects or GENETIC DISORDERS.

**amniotic band syndrome** (ADAM complex)    Term referring to a variety of anomalies associated with fibrous bands that entangle the fetus in the womb, interfering with fetal development. The fibrous bands are thought to result from ruptures of the amniotic membranes within the womb. The earlier and more severe the intrauterine damage, the greater the impact on the infant. It may simply constrict a portion of the fetus or cause more widespread problems by cutting off blood supply to a region of the body of the fetus.

In its most common form, only the limbs are involved, ranging from constriction rings that appear around digits or limbs to amputation of digits or limbs. There may be fusion of the ends of digits (distal pseudosyndactyly). The most severe form involves both limb malformations and craniofacial anomalies, and has been referred to by the acronym ADAM (Amniotic Deformity, Adhesions, Mutilations) Complex.

The craniofacial malformations may include cleft lip and palate, an increase in cerebral fluid causing enlargement of the head (HYDROCEPHALUS), gross clefts of the midface and protrusion of the brain through fissures in the skull (ENCEPHALOCELE). A number of ocular and nasal abnormalities may also be present.

Part of the intestine may protrude through the abdominal wall, covered only by a thin membrane. The failure of the abdominal wall to close is referred to as "gastroschisis."

This is a non-hereditary congenital condition estimated to occur in one in 5,000 to one in 10,000 live births, with at least 600 cases reported. While some genetic conditions may cause similar malformations, they tend to be symmetrical, that is, the limb defects are mirror images of each other.

PRENATAL DIAGNOSIS may be possible in severe cases, due to the association of elevated alpha-fetoprotein levels with ADAM complex, as well as by ultrasound examination. Simple cases may cause only cosmetic problems. Congenital limb amputations require prosthetic limbs, and MENTAL RETARDATION may be associated with cases involving craniofacial defects. Many cases of the ADAM complex may result in STILLBIRTH or death soon after birth.

**amniotic fluid**    The colorless, almost transparent fluid that surrounds the developing FETUS in the womb. Amniotic fluid is composed of fluid from the mother as well as fetal urine and other body secretions. It contains cells, for example, shed from the fetus's skin as well as fetal bladder cells excreted in the urine.

This protective fluid is rapidly recirculated throughout the mother's body, with a complete replacement requiring approximately three hours. The fetus swallows some of the fluid, and if there is, for example, an obstruction in the fetus's intestinal tract or the fetus has a neurologic disorder that impairs swallowing, the fluid accumulates. This condition of excess fluid is termed polyhydramnios. If the fetal kidneys are not working properly and no fetal urine is produced, there is a deficiency of amniotic fluid. This is termed oligohydramnios.

In the genetic testing procedure of AMNIOCENTESIS, amniotic fluid is withdrawn from the womb via a surgical needle for later examination.

**amyloidosis**    A rare metabolic disorder marked by deposition of amyloid, a starchlike protein, in organs and tissues, leading to slowly progressive deterioration of nerves (in adulthood) and ultimately death. AUTOSOMAL DOMINANT hereditary forms have been identified in isolated families and populations around the world.

**amyotrophic lateral sclerosis**    (ALS) Known as "Lou Gehrig's disease" after perhaps the best-known patient, ALS is a progressive and fatal degenerative disease of the neuromuscular system. The disease attacks the motor neurons, among the largest nerve cells, which reach from the brain to the spinal cord and from the spinal cord to muscles throughout the body. The destruction of these neurons leads to complete loss of voluntary muscle movement, and total paralysis.

It was first described by French neurologist Jean-Martin Charcot in 1869. The name is derived from Greek. "A" means "without" or "negative," "myo" refers to muscle, and "trophic" means nourishment. When a muscle has no nourishment, it withers and wastes away. "Lateral" refers to the area of the spinal cord (the lateral columns) where portions of the affected neurons are located. The degenerative changes produce scarring, or hardening, referred to as "sclerosis" of the muscle and nerve tissue.

Onset usually occurs between the ages of 40 and 70, though it may begin as early as the teen years. Early symptoms include tripping, dropping objects, abnormal fatigue of the arms or legs, slurred speech, muscle cramps and twitching and involuntary bouts of laughing or crying.

The hands and feet are usually affected first, progressing to the muscles of the trunk. It eventually affects chewing, breathing and swallowing, and requires permanent mechanical breathing assistance to maintain life.

Mental functions, and senses of sight, touch, hearing, taste, smell and muscles of the eyes and bladder are generally unaffected.

The basic cause of the disorder is unknown. While the majority of cases are sporadic, it's estimated that 5% to 10% of cases are familial, with a pattern suggesting autosomal dominant inheritance. One affected Pennsylvania Dutch family was locally said to have "Pecks disease." Currently, there is no method of prenatal diagnosis for ALS. Other inherited motor system diseases include SPINAL MUSCULAR ATROPHY, Werdnig-Hoffman disease and Kugelberg-Welander disease.

Once thought to be a rare disorder, some 5,000 people in the United States are newly diagnosed annually. An estimated 30,000 have the disease at any given time, with approximately 300,000 presently unaffected individuals expected to develop the disease in the future. Half live at least three years after diagnosis, 25% five years or more, and 10% survive for more than 10 years.

Other famous affected individuals include Vice President Henry A. Wallace, boxing champion Ezzard Charles, jazz musician Charlie Mingus, actor David Niven and U.S. Senator Jacob Javits.

For more information, contact:

The Amyotrophic Lateral Sclerosis
   Association
15300 Ventura Blvd., Suite 315
Sherman Oaks, CA 91403
(818) 990-2151

**Andersen disease**   See GLYCOGEN STORAGE DISEASE.

**anemia**   Not a disease, but a manifestation of a group of disorders of the red blood cells, which collect oxygen absorbed in the lungs and carry it throughout the body. Among the more prevalent causes: The blood cells themselves may be abnormal, as in spherocytosis (see below); the levels of HEMOGLOBIN, the pigment that carries the oxygen in the blood cell, may be abnormally low, as in THALASSE-MIA; the hemoglobin itself may exhibit abnormalities, as is the case in SICKLE-CELL ANEMIA; if hemoglobin production is normal, the red blood cells may be broken down (hemolyzed) in the body faster than they can be replaced (this is called a "hemolytic" anemia). There can be decreased production of red cells as in the hypoplastic anemias or the cells can be trapped and destroyed in an enlarged spleen, as in GAUCHER DISEASE.

Several conditions causing anemia are inherited, and it is also a feature of numerous hereditary disorders. These include ABETALIPOPROTEINEMIA, Gaucher disease, FANCONI'S ANEMIA, dyskeratosis congenita, METHYLMALONIC ACIDEMIA, CYSTINOSIS, osteopetrosis (see INFANTILE OSTEOPETROSIS), CHEDIAK-HIGASHI SYNDROME and thrombocytopenia—absent radius (TAR) syndrome. Anemia may also result from dietary or vitamin deficiencies (e.g., iron, folic acid), drugs or other disease processes. It tends to be highly variable in expression, ranging from mild to severe.

Regardless of the cause, the symptoms in all forms may include weakness, general malaise, headaches, drowsiness, sore tongue, loss of libido, slight fever, hunger for air and breathing difficulties (dyspnea), and heart palpitations. The skin, gums, eyes and nail beds may exhibit a pallor or paleness. In severe cases anemia may induce cardiac disease, resulting in chest pain or heart failure.

Although individuals with anemia exhibit a reduced number of functioning red blood cells within a given volume of blood, there is no precise definition for specific levels below which anemia is said to exist. The defined level must also take into account age and gender. If the onset is slow, the body may adjust so well that there is no functional impairment, despite extremely low levels of hemoglobin.

*Congenital Hemolytic Anemias.* These inherited chronic diseases are characterized by hemolysis (breakdown) of red blood cells at an accelerated rate. While symptoms are the same as in other forms of anemia, there may be jaundice or yellowing of the skin and eyes, as well. This results from an excess of bilirubin, a yellow pigment, which is released when red blood cells are hemolyzed. The spleen, which is where most hemolysis occurs, may become enlarged and is one of the signs of the disorder.

There is also a familial, non-congenital form of hemolytic anemia, as well as acquired forms. Hemolytic anemia is also a feature of numerous specific disorders, such as sickle-cell anemia and thalassemia, spherocytosis, elliptocytosis, glucose-6-phosphate dehydrogenase deficiency and other red cell enzyme deficiency disorders.

*Spherocytosis.* This is a hereditary form of hemolytic anemia that results from the red blood cells being abnormally small and round (that is, spherocytic; red cells are normally biconcave disks). It results from a defect in the red cell membrane and occurs as an AUTOSOMAL DOMINANT trait. Incidence has been estimated at 2.2 per 10,000 live births, with about one-quarter of the cases being sporadic.

Symptoms are the same as for congenital hemolytic anemia. In some cases, removal of the spleen may cure the accelerated destruction of red blood cells.

*Elliptocytosis.* This is characterized by abnormalities of the membrane imparting an oval or cigar shape to the red blood cells. Inherited as an autosomal dominant trait, incidence is estimated at approximately one in 2,500 live births. Most affected individuals are asymptomatic, though about 12% exhibit symptoms similar to spherocytosis.

*Hypoplastic, Congenital Anemia.* Symptoms, beginning with skin pallor, usually have onset within the first three months of life. The pulse becomes rapid as anemia increases, and cardiac enlargement and dilation may develop. Heart failure and pneumonia may ensue. This rare condition has been reported in both autosomal dominant and AUTOSOMAL RECESSIVE forms. The recessive form is the more common and is also known as Blackfan-Diamond syndrome, for U.S. physicians K.D. Blackfan and L.K. Diamond, who first described it in 1938. Some affected infants have also had two thumbs on one hand, or thumbs with an extra joint (triphalangeal thumbs). This latter entity is often referred to as Aase syndrome, named for physician J.M. Aase who published the first description in 1969.

Anemia may also be associated with pregnancy. A 1987 survey of lower income women by the Centers for Disease Control found that in the first three months of pregnancy, 13% of black women and 4% of white women had hemoglobin levels indicating anemia. In the second trimester the rates rose to

18% and 6%, respectively, and in the last trimester, 38% and 19%. Anemia during pregnancy increases the risk of premature birth, LOW BIRTH WEIGHT and fetal death.

**anencephaly**   A severe NEURAL TUBE DEFECT that results in absence of most of the brain and, in extreme cases, the spinal cord as well. Additionally, there are often multiple malformations of the skeleton and internal organs. The cranial vault, or top of the skull, is absent, and the brain tissue, if present, is exposed. Though the cerebral hemispheres are usually missing, the lower brain stem, which controls internal organs, is present. Almost all the bones in the skull are abnormal. Defects in skull formation cause characteristic facial anomalies. The eyes protrude, the nose is prominent and cleft lip/palate is often seen. Malformations of limbs, thoracic cage, the abdominal wall, gastrointestinal tract and genitourinary system are relatively common. The heart, lungs, kidneys and adrenal glands are also often malformed.

The disorder is thought to develop between the 23rd and 26th days following conception, due to a failure of part of the neural tube to close.

While there have been reports of cases believed to be transmitted in AUTOSOMAL RECESSIVE and X-LINKED patterns, anencephaly appears to be a MULTIFACTORIAL condition. Incidence in the United States is estimated at one in 1,000 live births, with 2,000 to 3,500 anencephalics born annually. However, prevalence varies with geography, racial and ethnic background, sex and socioeconomic conditions. In some areas of Ireland and Wales, incidence is as high as five to seven per 1,000 live births. (In South Wales, the disorder has been reported as high as one in 105 live births.) Neural tube defects as a whole have a low incidence among blacks, Ashkenazi Jews (those of Eastern European ancestry) and Asians. Affected females outnumber affected males by at least a two to one ratio. There is an approximately 5% risk of recurrence of a neural tube defect (either SPINA BIFIDA or anencephaly) in subsequent pregnancies, after the birth of a child with a neural tube defect.

Prenatal screening for elevated maternal serum alphafetoprotein levels, in conjunction with ULTRASOUND (and AMNIOCENTESIS) is thought to be capable of diagnosing 90% of cases.

Parents of infants with neural tube defects appear to have a higher than average incidence of defects of spinal cord development, including spina bifida occulata.

This condition is incompatible with life, and most anencephalic infants are either stillborn, or die within a few days of birth. Some anencephalic infants have been kept alive by artificial means in order to preserve their organs for transplant. Without life support, the organs deteriorate by the time these infants are legally dead. Typically, the organs sought are liver, heart, heart valves and corneas. It is estimated that 40% to 70% of children under two years old on waiting lists for organ transplants die before suitable organ donors are found.

The Loma Linda University Medical Center, in Loma Linda, California, developed the first guidelines in the United States for accepting anencephalic organ donors and keeping them alive. Though parents of anencephalic infants have requested that their infant's organs be donated in this manner, the practice raises troubling ethical and legal issues, and the program at Loma Linda was suspended soon after its inception.

**aneuploidy**   The state of having an abnormal number of chromosomes. (Normally, humans have 23 pairs of chromosomes in each cell.) A cell, or an individual, that has a number of chromosomes that is not an exact multiple of 23 (e.g., 47 instead of 46) is said to be aneuploid. Some CHROMOSOME ABNORMALITIES are characterized by aneuploidy. Conditions of aneuploidy include DOWN SYNDROME and TURNER SYNDROME.

**angioneurotic edema, hereditary**   See HEREDITARY ANGIONEUROTIC EDEMA.

**aniridia**   The absence of all or part of the iris, the pigmented circle that gives eyes their color. This condition affects both eyes (bilateral) and is usually detected at birth. Accompanying visual disturbances include cataracts, glaucoma and malformation of the cornea.

Affected individuals with isolated aniridia have acute visual problems but normal life expectancy and intelligence. However, it has been associated with disorders including partial or complete absence of the kneecap (patella), speech disturbances, psychomotor malfunction, CHROMOSOME ABNORMALITIES (deletions of the short arm of chromosome 11), WILMS TUMOR of the kidney and varying degrees of mental retardation.

The cause of this anomaly, which can be inherited as an AUTOSOMAL DOMINANT trait, is unknown. As an isolated condition, it occurs in approximately one in 50,000 live births. Prenatal diagnosis is theoretically possible in cases where aniridia is associated with Wilms tumor or chromosomal anomalies.

**ankyloglossia** (tongue-tie)   Movement of the tongue is severely restricted by this defect, also known as tongue-tie. It results from an abnormal shortness of the membrane that anchors the underside of the tongue to the floor of the mouth (frenulum linguae). An affected person cannot raise his or her tongue above the corners of the mouth when it is wide open. Efforts to make the tongue protrude reveal a central groove.

The cause is not known, but evidence suggests an AUTOSOMAL DOMINANT mode of inheritance in some cases. The defect occurs in about one in 330 live births. Male and female infants are affected equally. The defect can be identified at birth.

**ankylosing spondylitis (AS)**   A chronic arthritis involving the joints of the spine, it takes its name from the Greek terms for stiffening (ankylosing) and inflammation of the spinal joints (spondylitis). The joints may fuse and become immobile, causing a stooped posture. The disorder is variable in its expression, ranging from mild aches and pains to severe stooping posture. (In 20% of cases, joints of the pelvis, shoulders, hips and knees may also be involved.)

It has been identified in 4,000-year-old Egyptian mummies, and, as with other diseases characterized by inflammation of the joints (arthritic diseases), a strong familial link has been established. Previously thought to affect only males, females are now known to be equally at risk, though they are usually less severely affected.

Onset is gradual, typically beginning between the ages of 18 and 30 years, with episodes of lower back pain that may be acute at night. Frequently, the back pain improves with exercise and grows worse with rest, making it distinguishable from common lower back pain.

AS is the third most common form of chronic arthritis in the United States, affecting an estimated 500,000 individuals.

The basic defect that causes the inflammation of the joints is unknown. However, a genetic marker for the condition, HLA B27, has been identified. This particular variation of HLA antigen (see HUMAN LEUKOCYTE ANTIGEN), the "tissue type" marker on cell surfaces, is found in almost everyone with AS, and unaffected individuals with HLA B27 have 300 times the susceptibility to develop the condition as those without it. While there is no cure, proper diagnosis and treatment (generally consisting of nonsteroid anti-inflammatory drugs, to alleviate inflammation, and daily exercise for the joints) can minimize the effects of the disorder.

For more information, contact:

Ankylosing Spondylitis Association
511 N. La Cienega, Suite 216
Los Angeles, CA 90048
(213) 652-0609

**annular pancreas**    The pancreas is a gland that, in addition to secreting the hormone insulin, releases ENZYMES for the proper digestion of fats, proteins and carbohydrates. The pancreas is situated behind the stomach and connects to the duodenum, the first portion of the small intestine through which food passes from the stomach. Pancreatic juices are released into the duodenum through an opening in the wall of the duodenum. This opening also acts as the point of release for bile, a liver secretion that emulsifies fats in food.

In this condition, during development of the embryo, portions of the pancreas form an abnormal collar or ring encircling the duodenum. This can lead to an intestinal obstruction in the duodenum, symptoms of which can include intermittent vomiting, bile-stained vomit, failure to thrive, and in rare cases later in life, inflammation of the pancreas (pancreatitis) and biliary tract disease.

The intestinal obstruction can be corrected surgically. Life expectancy is normal, except in cases where pancreatitis or biliary tract disease occur.

Annular pancreas occurs in about one of every 10,000 live births and can be detected from birth on. The exact cause is unknown.

**anomaly**    An in utero developmental deviation from normal form or structure, such as a missing organ or limb, or an extra digit. Synonym: congenital anomaly.

Anomalies may be divided into two categories: malformations and deformations. A malformation occurs where the body part or organ etc., is different because of an intrinsically abnormal developmental process (e.g., a CONGENITAL HEART DEFECT or a CLEFT LIP). A deformation occurs when a previously normally formed body part is altered in shape or structure (e.g., a clubfoot or congenital hip dislocation) by mechanical forces, such as compression against the wall of the womb due to deficient AMNIOTIC FLUID. (See also BIRTH DEFECTS.)

**anonychia, hereditary**    See HEREDITARY ANONYCHIA

**anorchia**    See ABSENT TESTES.

**anosmia** (congenital anosmia)     The complete absence of the sense of smell (anosmia) and an abnormally decreased sense of smell (hyposmia) are, by themselves, quite rare among newborns. Risk, prevalence and the ratio of males to females are unknown for isolated cases. However, either condition may accompany certain congenital endocrine disorders, defects in head or facial shape, and hearing or visual disabilities. Failure to respond to parathyroid hormone (pseudohypoparathyroidism) and abnormally decreased activity of the gonads (hypogonadotropic hypogonadism) are two endocrine abnormalities often associated with anosmia. Loss or impairment of smell may also accompany USHER SYNDROME of congenital deafness, and both have been seen in infants with RETINITIS PIGMENTOSA (a progressive loss of response and wasting of the eye's retina leading to blindness). When no other abnormalities are present, anosmia and hyposmia are usually detected by clinical surveys during childhood. Neither condition, by itself, affects normal life span or intelligence.

While the cause of both conditions is unknown, it is believed that developmental abnormalities in the sense of smell (olfactory system) are to blame, particularly a lack of development of the olfactory bulb in the embryo. Other hypothesized causes are trauma to the fetus, inflammation and lack of vitamin A during gestation. There is no known treatment for either disorder, and therapy for associated endocrine imbalances does not restore olfactory function.

**antenatal diagnosis**     See PRENATAL DIAGNOSIS.

**anticonvulsants**     Some of these medications, used to control seizures, have been linked to birth defects when taken during pregnancy. It is not clear whether the association of anticonvulsants and congenital defects is due to the drugs, the underlying disease itself, other genetic factors or a combination of all of the above. Clearly, there is some evidence pointing to the drugs as a causative factor.

Hydantoins, such as phenytoin, prescribed for epileptic seizures, may cause fetal hydantoin syndrome characterized by distinctive facial malformations, such as a short nose, bowed upper lip, broad nose bridge, wide space between the eyes, and cleft lip or cleft palate. Underdeveloped fingertips, with small or missing nails are also common. Slow growth both before and after birth, an abnormally small head (MICROCEPHALY), MENTAL RETARDATION and heart defects are additional signs of the disorder.

About 10% of infants born to women taking hydantoins have the full-blown syndrome. An additional 30% show some of the abnormalities. Some facial deformities and heart defects may require surgical correction. There may be an underlying genetic/metabolic predisposition to develop the syndrome in those infants who manifest it.

The anticonvulsants trimethadione, paramethadione and primidone are known to cause birth defects, but are rarely prescribed to women during their childbearing years. In 20% to 50% of exposed infants, trimethadione and paramethadione have been linked to a syndrome characterized by INTRAUTERINE GROWTH RETARDATION, small head circumference, delayed development, mental retardation, deformed ears and heart defects. Other features include V-shaped eyebrows, a short nose with a broad, depressed bridge, a small jaw, and cleft lip or palate and hearing loss.

Children with primidone syndrome grow more slowly than normal and have an abnormally small head, jitteriness, a hairy forehead, deformed nostrils, a small jaw, underdeveloped fingernails and heart defects.

Valproic acid, another anticonvulsant, has been associated with an increase in neural tube defects. (See also TERATOGEN.)

**antitrypsin deficiency**     See ALPHA-1-ANTITRYPSIN DEFICIENCY.

**Apert syndrome** (acrocephalosyndactyly)     A form of CRANIOSYNOSTOSIS, a condition caused by the premature closure of the gaps, or sutures, of the skull bones, resulting in an abnormal shape of the head. This form is named for Eugene Apert (1868-1940), a senior pediatrician at the Hopital des Enfants Malades in Paris, who published the definitive description in 1906.

The most characteristic features are a peaked, pointed head (acrocephaly; turribrachycephaly) and webbed fingers and toes (SYNDACTYLY).

The deformities of the hands and feet are symmetrical; that is, both appendages exhibit similar abnormalities. The first and fifth finger are often partially attached to the fused three middle fingers.

As they age, the joints and fingers become more stiff, and the bones of the hands, feet and spine progressively grow together (synostosis).

Most affected individuals are mentally retarded. Facial acne is common. The eyes are wide-set (HYPERTELORISM), and the midface is often underdeveloped, with a depressed nasal bridge, making the jawbone appear large. One-third are reported to have cleft palate.

While this disorder is inherited as an AUTOSOMAL DOMINANT trait, most cases are sporadic. Increased paternal age has been noted, which may be a factor in the appearance of the new MUTATIONS that may cause these sporadic cases. More than 250 affected individuals have been reported, and the condition is estimated to occur in one of every 160,000 live births. Due to the high neonatal mortality rate, prevalence in the general population is estimated at one in two million.

PRENATAL DIAGNOSIS has been successful using FETOSCOPY to detect malformations of the hands and feet. These should also be identifiable by prenatal ULTRASOUND.

The exact trigger for the abnormal development (dysplasia) of the skull, hands and feet is unknown. Facial surgery can correct some abnormalities, and digits of the hands are often separated surgically.

For other forms of craniosynostosis, see CARPENTER SYNDROME, CROUZON DISEASE, PFEIFFER SYNDROME and SAETHRE-CHOTZEN SYNDROME.

**arachnodactyly** (spider fingers)     Abnormally long and slender fingers and toes. This is seen as several genetic conditions, MARFAN SYNDROME being perhaps the most well known.

**argininemia**     See UREA CYCLE DEFECTS.

**argininosuccinic aciduria**     See UREA CYCLE DEFECTS.

**arteriohepatic dysplasia**     See ALAGILLE SYNDROME.

**arthritis**     See RHEUMATOID ARTHRITIS.

**arthrogryposis** (arthrogryposis multiplex congenita; AMC)     The presence of multiple joint contractures at birth, and representing a large group of congenital disorders. A contracture is a limitation in the range of motion of a joint. There is a wide variability in the expression of this problem. In some cases only a few joints may be affected, and the range of motion will be nearly normal. In classic cases, hands, wrists, elbows, shoulders, hips, feet and knees are affected, and in the most severe cases, almost every body joint may be involved, including the jaw and back. Frequently, muscle weakness accompanies joint contractures, further limiting movement.

AMC was first described in 1841 by A.G. Otto, who referred to it as "congenital myodystrophy." The term "arthrogryposis" was first applied to the condition in 1923.

AMC is estimated to occur in approximately one of every 3,000 to 4,000 live births. Many varieties of hereditary arthrogryposis have been identified, including an X-LINKED recessive form, which resolves spontaneously, and AUTOSOMAL DOMINANT and RECESSIVE forms; it can be a feature of many multiple anomaly syndromes as well. The most common hereditary form, distal arthrogryposis (autosomal dominant), is characterized by overlapping fingers and clenched fist, which eventually opens with use, leaving a residual loss of movement in adults. There may also be foot deformities.

However, hereditary forms account for only 30% of all cases. The majority of cases are caused by non-genetic factors during fetal development. Non-genetic forms have their origin in several developmental aberrations. The most common of these forms is amyoplasia, and it is characterized by flexed wrists and extended elbows, as well as involvement of the shoulders and feet. All cases have been sporadic.

Anything that prevents normal joint movement during fetal development can result in joint contractures, even if the joint itself is normal. This can occur if there is insufficient room in the uterus for normal movement, due to low levels of AMNIOTIC FLUID or abnormal shape of the uterus. If movement is restricted, extra connective tissue may grow around the joint, fixing it in position. Additionally, tendons may lose their ability to stretch or contract.

Muscles responsible for joint movement may also fail to develop properly, due to muscle diseases (such as congenital muscular dystrophies) or environmental exposures such as viruses which can damage cells responsible for transmitting nerve impulses to the muscles. In some cases, tendons, bones, joint linings or joints themselves may develop abnormally for unknown reasons.

Arthrogryposis can also result from malformations of the central nervous system and spinal cord, though in these cases the condition is usually accompanied by a wide range of other disorders.

PRENATAL DIAGNOSIS for hereditary forms has been attempted for at-risk pregnancies using ULTRASOUND to monitor prenatal movement.

Physical therapy is the primary recommended treatment. Surgery is sometimes performed as an adjunct, most commonly on the ankles to assist in supporting weight and walking. These measures can provide substantial improvement in functional ability.

For more information, contact:

National Support Group for Arthrogryposis
Multiplex Congenita

P.O. Box 5192
Sonora, CA 95370
(209) 928-3688

National Foundation for AMC
P.O. Box 382
Chicago Heights, IL 60411

**arthrogryposis multiplex congenita, AMC**   See ARTHROGRYPOSIS.

**aspartyglycosaminuria**   The most distinctive physical feature of this rare disorder is the thick, sagging skin observed on the cheeks of affected infants, though it also causes severe MENTAL RETARDATION and susceptibility to frequent infections. Affected infants resemble those with MUCOPOLY-SACCHARIDOSES. Though the first symptoms occur in infancy, the course is slowly progressive, with death by the fourth decade. In Finland, where most affected individuals have been identified, incidence is estimated at one in 26,000 births. It is inherited as an AUTOSOMAL RECESSIVE trait. It is a lysosomal storage disease, resulting from a specific ENZYME deficiency. CARRIER testing and PRENATAL DIAGNOSIS by measurement of this enzyme is possible.

**asphyxiating thoracic dysplasia**   See JEUNE SYNDROME.

**asplenia syndrome** (Ivemark syndrome)   Affected individuals have no spleen and usually exhibit many internal abnormalities. A distinctive feature is a strong tendency for organs or pairs of organs that are normally asymmetric to develop symmetrically. This is a syndrome of bilateral "right-sidedness," i.e., left-sided organs or members of pairs of organs have the structural characteristics of their right-sided counterparts, but in mirror images.

In at least 90% of the cases, the left lung has three lobes, instead of the normal two. In 40% of the cases, the right and left lobes of the liver are equal in size. In about half the cases, the stomach is located on the right side instead of the midline. Usually the intestinal tract has failed to rotate normally, resulting in abnormalities of the position of the colon.

Children with this anomaly also have complex cardiovascular defects. Partial or complete obstruction to pulmonary arterial blood flow is found in at least 70% of the cases.

Symptoms are usually evident within days or weeks of birth and include blue discoloration of the skin (cyanosis), breathing problems, feeding difficulties and congestive heart failure. Prognosis is poor, with most infants dying during the first year. Infants who survive for any length of time often fail to thrive and suffer from infections.

The cause of this disorder is unknown. It is about twice as prevalent in males as in females. Though rare, it is being identified more often and is more common than originally thought.

**ataxia-telangiectasia** (AT; Louis-Bar syndrome)    Ataxia is derived from the Greek word *ataxis*, meaning without order or incoordination. Ataxia is a neurological disorder characterized by disturbances of muscular coordination and the inability to control muscular action and balance, caused by degeneration of the cells of the spinal cord and brain. There are several hereditary ataxias, such as Marie's ataxia (hereditary cerebellar ataxia), striatonigral degeneration (Joseph's or AZOREAN DISEASE) and FRIEDREICH'S ATAXIA, with AT being one of the more prevalent.

AT is a chromosomal fragility syndrome, inherited as an AUTOSOMAL RECESSIVE disorder. An inability properly to repair DNA damaged by ultraviolet radiation (such as found in sunlight) is thought to be responsible for chromosomal breakage and rearrangement, which results in characteristics of the disorder.

Along with progressive cerebellar ataxia and inability to control movement (apraxia) of the eyes, a striking characteristic is the development of "telangiectasias," vascular lesions formed by the dilation of small blood vessels that appear on the eyes, ears, face, chest, hands, feet and folds of the elbows and knees.

The telangiectasias usually become apparent by the age of five, appearing on parts of the body most exposed to the sun. Graying of the scalp hair is common, even in children. With continued exposure to the sun, the skin becomes hardened and mottled with hyperpigmented and depigmented areas.

Growth is greatly diminished in more than 65% of affected individuals. They tend to have thin faces, with a relaxed, dull or sad expression. The head is often held to one side, and individuals often present a stooped posture with drooping shoulders.

The loss of motor control is progressive, with speech becoming difficult due to loss of control over vocal cords and mouth. Drooling is frequent. Additionally, there is often endocrine malfunction, intellectual decline and development of immune deficiency disorders. Death in childhood or young adulthood is frequent. Few individuals have survived past the age of 20. Death typically results from infection or, less frequently, the development of malignant growths.

The condition can be diagnosed by chromosomal analysis, which can detect characteristic changes in the chromosomes of affected individuals.

Incidence of the disorder is thought to be between two and three per 100,000 live births. One percent of the population is thought to be CARRIERS. Carriers can be identified by deficiencies in DNA repair ability, and have a five-fold increase in tumors of all types. PRENATAL DIAGNOSIS may be possible by evaluating the sensitivity of cultured fetal cells, obtained via AMNIOCENTESIS, to ultraviolet radiation.

For more information, contact:

National Ataxia Foundation
600 Twelve Oaks Center
15500 Wayzata Blvd.
Wayzata, MN 55391
(612) 473-7666

**atypical cholinesterase**    A hereditary defect in the ENZYME necessary to reverse the effects of the skeletal muscle relaxant succinylcholine, often used as anesthesia during surgery. The result is a prolonged cessation of breathing (apnea) following administration of this anesthetic.

Succinylcholine acts at the neuromuscular junction to block the effects of acetylcholine, which transmits neural impulses across the nerve junction. Under ordinary circumstances, succinylcholine is a short-acting drug (about 10 minutes); plasma levels fall rapidly due to the action of plasma cholinesterase. However, if plasma cholinesterase levels are low, the effects of succinylcholine are greatly prolonged, and the ability to breathe without respiratory assistance is delayed.

Theoretically, diagnosis is possible at any time with laboratory tests. However, the condition will not be discovered unless a specific history is taken or tests are run before surgery. Often, it is not evident until prolonged apnea occurs after succinylcholine administration. Prognosis is good, provided the apnea is recognized and respiratory assistance is given.

Inherited as an AUTOSOMAL RECESSIVE trait, the most common form of atypical cholinesterase (dibucaine-resistant) is estimated to occur in approximately one in 2,000 to one in 4,000 live births in various populations. Two variations (fluoride-resistant and silent gene variant) are much rarer. PRENATAL DIAGNOSIS has not been achieved.

**auditory canal atresia**    Absence (atresia) of the auditory canal. It may take the form of a visible block where the canal would normally begin at the outer ear, or it may resemble a funnel leading down to a block farther within the canal. The outer ear may appear normal, or it may be set lower than normal on the side of the head with minor variations in shape. Persons with atresia of both auditory canals suffer complete hearing loss and impairment of speech development. The defect may be detected by careful examination at birth, or it

may escape detection until the hearing loss becomes apparent.

It is not known how the defect develops, but it is hypothesized that early in fetal development the primitive auditory canal fails to form properly.

Associated defects and malformations include excessive distance between paired organs, such as the eyes (HYPERTELORISM), skin folds covering the inner corner of the eyes (EPICANTHUS), small nose, flattened midface, cleft palate, webbing or fusion of fingers or toes (SYNDACTYLY) and clubfoot.

This condition is rare. The cause and the risk of occurrence are unknown. The life span of an affected person is generally normal if there are no serious associated defects.

**autism, infantile**    See INFANTILE AUTISM.

**autosomal dominant** (dominant)    A method of transmission of a hereditary trait. It is the confirmed mode of transmission of approximately 1,500 GENETIC DISORDERS or conditions, and the suspected mode of over 1,100 more. While popularly referred to as "dominant" traits, they are more properly termed "autosomal dominant," reflecting the location on the autosomes, any of the 22 non-sex chromosome pairs, of the aberrant GENES responsible for the disorders. (Genetic disorders involving the sex chromosomes, the 23rd chromosome pair, are termed X-LINKED, and they may also be dominant traits, though most X-linked disorders are recessive.)

Autosomal dominant disorders have their origins in MUTATIONS or defects in a single gene or a gene pair. They are called dominant due to their ability to override, or dominate, their normal gene counterpart. Hence, an individual who inherits a single copy of the gene for a dominant disorder will usually exhibit that disorder.

In general, autosomal dominant disorders show a wide variability of severity, and not all who inherit the defective gene will exhibit its associated disorder. The ratio of those who

**Figure I**

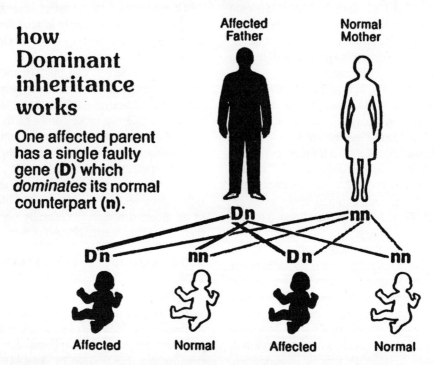

## how Dominant inheritance works

One affected parent has a single faulty gene **(D)** which *dominates* its normal counterpart **(n)**.

Affected Father    Normal Mother

Dn    nn

Dn    nn    Dn    nn

Affected    Normal    Affected    Normal

Each child's chances of inheriting either the **D** or the **n** from the affected parent are 50%.

Source: *Genetic Counseling* (January 1987), March of Dimes Birth Defects Foundation.

exhibit the disorder to those who inherit the gene for the disorder is referred to as PENETRANCE, and is expressed as a percentage. (For example, if half of those who possess the gene exhibit the disorder, penetrance is 50%.)

For an individual to have a dominant disorder, one parent is generally affected; unlike AUTOSOMAL RECESSIVE disorders, dominant conditions generally do not skip generations. The exceptions: (1) an individual may have unaffected parents, if that individual has the disorder as the result of a new mutation that has occurred in the sperm, egg or fertilized zygote that has gone on to produce that individual; and (2) as a result of

lack of penetrance, an individual who has inherited the gene for a disorder will not display the manifestations of the disorder and appears unaffected.

Among couples in which one individual has a dominant disorder, each child has a 50% chance of inheriting the gene, and therefore the disorder, from the affected parent, and a 50% chance of being unaffected. Affected individuals are said to be "heterozygotes," that is, the two genes in the gene pair are dissimilar—one is faulty and one is normal. "Homozygotes," those who have two identical faulty genes, are extremely rare in dominant disorders (both

## Table II
### Frequencies of the Most Common Dominant Disorders Found in a Survey Conducted in British Columbia*, Canada

| Dominant Condition | 1952-63 | | 1964-73 | | 1974-83 | | Total | |
|---|---|---|---|---|---|---|---|---|
| | N | Rate[1] | N | Rate[1] | N | Rate[1] | N | Rate[1] |
| Retina, malignant neoplasm | 6 | 13.7 | 14 | 40.6 | 16 | 41.3 | 36 | 30.8 |
| Neurofibromatosis | 34 | 77.7 | 33 | 95.7 | 32 | 82.5 | 99 | 84.6 |
| Other disorders of metabolism | 1 | 2.3 | 7 | 20.3 | 11 | 28.4 | 19 | 16.2 |
| Hereditary spherocytosis | 12 | 27.4 | 18 | 52.2 | 20 | 51.6 | 50 | 42.7 |
| Von Willebrand disease | 5 | 11.4 | 7 | 20.3 | 8 | 20.6 | 20 | 17.1 |
| Myotonic disorders | 14 | 32.0 | 8 | 23.2 | 6 | 15.5 | 28 | 23.9 |
| Hereditary retinal dystrophies | 13 | 29.7 | 0 | 0.0 | 0 | 0.0 | 13 | 11.1 |
| Nystagmus and other irregular eye movements | 14 | 32.0 | 2 | 5.8 | 3 | 7.7 | 19 | 16.2 |
| Sensorineural deafness | 3 | 6.9 | 15 | 43.5 | 4 | 10.3 | 22 | 18.8 |
| Congenital cataract and lens anomalies | 21 | 48.0 | 10 | 29.0 | 5 | 12.9 | 36 | 30.8 |
| Polydactyly | 6 | 13.7 | 16 | 46.4 | 14 | 36.1 | 36 | 30.8 |
| Other anomalies of upper limbs, including shoulder girdle | 3 | 6.9 | 2 | 5.8 | 9 | 23.2 | 14 | 12.0 |
| Anomalies of skull and face bones | 9 | 20.6 | 11 | 31.9 | 14 | 36.1 | 34 | 29.1 |
| Chondrodystrophy | 48 | 109.7 | 21 | 60.9 | 20 | 51.6 | 89 | 76.1 |
| Osteodystrophies | 24 | 54.9 | 31 | 89.9 | 29 | 74.8 | 84 | 71.8 |
| Other specified anomalies of muscle, tendon, fascia, etc. | 13 | 29.7 | 14 | 40.6 | 7 | 18.1 | 34 | 29.1 |
| Unspecified anomalies of musculoskeletal system | 2 | 4.6 | 8 | 23.2 | 0 | 0.0 | 10 | 8.5 |
| Other specified congenital anomalies of skin | 11 | 25.1 | 5 | 14.5 | 6 | 15.5 | 22 | 18.8 |
| Tuberous sclerosis | 13 | 29.7 | 23 | 66.7 | 22 | 56.7 | 58 | 49.6 |
| Other specified congenital anomalies | 17 | 38.9 | 16 | 46.4 | 9 | 23.2 | 42 | 35.9 |
| All other dominant conditions[2] | 110 | 251.4 | 85 | 246.6 | 81 | 208.9 | 276 | 235.9 |
| Total | 379 | 866.3 | 346 | 1,003.9 | 316 | 815.1 | 1,041 | 889.8 |
| Sum of highest individual rates | | | | | | | | 1,395.4 |

N- Number of patients.
[1]Per 1 million live births
[2]Each individual rate was used to determine the sum of the highest individual rates for these conditions.
*Statistics reflect local population bias.

Source: Patricia A. Baird, "A Population Study of Genetic Disorders in Children and Young Adults," *American Journal of Human Genetics*, 42 (1988): 677-693.

parents would also have to have the disorder), and homozygosity usually results in severe, lethal forms of dominant conditions. If both parents are affected, each child has a 25% chance of being homozygous for the condition and a 25% chance of being unaffected. (See Figure I; Table II.)

**autosomal recessive** (recessive)     A method of transmission of a hereditary trait. It is the confirmed mode of transmission of more than 625 GENETIC DISORDERS or conditions, and the suspected mode of over 850 more. While popularly referred to as "recessive"

traits, they are more properly termed "autosomal recessive," reflecting the location on the autosomes, any of the 22 non-sex chromosome pairs, of the aberrant GENES responsible for the disorders. (Genetic disorders involving the sex chromosome, the 23rd chromosome pair, are termed "X-LINKED"; most X-linked traits are recessive, though there are X-linked dominant disorders, as well.)

Autosomal recessive disorders have their origins in MUTATIONS or defects in both genes in a gene pair. They are called recessive because the influence of the faulty gene remains recessed, or suppressed, if paired with a normal gene. Hence, individuals must inherit a

**Table III**

**Frequencies of the Most Common Recessive Disorders Found in a Survey
Conducted in British Columbia**

| Recessive Condition | 1952-53 | | 1964-73 | | 1974-83 | | Total | |
|---|---|---|---|---|---|---|---|---|
| | N | Rate[1] | N | Rate[1] | N | Rate[1] | N | Rate[1] |
| Hyperaldosteronism | 13 | 29.7 | 7 | 20.3 | 1 | 2.6 | 21 | 18.0 |
| Adrenogenital disorders | 5 | 11.4 | 8 | 23.2 | 12 | 31.0 | 25 | 21.4 |
| Phenylketonuria | 26 | 59.4 | 18 | 52.2 | 31 | 80.0 | 75 | 64.1 |
| Other disturbances of aromatic amino acid metabolism | 22 | 50.3 | 19 | 55.1 | 16 | 41.3 | 57 | 48.7 |
| Glycogenosis | 3 | 6.9 | 12 | 34.8 | 8 | 20.6 | 23 | 19.7 |
| Lipidoses | 4 | 9.1 | 10 | 29.0 | 4 | 10.3 | 18 | 15.4 |
| Cystic fibrosis | 80 | 182.9 | 105 | 304.6 | 87 | 224.4 | 272 | 232.5 |
| Mucopolysaccharidosis | 8 | 18.3 | 11 | 31.9 | 2 | 5.2 | 21 | 18.0 |
| Deficiency of humoral immunity | 4 | 9.1 | 12 | 34.8 | 4 | 10.3 | 20 | 17.1 |
| Thalassemias | 15 | 34.3 | 7 | 20.3 | 16 | 41.3 | 38 | 32.5 |
| Cerebral lipidoses | 5 | 11.4 | 10 | 29.0 | 3 | 7.7 | 18 | 15.4 |
| Werdnig-Hoffmann disease | 6 | 13.7 | 19 | 55.1 | 15 | 38.7 | 40 | 34.2 |
| Other myoneural disorders | 18 | 41.1 | 4 | 11.6 | 0 | 0.0 | 22 | 18.8 |
| Hereditary progressive muscular dystrophy | 19 | 43.4 | 3 | 8.7 | 0 | 0.0 | 22 | 18.8 |
| Hereditary retinal dystrophies | 21 | 48.0 | 10 | 29.0 | 0 | 0.0 | 22 | 18.8 |
| Sensorineural deafness | 9 | 20.6 | 12 | 34.8 | 8 | 20.6 | 29 | 24.8 |
| Unspecified deafness | 1 | 2.3 | 8 | 23.2 | 7 | 18.1 | 16 | 13.7 |
| Cystic kidney disease | 11 | 25.1 | 10 | 29.0 | 7 | 18.1 | 28 | 23.9 |
| Osteodystrophies | 1 | 2.3 | 8 | 23.2 | 7 | 18.1 | 16 | 13.7 |
| Other specified congenital anomalies | 7 | 16.0 | 18 | 52.2 | 21 | 54.2 | 46 | 39.3 |
| All other recessive conditions[2] | 104 | 237.7 | 91 | 264.0 | 126 | 325.0 | 321 | 274.4 |
| Total | 401 | 916.6 | 406 | 1,178.0 | 372 | 959.5 | 1,179 | 1,007.8 |
| Sum of highest individual rates | | | | | | | | 1,655.3 |

N- Number of patients.
[1]Per million live births.
[2]Each individual rate was used to get the sum of highest individual rates for these conditions.
*Statistics reflect local population bias.

Source: Patricia A. Baird, "A Population Study of Genetic Disorders in Children and Young Adults," *American Journal of Human Genetics*, 42 (1988: 677-693.

faulty gene from both the mother and father for the associated condition to manifest itself.

Individuals who possess one recessive gene may pass the gene on to their offspring, but will rarely exhibit any symptoms of the disorder itself. (These individuals, who remain asymptomatic, are termed CARRIERS.) As a result, recessive disorders can skip one or more generations, and will appear only when two individuals, both possessing the faulty gene, have offspring. Even in those circumstances, all the offspring will not necessarily (that is, 100% of the time) inherit the condition unless both parents are actually affected by the disorder.

Carrier testing, when possible, can establish whether an individual possesses the recessive gene.

Among couples where only one member has a single recessive gene for a disorder, each offspring has a 50% chance of inheriting the gene and being a carrier, and a 50% chance of not inheriting the gene. If one parent has a recessive disorder (two faulty genes) and the other parent has no recessive genes for the disorder, all offspring will be carriers.

Among couples where both members have a single recessive gene, each child has a 25% chance of inheriting two recessive genes and

## Figure II

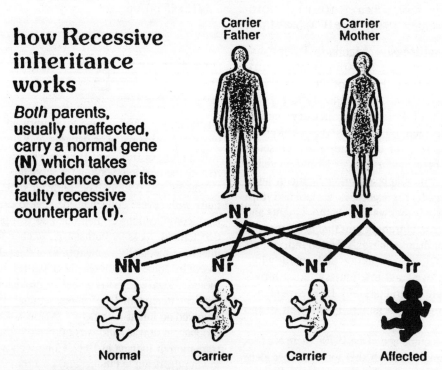

# how Recessive inheritance works

*Both* parents, usually unaffected, carry a normal gene **(N)** which takes precedence over its faulty recessive counterpart **(r)**.

The odds for each child are:
1. a 25% risk of inheriting a "double dose" of **r** genes, which may cause a serious birth defect
2. a 25% chance of inheriting two **N**s, thus being unaffected
3. a 50% chance of being a carrier as both parents are

Source: *Genetics Counseling* (January 1987), March of Dimes Birth Defects Foundation.

therefore inheriting the disorder, a 50% chance of inheriting one faulty gene and being a carrier, and a 25% chance of inheriting no recessive genes.

If one parent has a recessive disorder and the other a single recessive gene for it, each child will either be a carrier or have the disorder, with the chances for either being 50%.

If both parents have a recessive disorder, all their offspring will inherit the disorder.

Affected individuals are said to be "homozygotes," that is, the two genes in the gene pair are identical—both faulty. Carriers, those capable of transmitting the faulty gene without having the condition themselves, are said to be "heterozygotes"—the genes are dissimilar, one faulty, one normal. The unaffected parents or offspring of an individual with a recessive disorder are termed obligate heterozygotes, since they must have one copy of the recessive gene.

In general, autosomal recessive disorders tend to be less variable in expression and more uniformly severe than AUTOSOMAL DOMINANT disorders. (See Figure II; Table III.)

**Azorean disease**  (Machado-Joseph disease; Joseph disease; spinopontine atrophy)   A fatal disorder of the central nervous system that predominantly affects individuals of Portuguese ancestry, and is characterized by progressive weakening and spasticity of the extremities. Onset is usually between the ages of 15 and 35 years, though it may appear earlier or much later. The rate of progression is variable. Symptoms include awkward body movements and a staggering, lurching gait that is easily mistaken for drunkenness. Affected individuals have difficulty speaking and swallowing. Bulging eyes and involuntary facial movements are characteristic. Life expectancy following onset is generally between 10 and 30 years.

First documented in the 1970s, there is a lack of agreement over whether some of those identified as having this disorder may actually have some other form of ATAXIA. Two separate individuals have been identified as the "original" case: William Machado, a native of the Azores, a group of islands off the coast of Spain, and Antone Joseph, a Portuguese sailor, also from the Azores, who jumped ship in California in 1845. In fact, they may both have had a common ancestor, three generations back, who was the original case. It has also been suggested that the Joseph family may have been Sephardic Jews. Non-Portuguese cases have also been reported, including some Japanese families, thought to be the result of the early influence of the Portuguese in Japan.

Inherited as an AUTOSOMAL DOMINANT trait, there is currently no method of PRENATAL DIAGNOSIS or of identifying, prior to onset of symptoms, those who possess the gene for the disorder.

For more information, contact:

International Joseph Disease
  Foundation, Inc.

P.O. Box 2550
Livermore, CA 94550
(415) 455-0706

# B

**Baby Doe**   Name used to identify anonymous infants in several court cases involving the withholding of treatment from newborns who require medical intervention for survival.

Parents and doctors have allowed some infants with severe congenital defects to expire from complications of their conditions, a practice termed "passive euthanasia," rather than intervene medically to attempt to sustain their lives. In some situations, third parties have mounted legal efforts to compel the provision of medical treatment. One of the seminal cases involved an infant with DOWN SYNDROME and esophageal atresia who was allowed to die of starvation in Indiana in 1982. Controversy following the death led the federal government to define nontreatment of newborns with congenital anomalies as discrimination against the handicapped, making institutions involved at risk for losing federal funds. This federal policy was subsequently invalidated by the Supreme Court. Withholding treatment in these situations is not currently illegal under federal statutes, but courts continue to be asked to rule on individual cases, with the affected infants usually designated as Baby Doe.

**baldness**   See ALOPECIA.

**baldness, male-pattern**   See MALE-PATTERN BALDNESS.

**Bardet-Biedl syndrome**  (Laurence-Moon-Biedl syndrome)   Syndrome characterized by obesity, abnormally small genitals (hypogenitalism), extra fingers and toes (POLYDACTYLY), degenerative disease of the retina (pigmentary retinopathy) and psychological and neurological disorders.

It bears the name of George Louis Bardet (b. 1885), a French physician, and Arthur Biedl (1869-1933), a professor of experimental pathology at the University of Prague. It has also been identified with the names of John Zachariah Laurence (1829-1870), an English ophthalmologist, and Richard Charles Moon (1845-1914), his assistant.

Birth weight is usually above average, and by the age of one year nearly one-third of affected children are obese, with the extra weight typically found disproportionately within the trunk of the body. Tending toward shortness of stature, most exhibit infantile, unstable personalities (labile) and are mentally retarded.

They may experience kidney problems and nearly 35% of those afflicted with this syndrome die from kidney failure. Other problems include mild spasticity of the extremities, abnormalities in brain structures affecting body movements (extrapyramidal disorders), deafness, lack of eye coordination (nystagmus) and glucose intolerance. Urine shows decreased levels of gonad-stimulating hormones (gonadotropin).

Inherited as an AUTOSOMAL RECESSIVE trait, over 300 cases have been reported. Prenatal diagnosis is possible only if extra digits are observed by ultrasonic scanning (see ULTRASOUND), for example.

Though sometimes referred to as Laurence-Moon-Biedl syndrome, many authors prefer to use the Bardet-Biedl syndrome after the two authors who described this disorder in the 1920s. Laurence and Moon described a similar disorder in 1865, but those patients did not have polydactyly or obesity.

For more information, contact:

Lawrence-Moon-Biedl Syndrome (LMBS)
   Support Network
306 Mirfield Lane
Lexington Park, MD 20653
(301) 863-5658

**basal cell nevus syndrome**    See NEVOID BASAL CELL CARCINOMA SYNDROME.

**Bassen-Kornzweig syndrome**    See ABETALIPOPROTEINEMIA

**Batten disease** (neuronal ceroid lipofuscinosis; NCL)    A group of invariably fatal childhood neurologic nervous system disorders. The first symptoms are deteriorating vision or seizures, progressing to personality and behavior changes, loss of communication skills, increasing spasticity and loss of motor skills, facial grimacing, abnormal body movements and mental impairment. Affected children eventually become blind, bedridden and demented.

The disorder was first described in Norway in 1826 by Dr. Christian Stengel, but it is named for English neurologist F.E. Batten (1865-1918), who was the first to recognize the range of manifestations of the disease, publishing his findings in 1902.

Batten disease is associated with a buildup of fatty pigment (ceroid lipofuscin) in cells of the brain, nervous system and other parts of the body. This pigment is thought to be the end product of a combination of metabolic derangements that mark the progressive deterioration of brain function. The cause of the accumulation is unknown, but it is suspected there may be one or more missing enzymes, which are necessary to break down fats and their associated sugars and proteins in the normal way, allowing them to accumulate in tissue. This same pigment accumulates slowly during the normal aging process, but it is greatly accelerated in this disorder.

Diagnosis requires numerous tests for confirmation, including blood tests, biopsies, electrophysiological examination of the brain (via electroencephalogram), and computer tomography of the head (CT scan). Characteristic cellular deposits ("curvilinear bodies") are seen when cells from biopsy are examined under the electron microscope.

Currently there is no treatment available. Research on animal models is being conducted; a similar disease has been found in English setters, dalmatians and New Zealand sheep, and several colonies have been bred for research purposes.

Inherited as an AUTOSOMAL RECESSIVE trait, incidence has been estimated to be between one in 12,500 and one in 50,000 live births. PRENATAL DIAGNOSIS has been accomplished through electron microscope detection of curvilinear deposits in amniotic fluid cells.

While there are two very rare adult forms (Kuf's disease and Parry's disease), the great majority of cases appear in three childhood forms. Symptoms are similar, but age of onset and speed of progression vary.

*Infantile (Santavuori disease).* Age of onset is about eight months and progresses rapidly. Infants fail to thrive, head growth slows, resulting in an abnormally small head (MICROCEPHALY), and they exhibit shock-like muscle contractures (myoclonic jerks). Death usually occurs by age five, though some have survived a few years longer in a vegetative state.

*Late infantile (Jansky-Bielschowsky disease).* Onset occurs at about three years of age, beginning with loss of muscle coordination and seizures. Symptoms progress rapidly, and death usually occurs between the ages of seven and 12. This form is common in Newfoundland, with a birth frequency of one in 5,000.

*Juvenile (Spielmeyer-Vogt-Sjögren disease).* Age of onset is between five and 10 years. Progressive visual failure and seizures are the first signs. With a slower progression than the earlier-onset type, individuals survive into the late teens or early twenties. Some have lived longer.

For more information, contact:

The Children's Brain Diseases Foundation
350 Parnassus Heights Medical Building
Suite 900
San Francisco, CA 94117
(415) 566-5402

**Becker's muscular dystrophy**    See
MUSCULAR DYSTROPHY.

## Beckwith-Wiedemann syndrome

This condition includes a vast and varied constellation of congenital symptoms, most notably an enlarged tongue (macroglossia) that pushes out of the mouth, protrusion of a portion of the intestine through a defect in the abdominal wall (OMPHALOCELE), severe low blood sugar (hypoglycemia) that disappears within a year of birth, and large size. Other frequently seen characteristics include facial birthmarks, and grooves and pits on the ears and earlobes. Umbilical and INGUINAL HERNIA are common, as is intestinal malrotation. Mild to moderate MENTAL RETARDATION is frequent.

It bears the names of J.B. Beckwith and H.R. Wiedemann, who independently described it in 1964.

Mean weight at birth is generally high (3,900 g or 8.6 lb.), even though approximately 25% of births are premature. In general, gigantism is a feature of Beckwith-Wiedemann syndrome: Stature and weight eventually are above the 90th percentile, with advanced bone age. One half of the body may be noticeably larger than the other (HEMIHYPERTROPHY). The visceral organs are commonly enlarged, as is the clitoris in females. Cells of the adrenal cortex are large (cytomegaly), and the kidneys often develop abnormally.

Prognosis is fair. Most deaths in infancy occur due to complications of the syndrome, but later malignant tumors of the kidneys or adrenal cortex occur in approximately 5% of cases. Surgery can correct omphalocele, intestinal rotation and macroglossia.

The basic defect that causes Beckwith-Wiedemann syndrome is unknown, and most cases are sporadic. In those that are familial, there is no general agreement on the genetic basis. Abnormalities on the short arm of chromosome 11 have been suggested. The condition affects both sexes equally and is estimated to occur in one in 15,000 live births. Although there is no prenatal diagnostic test for Beckwith-Wiedemann syndrome, ULTRASOUND and ALPHA-FETOPROTEIN levels may detect the presence of omphalocele. Approximately 15% of infants with omphalocele have this syndrome.

**benign familial hematuria**   This benign disorder, inherited as an AUTOSOMAL DOMINANT trait, is characterized by the presence of blood in the urine. It is non-progressive and not associated with kidney failure.

**bent stick syndrome**   See PEYRONIE DISEASE.

**bifid uvula**   (split uvula; cleft uvula) The uvula is the small, soft tissue that hangs from the roof of the mouth over the root of the tongue. In approximately 1% of whites and 10% of American Indians and Japanese, the uvula is split by a central fissure. The frequency in SIBLINGS, parents and children (first degree relatives) of affected persons is reported to be about 18%. This defect can be considered a minor form of cleft palate, and, as in that anomaly, MULTIFACTORIAL inheritance is thought to be the cause of this benign condition. In persons with cleft uvula, the complete removal of the adenoids may produce hypernasal speech.

**biliary atresia**   This disease, seen in very young infants, is caused by inflammation and obstruction of the bile ducts, which carry bile from the liver into the small intestine. Due to the blockage, bile backs up into the liver, resulting in destruction of healthy liver cells and scarring of the liver (cirrhosis). The scarring interferes with blood flow through the liver, resulting in further damage.

The symptoms, which usually appear between two days and six weeks after birth, are a yellowing of the skin (jaundice), frequently accompanied by the enlargement and hardening of the liver, and a swelling of the abdomen. Stools are usually pale or grayish, resembling the color of clay. The urine appears dark. Some babies may develop intense itching (pruritus), which makes them extremely uncomfortable and irritable. As the disease progresses, it results in anemia, malnutrition and growth retardation.

Biliary atresia mimics the symptoms of other liver diseases, especially neonatal HEPATITIS, requiring several tests before the diagnosis can be made conclusively. These tests may include blood and urine tests, liver function tests, blood counts and clotting function tests, liver biopsy, liver scans using radioisotopes, and ULTRASOUND to determine the size of liver and bile ducts.

In the past, this condition was always fatal. Now some cases can be successfully treated with the surgical creation of a new bile duct fashioned from a piece of the small intestine. However, it must be performed in the first three months of life. Called the Kasai procedure, after Dr. Morio Kasai, a Japanese surgeon who developed it, it is successful in one-third to one-half of cases. An additional one-third continue to manifest signs of liver disease, but can lead relatively normal lives. Affected infants who do not respond to this treatment generally face increasing complications from cirrhosis, and may succumb by age two. Liver transplants are sometimes attempted if the Kasai procedure is ineffective. Liver transplantation has improved the outlook for children affected with biliary atresia; nearly 75% of recipients treated for this condition are alive and in good health five years later.

Biliary atresia is not a hereditary condition. Although the exact cause is not known, a viral infection near the time of birth may be responsible for the inflammation and obstruction of the bile ducts.

The condition occurs in an estimated one in 16,000 to one in 20,000 live births. There is an increased incidence in Japanese and Hawaiians of Chinese ancestry.

For more information, contact:

The American Liver Foundation
998 Pompton Avenue
Cedar Grove, NJ 07009

(201) 857-2626
(800) 223-0179

The Children's Liver Foundation
155 Maplewood Avenue
Maplewood, NJ 07040
(201) 761-1111

**biochemical assays**    A laboratory test for ENZYME activity that may be used for diagnosis of some hereditary disorders. An enzyme is a protein involved in chemical reactions in living matter. Hundreds of GENETIC DISORDERS are caused by lack of a certain enzyme or its reduced activity, which produces a biochemical imbalance. These include a form of ANEMIA, ALBINISM and TAY-SACHS DISEASE. (In the diagnosis of other genetic disorders the amount of non-enzyme biochemicals in body fluids may also be assayed or measured. These substances include amino acids and mucopolysaccharides.)

The deficiency or absence of an enzyme or other substance can often be determined either through biochemical assay of the individual's blood or prenatally, through analysis of cultured amniotic fluid cells gathered via AMNIOCENTESIS or CHORIONIC VILLUS SAMPLING.

**bird-headed dwarfism**    See SECKEL SYNDROME.

**birth control**    See CONTRACEPTIVE.

**birth defect**    A CONGENITAL abnormality. Literally thousands of types of birth defects have been reported and identified, ranging from mild conditions with only minor cosmetic significance, to lethal conditions, which may result in STILLBIRTH. About 2% to 3% of infants are born with a significant birth defect or defects, though not all are detected at birth or even soon after. For example, some congenital heart defects may be identified only during autopsy following a death they have precipitated. Conversely, some defects visible at birth may in some cases spontaneously correct themselves. For example, some

birthmarks called HEMANGIOMAS, red-colored marks that are composed of dilated blood vessels, may spontaneously fade during infancy.

Birth defects have been noted throughout recorded history. Official records of ancient astrologers of Nineveh and Babylon, dating to 2800 B.C., mention the birth of "monsters," severely deformed infants or aborted fetuses. These births were given great weight, and various deformities of specific limbs or other body parts were considered portents with highly specific meanings, heralding war, peace, natural disasters or the success or failure of a monarch's reign. Based on the specific nature of these prophesies, numerous congenital malformations must have been known to the Babylonians. Aristotle was also familiar with birth defects and wrote, in *On the Generation of Animals*, that "In man the male is more often born with deformity than the female," which appears to be the case for a number of congenital ANOMALIES.

Such has been the ubiquity of these conditions throughout history that laws have been passed and policies established dating at least to Roman times to deal with questions of inheritance, culpability for criminal acts and baptism among those born with significant deformities. (For example, while it is unclear if it was necessary to invoke these statutes, according to Roman law one member of a set of CONJOINED TWINS could not be put to death for a capital offense since it would require killing the innocent twin as well. Additionally, in the eyes of the church each individual head required a baptism; if a malformation resulted in two heads joined to a single trunk, two baptisms would be performed.) These canons have been referred to as "monster laws."

However, despite the recognition of various anomalous conditions, little effort was made by the medical community to study them until the 19th century. Among the first to apply scientific standards to the investigation of birth defects was zoologist Isidore Geoffroy Saint-Hilaire (1805-1861), who gave the name "teratology" from the Greek *teras*, for monster, to their study and classification.

## Table IV
## Congenital Anomalies Found in a Survey Conducted in British Columbia, Canada*

| Congenital Anolomy | 1952-63 N | 1952-63 Rate[i] | 1964-73 N | 1964-73 Rate[i] | 1974-83 N | 1974-83 Rate[i] | Total N | Total Rate[i] |
|---|---|---|---|---|---|---|---|---|
| Anencephaly | 74 | 169.1 | 60 | 174.1 | 89 | 229.6 | 223 | 190.6 |
| Spina bifida | 377 | 861.7 | 267 | 774.7 | 261 | 673.2 | 905 | 773.6 |
| Encephalocele | 12 | 27.4 | 26 | 75.4 | 46 | 118.6 | 84 | 71.8 |
| Congenital hydrocephalus | 182 | 416.0 | 273 | 792.1 | 347 | 895.0 | 802 | 685.5 |
| Other nervous system disorders | 158 | 361.1 | 268 | 777.6 | 372 | 959.5 | 798 | 682.1 |
| Eye | 382 | 873.1 | 507 | 1,471.0 | 603 | 1,555.3 | 1,492 | 1,275.4 |
| Ear, face, neck | 158 | 361.1 | 606 | 1,816.3 | 858 | 2,213.0 | 1,642 | 1,403.6 |
| Heart and circulation | 1,981 | 4,528.0 | 3,628 | 10,526.2 | 5,073 | 13,084.7 | 10,682 | 9,130.9 |
| Respiratory | 38 | 86.9 | 748 | 2,170.2 | 748 | 1,929.3 | 1,534 | 1,311.3 |
| Cleft palate and cleft lip | 812 | 1,856.0 | 757 | 2,196.3 | 809 | 2,086.6 | 2,378 | 2,032.7 |
| Pyloric stenosis | 38 | 86.9 | 900 | 2,611.2 | 1,063 | 2,741.8 | 2,001 | 1,710.4 |
| Hirschsprung disease, etc. | 16 | 36.6 | 81 | 235.0 | 89 | 229.6 | 186 | 159.0 |
| Other digestive system disorder | 212 | 484.6 | 667 | 1,935.2 | 1,277 | 3,293.7 | 2,156 | 1,842.9 |
| Hypospadias and epispadias | 174 | 397.7 | 788 | 2,286.3 | 990 | 2,553.5 | 1,952 | 1,668.6 |
| Other genito-urinary disorder | 421 | 962.3 | 2,866 | 8,315.3 | 3,369 | 8,689.6 | 6,656 | 5,689.5 |
| Clubfoot | 1,065 | 2,434.3 | 1,896 | 5,501.0 | 2,694 | 6,948.6 | 5,655 | 4,833.9 |
| Congenital disloca-tion of hip | 313 | 715.4 | 1,109 | 3,217.6 | 1,713 | 4,418.3 | 3,135 | 2,679.8 |
| Congenital dislocatable hip | 4 | 9.1 | 23 | 66.7 | 779 | 2,009.3 | 806 | 689.0 |
| Other musculo-skeletal disorders | 1,255 | 2,868.6 | 2,256 | 6,545.5 | 3,261 | 8,411.0 | 6,772 | 5,788.7 |
| Integument disorders | 227 | 518.9 | 678 | 1,967.1 | 1,165 | 3,004.9 | 2,070 | 1,769.4 |
| Chromosomal anomalies | 665 | 1,520.0 | 574 | 1,665.4 | 630 | 1,624.9 | 1,869 | 1,597.6 |
| Other | 137 | 313.1 | 248 | 719.5 | 424 | 1,093.6 | 809 | 691.5 |
| Total diagnoses | 8,701 | 19,887.8 | 18,671 | 54,171.4 | 26,660 | 68,763.6 | 54,032 | 46,186.2 |
| Total cases | 7,065 | 16,148.4 | 14,707 | 42,670.4 | 20,474 | 52,808.2 | 42,246 | 36,111.6 |

N- Number of patients
[i]Per 1 million live births.
*Statistics reflect local population bias.

Source: Patricia A. Baird, "A Population Study of Genetic Disorders in Children and Young Adults," *American Journal of Human Genetics*, 42 (1988): 677-693.

It has only been recently, perhaps since the 1960s, that classification and causes of birth defects have received extensive research attention, coinciding with the development of diagnostic procedures that can identify the chromosomal, molecular or chemical basis of some disorders. Prior to this time, medical authorities tended to lump birth defects together in broad categories such as DWARFISM or MENTAL RETARDATION, without concern for the subtle differences between many anomalies or the tremendous diversity of developmental defects that often exhibit almost identical characteristics. Additionally, little attention was given to the unexplained causes of death in early infancy following FAILURE TO THRIVE, which can now often be attributed to specific conditions. Thus there is a paucity of historical data on many genetic and congenital conditions.

Generally, defects that occur in one or more per 1,000 live births are considered common.

**Table V**
**Congenital Anomalies with Specific Genetic Etiology Found in a Survey**
**Conducted in British Columbia***

| Congenital Anomaly | 1952-63 | | 1964-73 | | 1974-83 | | Total | | Sum % of Highest Individual Rates | |
|---|---|---|---|---|---|---|---|---|---|---|
| | N | Rate[1] | N | Rate[1] | N | Rate[1] | N | Rate[1] | | |
| Dominant conditions | 202 | 461.7 | 198 | 574.5 | 181 | 466.8 | 581 | 496.6 | 741.5 | 2.8 |
| Recessive conditions | 52 | 118.9 | 71 | 206.0 | 74 | 190.9[1] | 197 | 168.4 | 290.3 | 1.1 |
| X-linked conditions | 10 | 22.9 | 13 | 37.7 | 20 | 51.6 | 43 | 36.8 | 66.4 | 0.2 |
| Autosomal chromosome conditions | 586 | 1,339.4 | 524 | 1,520.3 | 533 | 1,374.8 | 1,643 | 1,404.4 | 1,693.1 | 6.4 |
| Sex-chromosome conditions | 64 | 146.3 | 39 | 113.2 | 33 | 85.1 | 136 | 116.3 | 152.3 | 0.6 |
| Multifactorial conditions | ... | ... | ... | ... | ... | ... | ... | ... | 23,076.0 | 86.8 |
| Genetic unknown | 247 | 564.6 | 176 | 510.6 | 116 | 299.2 | 539 | 460.7 | 564.6[2] | 2.1 |
| Total | ... | ... | ... | ... | ... | ... | ... | ... | 26,584.2 | 100.0 |

N- Number of patients
[1]Per 1 million live births.
[2]Sum for the decade (1952-63) showing the highest rate.
*Statistics reflect local population bias.

Patricia A. Baird, "A Population Study of Genetic Disorders in Children and Young Adults," *American Journal of Human Genetics*, 42(1988): 677-693.

However, there is no consensus for what constitutes a rare condition. While there is ample documentation on conditions that have been seen in far fewer than 100 individuals worldwide, or in just one family, there is no way of knowing the true incidence of many of these or other rarely-reported disorders.

Birth defects can be caused in several ways. Genetically, they may be caused by the action of a single mutant GENE or gene pair, or may be due to abnormalities involving entire chromosomes or sections of them (see CHROMOSOME ABNORMALITIES). They may also be caused by the action of several genes in concert with an environmental trigger (MULTIFACTORIAL traits) or by the action of several genes alone (POLYGENIC).

Non-genetic causes include fetal exposure to TERATOGENS, substances that can have a harmful impact on fetal development. Birth defects may also result from mechanical forces within the womb. CLUBFOOT, for example, is the result of uterine crowding of a normally developed foot.

Due to their diversity in origin and expression, congenital anomalies are classified a number of ways. Birth defects caused by defective or abnormal development of an organ or body part are referred to as malformations. These include CONGENITAL HEART DEFECTS, SPINA BIFIDA and biochemical disorders that may manifest after birth, such as CYSTIC FIBROSIS, MUSCULAR DYSTROPHY and SICKLE-CELL ANEMIA. "Deformation" refers to a congenital anomaly caused by damage that occurs in the womb, to a normally developed part, such as clubfoot. "Dysplasia" refers to abnormal tissue development, and may involve skin, bones, nerves, organs or other tissue. Some anomalies, which may occur in isolation, are frequently seen together in a recognizable pattern. This group of defects is termed a syndrome.

More than 250 birth defects can now be detected prenatally. While the incidence of major birth defects has remained remarkably constant, improvements in prenatal detection and treatment, as well as societal attitudes about these conditions, continue to offer more options and opportunities for affected individuals and their families. (See also DATING; EDUCATION; GENETIC DISORDERS; HANDICAP; "INTRODUCTION.")

For more information, contact:

March of Dimes Birth Defects Foundation
1275 Mamaroneck Avenue
White Plains, NY 10605
(914) 428-7100

National Organization for Rare Disorders,
    Inc. (NORD)
P.O. Box 8923
New Fairfield, CT 06812
(203) 746-6518

Association of Birth Defect Children
3526 Emerywood Lane
Orlando, FL 32806
(305) 859-2821

National Center for Education in Maternal
    and Child Health (NCEMCH)
38th and R Streets, NW
Washington, DC 20057
(202) 625-8400

National Easter Seal Society
2023 West Ogden Avenue
Chicago, IL 60612
(312) 243-8400

**birth injury**    An injury to a newborn that
occurs during the birth process. It may result
from forces due to maternal factors, such as an
abnormal position of the newborn during
birth, or as a result of medical intervention,
such as the use of forceps to assist a prolonged
labor.

Injuries include hemorrhaging, damage to
organs and nerves, trauma that causes fluid
buildup in the tissues (edema), and fractures.

The most common fractures are of the collarbone (clavicle), and are most prone to occur
during delivery of large infants. Hemorrhaging of the retina is the most common birth
injury involving the eye, and may occur in as
many as 35% of all live births, though typically there is no lasting damage.

Injuries to abdominal organs and nerves
(most commonly facial nerves) are other
noted birth injuries. Facial nerve paralysis is
estimated to occur in one in 400 live births,

though it is usually a self-correcting condition.

The majority of serious birth injuries are
thought to be from trauma associated with
breech delivery, in which an infant emerges
from the womb feet, instead of head, first.
Spinal cord injuries are the most common
complication in these deliveries and may result in death. (Spinal cord injuries are extremely rare in deliveries where the infant
emerges head first.)

Kaiser Wilhelm II of Germany was delivered in a breech birth, and as a result of ensu-
ing nerve damage his left arm was atrophied.
It has been suggested that this birth trauma
may have contributed to World War I; the
psychological effects of his permanent injury
were said to have enhanced his aggressive
militaristic tendencies.

Statistics on birth injuries appear to be
somewhat unreliable, and while they indicate
a declining trend over the past several decades, trauma associated with delivery may be
underreported, particularly in the case of
minor injuries.

**birthmark**    Well-defined areas of colored skin present at birth to some degree on
most people.

In whites, birthmarks are usually dark
brown, the result of hyperpigmentation, and
may lighten and become slightly raised in
time. They may also be strawberry colored,
the result of vascular lesions consisting of
masses of small blood vessels (capillaries) just
below the surface of the skin. These lesions
are called HEMANGIOMAS.

Birthmarks are generally benign, though in
rare cases they may become cancerous. Additionally, large strawberry-colored birthmarks
may be associated with some hereditary disorders, such as STURGE-WEBER SYNDROME.
(See also NEVUS; PORT WINE STAIN.)

**birth palsy**    Paraplegia or hemiplegia
caused by a birth injury. (See PARAPLEGIA.)

**birth, premature**   See PREMATURITY; LOW BIRTHWEIGHT.

**Blackfan-Diamond syndrome**   See ANEMIA.

**bladder, exstrophy of**   See EXSTROPHY OF BLADDER.

**bleeder's disease**   See HEMOPHILIA.

**blindness**   The eye is particularly sensitive to genetic influences. A vast array of hereditary ocular disorders have been identified, some affecting the eyes alone and many others existing as part of more complex syndromes that affect other body systems as well. These disorders may be inherited as AUTOSOMAL DOMINANT, AUTOSOMAL RECESSIVE, X-LINKED, POLYGENIC or MULTIFACTORIAL conditions.

About 124,000 individuals in the United States under 45 years old are legally blind, and genetic aberrations account for almost half such cases. In addition, severe visual impairment or blindness in childhood affects about one of every 2,000 children in developed countries, and it is estimated that well over half such vision loss is attributable to genetic causes.

Some of the many eye findings that may indicate the presence of a hereditary disorder are: CATARACTS (any opacities in the lens that result in blurred vision); cherry-red spot; corneal clouding (opacity); nystagmus (rapid involuntary movement of the eyes from side to side, up and down, or in circular fashion); pain; pale or absent iris; photophobia (abnormal intolerance to light, causing intense eye discomfort accompanied by tight contractions of the eyelids or other attempts to avoid the light); PTOSIS (drooping of the upper eyelid); retinal detachment (frequently associated with severe myopia); small or malformed eye; STRABISMUS (any abnormal alignment of the two eyes accompanied by double vision).

Hereditary visual disorders include CONGENITAL GLAUCOMA, LEBER'S OPTIC ATROPHY and RETINOBLASTOMA.

Genetic disorders associated with visual defects include: ALBINISM, ANIRIDIA, BARDET-BIEDL SYNDROME, CROUZON DISEASE, DOWN SYNDROME, FABRY DISEASE, GALACTOSEMIA, HOMOCYSTINURIA, KNIEST DYSPLASIA, Lenz Syndrome, LOWE SYNDROME, MARFAN SYNDROME, MUCOLIPIDOSIS, MUCOPOLYSACCHARIDOSIS, MYOTONIC DYSTROPHY, NEUROFIBROMATOSIS, OSTEOGENISIS IMPERFECTA, Refsum disease, RETINITIS PIGMENTOSA, RIEGER SYNDROME, SPHINGOLIPIDOSIS, USHER SYNDROME, WAARDENBURG SYNDROME, WERNER SYNDROME, WILMS TUMOR, WILSON DISEASE and XERODERMA PIGMENTOSUM.

For more information, contact:

American Council of the Blind
1010 Vermont Avenue, NW
Suite 1100
Washington, DC 20005
(202) 393-3666
1-800-424-8666

National Federation of the Blind
1800 Johnson Street
Baltimore, MD 21230
(301) 659-9314

National Association For Visually
   Handicapped
305 East 24th Street, 17C
New York, NY 10010
(212) 889-3141

**Bloom syndrome**   Condition characterized by low birthweight and short stature, a characteristic facial appearance, development of skin rashes on the face during the first year of life, sun-sensitivity and a predisposition to develop CANCER. An immune defect is usually associated with Bloom syndrome, and frequently there are infections of the ear and respiratory tract as well. Physical growth remains stunted. Mild mental deficiency, though not a typical feature, has also been seen in a few individuals with this syndrome.

Since it was first described in 1954 by Dr. David Bloom, a New York City dermatologist with an interest in genetics, more than 300 affected individuals have been identified, almost half of them Ashkenazi Jews (those of eastern European ancestry). The genetic basis (AUTOSOMAL RECESSIVE inheritance) was identified in 1963. Approximately one in 120 Ashkenazim are estimated to be carriers of the defective gene.

Males average under five pounds (2.5 kg) at birth and females approximately four pounds (1.8 kg). The skin appears normal, but late in infancy or early childhood, reddish rashes (telangiectasias) appear, caused by dilated capillaries near the surface of the skin. These lesions most often appear on the face, primarily around the nose, lips and cheeks. In approximately half, the lesions appear on the forearms, backs of the hands, ears and neck as well. Exposure to the sun exacerbates the skin eruptions. At puberty, these areas of the skin scar, atrophy and become depigmented. Café au lait spots (irregularly shaped, coffee-colored splotches) frequently appear.

Body proportions, though normal, have a slender and delicate appearance. Affected individuals show a striking resemblance to each other. They have small, narrow faces. The nose is prominent, and the distance between the nose and the back of the head is greater than average. (This skull shape is referred to as dolichocephalic.) The ears protrude, and the voice tends to be high-pitched. Though they appear to be dwarfed in childhood, adolescent growth generally removes them from the category of true dwarfs, though height rarely reaches five feet. Infertility appears to be the rule in males. Life span is shortened due to the development of malignant cancers at an early age. About one in four has developed a malignancy, most commonly leukemia or digestive tract cancers.

The basic defect that causes this syndrome is unknown; however, it may be due to a defect of an enzyme involved in DNA replication, DNA-ligase I. Confirmation of the diagnosis based on physical characteristics is accomplished by findings of diminished immunoglobulin levels and cultured blood and skin cells showing chromosomal "instability," that is, the tendency of the chromosomes to break and rearrange themselves, which is a characteristic of this disorder. An increase is seen in sister chromatid exchange (exchange of DNA segments between the two parallel strands of a CHROMOSOME, each of which becomes a chromosome in the daughter cell during mitosis or cell division).

There is no method of carrier screening. Although there is no definitive prenatal diagnostic test, ULTRASOUND findings of a small fetus, tissue cultures taken via AMNIOCENTESIS revealing chromosomal instability, and increased sister chromatid exchange could be of use in at-risk pregnancies.

For more information, contact:

National Foundation for Jewish Genetic
    Diseases, Inc.
250 Park Avenue, Suite 1000
New York, NY 10177
(212) 682-5550

The National Tay-Sachs & Allied Diseases
    Association
92 Washington Avenue
Cedarhurst, NY 11516
(516) 569-4300

**blue baby (congenital cyanosis)**    Any infant with a cyanotic form of CONGENITAL HEART DEFECT causing poor oxygenation of the blood shortly after birth, and resulting in a blue tint of the skin. (See also PATENT DUCTUS ARTERIOSUS; CONGENITAL CYANOSIS.)

**bottled water**    A series of studies by the California Department of Health Services conducted in the Silicon Valley area found that women who reported drinking only bottled water while pregnant had a lower rate of miscarriage and birth defects in their children than did women who reported drinking tap water.

Over the course of four surveys involving 5,000 women, bottled water drinkers had miscarriage rates ranging from zero to 7.7%, while tap water drinkers had miscarriage rates within the normal range of 8% to 14%. Birth defects in children of the former group ranged from zero to 1.6%, and in children of the latter group, 2.6% to 6.2%, higher than the 2% to 3% national average.

Other factors such as smoking, alcohol consumption and exercise were taken into account in comparing the two groups. Researchers were unable to explain the findings and the results were noted mainly as a curiosity. It should not be taken as an advertisement for bottled water nor as evidence that tap water is dangerous. However, it does point out how difficult it can be to prove whether a drug or environmental exposure is safe or dangerous.

**bowleg**   A skeletal deformity in which the lower limbs bow outward. Synonyms: genu varum; bandy leg.


### Brachmann-de Lange syndrome
See CORNELIA DE LANGE SYNDROME.


**brachy**   Taken from the Greek *brachys*, meaning "short," this is a prefix used with a variety of terms to describe, among other conditions, abnormalities often associated with congenital anomalies and inherited conditions. Common terms using this prefix include:

*Brachycephaly*—Abnormally short head.
*Brachychelia*—Abnormally short lips.
*Brachydactyly*—Abnormally short fingers or toes.
*Brachygnathia*—An abnormally short lower jaw.


**brachycephaly**          See   CRANIOSYN-
OSTOSIS.

**brachydactyly**   Shortness of the fingers due to malformation of bones in the hand (metacarpals) or fingers (phalanges), from Greek *brachys*, meaning short, and *dactyl*, meaning digit. There are seven distinct genetic variations of the disorder, some of which cause shortness of the toes as well as fingers.

In Type A1, the middle phalanges (the middle of the three bones in each finger) are rudimentary and sometimes fused to the bones at the tips of the fingers (terminal phalanges). In the thumbs, the bones nearest the hand (proximal phalanges) are also short, as are the corresponding phalanges on the big toes.

In type A2, all the fingers are normal except the middle phalanges of the index fingers and second toes.

Type A3 is characterized by shortened middle phalanges of the little fingers.

In Type B, not only are the middle phalanges short, but the terminal phalanges are also rudimentary or absent altogether. Both fingers and toes are involved.

Type C is marked by shortened middle and proximal phalanges of the index and middle fingers. The middle phalanx of the fifth finger is also short. The index finger characteristically deviates away from the thumb.

In Type D, the terminal phalanges of the thumbs and big toes are short and broad.

In Type E, the bones of the hands and feet (metacarpals and metatarsals) are shortened. Short stature and a round face are also characteristic of this variation.

Types A3 and D are the commonest variations.

Brachydactyly may occur as an isolated malformation (unaccompanied by malformations of other parts of the body) or may occur as a part of a syndrome. For example, type A3 brachydactyly is seen in DOWN SYNDROME, type D in RUBINSTEIN- TAYBI SYNDROME and type E in TURNER SYNDROME. Isolated type D brachydactyly (stub thumbs) is common among Jews.

Isolated brachydactyly is generally inherited as an AUTOSOMAL DOMINANT trait. It may be detected at birth but often remains undiagnosed until late in childhood. Life span is not affected by the condition, and it is sometimes surgically correctable. Routine prenatal diagnosis is not currently available, but in severe cases brachydactyly may be detectable by prenatal ULTRASOUND.

**branchial cleft cysts or sinuses**   A painless cyst on the neck, which may be present at birth. It slowly enlarges, and may grow larger during infections, and subside afterward. Males are affected three times as frequently as females. The cause is unknown, but it is thought to result from a fetal developmental defect. The cyst can be removed surgically. Lifespan is normal, except in rare cases where the cyst becomes malignant.

**breast cancer**   See CANCER.

**brittle bone disease**   See OSTEOGENESIS IMPERFECTA.

**Bubble boy**   The popular designation given to a child named David in Houston, Texas, with severe combined immunodeficiency disease or SCID (see IMMUNE DEFICIENCY DISEASE); his story was dramatized in a made-for-television movie starring John Travolta, *The Boy in the Plastic Bubble*, first aired in 1976. The extremely rare disorder made his body unable to defend itself against viral, bacterial or parasitic agents, and his survival required a sterile environment completely sealed from the outside world. Hence, he lived in a plastic, room-sized "bubble" in a hospital.

An older sister was immunodeficient, and an infant brother died of a similar disorder before David's birth. Upon birth, David was placed in isolation, tested, found to be immunodeficient and remained in isolation throughout his life.

Efforts were made to find a suitable donor for a bone marrow transplant, which can sometimes enable recipients to produce components of the immune system that their own body is unable to manufacture. David died on February 22, 1984, at age 12, shortly after an unsuccessful bone marrow transplant procedure.

**Burkitt's lymphoma**   A lymph CANCER most commonly found in Central Africa, named for D.O. Burkitt, a contemporary physician posted in Uganda. Although the Epstein-Barr virus plays a role in its development, a specific translocation (see CHROMOSOME ABNORMALITIES), involving chromosomes 8 and either 14 or 22, the myc oncogene and the immunoglobulin genes, appears to be involved as a genetic trigger of the disease.

**Burton's agammaglobulinemia**   See IMMUNE DEFICIENCY DISEASES.

# C

**caffeine**   In laboratory studies, rats fed large quantities of caffeine—the equivalent of 80 cups of coffee daily—gave birth to offspring with below average birth weights and a higher incidence of bone abnormalities. Recent studies have also suggested a link between caffeine intake and infertility. However, there is lack of agreement on whether ingesting caffeine during pregnancy increases the risk of miscarriage, stillbirth or premature birth in humans (see ABORTION). It has not been directly linked to BIRTH DEFECTS.

In view of the uncertainties, the U.S. Food and Drug Administration has advised women during pregnancy to avoid coffee, tea, chocolate, cocoa, soft drinks and other foods that contain caffeine, as well as cold medicines, pain killers and weight control drugs that list caffeine among their ingredients. (See also TERATOGEN.)

**camptodactyly**   A permanent flexing of finger(s) or toe(s). It is most common in the little finger, though any finger or toe may be affected. Also, though any joint may be affected, it is most commonly seen in the middle joints.

As an isolated anomaly, it is inherited as an AUTOSOMAL DOMINANT trait with variable PENETRANCE. It is a feature of many genetic disorders, including syndromes with multiple contractures. (See also ARTHROGRYPOSIS.)

**camptomelic dysplasia**   (CMD; camptomelic dwarfism)   This condition, inherited as an AUTOSOMAL RECESSIVE trait, is a rare form of neonatal DWARFISM, characterized by congenital bowing of the bones of the legs (campomelia is the bending of the limbs), along with defects of the ribs and pelvis and facial anomalies. The bones of the arms are rarely bowed, but may be mildly short. The skull is large with a disproportionately small, flat face, low-set ears, small jaw (micrognathia) and wide-set eyes (HYPERTELORISM). Disarray of the hair (unruly hair) and cleft palate are sometimes present. There is generally a decreased number of ribs, which are slender in appearance, producing a small chest.

Death usually occurs soon after birth, generally due to respiratory distress caused by the decreased size of the rib cage.

The basic defect that causes this disorder is unknown. Twice as many female as male cases have been reported. This may be due to the external sex reversal that sometimes occurs in this condition (i.e., genetic males fail to develop masculine characteristics and thus have female external genitalia combined with XY chromosomal constitution).

PRENATAL DIAGNOSIS has been accomplished using ULTRASOUND to measure fetal long bone length.

**Canavan disease** (spongy degeneration of the brain)   A form of LEUKODYSTRO-PHY, a group of progressive, degenerative disorders of the nervous system. In Canavan disease, white matter in the brain is replaced by microscopic, fluid-filled spaces, hence its "spongy degeneration" appellation. It is

named for M.M. Canavan (1879-1953), who reported her patient in 1931.

Onset is in early infancy, beginning with feeding difficulties, poor muscle tone (hypotonia), progressive MENTAL RETARDATION, apathy and weakness, especially in the muscles supporting the head. As the disorder progresses, the head becomes enlarged as the brain enlarges, and the bones of the skull fail to fuse properly. Spasticity and paralysis develop. Vision, and sometimes hearing, deteriorate. Death usually occurs by three years of age. There is no cure.

The basic defect that causes this disorder has been identified as a deficiency of the EN-ZYME aspartoacylase. Although computerized axial tomography (CAT scan) can reveal severe changes in the white matter of the brain, previously the only way to confirm the disease was upon autopsy, with the finding of spongy degeneration of the gray and white matter of the brain. Now it has been demonstrated that affected individuals have deficient aspartoacylase and excrete excessive amounts of N- acetyl aspartic acid in their urine.

Inherited as an AUTOSOMAL RECESSIVE trait, Canavan disease is a rare disorder, though it has increased frequency in Ashkenazi Jews (those of Eastern European ancestry). Symptoms resemble TAY-SACHS DISEASE, another hereditary disorder exhibiting increased incidence in this ethnic group. (The latter stages of Canavan disease also resemble KRABBE DISEASE, another form of leukodystrophy.) With the identification of a biochemical defect, carrier detection and PRE-NATAL DIAGNOSIS are now possible for the first time.

For more information, contact:

United Leukodystrophy Foundation, Inc.
2304 Highland Drive
Sycamore, IL 60178
(815) 895-3211

The National Foundation for Jewish
   Genetic Diseases
250 Park Avenue, Suite 1000

New York, NY 10017
(212) 371-1030

**cancer**    Term describing more than 100 distinct disorders characterized by uncontrolled cell growth. Taken from the Latin for crab, cancer refers to the extension, like legs of a crab, of the neoplasm, or new growth, into adjoining tissue (though not all cancers exhibit this characteristic). If a neoplasm is not self-limiting and resists efforts to contain it, it is said to be malignant.

Cancers may be associated with chromosomal abnormalities, single mutant genes or exposure to viral or environmental agents. There are approximately 200 inherited disorders in which cancer has been reported as a regular or occasional feature, and the existence of some "cancer families" with a demonstrated predisposition to develop malignancies has long been recognized. Though the causes of cancer, either in general or in specific cases, are poorly understood, most are thought to result from a combination of genetic and environmental factors. However, when genetics are involved, the predisposition to develop a cancer, rather than the cancer itself, is what is inherited (see FAMILIAL DISEASE).

Assessing a genetic link in a given case may be difficult, though there are several characteristics associated with hereditary cancers: They tend to appear at an earlier age than would generally be expected for a given form of cancer and in approximately 50% of the cases, the cancer develops simultaneously in more than one area, whereas this only occurs in 3% to 5% of sporadic cases of cancer. Medical histories of family members may be useful in making a determination.

Currently, cancers caused by single gene mutations account for 5% to 7% of cases, with most of these inherited as AUTOSOMAL DOMINANT traits. About 25% of cancers are familial; though family members exhibit a greatly increased risk for developing cancer, affected individuals demonstrate no known pattern of inheritance. Typically, the risk of developing a cancer in these families is greater than within high-risk groups in the general population, such as heavy smokers or workers exposed to cancer-causing environmental agents.

In some cancers, exposure to toxic substances may trigger the development of neoplasms by transforming a normal gene into one that orchestrates uncontrolled cell growth. Genes that trigger the aberrant cell growth are called ONCOGENES, and approximately 50 have been identified. A number of anti-oncogenes have also been identified, which appear to inhibit the development of cancer. A MUTATION that inactivates an anti-oncogene results in neoplasia. It is thought that a number of cumulative errors must occur before cell growth becomes uncontrolled. It is likely that the actions of oncogenes and anti-oncogenes underlie most if not all cancers, and it is only how these are triggered that differs from situation to situation. Many oncogenes are located at the sites of the chromosome rearrangements seen in various cancers, such as the Philadelphia chromosome observed in many leukemia patients.

*Breast cancer.* This is the most common form of cancer among women, with more than 115,000 new cases and 30,000 deaths reported annually in the United States. In 1989, the National Cancer Institute of Canada estimated 12,300 new cases and 4,800 deaths that year. The average American woman has a lifetime risk of approximately 7% for developing breast cancer. Factors involved in its development include genetics, hormones, viruses and chemical agents.

Between 15% and 30% of all breast cancers are thought to be genetically determined and heterogeneous, that is, they represent various genetic disorders with a common symptomatic expression. A familial link was noted by the Romans as early as 100 A.D. Familial breast cancer may also be associated with other forms of cancer, particularly ovarian, uterine and colon cancer, and acute leukemias. The role of various oncogenes is presently under investigation.

Among the indications that a given case is familial are a family history of breast cancer, an earlier-than-average age of onset and the appearance of the cancer in both breasts (bilateral). If a woman's mother or sister had breast cancer, her risks are two to three times above average; if both mother and sister were affected, the risk rises to six times above average. If her mother had breast cancer and a sister had bilateral breast cancer prior to menopause, her risk is increased 40 times. It is suggested that women with increased risk undergo careful periodic examinations.

Breast cancer may also appear in males, and while rare, appears to have a strong genetic link.

Self-examinations and mammography are useful methods of early detection. Treatment generally consists of surgery to remove the growth, in conjunction with chemo-, hormonal or radiation therapy.

*Colorectal cancer.* Cancers of the colon and rectum are the second most common form of cancer behind lung cancer. Approximately 145,000 new cases and 60,000 deaths are recorded annually in the United States. In Canada, 14,600 new cases and 5,900 deaths were estimated for 1989. (The great majority are colon, rather than rectal cancers.) As in other forms of cancer, most are thought to be multifactorial, involving the action of several genes as well as environmental factors such as diet. A number of hereditary and familial forms have been identified and appear to be associated with the loss of material from chromosome 5. Among the most studied are various polyposis syndromes, so named due to the characteristic polyps that develop throughout the colon and, sometimes, the gastrointestinal tract. Polyps are small growths that in many cases may become malignant. Polyposis syndromes account for perhaps 5% of all cases of colon cancer.

*Familial polyposis of the colon (FPC).* Inherited as an AUTOSOMAL DOMINANT trait, FPC is characterized by the development of from hundreds to thousands of polyps throughout the colon, often beginning in childhood or early adulthood. The polyps frequently become malignant and spread rapidly.

It is estimated to occur in one in 8,000 births. This disorder has also been known as familial adenomatous polyposis (FAP) and accounts for perhaps 1% of colon cancers. The gene for this disorder has been mapped to chromosome 5.

*Gardner syndrome.* Named for E.J. Gardner (b. 1909), who described it in 1950, this autosomal dominant form of polyposis is also associated with cysts and tumors of the skin and bones, and dental abnormalities. Onset is usually at around age 20, with symptoms including mild diarrhea with mucous and blood. While some affected individuals remain asymptomatic, in the rest malignancies develop 15 to 20 years after symptoms first appear. Death from colon cancer usually occurs between the ages of 40 and 50. Incidence is estimated at one in 16,000 births. Some believe that it is a subset of and a specific form of FPC. Preliminary evidence from gene mapping indicates that this is so; the site of the gene seems to be the same.

*Peutz-Jeghers syndrome.* This autosomal dominant disorder is characterized by benign polyps found throughout the gastrointestinal tract and abnormal patterns of pigmentation, particularly about the lips. It bears the names of Dutch physician J.L.A. Peutz, who described it in 1921, and U.S. physician H. Jeghers, who described it in 1949. The polyps typically develop in adolescence, while the characteristic "black freckles" are present from birth.

Symptoms include severe, recurrent bouts of abdominal pain. However, the polyps become malignant in only 2% to 3% of those under medical attention. If all polyps are removed surgically in adulthood, no new ones develop.

*Non-polyposis syndromes with predisposition to colorectal cancer.* The majority of genetically determined colon cancers appear to be familial, without a clear MENDELIAN hereditary pattern. Families have been identified that are predisposed to developing bowel cancer and ulcerative colitis, an inflammatory bowel disorder that may lead to colon cancer. In these families, other family members may exhibit a variety of malignancies.

*Leukemia.* This cancer of the white blood cells is the most common childhood malignancy, though numerically it is much more common in adults. About 24,000 new cases are reported annually in the United States, with children accounting for an estimated 4,000 to 5,000 of them. It results in approximately 16,000 American deaths a year. In Canada, 3,000 new cases and 1,790 deaths were estimated for 1989.

The disorder is characterized by the production of abnormal white blood cells. Onset and progression may be rapid, as in acute leukemia, or may progress slowly, as in chronic leukemia.

Families with successive generations with leukemia (where affected individuals have had no contact) have been well-documented, establishing a strong genetic link in at least some cases. Additionally, many chronic leukemia patients exhibit a chromosome translocation, with a rearrangement involving chromosomes 9 and 22. This chromosome abnormality is referred to as "Philadelphia chromosome." Children with DOWN SYNDROME are also at increased risk for developing leukemia.

Previously a uniformly fatal disease, many affected individuals now survive.

*Lung cancer.* This is the greatest cause of cancer death in the United States and Canada, accounting for approximately 135,000 American, and 16,800 Canadian, deaths a year. While smoking is considered the major cause, genetic predisposition is also involved. The risk of developing lung cancer is thought to be 14 times above average for smokers with a close relative with lung cancer. A deletion of genetic material from chromosome 3 has been linked to small-cell lung cancer, a form that causes 35,000 to 40,000 fatalities annually in the United States.

*Skin cancer.* Skin cancer is the most common form of cancer in the United States, and the most easily treatable. The primary cause is thought to be exposure to ultraviolet radiation from sunlight, though again, genetic predisposition is a factor. However, unlike the majority of skin cancers, melanoma, a rapidly progressive form, is lethal. First noted by Hippocrates, a hereditary, "familial atypical mole melanoma," has been identified. It may have been described as early as 1820 by an English surgeon who observed multiple skin moles and melanoma in three generations of one family. (See also RETINOBLASTOMA, WILMS TUMOR, BURKITT'S LYMPHOMA, IMPRINTING.)

For more information, contact:

American Cancer Society, Inc.
4 West 35th Street
New York, NY 10001
(212) 382-2169

National Cancer Institute
805 15th Street N.W., Room 500
Washington, DC 20005
(205) 496-4070

Candlelighters Childhood Cancer
 Foundation
1901 Pennsylvania Avenue, NW
Washington, DC 20006
(202) 659-5136

Familial Polyposis Registry
Department of Colorectal Surgery
Cleveland Clinic Foundation
Building A-111
9500 Euclid Avenue
Cleveland, OH 44106
(216) 444-6470

**cannabis**     See MARIJUANA.

**carbamyl phosphate synthetase deficiency, CPS-I**     See UREA CYCLE DEFECTS.

**cardioauditory syndrome**     See JERVELL AND LANGE-NIELSEN SYNDROME.

**carnitine deficiency**     Carnitine helps to regulate the cellular rate of long-chain fatty acid oxidation. Deficiency of the carnitine protein can result in impaired oxidation of fat with episodes of coma or a muscle disorder related to increased lipid storage. Some patients may have mental retardation. Although the basic cause is often unknown, carnitine deficiency in the muscle may be due to defective absorption of carnitine by the muscle fiber, to defective carnitine synthesis in the liver, or to depletion of the body's stores of this compound. The diagnosis is based on finding decreased levels of carnitine in the blood.

The first carnitine deficiency disorder was identified by Dr. W. Engle in 1970, who published a description in the journal "Science." Symptoms generally appear during the 20s or 30s or earlier, and include muscle cramping following exercise. Affected individuals may have had prolonged fasts or may indulge in high-fat diets.

The long-term prognosis is uncertain. However, progressive muscle and liver damage may occur. Primary treatment may target avoidance of such exacerbating factors as strenuous exercise, severe dietary restriction and high-fat diets.

The mode of transmission of this very rare disorder is generally as AUTOSOMAL RECESSIVE traits.

Most carnitine deficiency is not primary, but rather occurs secondary to other diseases, mainly the organic acidurias, including propionic acidemia or the more recently described acyl-coA dehydrogenase deficiencies, primary disorders of fatty- acid breakdown. This implies that it is not the deficiency of carnitine that is the fundamental problem, but rather that deficiency occurs as a result of a primary defect of another ENZYME involved in fatty acid utilization.

**Carpenter syndrome**   (acrocephalopolysyndactyly)  A form of CRANIOSYN-OSTOSIS, skull malformations caused by premature closure of the gaps (sutures) between one or more skull bones. Head growth is thus directed in aberrant directions. Two sisters with this form were first described in 1901 by English pediatrician George Alfred Carpenter (1859-1910).

Carpenter's syndrome is distinguished by the presence of extra toes, which may be webbed. Cardiac abnormalities, obesity, poorly developed genitalia and mental retardation are sometimes present. Early surgical treatment may reduce incidence of mental retardation by relieving cranial pressure.

Inherited as an AUTOSOMAL RECESSIVE trait, about 35 affected individuals have been reported.

For other forms of craniosymostosis, see APERT SYNDROME; CROUZON DISEASE; PFEIFFER SYNDROME; and SAETHRE-CHOTZEN SYNDROME.

**carrier**   An individual with a single recessive gene for a particular disorder; a HETEROZYGOTE for a recessive disease. The term is often applied to a female who possesses a gene for an X-LINKED disorder. The carrier will usually not exhibit any signs of the disorder, but is capable of passing the gene to his or her offspring, or of having an infant with the disorder if he or she mates with another carrier. (See also AUTOSOMAL RECESSIVE.)

**cartilage-hair hypoplasia**   See METAPHYSEAL CHONDRODYSPLASIA.

**cataracts**   Opacities or clouding of the lens of the eye that can result in decreased vision and, in some cases, BLINDNESS. The severity of congenital cataracts varies greatly, ranging from functionally insignificant to blindness caused by a totally opacified lens.

An estimated one in 250 infants is born with a cataract, as a result of either genetics or other prenatal influence. Their formation is poorly understood. They account for 11.5% of blindness in preschool children. About 25% of congenital cataracts are believed to be genetically induced, most often the result of AUTOSOMAL DOMINANT inheritance. AUTOSOMAL RECESSIVE and X-LINKED inheritance is rare.

Additional ocular defects are seen in approximately 50% of all affected individuals. Congenital cataracts are also an associated feature of a number of GENETIC DISORDERS as well as of other systemic diseases or syndromes. These include GALACTOSEMIA, cerebral cholesterinosis, congenital ICHTHYSOSIS, CHONDRODYSPLASIA PUNCTATA, WERNER SYNDROME, LOWE SYNDROME and MYOTONIC DYSTROPHY, in addition to disorders such as congenital rubella, diabetes and chromosomal aberrations.

Total congenital cataracts, possibly with X-linked inheritance, have been observed in the We-Sorts, a triracial group of southern Maryland.

Management depends on the severity of the opacities, whether they are unilateral or bilateral and their association with other ocular defects or systemic problems. Early surgery is needed in bilateral, complete cataracts. This is followed by contact lens fitting, even in the infant.

**cat eye syndrome** Condition named for the vertical appearance of the pupil of those affected, caused by a fissure or cleft of the iris (coloboma). The two major features of the SYNDROME are this "cat eye" and an anus that has failed to open during fetal development (IMPERFORATE ANUS). Several other conditions are commonly seen in those with the syndrome. MENTAL RETARDATION of varying severity is present in between 55% and 80%. Forty percent have abnormally small heads (MICROCEPHALY), and cardiovascular anomalies occur in about 55%. CLEFT LIP or cleft palate occur in about 25% and genital and kidney malformations in about 20%.

Additional eye anomalies often associated include wide-set eyes (HYPERTELORISM), seen in about 40% and small eye(s) (microophthalmia), in 25%.

Cat eye syndrome is believed to be caused by a CHROMOSOMAL ABNORMALITY in which there is an extra segment or small fragment of a chromosome. However, cases have been reported in which no chromosome abnormality is present, and similar extra chromosome fragments are sometimes seen in normal individuals. Other chromosome abnormalities, e.g., trisomy 22, may have similar features.

PRENATAL DIAGNOSIS of a baby with cat eye syndrome is theoretically possible by finding the chromosome fragment in fetal cells collected via AMNIOCENTESIS or CHORIONIC VILLUS SAMPLING.

Surgery can correct the imperforate anus and other associated anomalies. Life span may be shortened in those individuals with cardiac and renal malformations associated with the syndrome.

**cats** Cats are believed to be a vector for transmitting the microorganism that causes TOXOPLASMOSIS, a disease that, if contracted during pregnancy, can cause fetal development anomalies that may result in mental retardation or death.

Evidence indicates that the feces of infected cats may harbor the microorganisms, thereby contaminating soil or litter boxes, which may remain infectious for weeks or months. It has been advised that all individuals wash their hands after handling or disposing of cat litter, and that pregnant women avoid contact with used cat litter.

**cebocephaly** See HOLOPROSENCEPHALY.

**celiac disease** See GLUTEN-INDUCED ENTEROPATHY.

**cell bank** A repository for collecting, storing and distributing CELL CULTURES for scientific research. The Human Genetic Mutant Cell Repository, at the Coriell Institute for Medical Research in Camden, New Jersey, for example, maintains a collection of human cells preserved for the study of genetic diseases. With some 5,000 donated samples from individuals affected with various hereditary disorders, this unit of the National Institutes of Health is the largest facility of its kind in the world.

About 500 to 600 new samples are received annually. In many cases, samples are donated by several family members exhibiting a hereditary disorder whose exact genetic cause has yet to be determined. Cells from donated tissue samples are cultured and then stored at minus 316° Fahrenheit. Portions of the repository's cell samples are thawed and sent to researchers around the world. Studies of these cells may help unravel the genetic secrets of hundreds of inherited disorders. Other institutions also maintain similar, often more specialized, collections.

For more information, contact:

Human Genetic Mutant Cell Repository
Coriell Institute for Medical Research
Copewood Street
Camden, NJ 08108
(609) 966-7377

**cell culture**  The growth of cells in vitro, that is, in glass, such as a test tube, for experimental purposes. The cells proliferate but do not organize into tissue. Cells taken from amniotic fluid or fetal tissue for use in prenatal diagnostic procedures are cultured prior to their analysis. Other types of cells (for example from skin) can be maintained in culture (see CELL BANK) for experimental studies. (See also AMNIOCENTESIS.)

**central core disease**  Characterized by weak muscles and lack of muscle tone (hypotonia), this rare AUTOSOMAL DOMINANT trait is a form of benign familial polymyopathy (disorders that affect skeletal muscles). Described in 1956, though not named until later, it was the first example of a stationary muscle disorder. (Stationary muscle disorders are non-progressive, as opposed to the MUSCULAR DYSTROPHIES.) It produces a "FLOPPY INFANT" and is usually observed in early infancy. In initial stages it resembles Duchenne muscular dystrophy, except for its non-progressive nature. Walking and muscular development are delayed.

It is caused by a biochemical abnormality of the muscle, involving liberation of phosphate from glucose 6-phosphate. The name is derived from the fact that when affected muscle fibers are stained and examined microscopically, there is a central "core" of fibers that do not stain the same way as the fibers at the margins.

**cerebral gigantism**  See SOTOS SYNDROME.

**cerebral palsy**  (CP; congenital cerebral palsy)  A group of disabling conditions resulting from damage to the central nervous system; "cerebral" refers to the brain, and "palsy" refers to a lack of muscle control that is a frequent feature of the disorders. Characteristics of CP may include spasms, involuntary movements and disturbances of gait and mobility, which may be accompanied by abnormal sensation and perception.

CP is best described as a group of chronic, nonprogressive disorders of movement and posture of early onset. That is, these disorders begin early in life and persist throughout life but do not get worse with time. Though primarily disturbances of movement, they may have associated abnormalities of vision or hearing, seizures or MENTAL RETARDATION. It was formerly named "Little's disease," for British physician William John Little (1810-94), who was among the first to study this disorder.

There are three major types of CP: spastic, characterized by stiff and difficult movement; athetoid, characterized by uncontrolled, abnormal movement; and ataxic, characterized by a disturbed sense of balance and depth perception. Individuals may exhibit characteristics of any combination of these types. (There are other, more rare types of movement disorders that are not really CP; for example, LESCH-NYHAN SYNDROME has been considered a severe form of cerebral palsy, but it is really an inherited metabolic disease that affects only males and is progressive in nature.)

There is great variability in the expression of CP, ranging from severe cases that result in total inability to control body movements and mental retardation, to mild cases that may result only in slight speech impairment. The severity of the condition is dependent on the part of the brain affected and the extent to which it has been damaged.

The cause of CP is not clearly or fully understood. Cerebral palsy is thought to be caused by damage to the brain before, during or shortly after birth. There are numerous possible ways for this damage to occur. For example, it is clear that maternal viral infections during pregnancy (such as German measles) can seriously affect fetal development. A blood type incompatibility conflict between the mother and the fetus can also cause damage to the fetus and result in CP, if Rh factor is absent from the mother's blood and present in the father's (see HEMOLYTIC DISEASE OF THE NEWBORN.) Lack of oxygen reaching the fetal or newborn brain may be a cause of CP, and may result from infant breathing problems associated with premature birth, or complications in pregnancy and labor. While in the past it was thought that most cases of CP were caused by oxygen deprivation related to the birthing process, such as awkward birth position, extended labor or interference with the umbilical cord, recent data is making it clear that this is not the case. Large studies in the United States and Australia have shown that most newborns with lack of oxygen at birth do not suffer from CP, and most children with CP were not deprived of oxygen at birth. Clearly, other poorly understood factors must occur before birth that play a role in causing CP. Because of this link to delivery, a growing number of lawsuits have been brought by parents of affected individuals, claiming obstetrical malpractice caused the condition in their child, though this is generally not the case.

An estimated 500,000 to 700,000 children and adults in the United States manifest one or more CP symptoms, with 5,000 to 7,000 infants born with the condition each year.

Improvements in treatments for affected individuals in recent years have lessened their isolation. Medication for controlling seizures, surgery for correcting some physical problems, counseling to assist emotional adjust-ment, and mechanical aids such as communication equipment, specially equipped cars and page turners, have helped increase opportunities for affected individuals. Additionally, an increase in available programs offering physical therapy, occupational therapy and speech therapy have assisted in helping these individuals become more integrated into society.

For more information, contact:

United Cerebral Palsy Association, Inc.
66 East 34th Street
New York, NY 10016
(212) 481-6300
(800) 872-1827

National Council on Independent Living
815 West Van Buren
Suite 525
Chicago, IL 60607
(312) 226-5900

United Together, Inc.
3111 Haworth Hall
Lawrence, KS 66045
(913) 864-4950

**cerebro-hepato-renal syndrome**
See ZELLWEGER SYNDROME.

**cerebro-oculo-facio-skeletal syndrome**
Rare AUTOSOMAL RECESSIVE disorder that typically leads to death from emaciation and respiratory failure, or from repeated respiratory infections within the first three years of life.

Affected infants are usually small; though typically born at term with normal birth weights, there is virtually no growth. Other features include a small head, often with a sloping forehead, CATARACTS or small eyes, high nasal bridge, large ears, overhanging upper lip and small jaw. There are also skeletal abnormalities, such as narrow pelvis, prominent heels, "rocker bottom feet" and, importantly, flexion contractures of the limbs and fingers. These congenital contractures (see

ARTHROGRYPOSIS) are due to an apparent neurologic degeneration occurring before birth.

**cesarean delivery**    (cesarean section; C section)    A method of childbirth in which the baby is surgically removed from the uterus through an incision made in the abdomen. Cesarean deliveries were practiced as early as 3000 B.C. in Egypt, and the name of the procedure is taken from a set of Roman laws, the *Lex Caesare*, dating to 715 B.C., which mandated the surgical removal of a fetus following maternal death. (Julius Caesar was also said to have been delivered this way, as was Macduff in Shakespeare's Macbeth.)

Historically, cesarean deliveries have been a high risk to both mother and infant, due to the likelihood of infection and the primitive surgical techniques employed. However, as these risks have dropped, the rates of cesarean childbirth have climbed dramatically, more than tripling in the decade from 1970 to 1980—from 5% to 16.5% of all births. Currently, first-time cesarean births represent about 17% of all deliveries.

Despite improved medical techniques, C sections are still associated with increased risks to both maternal and infant health. Maternal mortality is approximately one in 2,500 for cesarean deliveries, as compared with one in 10,000 for vaginal deliveries. Infants delivered by cesarean section are at increased risk for respiratory ailments and fetal distress caused by the anesthesia administered to the mother.

The continued high rates of cesarean deliveries are due to several factors: Since the procedure is safer than it once was, many infants who would be difficult to deliver vaginally due to complications of labor, termed dystocia, are instead delivered via C section. (Dystocia refers to a broad range of labor complications, including a mismatch between the size of the baby and that of the mother's pelvis or the position of the fetus.) The accepted notion that once a woman has had a cesarean she will always deliver by that method has also made it more common. (More than 98% of U.S. women who have had a cesarean delivery continue to deliver this way in subsequent childbirths.) Cesarean deliveries also allow more control over when an infant will be delivered.

The current consensus among maternal and childcare authorities is that the rates of cesarean deliveries should be reduced and that, where possible, vaginal delivery should be the method of choice. The American College of Obstetricians and Gynecologists, noting both the additional risks and costs of surgical delivery, has recommended that most women who have had a cesarean delivery try to have vaginal deliveries in subsequent births.

**cesarean section**    See CESAREAN DELIVERY.

**CF**    See CYSTIC FIBROSIS.

**Charcot-Marie-Tooth disease, CMT** (peroneal muscular atrophy; hereditary motor and sensory neuropathy)    A group of GENETIC DISORDERS characterized by degeneration of the motor and sensory nerves that control movement and feeling in the arm below the elbow and in the leg below the knee. There is progressive muscle atrophy and wasting, resulting in severe weakness in the wrists, hands and fingers, as well as in the feet, ankles and lower legs. Simple tasks requiring manual dexterity, such as buttoning buttons, picking up small objects and writing, may become difficult. In the legs, degenerative changes may limit mobility. Reflexes slow considerably.

It is named for French neurologists Jean M. Charcot and Pierre Marie and British neurologist Howard Tooth, who simultaneously described the disorder in 1866.

The severity of the disorder is highly variable, even among members of the same family. Some researchers believe a large number of mildly affected individuals are never diagnosed. Symptoms most frequently appear in adolescence. Typically it begins with weakness in muscles of the feet, progressing to the calf muscles and muscles of the lower arms. Due to atrophy of muscles in the foot, the toes become cocked and the foot becomes foreshortened and may develop a very high arch (pes cavus) or become uncommonly flat. Affected individuals develop a high-stepping drop-foot gait, with the foot raised well above the ground (stork leg), in order to prevent the forefeet from dragging on the ground and tripping them. The foot slaps as it hits the ground. Affected individuals cannot run very fast, and due to weakness in the ankles, they often have frequent sprains. Changes in the shape of the foot may lead to blistering of the toes and other problems due to the unaccommodating shape of normal shoes. Loss of feeling occurs to a variable degree.

The disorder is slowly progressive, may stabilize for long periods of time, and may stop progressing entirely at any time. Therefore, affected individuals can never be sure about the extent of the ultimate severity of their condition. Lifespan is unaffected. The majority of therapy is focused on care of feet and lower legs to ease mobility and to reduce problems caused by weakening and degenerative changes in the feet. Surgery can sometimes reduce hand, foot, ankle and toe problems.

An inherited disorder, CMT is transmitted in AUTOSOMAL DOMINANT, AUTOSOMAL RECESSIVE and X-LINKED recessive forms. Some cases appear to be the result of new MUTATION. The majority of cases are autosomal dominant, followed by the X-linked recessive form. One form of the disease has been linked to GENETIC MARKERS on CHROMOSOME 1. A form of the disorder linked with DEAFNESS has been reported to be unusually frequent in the hill country of western North Carolina.

One study in western Norway found the prevalence of autosomal dominant forms to be 36 in 100,000 people, of X-linked to be 3.6 in 100,000, and autosomal recessive, 1.4 in 100,000.

For more information, contact:

Charcot-Marie-Tooth International Assn., Inc.

34 Bayview Drive
St. Catherines, Ontario, Canada L2N 4Y6
(416) 937-3851

**CHARGE association** This rare syndrome results from defects in embryonic development summarized by the acronym CHARGE: fissure of the eye (COLOBOMA); Heart disease; a block in the nasal passages (Atresia choanal); Retarded growth and development; Genital anomalies; and deformed Ears or deafness. In addition, kidney anomalies, or abnormal connection between the windpipe and esophagus (TRACHEOESOPHAGEAL FISTULA), facial tremors, an abnormally small jaw (micrognathia), CLEFT LIP and CLEFT PALATE may occur. The abnormalities are believed to originate during the second month of gestation, when the differentiation of tissues and organs in the fetus takes place.

Most affected individuals are mentally deficient. Visual or hearing handicaps may also influence their ability to function. If the defects are severe, death may occur soon after birth.

The cause of this disorder is unknown, although it is believed to be genetically influenced, since certain abnormalities have recurred within families.

**Chediak-Higashi syndrome** A lethal metabolic disorder, named after M. Chediak, a Cuban physician who described it in 1952, and O. Higashi, a Japanese pediatrician who published a description in 1954. A form of ALBINISM, it is characterized by decreased pigmentation of hair and eyes, sensitivity to light (photophobia), constant, involuntary movement of the eyes (nystagmus), abnormal susceptibility to infection, and peculiar malignant lymphoma. Nerve damage is also present. There is muscle weakness, foot drop (a peculiar gait) and decreased muscle stretch reflexes. Affected infants may have convulsions and MENTAL RETARDATION, and often have frequent recurring infections, especially of the gastrointestinal tract, skin and respiratory tract, and fevers of unknown origin.

Inherited as an AUTOSOMAL RECESSIVE trait, it is very rare. Most cases have been of European ancestry, especially Spanish, and most have died in childhood due to infection, often before the age of seven. Those that survive beyond infancy generally die of a rapidly developing malignancy.

CARRIER detection is possible in some cases by the presence of abnormally large granules in the blood cells. A similar or identical blood cell disorder has been found in Aleutian mink, Hereford cattle, Beige mice and a killer whale.

**cherry-red spot**    An abnormal red circular area in the retina of the eye. It is one of the hallmarks of TAY-SACHS DISEASE. It results from swelling of the nerve cells around the macula of the retina (the central area of vision on the retina) that makes the macula stand out as a red circle. It can also be seen in other storage diseases, though Tay-Sachs is the most common disorder causing it.

**chicken pox**    See VARICELLA.

**chimera**    Taking its name from the mythological hybrid beast with a lion's head, goat's body and serpent's tail, this is an individual with, or the condition of having, genetic material from two different embryos. It is most common in the blood of fraternal twins due to the mixing of the fetal blood cells during embryonic development. True HERMAPHRO-DITES with an XX/XY chromosomal constitution also may be chimeras. Additionally, individuals who have had transplants, in particular, bone marrow transplants, are often referred to as chimeric, as their blood cells are thereafter derived from another individual, and therefore from a different embryo.

**Chinese restaurant syndrome**    (monosodium glutamate sensitivity)    An estimated 25% of the general population may be sensitive to MSG (monosodium glutamate), a chemical used as a flavor enhancer. Its heavy use in some Chinese foods is the reason these individuals often experience a characteristic reaction following a meal in a Chinese restaurant. Symptoms include a tightening in the back of the neck, pressure around the eyes, headache, flushed face and nausea. So-called "hot dog headache" and migraine headaches triggered by diet may be similar sensitivities. (Individuals who think they are allergic to MSG actually have this inherited sensitivity [see ALLERGY].)

The sensitivity may be inherited as an AUTOSOMAL RECESSIVE trait, though this is not proven. The basic defect involved in the reaction is unknown, but may be due to an inborn error of metabolism.

**choanal atresia**    See POSTERIOR CHOANAL ATRESIA.

**choledochal cyst**    A congenital cyst found in the bile duct, which manifests itself as a mass in the right upper quadrant of the abdomen, frequently accompanied by jaundice and pain due to blockage of the flow of bile. It affects females four times as often as males, and appears most commonly in the Japanese. The exact cause is unknown and appears to be non-genetic.

Without treatment, this defect is lethal due to inflammation of the bile ducts (cholangitis) and prolonged jaundice caused by chronic retention of bile (biliary cirrhosis). It can be treated by surgery, often biliary-intestinal drainage, or complete removal of the cyst.

It is detected in the first year of life in approximately 20% of cases, and between the ages of one and 10 years in an additional third. Eighty percent of all cases are identified in the first 30 years of life. Over 500 cases have been reported.

PRENATAL DIAGNOSIS may be possible by identifying the cyst via ULTRASOUND.

**cholesteryl ester storage disease**    An extremely rare hereditary condition, apparently caused by a deficit of acid lipase, an ENZYME that breaks down cholesteryl esters (a particular form of fat). As a result, abnormally high levels of cholesteryl esters and trigylcerides accumulate in the liver, spleen and intestine. The liver is enlarged (hepatomegaly), and the spleen may be as well (splenomegaly). Lipid levels in blood, plasma and bone marrow are extremely high. There is also an indication that premature coronary vascular disease may be a part of this condition.

Transmitted as an AUTOSOMAL RECESSIVE trait, very few cases have been documented. Females may be more often affected than males. The disease can be detected at birth by measuring levels of the affected enzyme. There is no treatment. PRENATAL DIAGNOSIS has been accomplished. Life expectancy appears shortened, though the exact cause of death has not been fully established.

It appears that this disorder is related to WOLMAN DISEASE, which also has as its cause deficiency of the enzyme acid lipase. However, that disease causes more serious manifestations, earlier in life, with death within a few months after birth.

**cholinesterase, atypical**   See ATYPICAL CHOLINESTERASE.

**chondrodysplasia punctata**   A group of dwarfing conditions characterized by multiple abnormalities in the development of the bones, especially the bones of the upper leg (long bones) and the bones in the fingers. "Chondro" refers to cartilage, "DYSPLASIA" to abnormal development and "punctata" refers to the characteristic pinpoint spots of calcification found by X rays in cartilage of developing bones. In addition, affected individuals may have a characteristic facial appearance and other defects as well. Scalp hair tends to be sparse and coarse, and the skin tends to be dry and scaly.

There are several forms of chondrodysplasia punctata. The majority are genetically determined. As a hereditary disorder, it occurs in AUTOSOMAL DOMINANT, AUTOSOMAL RECESSIVE, X-LINKED dominant and recessive forms. Maternal ingestion of certain drugs

(e.g., anticoagulants such as warfarin) during pregnancy has also been associated with this disorder. The punctate calcifications have also been seen in other disorders, such as ZELLWEGER SYNDROME.

Theoretically, detection of the abnormal skeletal development with ULTRASOUND could be used as a method of prenatal screening, but this has not yet been accomplished in early pregnancy. Identification of a specific underlying biochemical abnormality has made prenatal diagnosis of the recessive form possible (see below).

*Conradi-Hunermann type.* This is the autosomal dominant form of chondrodysplasia punctata. It bears the name of E. Conradi and C. Hunermann, who published descriptions in 1914 and 1931, respectively. The skeletal dysplasia is marked by asymmetry of the limbs. The face appears flat, with a depressed nasal bridge. Other common characteristics include scoliosis (often developing in the first year of life) and contractures of the large joints. Dry scaly skin or loss of hair (ALOPECIA) occur in about 25% of cases. CATARACTS occur in less than 20% of cases. CONGENITAL HEART DEFECTS are sometimes present.

There is a wide variability in this form. Though severe cases may be stillborn, for those who survive beyond the first weeks of life, life expectancy and mental development are normal.

Most cases are thought to be the result of new mutation.

*Rhizomelic type.* Rhizomelic is a term denoting disproportionate shortening of those parts of the limbs closest (proximal) to the body (i.e., the upper arm and thigh). This is the autosomal recessive form of chondrodysplasia punctata. It is rare and usually fatal. Infants fail to thrive and die in the first weeks of life from respiratory difficulties. Those who survive the first year of life are severely retarded and usually die in early childhood.

In addition to the disproportionate shortening of the proximal portions of the limbs, other findings may include a small head (MICROCEPHALY) and CLEFT PALATE. Swelling of the cheeks due to blockage of the lymph glands (lymphedema) give the cheeks a "chipmunk" appearance. Cataracts in both eyes (bilateral) are found in 70% to 80% of cases. In Australia, the depressed bridge of the nose (saddle nose) seen in many cases led to the designation "koala bear syndrome" for this disorder in 1970.

As in other rare recessive disorders, the frequency of CONSANGUINITY appears high in the parents of infants with this disorder.

Rhizomelic chondrodysplasia punctata has recently been found to be due to a defect in the function of the subcellular organelles called peroxisomes. The peroxisomal disorders are a newly recognized group of disorders with dysfunction of this organelle. The disorders include the Zellweger syndrome, ADRENOLEUKODYSTROPHY. Refsum disease and rhizomelic chondrodysplasia punctata. There are specific biochemical abnormalities identifiable now in rhizomelic chondrodysplasia punctata that not only shed light on the origin (pathogenesis) of this disorder but also permit precise prenatal (by CHORIONIC VILLUS SAMPLING or AMNIOCENTESIS) and postnatal diagnosis.

*X-linked.* The X-linked dominant form accounts for perhaps approximately one-quarter of all cases. It is lethal in males. Affected females have markedly asymmetric bone and eye involvement. The skin and scalp manifestations are characteristically patchy. MENTAL RETARDATION does not seem to occur in this form, and the prognosis is generally favorable.

An X-linked recessive form has been described with mild physical symptoms and mental deficiency.

For more information, contact:

Parents of Dwarfed Children
11524 Colt Terrace
Silver Spring, MD 20902
(301) 649-3275

Little People of America, Inc.
P.O. Box 633
San Bruno, CA 94066
(415) 589-0695

**chondrodystrophy**　　See ACHONDROPLASIA.

**chondroectodermal dysplasia**　　See ELLIS-VAN CREVELD SYNDROME.

**chorea, hereditary benign**　　See HEREDITARY BENIGN CHOREA.

**chorea, Huntington's, chronic**　　See HUNTINGTON'S DISEASE.

**chorion**　　One of the membranes surrounding the fetus and containing another membrane, the amnion, the sac that holds the fetus and the AMNIOTIC FLUID. The placenta develops from this membrane. In early gestation the chorion contains finger-like projections, the chorionic villi. Sampling of these pieces of tissue (CHORIONIC VILLUS SAMPLING or CVS) allows for early prenatal diagnosis of some genetic conditions in the first trimester of pregnancy.

**chorionic villus sampling (CVS)**　　An invasive prenatal diagnostic procedure. First introduced in the United States in 1983, an advantage over the older and more widely used AMNIOCENTESIS procedure is that CVS can be performed much earlier in a pregnancy—usually about the ninth week—thus providing diagnostic information during the first trimester.

The CHORION is a membrane that forms early in pregnancy and later develops into the placenta, through which the fetus is nourished. At the edge of the chorion are villi, tiny frondlike projections containing blood vessels. The villi connect the chorion to the lining of the uterus and contain many fetal cells, which can be analyzed in the laboratory to aid in prenatal diagnosis of possible genetic defects and CHROMOSOME ABNORMALITIES.

In chorionic villus sampling, a small piece of villus tissue is removed by one of two methods. In the first, which was the original technique employed, a catheter is inserted into the mother's vagina and, with the aid of ultrasound imaging, the catheter is guided through the cervix and into the uterus to the chorionic villi. A syringe is then used to suction out the required tissue sample. In the second method, a needle is inserted through the mother's abdominal wall, as in amniocentesis, and the chorionic villus sample is obtained in this manner.

Once removed, the tissue sample can be analyzed quickly. Fetal cells from chorionic villi may not require extensive culturing in the laboratory, as do cells obtained from the amniotic fluid in amniocentesis, and test results can often be available in about a week. Prenatal diagnosis becomes a more private issue as the woman is not yet "showing," and a termination of pregnancy, if such an option is chosen, is safer (see ABORTION). Chorionic villus sampling can aid in prenatal diagnosis of a range of genetic disorders including DOWN SYNDROME and Duchenne MUSCULAR DYSTROPHY.

A major disadvantage of chorionic villus sampling is that risks of miscarriage and fetal death seem to be somewhat greater than with amniocentesis, on the order of 1-2%. The decision as to whether to use chorionic villus sampling, therefore, is made only after careful consideration of all factors involved.

**choroideremia**    A rare X-LINKED hereditary vision disorder. It affects the choroid, the dark brown vascular coat of the eye between the white of the eye (sclera) and the retina. Females are rarely affected.

Early symptoms are night blindness and a gradual constriction of the visual field. As the condition progresses, the choroid and the retina undergo complete atrophy, resulting in blindness.

Vision is usually normal in female carriers, but they may exhibit striking changes in the pigmentation of the eye.

The gene for this disorder has been localized to a particular site on the X-chromosome, and linked DNA markers may be useful in CARRIER detection and prenatal diagnosis.

**Christmas disease**    Hemophilia B. It takes its name from the surname of the first patient with the disease who was studied. (See also HEMOPHILIA.)

**chromosome**    Strands of genetic material that contain our entire genetic heritage, and are responsible for the expression of hereditary traits that distinguish us as individuals and as members of a particular species. They are found in the nucleus of all cells, with the exception of red blood cells.

In the 1880s, German biologist Walther Flemming, using synthetic dyes, discovered a staining technique that revealed tiny threadlike bodies within the nucleus of the cell. In 1882, he published drawings of his observations, showing a cycle of positions in which these bodies regularly aligned themselves. He was observing, for the first time, the process of mitosis, whereby chromosomes replicate.

Due to their ability to absorb dye, these structures were called chromosomes, colored bodies. In 1903, American Walter S. Sutton and German Theodor Boveri independently suggested that chromosomes were the carriers of genetic information, and that they occurred in pairs, one from the mother and one from the father. Proof of their importance to heredity came in 1944 with the experiments of Oswald Avery at Rockefeller University in New York. He demonstrated that chromosomal material could, when transferred into the nucleus of a cell, transmit characteristics from one strain of bacteria to another.

Chromosomes are composed of a double helix of DEOXYRIBONUCLEIC ACID (DNA), a shape reminiscent of a twisted ladder, constructed of pairs of genes, locked together rung by rung. (There are between 50,000 and 100,000 gene pairs in human chromosomes.) The chromosomes can be visualized as strings of individual genes, one after another. Chromosomes occur in pairs (except in sperm and egg cells), and humans have a normal complement (karyotype) of 23 chromosome pairs. Twenty-two of the chromosomes or chromosome pairs are referred to as "autosomes" or "somatic chromosomes." The 23rd chromosome or chromosome pair are the sex chromosomes, or X and Y chromosomes, and determine gender. (Males have an X and a Y chromosome, females have two X chromosomes.) It is estimated that if the chromosomal material found in a single human cell were uncoiled and stretched out, it would measure approximately six feet in length.

Aberrations in mitosis and meiosis, the process whereby chromosomes replicate themselves, are responsible for many genetic disorders. (See also CHROMOSOME ABNORMALITIES; X CHROMOSOME; Y CHROMOSOME.)

**chromosome abnormalities**    As high resolution microscopy and cytogenetic examination capabilities have increased (see CYTOGENETICS), it has become apparent that many CONGENITAL disorders previously regarded as being of unknown origin are in fact the result of specific chromosomal abnormalities.

Normally, humans possess 46 CHROMOSOMES, divided into 23 pairs. Each parent provides one chromosome of each pair. (There are 23 chromosomes in the female ovum, or egg, and 23 in each of the male sperm. When sperm and egg unite at conception, the resulting fertilized egg has 23 pairs of chromosomes.) Twenty-two of these chromosome pairs are called autosomes. The 23rd is composed of what are called SEX CHROMOSOMES. Each individual chromosome consists of a double strand that appears joined at an off-center point (the CENTROMERE), resembling a narrowed X with a misplaced intersection. Each autosome pair is numbered (1 through 22) and the individual sex chromosomes are identified as "X" or "Y" chromosomes. (Females have a pair of X sex chromosomes; males have one X sex chromosome and one Y sex chromosome; the presence of a Y determines "maleness." See X CHROMOSOME and Y CHROMOSOME.) Any disruption of the normal arrangement or number of chromosomes is considered a chromosomal aberration. While some aberrations are be-

nign, others can have severe consequences. (See Tables VI and VII.)

The abnormality may be in the number of chromosomes (ANEUPLOIDY), the loss of chromosomal material (deletion), duplication of chromosomal material, or the transfer of chromosomal material to another chromosome or to a different part of the same chromosome.

Chromosomal abnormalities may be inherited, they may occur before conception, during the formation of the sperm or egg, or they may occur early in embryonic development. (In this last case, some cells will have the normal complement of chromosomes, and some will not, a condition referred to as MOSAICISM.) In some cases of infants with chromosomal abnormalities, the chromosomal change is found in one of the parents, as well. If both parents exhibit normal KARYOTYPES (chromosomal arrangements), the abnormality in their offspring is said to have occurred "de novo" in the sperm or egg.

About one in every 200 liveborn infants has a detectable chromosomal abnormality. In about half of these cases, the abnormality is basically benign. In the other half, the aberrant condition causes congenital malformations, MENTAL RETARDATION or abnormalities that develop later in life. An estimated 12% of mentally retarded children have chromosomal abnormalities.

Chromosomal abnormalities are also found in approximately half of all spontaneously aborted fetuses, and in an estimated 7% of STILLBIRTHS and cases of perinatal death (see ABORTION). (Perinatal refers to the period from the 28th week of pregnancy to 28 days after birth.)

### General Terms

*Aneuploidy.* Any deviation from the normal number (46) of chromosomes in a cell. These include triploidy and tetraploidy, monosomy and trisomy. These most commonly result from nondisjunction, an abnormality in the

## Table VI
### Frequencies of Autosomal Chromosome Conditions Found in a Survey Conducted in British Columbia, Canada*

| Autosomal Chromosome | 1952-63 | | 1964-73 | | 1974-83 | | Total | |
|---|---|---|---|---|---|---|---|---|
| | N | Rate[1] | N | Rate[1] | N | Rate[1] | N | Rate[1] |
| Down syndrome | 571 | 1,305.1 | 460 | 1,334.6 | 394 | 1,016.2 | 1,425 | 1,218.1 |
| Patau syndrome (trisomy 13) | 3 | 6.9 | 15 | 43.5 | 22 | 56.7 | 40 | 34.2 |
| Edward syndrome (trisomy 18) | 1 | 2.3 | 31 | 89.9 | 57 | 147.0 | 89 | 76.1 |
| Autosomal deletion syndromes | 4 | 9.1 | 4 | 11.6 | 26 | 67.1 | 34 | 29.1 |
| Other conditions due to autosomal anomalies | 6 | 13.7 | 14 | 40.6 | 31 | 80.0 | 51 | 43.6 |
| Anomaly of unspecified chromosome | 1 | 2.3 | 0 | 0.0 | 3 | 7.7 | 4 | 3.4 |
| Total | 586 | 1,339.5 | 524 | 1,520.3 | 533 | 1,374.8 | 1,643 | 1,404.4 |
| Sum of highest individual rates | | | | | | | | 1,693.2 |

N- Number of patients.
[1]Per 1 million live births.
*Statistics reflect local population bias.

Source: Patricia A. Baird, "A Population Study of Genetic Disorders in Children and Young Adults," *American Journal of Human Genetics*, 42 (1988): 677-693.

## Table VII
### Frequencies of Sex Chromosome Conditions Found in a Survey Conducted in British Columbia.*

| ICD9, Sex-chromosomal Condition | 1952-63 | | 1964-73 | | 1974-83 | | Total | |
|---|---|---|---|---|---|---|---|---|
| | N | Rate[1] | N | Rate[1] | N | Rate[1] | N | Rate[1] |
| Gonadal dysgenesis | 33 | 75.4 | 26 | 75.4 | 23 | 59.3 | 82 | 70.1 |
| Klinefelter syndrome | 28 | 64.0 | 11 | 31.9 | 5 | 12.9 | 44 | 37.6 |
| Other sex-chromosome anomalies | 3 | 6.9 | 2 | 5.8 | 5 | 12.9 | 10 | 8.5 |
| Total | 64 | 146.3 | 39 | 113.2 | 33 | 85.1 | 136 | 116.3 |
| Sum of highest individual rates | | | | | | | | 152.3 |

N- Number of patients.
[1]Per 1 million live births.
*Statistics reflect local population bias.

Source: Patricia A. Baird, "A Population Study of Genetic Disorders in Children and Young Adults," *American Journal of Human Genetics*, 42(1988):677-693.

normal process whereby the pair of chromosomes split to form sperm and egg, each of which contain only a single copy of each chromosome. In nondisjunction, both copies of the pair go into a single daughter cell.

*Triploidy.* This is the condition of having three copies, rather than the normal complement of two of each chromosome. Instead of having a total of 46 chromosomes (2 X 23), individuals with triploidy have 69 (3 X 23). (See also TRIPLOIDY.)

*Tetraploidy.* This is the condition of having four copies of each chromosome, instead of the normal number of two. Individuals have 92 chromosomes in all (4 X 23). This is caused by the abnormal cell division of a normal fertilized egg. This condition is extremely rare, and infants generally die within six weeks of birth.

*Monosomy.* In this condition, one chromosome of one particular pair is missing. The total number of chromosomes is 45 (22 pairs, plus one unpaired chromosome). It is usually caused by abnormalities during the formation of sperm or egg cells (meiosis). TURNER SYNDROME is the only common condition that results from monosomy. All other forms of monosomy are extremely rare and generally lethal. Only monosomy X (Turner syndrome) usually survives to the stage of a recognizable pregnancy among non-mosaic monosomies.

*Trisomy.* In this condition, there is an extra, third chromosome in what would normally be a pair. The total number of chromosomes is 47 (22 pairs, plus three chromosomes where there should be only two). This is the result of nondisjunction during meiosis. DOWN SYNDROME is a form of trisomy.

While the origin of the extra chromosome may be either maternal or paternal, it is believed to be contributed by the mother in 75% of cases. The frequency of trisomy increases with maternal age.

### Rearrangements

In addition to abnormalities involving entire chromosomes, many abnormalities involve only portions of a single chromosome, as a result of chromosomal breakage that does not properly repair itself. These rearrangements can also have severe consequences. The more common forms of chromosomal rearrangement include:

*Deletion.* A section of one chromosome in a pair is absent. This is sometimes referred to as "partial monosomy."

*Duplication.* An extra section of one chromosome in a pair is present. This is sometimes referred to as "partial trisomy."

*Translocation.* A section of one chromosome is interchanged with a section of another chromosome (reciprocal translocation) or with a section of the same chromosome.

*Inversion.* A broken section of a chromosome has reattached in the same place on the same chromosome but in reverse direction ("upside-down" or inverted).

High resolution microscopy techniques recently identified several well-known hereditary conditions as also exhibiting chromosomal rearrangements, generally small deletions. These conditions include PRADER-WILLI SYNDROME, RETINOBLAS-TOMA, ANIRIDIA-Wilm's tumor syndrome, DIGEORGE SYNDROME, LANGER-GIEDION SYNDROME and Miller-Diecker lissencephaly.

There is a particular nomenclature for describing the position of chromosome abnormalities. The syndromes are designated by the chromosome that exhibits the abnormality, the location on the chromosome of the abnormality (based on the centromere, the off-center point at which the individual chromosome strands join) and the kind of abnormality. The letter "q" designates a position on the longer arm of a chromosome. The letter "p" designates the shorter arm. A "+" sign indicates a duplication and a "-" sign indicates a deletion. Thus, the syndrome "18q-" indicates a deletion of a section of the long arm of chromosome 18. "4p+" is a syndrome associated with a duplication of a section of the short arm of chromosome 4. "Trisomy 21" (Down syndrome) indicates the presence of an entire extra chromosome 21. "X monosomy" (Turner syndrome) indicates that there is only one sex chromosome. (Y monosomy would be lethal in utero.)

Even within recognized syndromes caused by duplication or deletion of portions of a chromosome, there may be a high degree of variability of expression, due to the variability of the length, or the exact position, of the section that is duplicated or deleted.

### Syndromes

Listed below are some of the most documented chromosome syndromes; other common or important syndromes have separate entries.

*3q+.* Birthweight is usually somewhat below average. Infants have poor muscle tone (hypotonia), presenting a "floppy infant" appearance. The head is small (MICROCEPHALY), and the face tends to be square-shaped. Characteristic facial features include wide-set eyes (HYPERTELORISM), dense eyebrows that join above the nose (SYNOPHRYS), upturned nose (anteverted nares), downturned corners of the mouth and low-set or malformed outer ears. Hirsutism (excessive hair) is common.

Nearly all exhibit a high-arched or CLEFT PALATE or BIFID UVULA. The neck is short and the chest is often deformed, with widely-spaced nipples. The extremities are usually short, and some of the toes may be fused together (SYNDACTYLY). Over 75% of cases have congenital heart abnormalities, and malformations of the urogenital tract are common.

Infants often have a low-pitched, growling cry. Almost half die before one year of age. Those that survive exhibit severe mental and growth retardation. These children resemble those with de Lange syndrome; recurrent cases of this syndrome may be due to familial translocation leading to 3q+.

4p-. See WOLF-HIRSCHHORN SYNDROME.

*4p+*. This condition results in mental and motor retardation and a characteristic facial appearance.

Infants have small heads (MICROCEPH-ALY) with wide-set eyes (HYPERTELORISM), a short, large nose with a rounded fleshy tip ("boxer nose") and prominent chin. The eyebrows are dense and may be joined above the nose (synophrys). The ears may be unusually large and rotated slightly backward. The neck is short and the hairline low.

Over 35 cases have been reported. Growth is retarded in about half of affected infants. About one-quarter to one-third have died by two years of age due to infections, respiratory complications or heart disease. Puberty appears to be delayed in those who survive. IQs are in the 20 to 65 range. Most cases have resulted from a familial translocation.

*4q-*. This condition is marked by mild early growth retardation, and mild to moderately severe mental retardation.

Birthweight is normal. Facially, the eyes are wide-set (HYPERTELORISM), the nasal bridge is depressed and the nose upturned (anteverted nares). The ears are low-set and rotated slightly backward. The chin is small (micrognathia), and cleft palate, with or without CLEFT LIP, is frequent. Deformities

of the hands and feet and cardiac anomalies are seen in about one quarter of the cases.

Over two-thirds of infants succumb within two years of birth to respiratory infections or congenital heart disease. Approximately 12 cases have been reported.

*4q+*. Severe mental and motor retardation, often accompanied by cardiac and genitourinary abnormalities, are hallmarks of this syndrome. IQ is generally below 50.

While the facial features are variable, they may include a small head (MICROCEPH-ALY) with sloping forehead, bushy eyebrows, mouth with downturned corners and a horizontal dimple below the lower lip, or a "pursed mouth." There may be anomalies of the hands and feet, as well.

The prognosis for survival for these infants is poor, due to the severe mental and motor retardation.

5p-. See CRI DU CHAT SYNDROME.

*7q+*. At least 25 cases of this syndrome have been reported. The skull is usually asymmetrical, with a bulging forehead. The scalp hair is fuzzy. The eye slits (palpebral fissures) are long and narrow, and have been described as "almond-shaped." The nose is small and becomes pointed as infants age. The tongue may be large (MACROGLOSSIA) and the upper lip may overhang the lower. The ears are low-set and rotated slightly backward.

The prognosis for affected individuals is based on the section of the long arm of the chromosome that is duplicated. Duplications of larger segments may be associated with malformations of brain, heart and kidneys. While some infants die by the age of one year, generally this condition is not incompatible with life.

*Trisomy 8*. This condition is one of the more common autosomal chromosomal abnormalities. At least 80 cases have been confirmed, and incidence is estimated at between one in 25,000 and one in 50,000 live births. Males are affected three to five times as frequently as females.

At birth, the forehead is prominent, the nose bulbous and the lower lip is thick and turned outward. The eyes are deep set. The jaw is small (micrognathia), the ears are low-set, prominent and malformed. The skull itself is abnormally long and narrow (scaphocephaly; see CRANIOSYNOSTOSIS). Individuals have been described as having a "what-me-worry?" face.

Contractures of the fingers and toes, and restricted mobility of joints, are frequent, as are abnormalities of the spinal column. Undescended testes (CRYPTORCHIDISM) occur in about half of affected males. Obstruction of urinary outflow and kidney and ureter malformations are characteristic. One-quarter have congenital heart disease. Approximately 90% exhibit mild mental retardation.

This condition is compatible with a normal lifespan. However, language development may be severely affected. The joint contractures become more pronounced with age, and may require treatment.

There is a very high frequency (approximately 85%) of mosaicism. It is the most common autosomal aneuploidy after trisomies 21, 13 and 18.

*9p-*. All reported cases exhibit mental retardation and mild skull abnormalities. Facial features, while characteristic in childhood, become less so as individuals age. The head is triangular in shape from early suture closure. The eye slits (palpebral fissures) are short and down-slanting toward the nose (mongoloid obliquity). The nasal bridge is flat and the nose is upturned (anteverted nares). The mouth appears small, with a narrow upper lip. The ears are low-set and may exhibit external and internal malformations.

The neck is short, the hairline is low and the nipples are widely spaced. The fingernails are characteristically square-shaped, and the fingers long and thin (ARACHNODACTYLY).

Lifespan is generally normal, as is adult height, though no affected individuals have IQs above 50. They tend to be friendly, affectionate and sociable. Adults tend toward obesity in their trunks, though the extremities remain thin.

*9p+*. This condition appears to be somewhat common, with twice as many affected females as males. Various sections of the short arm of chromosome 9 may be duplicated. Over 100 cases have been reported. It is characterized by variable mental retardation, typical facial appearance and maldevelopment of the fingers at their tips.

Facially, the forehead is high and broad. The skull is short. The eye slits (palpebral fissures) are slanted down away from the nose (antimongoloid obliquity). The nose is large and bulbous, as is the mouth, which angles downward, with a turned-out lower lip. The philtrum (the groove from the bottom of the nose to the top of the lip) is extremely short. The ears are large and low set. Affected individuals have a "worried look."

The neck is short, and the hairline low. Shoulders may be underdeveloped, there may be anomalies of the spinal cord, and individuals may be knock-kneed (genu valgum). The nipples may be darkly pigmented.

Growth retardation is sometimes noted, as is delayed sexual development. There is also severe speech delay. Mental retardation is generally in the IQ range of 30 to 65. Lifespan is normal.

*Trisomy 9*. Both mosaic and homogeneous trisomies of chromosome 9 have been seen. Characteristic features include small head (microcephaly) with sloping forehead. The eyes are deep-set and the palpebral fissures (eye slits) are small. The nose has a bulbous tip, the ears are low set and malformed. The jaw is small (micrognatia) and the upper lip covers the receding lower lip. Joint anomalies are common and characteristic, including hip dislocation, dislocation of knees or elbows, and contractures. Congenital heart defects are found in about two-thirds of cases. Brain, kidney or digestive malformations may also be seen. Most die in the first few months of life. Those who survive exhibit severe failure to thrive and mental retardation.

*10p+.* This syndrome is characterized by severe mental and psychomotor retardation, growth retardation, seizures, poor muscle tone (hypotonia) and hyperextensibility of joints.

The skull tends to be long and narrow (dolichocephaly; see CRANIOSYNOSTOSIS), with a high, prominent forehead and low hairline. The cheeks are prominent, the nose upturned (anteverted nares), with a long philtrum (the groove extending from the bottom of the nose to the top of the upper lip). The mouth has been described as triangular or as appearing like a "turtle's beak," with a protruding upper lip. Ears are large, low-set and rotated slightly backward. CLEFT LIP or cleft palate is present in about half the cases. Elbows, wrists, fingers and ankles may be permanently bent (flexion contractures). The feet may be clubbed (talipes equinovarus).

Approximately half die early in life, and those who survive are severely retarded (IQ is approximately 20).

*10q+.* This condition is marked by extreme mental retardation. Height, weight and head size are well below average (typically below the third percentile).

The face appears flattened and wide. The eye slits (palpebral fissures) are unusually small, the eyebrows are arched and fine. The nose is small and beaked, the cheeks are prominent and the mouth is bow-shaped with a protruding upper lip.

The eyelids have a tendency to droop (ptosis) in about half of the reported cases, and the same percentage have cleft palate. The hands and feet may be deformed, with digits abnormally flexed (CAMPTODACTYLY) or curving inward (CLINODACTYLY). The bottom of the foot may be convex (rockerbottom foot). About half of those under medical care exhibit congenital heart defects. Several kidney (renal) abnormalities have also been associated with this disorder.

Death usually occurs prior to four years of age in about half of the cases, due to cardiac, renal or respiratory complications. Individu-als who survive are severely retarded, usually bedridden, and without the ability to communicate.

*11p-* Associated with ANIRIDIA-Wilms tumor syndrome.

*12p+.* The severity of this syndrome is dependent on the amount of chromosomal material that is duplicated on the 12th chromosome. There may be severe congenital malformations of the brain, heart, intestinal tract and kidneys. Additionally, various abnormalities of skull development are frequent features.

In general, the head is broad, with a high forehead. The face tends to be rectangular and flat. Eyebrows are thick, high and arched, and slanted downward. The nasal root is broad, the nose short and upturned (anteverted nares). The upper lip is thin, the lower lip wide and turned outward. The ears may be low-set and rotated slightly backward. The neck is short and cloaked in folds of skin. The nipples may be misplaced, and there may be more than two of them. Hands and feet often show abnormalities, such as short, broad, overlapping and malformed digits.

Mental retardation is a constant feature. Those manifesting severe congenital abnormalities rarely survive the first six weeks of life (neonatal period). Those who survive have normal life expectancies, though there is severe delay of motor development, such as head control, sitting and standing, and poor speech development. Growth is also retarded, and most individuals are of short stature.

*13q-.* At least 100 cases of this condition have been reported. Affected individuals exhibit psychomotor retardation, poor muscle tone (hypotonia) and small heads (MICROCEPHALY). Birthweight is usually low.

The characteristic facial features include a triangular shape of the forehead (trigoncephaly), large, low-set ears and several defects of the eye, such as drooping lids (PTOSIS), fissures of the iris (COLOBOMA) and abnormal smallness of the eye (microphthalmia). The upper incisor teeth are large and protruding and described as "rabbit-like," the chin is small (micrognatia) and the neck is short and webbed. In some cases, the thumbs may be absent.

About one-third of those affected have CONGENITAL HEART DEFECTS. Over half the males have genital abnormalities, including undescended testicles (cryptorchidism), micropenis and an abnormal opening in the subsurface of the penis that connects with the urethra (HYPOSPADIASIS). RETINOBLASTOMA, a malignant eye tumor, is seen with deletion of the band 13q 14; a "retinoblastoma gene" has been found in this region.

*Trisomy 13.* See PATAU SYNDROME.

*15q-.* Associated with PRADER-WILLI SYNDROME and HAPPY PUPPET SYNDROME.

*18q-.* At least 65 cases have been reported of this disorder. The condition is marked by mental retardation and characteristic facial features, including a bulging forehead (bossing), deeply set eyes, poor development of the midface area, a "carp-shaped" mouth, a prominent chin and short neck. There may be subcutaneous nodules in the cheeks at the usual site of dimples.

A number of defects of the eyes may also occur, and the ears may be somewhat deformed. (About half of the individuals have impaired hearing.) Additionally, there may be genital abnormalities, clubbed feet (talipes equinovarus) and minor anomalies of the fingers and toes. Congenital heart defects are frequent, and infants have poor muscle tone (hypotonia) and seizures. Life expectancy is greatly reduced; only a few have survived to adulthood.

*Trisomy 18.* See EDWARD SYNDROME.

*Trisomy 21.* See DOWN SYNDROME.

For other chromosome syndromes, See CAT EYE SYNDROME; FRAGILE X SYNDROME (X-linked mental retardation); KLINEFELTER SYNDROME (XXY); TRIPLOIDY; TURNER SYNDROME; XXXXY SYNDROME; XXXXX SYNDROME; and XYY SYNDROME.

**chromosome banding**    A laboratory technique for staining chromosomes with a chemical dye to delineate various regions or bands of the chromosomes so that they may be examined and analyzed. The word chromosome means "colored body," and it is so named due to its ability to darken dramatically when dyed. Each chromosome or chromosome fragment has a unique identifiable pattern of bands observable under a microscope after it has been stained, and these serve as reference points for identifying the different chromosomes (e.g., 13 vs. 14 vs. 15) as well as the positions of specific genes on individual chromosomes.

The development of improved banding techniques, which underwent significant advances in the 1970s, has had a major impact on genetic research, greatly assisting in the mapping of individual genes and linked genes to specific points on the chromosomes. Using high-resolution banding techniques, it is possible to visualize as many as 5,000 bands on the 23 pairs of human chromosomes. (See "INTRODUCTION.")

**chronic granulomatous disease**    See IMMUNE DEFICIENCY DISEASE.

**cigarettes**    Smoking cigarettes during pregnancy has not been linked to physical abnormalities in the fetus. However, the more a pregnant woman smokes, the lower the weight of her child at birth; LOW BIRTH WEIGHT infants are prone to numerous health problems. Also, smokers have twice as many premature deliveries as nonsmokers, and an increased risk of miscarriage, stillbirth and infant death. The cause of this association is unknown, but may be due to carbon monoxide in the smoke, which is absorbed through the placenta, reducing levels of oxygen in the fetus and therefore interfering with proper development.

**cirrhosis, familial**    See FAMILIAL CIRRHOSIS.

**citrullinemia**    See UREA CYCLE DEFECTS.

**clawfoot**   A deformity of the foot in which the arch is abnormally high and the toes are long and permanently bent (flexion contracture). It may be present at birth or may occur as a result of nerve or muscle disease.

Synonyms: pes cavus; gampsodactyly; griffe des orteils; talipes cavus.

**cleft**   A split or fissure in a body part caused by improper union during fetal development. Cleft lip and palate are the most common forms, though clefts may appear on many parts of the body. Among the more common sites of clefting besides the lip and palate are the hand, foot or cheek. (See also CLEFT LIP, CLEFT PALATE AND ASSOCIATED CLEFTING CONDITIONS.)

**cleft lip, cleft palate and associated clefting conditions**   Cleft lip and cleft palate are the most common CONGENITAL clefting conditions, and may occur individually or together. However, cleft lip, which may be seen with or without cleft palate, is a separate and distinct condition from cleft palate alone. In about 25% of those affected, cleft lip alone occurs; cleft lip with cleft palate is seen in about 50%, and cleft palate alone in 25%.

Cleft lip is caused by the incomplete closure of the primary palate, which forms the lip and gum. Closure usually occurs by the 45th day of fetal development, and if it has not occurred by then, the infant will have a cleft lip. Cleft palate is caused by the incomplete closure of the secondary palate, which occurs by the ninth week of pregnancy. Where both cleft lip and cleft palate are present, the clefting of the primary palate is blamed for interfering with the closure of the secondary palate.

The causes of these conditions are unclear. The majority are thought to be MULTIFACTORIAL, that is, caused by the action of several GENES in concert with environmental factors. They may also be caused by single gene (MENDELIAN) disorders, CHROMOSOME ABNORMALITIES or environmental agents, and are seen in association with almost 200 genetic syndromes.

### Cleft lip with or without cleft palate (CL/P)

The frequency of CL/P varies widely across population groups, and its severity is highly variable, as well. Cleft lip alone occurs in one-third of the reported cases, with the remaining two-thirds being both cleft lip and cleft palate. The lip may be clefted on one side (unilateral, 80%) or both (bilateral, 20%). If the cleft of the lip is bilateral, the cleft of the palate may be bilateral as well.

An estimated 7% to 13% of those with cleft lip alone have additional congenital defects, a proportion that rises to between 11% and 14% for those with both cleft lip and cleft palate.

Various races exhibit substantially different frequencies of CL/P, frequencies that persist in differing geographical areas. Among Orientals, it is estimated at one per 600 births. Whites have a frequency of one per 1,000 and blacks of one per 2,500. Among blacks, females are more often affected, while males are more commonly affected in whites.

Children and SIBLINGS of affected individuals have an approximately 4% risk of CL/P. If both a parent and child have CL/P, risk to a subsequent child is estimated at approximately 15% to 17%. If two children (but no parent) are affected, risk to a third is placed at 9%. Second-degree relatives (nieces, nephews, uncles and aunts) have a 0.7% risk and cousins a 0.4% risk. (See Table VIII.)

Affected infants may have feeding difficulties. Speech therapy, orthodontic treatments and psychosocial counseling may be helpful. CL/P can be repaired surgically. An interdisciplinary team of specialists is usually required for optimal management of these individuals.

### Cleft Palate

The palate is the structure that forms the roof of the mouth. Cleft palate is a more rare

## Table VIII

### Estimated Risks for Isolated Clefts

|  | CL With or Without CP (%) | Isolated CP (%) |
|---|---|---|
| General population | 0.1 | 0.04 |
| One affected sibling | 4-7 | 2-5 |
| One affected parent | 2-4 | 7 |
| One affected parent and one affected sibling | 11-14 | 14-17 |
| Two affected siblings | 9-10 | 10 |

A careful check of other family members may reveal or rule out subtle signs, such as a sub-mucous cleft or a high arched palate, allowing more precise risk estimation.

Key: CL = cleft lip; CP = cleft palate

condition than CL/P, and is a separate and distinct condition. Cleft palate may involve the hard palate (the tissue toward the front of the mouth), the soft palate (the tissue toward the back of the mouth) or both. There may be one cleft (unilateral) of the palate or it may appear on both sides (bilateral). The fissure may be complete, extending through the palate, or incomplete.

As with CL/P, frequency varies with race. The condition occurs in Native Americans as frequently as 80 per 1,000 live births. Orientals have an incidence of one in 1,500 births. Among whites, frequency is one per 2,500 births, and in blacks, one per 5,000 births. Females appear to be affected slightly more often than males.

Siblings of affected individuals have about a 2% recurrence risk, while individuals with an affected sibling and parent have approximately a 7% risk. Among whites, recurrence risk in an infant with an affected sibling and parent is close to 15%.

Babies with cleft palate often have difficulty in feeding, swallowing and respiration. Their heads are usually smaller than those of unaffected individuals. Approximately one-third to one-half exhibit additional abnormalities, including CLUBFOOT, deformities of the limbs and ears, and umbilical hernia.

There is evidence that many cases go unreported and that the actual incidence may be more than 50% higher than present statistics indicate.

Cleft palate can be treated surgically, and speech therapy, orthodontic treatments and psychosocial counseling can also be helpful.

For more information, contact:

National Cleft Palate Association
1218 Grandview Avenue
Pittsburgh, PA 15211
800-24-CLEFT

Prescription Parents, Inc.
P.O. Box 426
Quincy, MA 02269
(617) 479-2463

**cleft palate**    See CLEFT LIP, CLEFT PALATE AND ASSOCIATED CLEFTING CONDITIONS.

**cleft uvula**    See BIFID UVULA.

**cleidocranial dysplasia**    A hereditary disorder that affects the formation and development of cartilage and bone. The most obvious symptom, recognized early in infancy, is a missing or incompletely developed collarbone (clavicle). Affected individuals appear to have a long neck and narrow shoulders. They also have a wide range of motion of the shoulders; some can bring their shoulders together in front of the chest.

Additional symptoms are a protruding forehead or top of the head (bossing), causing the face to appear small. The skull may appear to be short or broad (brachycephalic), and often the bones of the skull do not fuse together. The nasal bridge is broad, and the eyes are set far apart (HYPERTELORISM). Other skeletal malformations include fingers of asymmetric length, knock knees (genum valgum), SCOLIOSIS and deformed teeth.

The severity of expression of the disorder varies widely. Affected individuals live a normal life span and have normal intelligence. Hearing and dental problems may occur. Because of a pelvic deformity, affected females may have to give birth by CESAREAN SECTION.

The basic defect in this rare disorder, transmitted as an AUTOSOMAL DOMINANT trait, is unknown. Approximately one-third of cases represent new mutations.

**clinodactyly**  The permanent sideways curvature of one or more fingers or toes. It most commonly affects the fifth finger, and is often caused by lack of development of the middle of the three bones in the digit. It is associated with many congenital and genetic anomalies.

**clomiphene citrate**  A non-steroidal drug used to stimulate ovulation in women who have had difficulty conceiving, though they have potentially functioning pituitary and ovarian systems. Women who become pregnant as a result of this treatment have an increased incidence of multiple births.

**cloverleaf skull**  See  KLEEBLATT SCHADEL ANOMALY.

**clubfoot**  Misalignment of the bones in the front part of the foot resulting in an abnormal shape. The general medical term for this condition is talipes, and it is further delineated by direction of the misalignment. In the great majority of cases (approximately 95%) the front of the foot turns inward and downward (talipes equinovarus). In the remaining cases, the front of the foot turns outward and upward (talipes calceneovalgus; talipes calceneo-'varus).

As an isolated malformation, the condition often results from crowding in the uterus. It may be corrected surgically, or with splints and casts during infancy. Left uncorrected, affected individuals will usually develop an awkward gait. Clubfoot is also associated with many genetic syndromes.

George Gordon, Lord Byron (1788-1824), the English Romantic poet, had this condition.

Clubfoot is caused by MULTIFACTORIAL inheritance (the action of several genes in concert with environmental influence). It occurs in from one to three in 1,000 live births. Talipes equinovarus is the more severe form and occurs most often in males (two to one). The risk for siblings is around 3%, with the risk for siblings of a female patient being higher (5%) than for those of a male patient (2%).

**CMT**  See CHARCOT-MARIE-TOOTH DISEASE.

**CMV**  See TORCH SYNDROME.

**cocaine**  An alkaloid refined from the leaves of the coca plant, this stimulant is thought to be the illegal drug most widely abused by pregnant women. A 1985 study estimated 1.1 million women of childbearing age were regular users of cocaine.

Maternally ingested cocaine flows through the placenta into the fetus, causing a decrease in fetal blood supply and resulting in abnormalities of fetal development. Use during pregnancy increases the risk of miscarriage, premature birth and STILLBIRTH (see ABORTION, LOW BIRTH WEIGHT). Infants exposed before birth also tend to be smaller than average and exhibit higher-than-average incidence of central nervous system defects, abnormal development of the small intestine, and genital and urinary tract anomalies, including seriously malformed kidneys. A survey of 5,000 infants born with birth defects in the Atlanta area, conducted by the federal Centers for Disease Control from 1968 to 1980, found the risk of urinary tract defects was 4.8 times higher in infants whose mothers reported using cocaine from one month prior to conception through the first trimester of pregnancy. (The normal risk for urinary tract defects is 1.5 per 1,000 live births; among the infants exposed to cocaine in utero, these defects occurred in 7.2 per 1,000 births.) Since some people do not admit cocaine use, these statistics may be conservative, and the true increased risks actually may be higher.

Other research indicates SUDDEN INFANT DEATH SYNDROME occurs 10 times more frequently than the norm in these infants.

As they grow, these infants are often hypersensitive and irritable, and have motor difficulties that make their limbs stiff and interfere with learning to crawl and walk. It has been suggested that as these children grow older their neurological problems will be manifested as learning disabilities, hyperactivity and attention deficits. Studies of infants exposed before birth to crack, a concentrated, smokable form of cocaine, have found they exhibit subnormal emotional development, though these infants are capable of achieving normal intelligence.

**Cockayne syndrome**   A rare AUTOSOMAL RECESSIVE condition characterized by DWARFISM, precociously senile appearance, ocular abnormalities, and MENTAL RETARDATION, in addition to other common features. It bears the name of Edward A. Cockayne (1880-1956), a senior dermatologist at the Hospital for Sick Children in London, who described it in 1936.

At birth, weight is appropriate and affected infants appear normal. Symptoms begin to manifest themselves in the second year of life. Growth slows, and mental and motor development become abnormal. Dwarfing

and mental retardation become more pronounced with time.

As the condition progresses, there is retinal degeneration, optic atrophy and cataracts, leading to BLINDNESS. Hearing loss leads to DEAFNESS. The head is abnormally small (MICROCEPHALY) and the face takes on a strikingly senile appearance due to the absence of a subcutaneous layer of fat. Hair is sparse, and the nose is thin and beaked. There may be absence of some permanent teeth. There is also sensitivity to sunlight, causing severe skin rashes (photosensitive skin rash), and deficient perspiration. Susceptibility to infections is increased.

Arms and legs appear disproportionately long, and hands and feet are large. Joints of the ankles, knees, hands and elbows may become permanently bent (flexion contractures), eventually leading to total immobility.

By the late teens affected individuals are unable to care for themselves, with death occurring from respiratory infection or from a debilitated condition due to lack of nutrition (inanition). No reported cases have survived beyond the age of 31. Despite the bleak outlook for all affected individuals, a wide variability of expression has been reported.

The basic cause of Cockayne syndrome is unknown. Among the approximately 60 reported cases, males have outnumbered females by a ratio of three to one, though the reason for this preponderance is unknown.

Identification of CARRIERS of this recessive trait is not yet possible.

Fetal cells have shown a reduction in the ability to form colonies and decreased synthesis of DNA and RNA (see RIBONUCLEIC ACID) after exposure to ultraviolet light. Thus PRENATAL DIAGNOSIS might conceivably be accomplished by exposing cultured cells from the amniotic fluid to ultraviolet light to test for reduction in their DNA and RNA synthesis or ability to grow.

**codon**   A sequence of three nucleotides (the individual molecules making up nucleic acids) in the DNA or RNA (see RIBONUCLEIC ACID) chains that provides the code for a specific AMINO ACID or step required for the production of a protein. There are 64 of these nucleotide triplet sequences. Sixty-one codons "coded" for the 20 amino acids found in proteins, and three "termination" codons that signal a halt to the formation of the sequence of amino acids producing the protein.

If the codon is changed (a MUTATION) the result may be that the wrong amino acid is incorporated into the protein or the protein chain may be prematurely terminated. For example, a change in just one of the three nucleotides in just one codon of the hundreds encoding HEMOGLOBIN (the oxygen-carrying pigment in red blood cells) results in SICKLE-CELL ANEMIA.

**Coffin-Lowry syndrome**   First identified by Grange S. Coffin, a pediatrician in San Francisco, in 1966, and R. Brian Lowry, professor of medical genetics at the University of Calgary, Canada, in 1971. Coffin-Lowry syndrome features a characteristic facial appearance, severe MENTAL RETARDATION, anomalies of the hand, and short stature. Males are much more severely affected than females.

In early childhood, males display a prominent square forehead, coarse, straight hair, wide-set eyes (HYPERTELORISM) that slant down and away from the nose (antimongoloid obliquity), a short, broad, upturned nose (anteverted nares), prominent chin (prognathism), large, protruding ears, thick lips and open mouth. A variety of oral deformities, including malocclusion and absent permanent teeth are also characteristic. The facial features become more pronounced with age.

The hands appear large and soft, with thick, tapering fingers. The skin is loose and easily stretched. Skeletal features include either a protruding "pigeon breast" (PECTUS carinatum) or a depressed chest (pectus excavatum) and curvature of the spinal column (kyphoscoliosis).

Affected individuals also have a characteristic clumsy gait. All males are severely retarded, with IQs below 50. Most females exhibit mild mental retardation and tend toward OBESITY.

The basic defect that causes this syndrome is unknown, and PRENATAL DIAGNOSIS is not yet possible.

Coffin-Lowry syndrome is believed to be transmitted as an X-LINKED dominant trait. Life span is normal, though the condition may be lethal in severely affected males. Fewer than 50 cases have been reported.

**coloboma**   An ocular defect in which there is a fissure or cleft in the eyeball, usually in the iris or choroid, or in the eyelid. It is associated with many CONGENITAL and genetic anomalies. As an isolated defect it may be inherited as an AUTOSOMAL DOMINANT trait, with the fissure usually located in the lower part of the iris.

**colon aganglionosis**   See HIRSCHSPRUNG DISEASE.

**color blindness**   A group of visual disorders more properly termed "color deficiencies" characterized by inability to distinguish various wavelengths of light. There are approximately one dozen of these CONGENITAL conditions. Most are inherited as X-LINKED traits, affecting males almost exclusively. A familial link had been noted for several centuries before PEDIGREES of color-blind families, documented by Swiss ophthalmologist J.F. Horner (1831-1886), established its hereditary nature for the scientific community. In 1876 he first demonstrated that a man with red-green color blindness transmitted the trait to his male grandchildren through his unaffected daughter. Color blindness was the first gene to be assigned to a specific CHROMOSOME (on the X chromosome, as this is an X-linked trait) in a pioneering example of GENE MAPPING by E.B. Wilson in 1911.

Normal human vision is trichromatic, or three-colored; color is perceived by the response of red, green and blue visual pigments, or light absorbing proteins, to wavelengths of light falling on the retina, the interior surface of the back of the eyeball. The mixture of these three primary color pigments determines how color is seen. A defect or deficiency of any of the three pigments (or the cones from which they are produced) will result in abnormal color vision.

*Daltonism.* The majority of color defects are in red/green vision, affecting approximately 8% of Caucasian males and 0.5% of females. These defects are popularly known as "color blindness," in which males are unable to distinguish various colors. The group of conditions has also been called "Daltonism," for John Dalton (1766-1844), the English chemist and physicist considered the father of atomic theory. In 1794 he published a paper, "Extraordinary Facts Relating to the Vision of Colours," in which he reported that he did not perceive colors as others do.

*Protanopia* (red blindness). Marked by the inability to distinguish certain pastel shades and by a reduced sensitivity to red light. Affected individuals may, when driving, have difficulty ascertaining whether traffic lights are operating, and may confuse red and green lights. (Partial red blindness is called protanomaly.)

*Deuteranopia* (green blindness). Often renders individuals unaware they have defective color vision. Visual acuity is normal, but they may exhibit atypical color combinations in their clothing. Red and green are perceived as varying shades of yellow. Once identified, experience and education can help them adjust to chromatic deficiencies, though they may be unsuitable for occupations requiring proper identification of colors within this spectrum, such as with color-coded electronic wiring. (Partial green blindness is called deuteranomaly.)

*Tritanopia* (blue blindness). Rare, inherited as an AUTOSOMAL DOMINANT trait. The gene for blue pigment is located on chromosome 7. As well as the red and green pigment genes, located on the long arm of the X CHROMOSOME, it has been identified and cloned.

*Achromatopsia* (total color blindness). Very rare, and inherited as an AUTOSOMAL RECES-SIVE condition, affecting males and females equally. Color is perceived as various shades of gray, as on a black and white TV. These individuals generally also have poor visual acuity and extreme sensitivity to light (photophobia), restricting their vision and requiring squinting in even ordinary light. It is also called "day blindness" because vision is better at night. They can learn to interpret color to some degree by differences in brightness. Its estimated incidence is one in 30,000 live births, though on Pingelap, a Caroline Island in the South Pacific, incidence may be as high as six per 100.

English physicist John William Strutt, Lord Rayleigh (1842-1909), developed the anomaloscope, a device that remains the primary tool for testing color vision. However, no single instrument or test is totally reliable in detecting visual color deficiencies, and standard color vision tests are only effective in screening vision that deviates from normal; they cannot properly classify specific abnormalities.

**color deficient**    A term sometimes preferred for COLOR BLINDNESS, the inability to identify one or more of the primary colors. It has been noted that affected children may become alarmed by hearing the word "blindness," and therefore the more technically correct color "deficient" is used.

**colorectal cancer**    See CANCER.

**combined hyperlipidemia**    See CORONARY ARTERY DISEASE.

**common variable immunodeficiency**    See IMMUNE DEFICIENCY DISORDERS.

**complete androgen insensitivity**    See TESTICULAR FEMINIZATION SYNDROME.

**concordance**    The expression of a specific trait in both members of a pair of twins. (See also DISCORDANCE.)

**congenital**   A condition or abnormality that is present at birth. See BIRTH DEFECTS; ANOSMIA; BLUE BABY; CONGENITAL GLAUCOMA; CONGENITAL HEART DEFECTS; CONGENITAL DISLOCATION OF THE HIP; CONGENITAL HYPOTHYROIDISM; CONGENITAL INFANTILE LACTIC ACIDOSIS; CONGENITAL NEPHROSIS.

**congenital absence of the pituitary**   See PITUITARY DWARFISM SYNDROMES.

**congenital adrenal hyperplasia**   See ADRENOGENITAL SYNDROMES.

**congenital agammaglobulinemia**   See IMMUNE DEFICIENCY DISEASE.

**congenital analgesis**   See INDIFFERENCE TO PAIN.

**congenital anomaly**   See ANOMALY.

**congenital cerebral palsy**   See CEREBRAL PALSY.

**congenital cyanosis**   See BLUE BABY.

**congenital dislocation of the hip**   A congenital defect of the hip joint most likely due to MULTIFACTORIAL inheritance (the action of several genes in concert with environmental influence), though it is often noted following breech delivery. It is approximately three to four times more common in females than in males. Joint laxity, which is normally greater in females than in males, probably accounts for some of the preponderance of affected females.

Incidence is estimated at between one and five per 1,000 live births. Risk of recurrence when a SIBLING is affected is estimated at 1% for males and 11% for females. If a parent is affected, risk of recurrence is 5% for males and 17% for females. If one parent and one child are affected, risk for recurrence in future births is estimated at 36%. Congenital hip dislocation is also associated with single gene

disorders of bone and connective tissue, including MARFAN SYNDROME, EHLERS-DANLOS SYNDROME and LARSEN SYNDROME.

This condition occurs with high frequency in German shepherd dogs.

**congenital erythropoietic porphyria**   See PORPHYRIA.

**congenital facial diplegia**   See MOEBIUS SYNDROME.

**congenital glaucoma**   Elevated pressure in the eyes due to a blockage in the trabecular meshwork (supporting connective tissue in the eye), preventing the eye fluid (aqueous humor) from flowing normally. It results in clouding or enlargement of the cornea, tiny rips in the inner corneal lining (COLOBOMA), excessive tear production and abnormal reaction to light. In 75% of cases, both eyes are affected (bilateral). It is diagnosed within the first year of life in four out of five cases. MENTAL RETARDATION may be associated.

If eye pressure is elevated at birth, there is less chance of cure than if the symptoms appear after the second month. Surgery (most often trabulectomy, the removal of the trabecular meshwork) successfully saves the eyes in 80% of the latter cases, though vision may remain poor. Rare spontaneous remissions have been reported.

More males than females develop congenital glaucoma. It may be inherited as an AUTOSOMAL RECESSIVE trait or, more commonly, it occurs in a seemingly sporadic fashion. At present, CARRIERS of the autosomal recessive trait cannot be identified. The defect occurs in approximately one of 10,000 births.

It may also be associated with other generalized eye problems, e.g., RETINOBLASTOMA or STURGE-WEBER SYNDROME.

**congenital heart defects (CHD)**   A variety of structural malformations of the heart and its major blood vessels resulting from abnormal embryonic development. They may appear as individual ANOMALIES or as part of a large number of specific SYNDROMES.

Although they exist as isolated malformations in most of those who come to medical attention, affected individuals are 10 times more likely than the general public to have a non-CHD major birth defect. The estimated frequency of the presence of non-cardiac associated disorders ranges from less than 10% to more than 40%, with the presence of major non-cardiac malformations put at about 25%.

CHDs may result from hereditary, environmental and/or unknown factors. Approximately 3% are thought to be caused by single GENE disorders and 5% by CHROMOSOME ABNORMALITIES (primarily DOWN SYNDROME). The remainder are thought to be caused by the action of several genes in concert with environmental factors (MULTIFACTORIAL inheritance). Environmental factors include chemicals (drugs and toxic substances such as alcohol or some ANTICONVULSANT medications), biological agents (viruses such as rubella) and maternal conditions (2%), such as PHENYLKETONURIA and DIABETES (see TERATOGEN).

In families in which an individual has been diagnosed as having CHD, GENETIC COUNSELING and diagnostic procedures can help establish the origin of the disorder, evaluate asymptomatic family members and determine the risk of recurrence in future pregnancies. In defined syndromes, the recurrence risk may be as high as 50%, while if the defect occurred as the result of an environmental insult the recurrence risk can be minimal. After the birth of an affected child with an isolated CHD of a presumably multifactorial basis, the risk of recurrence in a subsequent child is estimated to be about 2% to 5%.

Pregnant women with CHDs face potential health complications and increased risks for their infants: Not only may it put an additional strain on the heart, but in some studies, affected females have been found to have a higher probability of transmitting CHDs to their offspring than affected males have. In addition, drugs taken for management of their CHDs may pose teratogenic risks.

A number of prenatal diagnostic procedures are available, depending on the particular form of CHD. Fetal cardiac ultrasonography (echocardiography) may detect certain abnormalities *in utero*, and is becoming more widely available. Analysis of fetal chromosomes obtained via AMNIOCENTESIS may be useful in establishing diagnosis of CHDs associated with chromosomal abnormalities. ULTRASOUND may be used to look for associated malformations in syndromic cases.

CHDs occur in about eight per 1,000 births and account for approximately half of all deaths caused by congenital malformations and 15% of all infants deaths, affecting all ethnic groups about equally. Each year in the United States approximately 30,000 infants are born with a CHD. Many forms of CHDs have been reported, though approximately 10 to 15 varieties account for the majority of cases. These individual malformations may occur alone or in complex combinations.

Symptoms of CHD in the infant include cyanosis (the bluish color of the skin resulting from poor oxygenation), shortness of breath, feeding difficulties, excessive sweating, failure to grow appropriately or recurrent infections. A heart murmur may be heard on examination.

*Ventricular septal defect* (VSD). The most common form of isolated CHDs, these account for about 20% to 25% of all cases, occurring in about 22 to 25 per 10,000 live births. An abnormal opening in the wall (septum) between the bottom two chambers (ventricles) of the heart allows blood to flow directly from the left to right ventricle, and recirculate through the pulmonary artery and lungs. Recirculation of this already oxygenated blood puts a strain on the heart.

Severity is variable. There may be single or multiple openings, ranging in size from 1mm. to several centimeters across. Individuals with mild defects may be asymptomatic, and the septal defect may spontaneously heal. In more severe cases, symptoms include congestive heart failure, pneumonia, rapid breathing, failure to thrive, and restlessness and irritability. Surgery is required in about 20% of cases, and mortality rate in these situations is estimated at between 1% and 2%.

VSDs may be associated with chromosome abnormalities, particularly trisomy 18.

*Atrial Septal Defects* (ASD). These consist of an abnormal opening in the wall (septum) separating the two upper chambers (atria) of the heart. This causes an increased flow of oxygenated blood into the right side of the heart, and thus to the lungs. This may lead to heart failure. The severity of the condition is variable, and may be corrected surgically in most cases. ASDs account for 10% to 15% of all cases of CHD, occurring in approximately six to seven per 10,000 live births. In about 85% of all cases, it is an isolated malformation. It is the third most common defect after VSD and PATENT DUCTUS ARTERIOSUS.

An autosomal dominant form of the disorder has been documented.

It is also a feature of the HOLT-ORAM and ELLIS-VAN CREVELD SYNDROMES and thrombocytopenia-absent radius syndrome (see TAR SYNDROME).

*Aortic stenosis* (AS). A narrowing of the aorta, the major artery leading from the heart, resulting in a reduced ability of the aorta to circulate blood from the left ventricle. The condition is classified by the site of the narrowing, which also determines the severity of the condition. Congestive heart failure, chest pain and fainting spells may result.

Valvular AS involves the point at which the aortic valve admits blood from the heart. It is often asymptomatic, but may lead to sudden death, due to abnormalities in the electrical impulses that control the valve's operation (conduction abnormalities). It accounts for about 5% of CHD.

Supravalvular AS involves the section of the aorta that rises (ascending aorta) from the heart. There is an increased pressure due to the narrowing, increasing the risk for arteriosclerosis. It is also associated with WILLIAMS SYNDROME, a disorder characterized by coarse facial features, mental retardation and dental abnormalities. High calcium levels in the blood may be found. Males and females are equally affected.

Subvalvular AS is an often asymptomatic disorder caused by a fibrous ring that encircles the left ventricular outflow tract at the point immediately before blood enters the aorta. Occurring twice as often in males as in females, it is suspected of being a rather common anomaly, possibly inherited as an autosomal dominant characteristic.

*Pulmonic Stenosis.* Like aortic stenosis, this condition may be subvalvular, valvular or supravalvular. It involves narrowing of the pulmonary artery, leading from the right ventricle to the lungs. The severity depends on the degree of narrowing, and whether or not there are accompanying septal defects. It may be asymptomatic, or the obstructions may result in heart failure and cyanosis by two to three years of age. In these cases, surgical intervention is usually required.

Pulmonic stenosis may be associated with fetal rubella syndrome (see TORCH SYNDROME), LEOPARD SYNDROME and NOONAN SYNDROME.

*Endocardial cushion defects* (ECDS; atrioventricular canal). A variety of abnormalities resulting from defective development of the atrioventricular cushions, embryonic structures from which the walls (septa) and valves of the upper heart chambers (atria) develop. Severity is variable. About one-third of cases are associated with trisomy 21 (Down syndrome), with the majority of the remainder due to multifactorial inheritance. They may also be associated with rare syndromes in which asplenia or polysplenia are features.

*Mitral valve prolapse* (MVP). A common but often undiagnosed condition in which the mitral valves fail to close properly, collapsing back into the upper left chamber (left atrium) of the heart when the lower chamber (ventricle) contracts during the cardiac cycle, allowing blood to flow back into the atrium. The condition is usually asymptomatic, though it may cause chest pains or an irregular heartbeat. The condition is not always present at birth. Incidence is estimated at 5% to 10% in the general population and a prevalence of 1% to 2% in children. The valve is also susceptible to infection and affected individuals need to take prophylactic antibiotics at the time of dental manipulations, for example, to prevent the development of infections.

As an isolated defect, MVP appears to follow an autosomal dominant hereditary pattern. It is also associated with MARFAN SYNDROME, OSTEOGENESIS IMPERFECTA, EHLERS-DANLOS SYNDROME, MUSCULAR DYSTROPHY and FRAGILE X SYNDROME.

*Hypoplastic left heart syndrome.* Perhaps the most common cause of heart failure in the first week of life, this condition is characterized by the failure of development (hypoplasia) of the left ventricle. It may occur in conjunction with abnormalities of the aorta and mitral valves. Symptoms of the cardiac abnormalities, difficulty in breathing and failure to thrive, usually become apparent within 48 to 72 hours of birth. Prognosis is poor, though surgical repair is now attempted in some cases.

*Coarctation of the aorta.* This is thought to be the most common cause of congestive heart failure from the second through fourth weeks of life, though most patients are asymptomatic. It consists of a constriction of the aorta, causing higher blood pressure on one side of the defect, and lower blood pressure on the other. This may result in an infant having high blood pressure in the arms and head, and low blood pressure in the legs. It is often associated with other CHDs, including patent ductus arteriosus and ventricular septal defects. It is three to four times more common in males. It accounts for about 5% of CHD, with a frequency of about five in 10,000 births.

Those who become symptomatic in childhood or later in life may exhibit dizziness, headaches, muscle cramps following exercise, nosebleeds and fainting. Surgery is usually recommended during childhood, due to life-threatening complications that may arise if left untreated, which include brain hemorrhage, heart failure, ruptured aorta and infections of lining of the heart (endocarditis). It is

the most common heart defect in TURNER SYNDROME.

*Congenital heart block.* Heart block results from abnormalities in the nerves responsible for conducting the electrical impulses that govern the heart beat. This results in altered rhythm of the heart (arrhythmia). The condition may be present at birth as a result of defective fetal development, though it may also be caused by degenerative changes in the tissue wrought by toxins or infections. It is frequently seen in offspring of mothers with systemic LUPUS erythematosis. Conduction defects can also be caused by single-gene disorders such as the Romano-Ward syndrome (see Q.T. INTERVAL, PROLONGED) and the JERVELL AND LANGE-NIELSON SYNDROME.

Other important CHDs include transposition of the great vessels (in which the aorta originates from the right ventricle instead of the left, and the pulmonary artery from the left instead of the right), truncus arteriosus (in which a single great vessel originates from the heart and gives rise to both the aorta and pulmonary artery), anomalous pulmonary venous return (where the blood from the lungs returns to the right side of the heart rather than the left) and tricuspid atresia (where the valve separating the right-sided chambers fails to perform properly). (See also EBSTEIN ANOMALY; PATENT DUCTUS ARTERIOSUS; TETRALOGY OF FALLOT.)

For more information, contact:

American Heart Association
7320 Greenville Avenue
Dallas, TX 75231
(214) 373-6300

Mended Hearts
7320 Greenville Avenue
Dallas, TX 75231
(214) 750-5442

Heartlife/A.H.P. (Assoc. of Heart
  Patients)
P.O. Box 54305

Atlanta, GA 30308
(404) 523-0826 or 800-241-6993

**congenital hemolytic anemias** See
ANEMIA.

**congenital hyperammonemia** See
UREA CYCLE DEFECTS.

**congenital hypothyroidism** In affected infants the thyroid gland is absent, malpositioned and poorly formed, or unable to properly synthesize thyroid hormones. The condition is asymptomatic at birth; however, unless detected and treated prior to one month of age, brain development and growth will be severely retarded. ("Cretinism" was the term previously used to describe the condition.) Screening involves a blood test to detect levels of thyroid hormones (blood thyroxine) in newborns, a relatively simple procedure. Every state in the United States and every province in Canada mandates that all newborns be screened for this condition.

Most cases occur sporadically. The incidence of thyroid dysgenesis is estimated at one in 5,000 births. Defects in thyroid hormone production occur in an estimated one in 30,000 births. Defects in the function of the hypothalamus and pituitary glands, which also cause congenital hypothyroidism, are estimated at about one in 20,000 births.

In PENDRED SYNDROME, hypothyroidism is associated with nerve deafness. It is an autosomal recessively inherited trait, and there may be other recessive forms of hypothyroidism as well.

**congenital infantile lactic acidosis**
Lactic acid, a byproduct of glucose metabolism, is an organic acid normally found in the tissues of the body. In this disorder, which occurs in both hereditary and non-hereditary forms, lactic acid accumulates in the blood. Exact symptoms of the inherited form can vary from family to family, but may include convulsions, MENTAL RETARDATION, OBESITY and poor muscle tone (hy-

potonia), possibly leading to death. As a hereditary disorder, it is transmitted as an AUTOSOMAL RECESSIVE trait.

The accumulation of lactic acid that characterizes this rare disorder is believed to have numerous causes, including pyruvate carboxylase and dehydrogenase deficiencies and other disorders of the mitochondria, the energy-generating organelle of the cells. Lactic acidosis is also a feature of GLYCOGEN STORAGE DISEASE.

**congenital myodystrophy** See ARTHROGRYPOSIS.

**congenital nephrosis** (congenital nephrotic syndrome, Finnish type) A fatal congenital kidney disease. Affected infants typically exhibit low birth weight and size, as well as an abnormal pooling of fluid in the tissues (edema). Diagnostic tests usually reveal a decrease or abnormally low level of the amount of protein in the blood (hypoproteinemia), decreased albumin in the blood (hypoalbuminemia), excessive blood cholesterol (hypercholesterolemia) and large amounts of protein in the urine (proteinuria).

This disease in generally fatal, with most infants dying within one year of birth, usually as the result of infection or kidney failure. Recent advances in kidney dialysis and transplantation may alter the previously gloomy outlook for these infants.

The greatest number of reported cases have occurred in Finland (approximately 200 cases) or in areas of other countries where there is a large population of Finnish extraction, though the prevalence of the condition is unknown.

It is believed to be inherited as an autosomal recessive trait. Mothers at risk of bearing a child with this condition exhibit a high level of ALPHA-FETOPROTEIN after the 15th week of pregnancy.

Other disorders may also cause nephrotic syndrome in newborns, such as neonatal SYPHILIS (as well as other TORCH infections),

NAIL-PATELLA SYNDROME, and kidney disease associated with brain malformations.

**congenital nephrotic syndrome, Finnish type**   See CONGENITAL NEPHROSIS.

**conjoined twins**   (Siamese twins)   Twins physically united at birth as a result of the incomplete separation of a single ovum that has split in the process of twinning. (The splitting of the ovum that produces identical twins occurs on about the 20th day of gestation.) This condition is commonly referred to by the public as "Siamese twins" and has been seen throughout history. There is an illustration of conjoined twins *in utero* in the first printed treatise on obstetrics, the *Rosengarten*, by Rosslin, printed in 1513; grown conjoined twins, united at the head (craniopagus), appear in a German woodcut dated 1510. Historical accounts of conjoined twins are rather common, and many of these united individuals achieved considerable notoriety. In addition, there are also many reports of individuals to whom a partially formed body, or "parasitic" twin, was attached from birth, and who lived their lives in permanent union with this bodily encumbrance.

The popular contemporary appellation "Siamese twins" dates to Chang and Eng (1811-1874), conjoined Chinese twins born in Siam and exhibited as a circus attraction by P.T. Barnum. He touted them with the following quatrain:

> The Twins of Siam
> Rarest of Dualities
> Two Ever Separate
> Ne'er Apart Realities

Joined by tissue at the trunk, an autopsy following their deaths (they died hours apart) revealed that they could most likely have been separated by surgical means. Other conjoined twins have also gained attention in modern times, exhibiting, for example, musical talents in addition to their anatomical abnormalities.

Conjoined twins may be joined at various parts of the body, and there are designations for various forms. Frequently these conditions are not compatible with life, and many conjoined twins die at birth or soon after.

*Craniopagus*. Two complete twins joined at the head. This accounts for approximately 2% of cases.

*Dicephalus*. A single body with two heads.

*Dipygus*. Twins joined at the hip with one head, thorax and abdomen with two pelves and four legs.

*Omphalopagus*. Two complete twins joined at the abdomen.

*Pyopagus*. Twins joined at the lower back. This accounts for about 19% of conjoined twins.

*Rachiopagus*. Twins joined at the upper back.

*Syncephalus*. A single head, with the body separated into twins at some point below.

*Thoracopagus*. Twins joined at the chest. This accounts for approximately 74% of cases.

Conjoined twins have lived far into adulthood without being separated. However, surgical separation is the treatment of choice whenever possible, though both individuals may not survive when certain organs are shared. Conjoined twins with one heart have never survived with or without surgery. In 1987, twins joined at the head who shared part of their cerebral blood supply and brain tissue were separated at Johns Hopkins University, the first time this surgery had been accomplished without causing severe brain damage or death.

Varying statistics on incidence have been reported, ranging from approximately one in 30,000 to one in 100,000 live births. Conjoined twins occur in six out of every 100,000 live births in India and Africa, and four of every 100,000 live births in Europe and the Americas. It affects seven females to every three males. No case of recurrence has ever been reported, either in parents of

## Table IX

### Proportion of Genes Shared by Relatives

| Relationship | Genes (%) |
|---|---|
| First-degree relatives | |
| Sibs | 50 |
| Parent-child | 50 |
| Second-degree relatives | |
| Half-sibs | 25 |
| Grandparents | 25 |
| Uncle, aunt-niece, nephew | 25 |
| Third-degree relatives | |
| First cousins | 12.5 |
| Half uncle, half aunt-niece, nephew | 12.5 |
| Fourth-degree relatives | |
| First cousins once removed | 6.25 |
| Fifth-degree relatives | |
| Second cousins | 3.12 |

Repoduced with permission of the National Genetics Foundation, Inc., from R.B. Berini and E. Kahn (eds.), *Clinical Genetics Handbook* (Oradell, N.J.: Medical Economics Co. Inc., 1987). All rights reserved.

conjoined twins, or a child of a conjoined twin. Prenatal diagnosis is possible by X-ray or ULTRASOUND techniques.

## Conradi-Hunermann-type chondrodysplasia    See CHONDRODYSPLASIA PUNCTATA.

## consanguinity    The mating of two individuals with recent common ancestors. Consanguinity is often associated with an increased risk of GENETIC DISORDERS or birth defects in offspring, due to the potential for expression of aberrant recessive hereditary characteristics, and a slightly increased risk for MULTIFACTORIAL disorders requiring a combination of several genes for expression.

It is estimated that the average individual has about five to seven mutant recessive genes. While any particular mutation, or combination of mutations, would be extremely rare in the general population, the chances that a close relative shares the same mutation are much greater. (First cousins share an average of one-eighth of their genes.) Thus the offspring of close relatives would be more likely to have two copies of the recessive gene and be affected with the disorder that this gene

causes. Yet, unless there is a known aberrant genetic condition in the family, the risk for a genetic disorder in the offspring of first cousins is only approximately 3%, as compared to 2% in the general population. (See Table IX.)

In families with a history of known recessive genetic disorders the risk of having an offspring with the condition rises dramatically. For example, an individual with a first-degree relative (parent, child or sibling) with a rare autosomal recessive disorder might have a one in 600 chance of having a child with the condition. However, in a marriage with a third-degree relative (e.g., first cousin), the risk of having an affected infant could be as high as one in 12.

Consanguinity is found with increased frequency in parents of individuals diagnosed as having genetic disorders, congenital anomalies and mental retardation. Infants resulting from incestuous matings clearly have a higher incidence of hereditary or congenital anomalies.

Consanguinous relationships are common in some cultures and isolated populations, and have historically been associated with royal families, where a desire to cement strategic relationships and assure alliances frequently resulted in intermarriage.

Acceptance of consanguinous relationships varies. For example, marriages of third-degree relatives (first cousins, half-uncle, half-aunt etc.), relatively common in some cultures, are illegal in some states in the United States.

Consanguinuous unions are also more likely to produce offspring affected with disorders associated with specific ethnic groups, such as TAY-SACHS DISEASE among Ashkenazi Jews and SICKLE-CELL ANEMIA among blacks.

**constitutional disease** Any disease that results from one's hereditary constitution. These can include not only single GENE disorders (i.e., disorders inherited in AUTOSOMAL DOMINANT, RECESSIVE or X-LINKED manner, like HUNTINGTON'S DISEASE, CYSTIC FIBROSIS or HEMOPHILIA) but also MULTIFACTORIAL diseases, such as MANIC-DEPRESSION or PYLORIC STENOSIS, and CHROMOSOME ABNORMALITIES such as DOWN SYNDROME.

**contraceptive** Any method of preventing conception and pregnancy; birth control.

Some couples whose offspring are at risk of inheriting a GENETIC DISORDER (or those couples in which the female has a genetic or other condition that may be complicated by pregnancy) practice contraception. The decision to avoid pregnancy in these cases is usually made after consultation with a medical geneticist or other appropriate specialist and a thorough review of probability figures for infant abnormalities or health risks for the mother. Once they understand these figures, couples who choose to avoid having children may practice any of several methods of contraception. These methods include oral contraceptives, spermicides, condoms, diaphragms, cervical caps, intrauterine devices (IUDs), sponges, implants and injectable contraceptives, vasectomies, tubal ligation and natural methods.

Oral contraceptives are synthetic steroids that mimic natural hormones (estrogen or progesterone), thus preventing ovulation. These include what is commonly called "the pill"

and "morning after" contraceptives, though the latter are most commonly used in cases of rape. (RU 486, a pill manufactured and approved for use in France, usually can induce ABORTION when taken before the seventh week of pregnancy. It is used in conjunction with prostaglandin, a synthetic hormone that causes uterine contractions.) Depending on the type of oral contraceptive used, their failure rate is estimated to result in 1 to 10 pregnancies per 100 users over the course of a year.

Spermicides in the form of jellies, foams, creams and vaginal suppositories act by killing sperm. Inserted into the vagina prior to intercourse, they have a failure rate estimated to result in 10 to 25 pregnancies per 100 users over the course of a year.

Condoms are thin-skinned rubber or natural membrane tubes, closed at one end. Fit over the penis, the condom prevents sperm from entering the vagina. Over the course of a year, they are estimated to have a failure rate resulting in 3 to 15 pregnancies per 100 users.

The diaphragm is a circular, domed-shaped rubber cup. Inserted in the vagina prior to intercourse, it covers the cervix, the entrance to the uterus, preventing sperm from reaching the egg. It is used in conjunction with a spermicide. Failure rate is estimated to result in 4 to 25 pregnancies per 100 users over the course of a year.

The cervical cap is similar to the diaphragm but smaller. Although it can be difficult to learn to use, it can be left in place for several days. Its failure rate is similar to that of the diaphragm.

IUDs are small plastic or metal devices inserted into the uterus, where they may be left in place for several years. They are believed to work by preventing the fertilized egg from attaching itself to the uterine wall. Use of IUDs has declined significantly since some (particularly the Dalkon Shield) were found capable of causing uterine infections resulting in scarring, pain and infertility. In 1983 IUDs were the method of choice of an estimated 7% of women practicing birth control. By 1988 the percentage had declined to an estimated

3%. IUDs are thought to have a failure rate resulting in 1 to 5 pregnancies per 100 users over the course of a year.

The sponge acts as a barrier and releases a spermicide. Though convenient, its failure rate is high, resulting in 15 to 30 pregnancies per 100 users over the course of a year.

Implants and injectable contraceptives were in use in almost 100 countries around the world by the end of the 1980s, though none were approved for use in the United States at that time. These operate on the same principle as oral contraceptives, but over a much longer period of time and at lower doses, since they are absorbed directly into the body rather than being ingested. Capsules surgically implanted under the skin may be effective for as long as five years. The Norplant is one such implant. Failure rates for these forms of birth control are low, typically resulting in one or fewer pregnancies per 100 users over the course of a year.

The vaginal ring, a new contraceptive technology, is a doughnut-shaped device inserted like a diaphragm, though it remains in the vagina between periods. It releases a low level of hormones similar to those used in oral contraceptives.

Natural methods of birth control include avoiding intercourse during the female's monthly fertile period (the "rhythm" method) and withdrawal of the penis during intercourse prior to ejaculation. Neither of these natural methods is considered reliable.

Permanent birth control methods include vasectomies for men (which may be reversible), in which the ducts that bring sperm from the testicles to the penis are tied or severed, and tubal ligation for women, in which the fallopian tubes that bring the eggs from the ovaries to the uterus, are tied closed.

**Cooley's anemia**   See THALASSEMIA.

**coproporphyria**   See PORPHYRIA.

**cordocentesis** (percutaneous umbilical blood sampling; PUBS)   A relatively new technique for fetal blood sampling, gen-erally performed anytime after the 16th week of pregnancy. It can be used for PRENATAL DIAGNOSIS in a variety of situations, including obtaining blood for chromosome analysis when results are needed more quickly than can be provided by AMNIOCENTESIS (in about three days rather than three weeks) or when there have been previously unclear chromosome results from either amniocentesis or CHORIONIC VILLUS SAMPLING. It is also used in the evaluation of potential fetal blood disorders (such as HEMOPHILIA), infection (such as TORCH SYNDROME) or other situations where fetal blood must be tested. It has been used not only to take blood from the fetus but also for transfusions or to administer drugs directly into fetal circulation.

After administration of local anesthesia, a needle is placed through the mother's abdominal wall and uterus directly into a fetal blood vessel in the umbilical cord, guided by ULTRASOUND.

PUBS is not a replacement for amniocentesis; rather it is an alternative in specific, well-defined situations. The procedure is more difficult to perform and carries a higher risk to the fetus (about 1%) of inducing a miscarriage than amniocentesis.

**Cori disease**   See GLYCOGEN STORAGE DISEASE.

**corneal dystrophy**   The cornea is the transparent membrane covering the eye. Several forms of hereditary disorders of the cornea have been documented. The degree of vision problems they create is variable as is their age of onset. Most are inherited as AUTOSOMAL DOMINANT traits, though at least two AUTOSOMAL RECESSIVE forms are reported. Though they may be slowly progressive, most forms rarely cause severe vision problems.

Typically, opacities will form on the cornea, clouding the vision. These opacities can often be removed surgically.

Corneal dystrophies may also be found as part of other disorders, for example, the MUCOPOLYSACCHARIDOSES.

**Cornelia de Lange syndrome** (de Lange syndrome; Brachmann-de Lange syndrome) A syndrome consisting of growth deficiency, mental retardation, anomalies of the extremities and characteristic facial appearance. It is named for pediatrician Cornelia de Lange (1871-1950), professor of pediatrics at the University of Amsterdam, Holland, who described two girls with the syndrome in 1933. It is sometimes called Brachmann-de Lange syndrome, as Dr. W. Brachmann described a patient with similar symptoms in 1916.

Infants have LOW BIRTH WEIGHT, typically under five pounds. Height and weight remain below the third percentile for their age. Other common features include recurrent respiratory infections and gastrointestinal problems, diminished sucking and swallowing ability, CONGENITAL HEART DEFECTS, CLEFT PALATE and bowel abnormalities. Permanent bending (flexion contractures) of the elbows are reported in 80% of cases. Hands are small and spadelike, with tapering fingers, a curved fifth finger and a single deep transverse crease across the palm (SIMIAN CREASE). There may be shortening of the limbs. In severe cases, there may be missing limbs or fingers.

The characteristic facial appearance consists of a small head (MICROCEPHALY), excessive hair (hirsutism), thick, bushy eyebrows that meet above the nose (SYNOPHYRYS), unusually long eyelashes, small nose with upturned nostrils (anteverted nares), small, widely spaced teeth, and low-set ears. The lips are thin and the mouth is turned down. There is a small "beak" in the middle of the upper lip and a corresponding notch in the lower lip. These features may not all be visible during the first year of life.

All cases exhibit moderate to severe mental retardation. The IQ is usually below 50. There is significant developmental delay, particularly in speech, even among those only mildly affected by the disorder. Life expectancy is diminished due to susceptibility to infections.

Diagnosis is made by a thorough medical evaluation, which includes X rays and chromosome analysis. This is because duplication of a band on the long arm of chromosome 3 leads to a pattern of abnormalities similar to de Lange syndrome (see CHROMOSOME ABNORMALITIES).

The cause for the disorder is unknown. Although it is believed to be transmitted as an AUTOSOMAL DOMINANT trait, most cases are sporadic, the result of new mutation. There have also been cases of multiple SIBLINGS of normal parents being affected with this disorder. The incidence is estimated at one in 20,000 live births. Currently, PRENATAL DIAGNOSIS of this condition is not possible.

For more information, contact:

Cornelia de Lange Syndrome
  Foundation, Inc.
60 Dyer Avenue
Collinsville, CT 06022
(203) 693-0159
(800) 223-8355

**coronary artery disease (CAD)**
Encircling the heart like a crown, the coronary arteries bring oxygenated blood to heart muscle. Disease of the coronary arteries is the consequence of atherosclerosis, the accumulation of fats, carbohydrates, components of blood, fibrous tissue and calcium into plaques on the artery's inside wall. According to one theory, the plaque develops at a site where the lining of the artery has been damaged or roughened by a mechanical, chemical or toxic factor or substance. As the plaque enlarges, it restricts or shuts off completely the flow of blood to an area of the heart, injuring or even killing heart-muscle fibers. This event is called a myocardial infarction or, popularly, a "heart attack." It may also cause extreme pain (angina pectoris), loss of normal heart beat (fibrillation) and death. As of 1989, CAD was responsible for more than 550,000 deaths in the United States each year and for more deaths than all types of CANCER combined. It was also estimated that there were over 5.4 million people in the

United States with CAD symptoms as well as a huge number whose disorder was as yet undiagnosed. Direct and indirect costs of CAD in the United States were estimated to approach $60 billion a year.

Perhaps the first to recognize a familial link in coronary artery disease was English poet and essayist Matthew Arnold (1822-1888). While visiting the United States in 1887, he experienced severe chest pains (angina pectoris), and wrote to a friend, "I began to think that my time was really coming to an end. I had so much pain in my chest, the sign of a malady which had suddenly struck down in middle life, long before they came to my present age, both my father and my grandfather." Arnold died less than a year later. The noted English physician Sir William Osler (1849-1919) cited the Arnold family in 1897 in proposing a genetic factor in the development of coronary disease.

People who smoke, have high blood pressure or high levels of fat-related substances in their blood, such as cholesterol and triglycerides (also termed lipids, or lipoproteins), are more likely than others to develop coronary artery disease. Some inherit a tendency to have high levels of these substances in the blood. These hereditary disorders include familial hypercholesterolemia and familial hypertriglyceridemia, as well as other familial forms of hyperlipoproteinemia.

## Familial Hypercholesterolemia

A characteristic sign is development of yellowish fat-laden nodules (xanthomas), particularly on the Achilles tendon or tendons of the hand. It is the result of a dominant mutation in the gene coding for a cell surface receptor for low-density lipoproteins (LDLs). As a result of the mutation LDLs continue circulating in the blood instead of being picked up and carried off for disposal. Low-density lipoproteins are about 75% lipid, and about two-thirds of the lipid is cholesterol. The accumulation of LDL in arterial pathways leads to formation of plaques.

This disorder occurs in about one in every 200 persons. It should be suspected if the blood level

of cholesterol is higher than 350 mg/dl, but in some cases the blood level may be lower. The disorder does not account for all instances of elevated cholesterol, some of which are likely to be due to other polygenic and environmental factors. The Nobel prize in medicine was shared in 1985 by molecular geneticists Joseph Goldstein (b. 1940) and Michael Brown (b. 1941) of the University of Texas for their discovery of the LDL receptor and its role in the regulation of cholesterol levels.

About one in one million people inherits two copies of a mutant LDL receptor gene. In these individuals with homozygous familial hypercholesterolemia, plasma levels of cholesterol are enormous and heart attacks occur in childhood and adolescence.

## Familial Hypertriglyceridemia

Triglycerides are fatty substances that, like cholesterol, can contribute to the formation of atherosclerotic plaques. Low-density lipoproteins are rich in triglycerides. The genetic defect and the cause of development of this disorder are not known, but family data on its appearance are consistent with an AUTOSOMAL DOMINANT mode of transmission. Frequency is estimated at about two or three of every 1,000 persons. Only 10% to 20% of carriers of the gene for familial hypertriglyceridemia show signs of the disorder before 20 years of age. Most affected persons exhibit OBESITY.

Other genetic disorders associated with an increased frequency of coronary artery disease include HOMOCYSTINURIA and the MUCOPOLYSACCHARIDOSES. (See also TANGIER DISEASE.)

## Combined Hyperlipidemia

Combined hyperlipidemia is frequently found in young to middle-aged adults recovering from heart attacks caused by clogged arteries (coronary atherosclerosis). It is diagnosed by elevated levels of plasma cholesterol and triglycerides—fatty substances associated with clogged arteries—in the blood.

Many of these individuals exhibit impaired glucose tolerance and obesity, and may succumb to coronary heart disease between the ages of 30 and 60.

Some studies suggest this disorder may be inherited as an AUTOSOMAL DOMINANT trait. Risk of occurrence is from approximately one per 500 to one per 1,000 in the general population. The cause is uncertain, but dietary modification is a generally effective treatment.

### Type III Hyperlipoproteinemia.

Hyperlipoproteinemia III rarely appears before 30 years of age. Cholesterol levels are high, ranging from 400 mgs. to 600 mg/dl and triglycerides range from 175 mgs. to 1,500 mgs., though individuals have usually consumed a regular diet. Low- density lipoproteins have an increased ratio of cholesterol compared to triglycerides. The defect lies in the structure of a protein named apolipoprotein E. Lipoprotein deposits in skin creases of the palm (xanthomata) may appear after age 25. Coronary disease and peripheral vascular disease may appear in males over 45 years of age and in females over 55 years of age.

Glucose tolerance is abnormal in about 40% of those brought to medical attention. The mode of transmission of this inherited disorder is not completely understood, but the risk of occurrence is considered infrequent. Rarely appearing before 30 years of age, it is usually seen in individuals between 40 and 60 years old. It can be managed with dietary restriction and lipid lowering drugs.

For more information, contact:

American Heart Association
7320 Greenville Avenue
Dallas, TX 75231
(214) 373-6300

Mended Hearts
7320 Greenville Avenue
Dallas, TX 75231
(214) 750-5442

Heartlife/A.H.P. (Assoc. of Heart Patients)
P.O. Box 54305
Atlanta, GA 30308
(404) 523-0826 or 800-241-6993

**Coxsackie virus**   This virus takes its name from Coxsackie, New York, the home town of the patients in whom it was first isolated. Though the illness produced by the virus is mild, infection during first trimester of pregnancy has been associated with an increased incidence of congenital heart lesions in newborns. (See also CONGENITAL HEART DEFECTS.)

**craniocarpotarsal dysplasia**   See WHISTLING FACE SYNDROME.

**craniodiaphyseal dysplasia**   A very rare disorder characterized by severe developmental defects of the skull and short stature. This is the condition that affected the youth who became the subject of the popular 1985 movie *Mask*. The skull bones thicken, resulting in severe facial deformities, which in turn cause nasal obstruction and cranial nerve compression that often leads to blindness, deafness, facial paralysis and seizures. Most affected individuals have exhibited MENTAL RETARDATION. Inherited generally as an AUTOSOMAL RECESSIVE trait, it is progressive, leading to death in the second or third decade of life.

**craniometaphyseal dysplasia**   There are two genetic forms of this disorder: one transmitted by a recessive gene and the other by a dominant gene. The dominant form is less severe and more common (see AUTOSOMAL DOMINANT and AUTOSOMAL RECESSIVE). Both forms can be recognized during the first year of life and display the same facial abnormalities, which include a long and narrow skull (scaphocephaly), swelling of the frontal and side skull bones, with wide-set eyes (HYPERTELORISM) that may bulge outward (proptosis), broadening of the root of the nose and a depressed nasal bridge, imperfect positioning and contact of the upper and lower teeth (dental malocclusion) and mouth breathing caused by narrowed nasal passages.

Other manifestations include facial paralysis, difficulties with eye movement and defective vision caused by wasting of the optic nerve (optic atrophy), as well as poor hearing caused by alterations in the bone structure around the eyes and ears. The latter may lead to sound distortion in the inner ear (sensorineural DEAFNESS), which occurs before puberty. The alterations in bone structure result in narrowing of the passage through which the nerves to the face, ears and eyes traverse, compressing them and disturbing their function.

X-ray examination discloses hardening and thickening (sclerosis) and abnormal growth (hyperostosis) of bone tissues of the front and back of the skull, increased bone growth in the skull spaces around the nose (paranasal sinuses) and below the ears, and a club-shaped thickening (flaring) to the tubular shafts of the long bones, especially in the upper extremities.

The basic defect causing this disorder is not known. It tends to be progressive, and some of the complications may require neurosurgery. Intelligence is not affected. Currently, there is no method for PRENATAL DIAGNOSIS.

**craniosynostosis** Deformities of the skull resulting from premature closure of the gaps, or sutures, between the skull bones. Normally, the bones of the skull are not joined at birth, allowing the head to grow evenly. In individuals with craniosynostosis, the sutures where the skull bones meet have closed, or close prematurely. ("Synostosis" means a union of adjacent bones.) As a result, the expanding skull bones grow abnormally, and the abnormal skull shape becomes more pronounced as the infant grows. The shape is dependent on which sutures have closed, and various abnormalities have specific names.

*Acrocephaly; oxycephaly; turricephaly.* These denote a pointed (high) head, caused by the premature closure of all sutures.

*Brachycephaly.* This denotes an abnormally short, squat skull, caused by the premature closure of the two coronal sutures, which cross the top front portion of the skull, widthwise.

*Dolichocephaly; scaphocephaly.* These denote an abnormally long front-to-back distance of the skull, caused when the sagittal suture, which runs lengthwise along the top of the skull, is closed.

*Plagiocephaly.* This denotes a somewhat lopsided, asymmetric, pointed appearance, caused by premature closure of sutures that cross the top of the skull widthwise (coronal sutures in the front, lambdoidal sutures in back), on only one side (unilateral).

*Trigonocephaly.* This denotes a triangular shape at the top of the skull, caused by the closing of the metopic suture, which runs lengthwise along the top front of the skull, forward of the sagittal suture and anterior fontanelle (the "soft spot" at the top front portion of an infant's skull).

The sagittal sutures are involved in over 50% of craniosynostosis cases. The coronal sutures are involved in between 20% and 30%. Least frequently involved are the metopic suture and labdoidal sutures. Mental retardation may occur in these disorders, and is more likely in cases where the closure of the sutures is greatest.

More than 50 craniosynostosis syndromes and more than 20 conditions in which craniosynostosis is a secondary or occasional feature have been described.

Most cases are sporadic with MULTIFACTORIAL inheritance, but AUTOSOMAL DOMINANT and AUTOSOMAL RECESSIVE forms have been reported. About 10% of cases are familial (see FAMILIAL DISEASE). Craniosynostosis is estimated to occur in from one in 1,000 to one in 2,500 live births. Prenatal diagnosis has been achieved by X rays in late pregnancy, revealing closed sutures, and by ULTRASOUND, indicating the unusual shape of the head.

Among those who don't exhibit mental retardation, there are few complications caused by this disorder other than cosmetic and sociopsychological problems. The craniosynostoses are treated surgically by removing the affected suture(s). (See also APERT SYNDROME; CROUZON DISEASE; SAETHRE-CHOTZEN SYNDROME; CARPENTER SYNDROME and PFEIFFER SYNDROME.)

For more information, contact:

The National Association for the
   Craniofacially Handicapped
P.O.B. 11082
Chattanooga, TN 37401
(615) 266-1632

Let's Face It
Box 711
Concord, MA 01742
(214) 371-3186

The Foundation for Craniofacial
   Deformities
3100 Carlisle, Suite 215
Dallas, TX 75204
(214) 871-1399

**cri du chat syndrome** CHROMOSOME ABNORMALITY that takes its name from the distinctive, mewing cry of affected infants, which has been likened to a kitten in distress. Birthweight is low, and infants exhibit FAILURE TO THRIVE and short stature. The condition is also referred to as monosomy 5p, as the cause has been traced to the deletion of a small section of the short arm of chromosome 5. All affected individuals are severely retarded, though survival into adulthood is common.

While facial features do not show any signature abnormalities, the head is small (MICROCEPHALY), eyes wide set (HYPERTELORISM), chin receding and the face round, with a paradoxically alert expression. The hair may gray prematurely. About 20% have CONGENITAL HEART DEFECTS.

The incidence is estimated at approximately one in 50,000 in the general population. PRENATAL DIAGNOSIS is possible by analysis of fetal chromosomes obtained by AMNIOCENTESIS. In about 10% to 15% of cases the syndrome results from an inherited translocation and thus is associated with an increased recurrence risk.

For more information, contact:

5P- Society (Cri du Chat Syndrome)
11609 Oakmont
Overland Park, KS 66210
(913) 469-8900

**Crohn disease** (regional ileitis) An inflammatory bowel disease characterized by abdominal distress, which slowly progresses to more severe bowel symptoms. Exhibiting a slightly increased prevalence in Jewish males, it is named for U.S. physician B.B. Crohn (b. 1884), who first described it in 1932.

Although the cause is unknown, familial cases have been reported (see FAMILIAL DISEASE). Recurrence risks in such families are low; they have been estimated at about one in 250 over all, with about a one in 100 risk for first-degree relatives (parent, child, SIBLING) of patients with Crohn disease. Prevalence in the general population is about one in 5,000.

**Crouzon disease** A form of CRANIOSYNOSTOSIS, anomalies of skull development characterized by oddly-shaped heads. In this form, the head is pointed and there is defective development (hypoplasia) of the mid-face. It is named for French neurologist Octave Crouzon (1874-1938), a neurologist at the Saltpetriere Hospital in Paris, who noted the disorder's familial occurrence in 1912 when he first described the syndrome.

The pointed head is caused by premature closure of sutures of the skull, forcing the bones to grow abnormally. The eyes are large and wide-set (HYPERTELORISM), with shallow orbits, so that they appear somewhat bulging. Approximately half of affected individuals have vision problems, and progressive vision loss may require surgical intervention in some cases.

The mouth is small, the nose beak-like. Deviated septum and obstruction of the nasal passages is common. The ears, depending on the degree of skull malformation, may be displaced downward. There are often defects of the middle and inner ear, as well. Defects in formation of the bones of the inner ear (ossicles) lead to conductive hearing loss in over half of those under medical treatment. Spine anomalies are present in almost one-third. Some affected individuals are mentally retarded.

The abnormal growth of the head begins during the first year of life and is usually complete by three years of age. It is inherited as an AUTOSOMAL DOMINANT trait, with new mutations responsible for perhaps 33% to 50% of cases. Increased paternal age has been associated with these sporadic cases. While there is currently little published data regarding PRENATAL DIAGNOSIS, theoretically it should be possible to detect severe cases by FETOSCOPY or, more commonly, ULTRASOUND.

No estimate of incidence per se has ever been given but Crouzon disease comprises about 3% to 7% of craniosynostoses patients.

Life expectancy is normal, and facial surgery can correct some of the cosmetic aspects of the disorder. However, effective treatment takes many years and requires a team of specialists.

**cryptophthalmos**  (also ABLEPHARIA) The congenital absence or reduction in size of the eyelids. The most severe cases are bilateral, that is, involve both eyes, and there may be no recognizable differentiation of the lids (e.g., the lids are completely fused or absent). Eyelashes and eyebrows are also absent. Less severe forms may be unilateral or incomplete, with only the upper or lower lid lacking. Pliny the Elder in the first century described the Lepidus family in which three children were born with a membrane over the eye, typical of this rare ANOMALY. In mild cases fused eyelids can be separated surgically, allowing normal vision. However, in more severe cases there may be malformations of ocular structures as well, resulting in BLINDNESS.

Other multiple malformations may be associated. In 1962, G.R. Fraser described a distinctive "cryptophthalmos syndrome." This AUTOSOMAL RECESSIVE condition includes ear anomalies, genital abnormalities and SYNDACTYLY (webbed or fused digits). In fact, cryptophthalmos is not always a feature of the "cryptophthalmos syndrome" and thus the eponymic Fraser syndrome is preferable for the condition.

**cryptorchidism**  See  CRYPTORCHISM.

**cryptorchism** (cryptorchidism)  T h e condition of having undescended testicles, or the failure of the testicles to descend into the scrotum. It is seen in many GENETIC DISORDERS. Individuals with cryptorchism exhibit much higher rates of testicular malignancies than unaffected individuals.

**C section**  See CESAREAN DELIVERY.

**cutis laxa**  A group of inherited conditions characterized by excess skin that hangs loosely in folds, about the face and body, often giving affected individuals a prematurely aged appearance. The Latin cutis laxa means "loose skin." The skin is inelastic and, if pulled, does not spring back upon release. It is not fragile, and the joints are not loose and hypermobile. It appears to be caused by a defect in elastin, a protein substance in the skin, though the exact nature of the defect has been identified in only one form.

While it is usually evident at birth, there have been reports of a few late-onset cases. Affected individuals are said to have "hound-dog faces," and are often described as appearing "mournful." They have a beaked nose and long upper lip. Frequently, other abnormalities are associated with cutis laxa.

These disorders are very rare, with approximately 40 cases reported. Four types are recognized:

*Type I.* In this relatively benign form, the laxity of skin is the only abnormality exhibited. Though the excess of skin is mildest in this form, adolescent children may appear older than their unaffected parents. It is inherited as an AUTOSOMAL DOMINANT trait.

*Type II.* This, the most common form, is severe or lethal. Affected individuals also have emphysema, which interferes with their ability to breathe, as well as other cardiopulmonary problems. There may be mild malformations of the gastrointestinal and genitourinary tracts. Infants typically have hoarse, harsh, deep and resonant voices caused by the laxity of vocal cords.

This form is Tinherited as an AUTOSOMAL RECESSIVE trait. Death usually occurs by age three years due to complications from emphysema.

*Type III.* In addition to loose skin, individuals exhibit retarded physical development, with height typically below the 10th percentile for age. Mild MENTAL RETARDATION is also common. Joint laxity and congenital hip dislocation are seen. It is thought to be inherited as an AUTOSOMAL RECESSIVE trait.

*Type IV.* This is the only form in which the basic defect causing the disorder has been identified. A deficiency of lysyl oxidase interferes with the normal activity of collagen, an important component in the formation of skin. This form is inherited as an X-LINKED recessive trait.

This is the same entity as EHLERS-DANLOS SYNDROME, Type IX. It is also known as occipital horn syndrome, because of the nubby protuberances at the back of the skull (occiput). These individuals have lax skin, hypermobile joints and other bony abnormalities. It appears as a result of a fundamental abnormality of copper metabolism, copper being necessary to lysyl oxidase activity.

**CVS**     See CHORIONIC VILLUS SAMPLING.

**cyanosis, congenital**     See CONGENITAL CYANOSIS.

**cyclopia** (cyclops)     The most extreme form of HOLOPROSENCEPHALY, a group of rare anomalies caused by maldevelopment of the forebrain in the embryo resulting in various degrees of brain defects and fusion of the optic nerves. In cyclopia there is a single eye, and typically no nose, though there may be a proboscus-like structure above the eye.

Cyclops have been a staple of legend since antiquity. Perhaps the most well-known is the giant cyclops in Homer's epic poem *The Odyssey.* There was also a belief dating to early Western civilization that certain tribes in Scythia (the area north of the Black Sea), Ethiopia and India existed that had but one eye in the middle of their heads. According to Pliny, the Roman scholar of the first century, there was a nation of these people called Arimaspi. The true condition of cyclopia, however, is incompatible with life. Most affected infants die at birth or within a few hours, although one was reported to have lived for 10 years. The cause of this extremely rare disorder is unknown, although it has been associated with various CHROMOSOME ABNORMALITIES (e.g., Trisomy 13).

**cyclops**     See CYCLOPIA.

**cystic fibrosis (CF)**     Cystic fibrosis is among the most common GENETIC DISORDERS in white populations. Inherited as an AUTOSOMAL RECESSIVE disorder, CF is a disorder of the exocrine (outward-secreting) glands, which causes the body to produce an abnormal amount of excessively thick, sticky mucus that clogs the lungs and pancreas, interfering with breathing and digestion. In some people, the respiratory system is primarily affected, while in others the digestive system is more affected.

Respiratory complications arise from the blockage of bronchial passages. Eventually, cilia, the small hairs lining the respiratory tract and responsible for clearing mucus, are destroyed. Additionally, CF mucus traps bacteria, which leads to lung infections and lung damage. In the digestive system, mucus may block ducts of the pancreas, which provides the enzymes necessary to help digest food. If the ducts become blocked, the enzymes are unavailable to assist in digestion, and nutrients cannot be absorbed.

Females may experience delayed puberty and infertility. More than 95% of males are sterile.

CF was first identified as a specific disease in 1938. The disorder occurs in about one in 2,000 to one in 1,600 live births among American whites. There are approximately 30,000 people in the United States with CF, and it's estimated that about one in 20 persons carries the recessive gene that causes CF. The incidence among American blacks is estimated at one in 17,000 live births.

The disorder usually appears in infancy, though rare mild cases may not become apparent until adulthood. Symptoms include persistent coughing, recurrent wheezing, more than one bout of pneumonia, excessive appetite with poor weight gain, salty-tasting skin, and bulky, foul smelling stools. However, the symptoms show a great variability, and often mimic other childhood diseases. Respiratory symptoms may initially be diagnosed as asthma, pneumonia or other respiratory conditions. Digestive symptoms of CF (malabsorption and malnutrition) may be confused with celiac disease or other digestive disorders. Ten percent of newborns with CF have obstruction of their small bowel because the meconium (the dark green intestinal contents that constitute the newborn's first bowel movement) that these infants produce is overly thick and sticky and "plugs up" their intestine (a process called "meconium ileus"). Liver disease is also seen in some individuals with CF.

Sweat glands of affected individuals produce perspiration with an abnormally high level of salt. A finding of excessive levels of salt in sweat is the primary method for diagnosing CF.

Physical therapy and medication can help alleviate respiratory and digestive problems associated with the disorder. Bronchial drainage (also called postural drainage), a form of physical therapy, helps break up mucus accumulations in small airways and move them into larger passages where they can be coughed up. Antibiotics are used to treat infections in the lungs. For digestive problems, regulated diet, pancreatic ENZYMES and nutritional supplements are usually prescribed. Heart-lung transplants have also been performed on a very limited basis.

The gene that causes CF has been identified, located on the long arm of chromosome 7 (see CHROMOSOME). The gene codes for a protein termed the CF transmembrane regulator, and an abnormality in this protein has been found to account for almost 70% of the MUTATIONS causing CF. A single AMINO ACID is deleted from this protein in these mutations. As of early 1990, other identified mutations have not been found to be present in a large percentage of affected individuals. As more mutations are identified, screening may become more feasible. There is no method of prenatal screening or CARRIER detection for the general population.

In families in which a previous pregnancy resulted in CF, both carrier and PRENATAL DIAGNOSIS are possible, through the use of linked DNA GENETIC MARKERS. Pilot studies of neonatal screening are underway based on blood tests for immunoreactive trypsin. The trypsin is elevated in the newborn's blood because of pancreatic disease. Studies of the reliability of the screening are ongoing as is much research aimed at identifying the fundamental defect in the disease. This may in turn lead to improved diagnosis and therapy for the disease.

CF is among the most common fatal inherited diseases. Yet the prognosis for CF has grown much more favorable than when it was first identified. In the early 1950s, children born with the disorder typically died before reaching elementary school age. Today, half live beyond the age of 21. For all ages, prognosis is poorer for females than for males. Repeated lung infections and blocked air passages eventually leading to respiratory failure are the major causes of death.

For more information, contact:

Cystic Fibrosis Foundation
6931 Arlington Road
Bethesda, MD 20814
(301) 951-4422

International Cystic Fibrosis Association
3567 East 49th St.
Cleveland, OH 44105
(216) 271-1100

**cystic hygroma**   A tumor consisting of enlarged lymphatic vessels or channels that usually appear in various locations on the neck. These structures consist of intact and collapsed cysts held together by connective tissue (stroma) and containing a clear or cloudy fluid. In most of the cases, the cyst is present at birth; in the remainder, it nearly always becomes apparent by the age of two. The cysts vary in size from 2.5 to 15 cm. (1 to 6 inches), and may grow rapidly or slowly. They are not painful unless they become infected. Skin may be stretched thin over this underlying sac, and may have a bluish hue. Large cysts, especially those in CONGENITAL cases (present at birth), may also involve the armpit, structures within the chest, tongue or mouth. Respiratory obstruction is common because of displacement of the windpipe (trachea). Cystic hygromas may be diagnosed before birth by ULTRA SOUND.

The cause of the condition is not believed to be genetic. Cystic hygromas are frequently found, however, in association with CHROMOSOME ABNORMALITIES (particularly, TURNER'S SYNDROME). Cystic hygromas in utero, which later resolve (with the fluid being reabsorbed), lead to redundant skin and are the cause of the webbed neck in disorders such as Turner syndrome, NOONAN SYNDROME and FETAL ALCOHOL SYNDROME.

**cystine storage disease**   See CYSTINOSIS.

**cystinosis** (cystine storage disease)   A genetic metabolic disorder, inherited as an AUTOSOMAL RECESSIVE trait and first described in 1903, that causes abnormal amounts of cystine, an AMINO ACID, to accumulate in various cells in the body. Primary sites of accumulation are the eyes, liver, white blood cells, muscles and the kidneys; most of the damage occurs in the kidneys, ultimately leading to kidney failure and death.

Cystine enters the cells normally and is stored in lysosomes, small digestive organelles found within each cell. However, it is unable to be transported out of the lysosomes, and reaches from 10 to 1,000 times the normal level, disrupting cellular activity and eventually destroying the cell itself.

The disorder is estimated to occur in one in 150,000 live births in the United States. For unknown reasons, the incidence is on the order of one in 30,000 in Brittany, France. Affected individuals tend to look younger than their age, and most are fair-skinned and blond, even though their parents may have dark complexions and hair.

Although present at birth, there is a variability in age of onset and progression. Typically, it is diagnosed between nine and 18 months of age. Symptoms are excessive thirst, excessive urination, fever, vomiting, failure to thrive, failure to walk or the development of rickets. Individuals are short statured and usually thin, with small pot bellies. Accumulation of cystine in the eye causes progressive sensitivity to light (photophobia), and ocular defects of the retina and cornea may also result. As cystine does not accumulate in the brain, intelligence is normal.

The finding of sugar in the urine leads to frequent misdiagnosis of diabetes (see DIABETES MELLITUS). Further testing reveals other hallmarks of cystinosis, such as excess waste products and acid in the body, anemia and a loss of alkali in the urine. X rays reveal bone disease. Cystine crystals in the eyes, or cystine in the white blood cells, provide confirmation of the presence of the disorder.

Ultimately, kidney (renal) failure results, generally between the ages of nine and 12 years, and the condition is usually fatal by age 16. Dialysis and kidney transplants are prolonging life among a growing number of affected individuals. However, complications, including possible nervous system disorders, result from the continued accumulation of cystine.

PRENATAL DIAGNOSIS in at-risk pregnancies is possible via CHORIONIC VILLUS SAMPLING. CARRIER detection is possible in families with an affected family member. However, this test is not widely available.

For more information, contact:

Cystinosis Foundation, Inc.
477 15th Street, Suite 200
Oakland, CA 94612
(415) 834-7897

**cystinuria**   An inherited inborn error of AMINO ACID metabolism leading to the formation of pebble-like deposits of the amino acid cystine in the kidney, ureter or bladder.

Symptoms of the kidney stones may include increased volume of urine excreted, pain to the back or flank from the kidney or ureter, blood in the urine and difficult or painful urination. Urinary tract infections are common. Because of poor kidney function, toxic wastes may accumulate in the blood.

An increased incidence of MENTAL RETARDATION or psychiatric disturbance has also been associated with the disorder, possibly due to impaired intestinal absorption of the amino acids cystine, lysine, arginine and ornithine, but the reason for this is unclear. Diagnosis is made by finding increased cystine or cystine crystals in the urine.

Life span is shortened by more than 10 years in affected males and less than 10 years in females, with death due to kidney failure.

Occurring in about one in 10,000 live births, this disorder is inherited as an AUTOSO-MAL RECESSIVE trait. There are at least three variants due to mutations: Types I, II and III. About two-thirds of all carriers are Type I HETEROZYGOTES (heterozygotes have only one of the two recessive genes required for expression of a recessive trait), whose condition can be detected only by studies of intestinal absorption or transport of cystine. Type II and Type III heterozygotes excrete increased amounts of cystine in urine.

Treatment includes a high fluid intake, treatment with sodium bicarbonate to keep the urine alkaline, or treatment with certain drugs. Without treatment kidney obstruction from the stone deposits can lead to kidney failure.

**cytogenetics**   The visualization and study of CHROMOSOMES. Examining chromosomes for abnormalities in size, structure and other aspects provides the means for diagnosing many GENETIC DISORDERS in the fetus. This field of research has led, for example, to identification of the cause of DOWN SYNDROME (an extra chromosome 21) and other genetic conditions caused by CHROMOSOMAL ABNORMALITIES. Use of the term "cytogenetics" has been dated to "The Chromosomes in Heredity," a paper published in 1903 by Walter S. Sutton of the United States, predating by three years William Bateson's formal proposal to name the study of heredity "genetics."

Cytogenetic analysis for PRENATAL DIAGNOSIS begins with the extraction, primarily through AMNIOCENTESIS, of sufficient fetal cells for study. The cells are cultured and prepared in the laboratory and stained by a variety of methods to allow effective visualization under a microscope. A photograph of the microscopic image (KARYOTYPE) of the chromosome complement of a cell allows the 23 chromosome pairs each human cell possesses to be arranged in descending order of size and studied for abnormalities that will indicate genetic defects.

An additional aspect of cytogenetic analysis is that the sex of the fetus can be determined by the X and Y chromosome makeup of the fetal cell being examined through the karyotype. A male child will have one X and one Y chromosome; a female will have two X chromosomes. Such information will be of value in diagnosing any sex-linked genetic defects.

Cytogenetic analysis may be performed for prenatal diagnosis of chromosome abnormalities primarily among pregnant women 35 years of age or older or among those who have had a previous child with a documented chromosome anomaly. Cytogenetic studies are also done on blood (or other tissues) for a variety of other indications. These include individuals who have manifestations suggesting a chromosomeabnormality or have multiple malformations, especially when associated with disturbances of growth or MENTAL RETARDATION, newborns with AMBIGUOUS GENITALIA (that is, whose sex is unclear), certain individuals with INFERTILITY, couples who have had multiple miscarriages (see ABORTION) and individuals with leukemias (see CANCER) and certain other tumors where chromosome anomalies have been described and may help determine the prognosis of the disorder. (See also "INTRODUCTION.")

**cytomegalovirus**  See TORCH SYNDROME.

# D

**Daltonism**  See COLOR BLINDNESS.

**Darwin tubercle**  A small, visible thickening or protuberance of the cartilage of the rim of the outer ear, common in many populations. Inherited as an AUTOSOMAL DOMINANT trait, it is a benign condition, of interest mainly as a genetic curiosity. It is estimated to occur in about 50% of the population in England and Finland, and about 20% in Germany.

**dating**  While conditions associated with many genetic anomalies and BIRTH DEFECTS have restricted social interactions for many affected individuals, the importance of developing social and sexual relationships for their emotional well-being is increasingly recognized.

For more information, contact:

Dating for Disabled
P.O. Box 452
Katonah, NY 10536
(914) 232-8881

Handicap Introductions
P.O. Box 232
Coopersburg, PA 18036
(215) 282-1577

Peoplenet
257 Center Lane
Levittown, NY 11756

**deafness**  The complete or partial loss of hearing. CONGENITAL deafness or early profound hearing loss occurs in approximately one in 1,000 infants in the United States, and an equal number become deaf or have severely impaired hearing by the age of 16. About half of these conditions of deafness are thought to be genetically caused. Over 175 hereditary syndromes featuring or associated with serious hearing loss have been identified. As an isolated problem, congenital deafness may be inherited in AUTOSOMAL DOMINANT (20% to 30%), AUTOSOMAL RECESSIVE (40% to 60%), MULTIFACTORIAL (20% to 30%) or X-LINKED (2%) forms, though they may be indistinguishable. Even if the mode of inheritance is known, it may be impossible to specify the type of deafness in a given situation.

Deafness at birth may also be the result of birth injuries, maternal infections or exposure to drugs. Rubella was a major cause of congenital hearing impairment until a vaccine for the virus was developed. Exposure to cytomegalovirus and herpes simplex type 2 virus can also result in congenital hearing loss.

Malformations of the ears may also cause deafness, and are reported in approximately 35 per 10,000 live births. These may accompany significant malformations of the middle or inner ear, and are thought to account for about 2% of conductive hearing loss.

Hearing disorders are classified as either conductive or sensorineural. Conductive hearing loss is caused by abnormalities in the hearing organs; sensorineural hearing loss involves defects in the nerves that transmit auditory impulses to the brain. However, even in these latter cases, some hearing, particularly of low tones, may be possible.

Severe congenital or early childhood deafness is most likely to be sensorineural and affect both ears (bilateral).

As an isolated disorder, affected infants may go undiagnosed for some time, especially since they make sounds until about nine months of age. It is important to detect hearing disorders as early as possible in order to begin and maximize the effectiveness of communication therapy.

Genetic conditions of deafness with onset after childhood are more likely to be inherited as AUTOSOMAL DOMINANT disorders, and more likely to be conductive. These are classified by the age of onset, rate of progression, frequencies involved and severity. Beyond this, it is often impossible to identify or attach a specific designation to them. Additionally, in familial cases there may be a wide variability of expression, such that members may be unaware of a common problem.

If parents with normal hearing have more than one deaf child, the condition is usually an AUTOSOMAL RECESSIVE disorder. If two generations are affected, it is usually dominant. If only one child has congenital deafness and careful investigation has eliminated syndromic or environmental causes, the estimated risk for recurrence in a SIBLING is one in six. If only one parent is affected the estimated risk is 5%.

If two congenitally deaf people marry, there is a 70% to 80% chance that all their offspring will have normal hearing. Even if the parents both have autosomal recessive hearing disorders, unless the disorders are identical, children will be CARRIERS of the disorders, rather than affected by them. Only 5% to 14% of the offspring of two congenitally deaf individuals are deaf children.

Historically those with severe hearing disorders were often thought to have low intelligence, and the word dumb, from the Old English root meaning mute or unable to speak, a condition exhibited in many with congenital deafness, gradually came to mean unintelligent. However, efforts in the late 19th century to improve education and opportunities for those with hearing disorders have helped reverse this misconception.

Hearing-impaired individuals now have a cohesive and structured social system of their own, in addition to an increased integration into society at large, and many do not regard their condition as a deficit. It has been reported by genetic counselors that some deaf couples or individuals would prefer to have a hearing-impaired child than a child with normal hearing whom they might not be able to cope with.

For syndromes associated with deafness, see ALPORT SYNDROME; MIDDLE-EAR INFECTIONS; OTOSCLEROSIS; PENDRED SYNDROME; TREACHER-COLLINS SYNDROME; USHER SYNDROME; and WAARDENBURG SYNDROME.

For more information, contact:

National Information Center on Deafness
Gallaudet College
800 Florida Avenue, NE
Washington, DC 20002
(202) 651-5000

American Society for Deaf Children
814 Thayer Avenue
Silver Spring, MD 20910
(301) 585-5400

National Fraternal Society of the Deaf
1300 W. Northwest Highway
Mount Prospect, IL 60056
(312) 392-9282

American Speech-Language-Hearing
    Association
10801 Rockville Pike
Rockville, MD 20852
(301) 897-5700
(800) 638-8255

**deafnesss and functional heart disease**
See JERVELL AND LANGE-NIELSEN SYNDROME.

**deformity**    See ANOMALY.

**de Lange syndrome**    See CORNELIA DE
LANGE SYNDROME.

**deoxyribonucleic acid (DNA)**    The su-
permolecule from which CHROMOSOMES are
made, and which carries the GENETIC CODE.
Nucleic acid was found in the nucleus of the
cell by Swiss chemist Friedrich Miescher in
1871, and DNA, its major component, was
isolated by English taxonomist Fred Griffith,
which he reported in 1928. While many geneticists suspected it played an important part in
heredity, this was not proved until 1944, when
Oswald Avery of Rockefeller University, New
York, used DNA to transmit characteristics from
one strain of bacteria to another.

Its structure remained a mystery until James D.
Watson and Francis H.C. Crick, of the Medical
Research Council Laboratories in Cambridge,
England, working with physicist Maurice Wilkins, defined its structure. Wilkins had taken X-
ray photographs of the molecule revealing a
helical shape. In 1953, Watson and Crick published their paper, "Structural Implications of
Deoxyribonucleic acid," in which they proposed
the double helix model of the molecule and its
functioning, and Wilkins simultaneously published his X-ray photographs. (The three shared
the Nobel prize for their work in 1962.)

As described by Watson and Crick, DNA
consists of two long, linked strands, resem-

bling a tightly coiled spiral staircase. Each
strand is composed of smaller units called
nucleotides which, in turn, are made of a sugar
molecule, a phosphate and any one of four
nitrogen bases: adenine, thymine, guanine or
cytosine. Nucleotides on each strand are
linked with a nucleotide on the opposite strand
by the nitrogen bases; each nitrogen base joins
only with a complementary nitrogen base, and
these are called "base pairs." Adenine always
joins with thymine, and guanine always pairs
with cytosine. A sequence of three nucleotides
is called a CODON.

When the DNA replicates during cell division, the two strands divide down the middle,
with the base pairs unlocking, and each strand
becomes a template, attracting mirror-image
segments of nucleotides. When the entire new
chain of nucleotides is complete, there is a
new, identical double helix of DNA.

DNA controls protein synthesis in a similar
fashion: DNA forms a template for
RIBONUCLEIC ACID (RNA). The assembled
RNA chain exits the nucleus, and itself becomes a template for the construction of the
AMINO ACID chains that form proteins and
ENZYMES. Thus, genes may be considered a
series of codons that give the instructions for
assembling a specific protein.

Changes or MUTATIONS of individual nucleotides may result in defective formation of
proteins and enzymes, and are the basis of
many GENETIC DISORDERS. (See also "INTRO-
DUCTION.")

**dermoid cyst (teratoma) of head and
neck**    Rare condition, marked by cysts or
sacs, containing skin-type tissue (dermoids)
or more complex benign tumors composed of
tissue not usually found at that site (teratomas). Dermoid cysts occur almost exclusively
in infants and young children. The signs and
symptoms depend upon the size and location
of the cyst or tumor.

Nasal dermoids, which may appear as a
small pit or depression on the bridge of the
nose with a hair protruding from it, are usually
detected shortly after birth. They are slightly

more prevalent in males and may be associated with obstructed nasal passages and mucus in the nose.

Infants born with nasopharyngeal teratomas may also have respiratory problems. These tumors, located in the airway between the nose and throat, are six times more prevalent in females than males.

With a teratoma of the orbit (eye), the infant is usually born with a mass behind one eye. This may cause the eye to bulge and may decrease vision. The tumor may extend through defects in the orbit or skull into the brain or nasal cavity.

Tumors that occur in the neck region (cervical teratomas) are usually present at birth and are rare after age one. Symptoms may include noisy or temporary cessation of breathing, a bluish tinge to the skin, and difficulty swallowing.

Surgical removal of all tumors is necessary to prevent recurrences and other complications, though tumors rarely become malignant. If the tumor is completely removed a normal life span can be expected.

The cause of these tumors and cysts is uncertain. They contain bizarre mixes of malplaced tissues. For example, teratomas often contain skin, hair, bone, teeth and even liver or kidney tissue. Inheritance patterns have not yet been determined.

**DES**    See DIETHYLSTILBESTROL.

**deuteranomaly**    See COLOR BLINDNESS.

**deuteranopia**    See COLOR BLINDNESS.

**developmental disability**    Any condition resulting from a CONGENITAL abnormality, trauma, disease or deprivation that interrupts or delays normal growth and development. Children with developmental disabilities may have multiple handicaps with or without MENTAL RETARDATION.

**diabetes mellitus**    A group of disorders that are caused by the absence of, or the body's inability to use, insulin. Insulin is a hormone necessary for regulating the blood levels of glucose (blood sugar), which is the body's main source of energy.

The condition known as diabetes has been recognized for millennia. Described in the Egyptian Ebers Papyrus, written about 1500 B.C., it was named by early Greek physicians, who called it *diabetes*, Greek for fountain or siphon, due to the copious urination that is one of the hallmarks of the disorder in its early, untreated state. They also noted that the urine had a sweet odor and taste, hence the term *mellitus*, which comes from the Latin word for honey. The familial nature of this disorder has been recognized for at least 300 years.

The primary symptoms are elevated blood sugar levels (hyperglycemia), frequent urination, excessive thirst, increase in appetite and weight loss. There can be emaciation, weakness, debility and a low resistance to infections as well as leg cramps, pins and needles sensations in the fingers and toes, and blurred vision. Sugar is excreted in the urine. Unsuspected cases of diabetes may first be recognized in a routine urine test. (Sugar in the urine is not always a sign of diabetes; it may merely indicate the kidneys are unable to process normal amounts of sugar. Conversely, sugar is not always present in the urine of diabetics. A glucose tolerance test, which measures the body's reaction to large amounts of sugar or glucose, is another diagnostic test, though individuals who display glucose intolerance do not always develop diabetes.)

If diabetes is undiagnosed and untreated, the body may accumulate incompletely metabolized fats, called ketones, leading to ketoacidosis. This condition is marked by fruity, sweetish breath odor, tremendous thirst and dryness of the tongue and skin, weakness and vomiting. If untreated, ketoacidosis can progress to diabetic coma and death.

Other complications of diabetes may affect the heart, kidneys, eyes, circulatory and nervous systems. Individuals are two to four times more likely to die of heart disease, and their incidence of strokes is two to six times higher than average. Kidney failure and kidney infections are common. Circulatory problems may lead to gangrene in the limbs, sometimes requiring amputation. Diabetes can damage any part of the eye, and is now the leading cause of new adult blindness in the United States, with 6,000 new cases a year developing. Over 90% of those who've had diabetes for 20 years or longer have damage to the blood vessels in the retina. In the nervous system, diabetes can slow reflexes, cause pain, impotence and loss of sensation.

Diabetes is also a feature of many GENETIC DISORDERS, for example, CYSTIC FIBROSIS, HEMOCHROMATOSIS, PRADER-WILLI SYNDROME.

The exact mechanism by which diabetes leads to complications in organ systems is unclear, but high blood glucose levels are thought to play a part. In addition to physical complications, diabetes takes a high emotional toll on individuals. Besides the mood swings wrought by changing blood sugar levels, the necessity of lifelong daily management of this disorder may result in anger, depression and anxiety.

As a group, this is among the most common disorders, estimated to affect 5% of the adult population of the western world. Approximately 11 million Americans and 379,000 Canadians have been diagnosed with the disorder, and it's estimated there may be an equal number of undiagnosed cases. It is a major cause of death, with approximately 150,000 to 300,000 people in the United States dying from diabetes and its complications annually.

Though it is impossible to calculate the suffering and toll exacted by any disorder, one comprehensive study of diabetes estimated the cost of medical services and lost productivity due to disability and premature death at $20.4 billion in 1987.

The disorder is centered in the islets of Langerhans, small clusters of hormone-producing tissue in the pancreas. The islets contain beta cells, which produce insulin.

There are two major types of diabetes: juvenile, insulin-dependent (IDDM) or Type I diabetes; and maturity-onset, non-insulin-dependent (NIDDM) or Type II diabetes.

*Juvenile diabetes; insulin-dependent diabetes mellitus, IDDM, or Type I.* This is the more severe form and accounts for nearly 10% of diagnosed cases of diabetes. Though most commonly diagnosed from infancy to the late 30s, it can appear at any age. Symptoms usually develop rapidly.

Juvenile diabetes is thought to be an autoimmune disorder (see IMMUNE DEFICIENCY DISEASES). Antibodies, proteins that destroy bacteria and other foreign tissue within the body, perhaps triggered by some infections, attack and destroy the beta cells that produce insulin. Individuals must take daily insulin injections to stay alive.

Familial aggregation has long been noted. However, the disease is not inherited; what is inherited is a susceptibility to develop the disease. Environmental factors are thought to play a role, and more than one gene may be involved in this predisposition. The HLA genes appear to play a major role in determining the susceptibility to develop diabetes. The risk that a sibling of an individual with the disorder will develop it is estimated at between 5% and 10%. The risk that a child of an individual with the disorder will develop it is 2% to 5%.

*Maturity-onset, non-insulin dependent (NIDDM), or Type II diabetes.* This milder form primarily affects people over the age of 40. Insulin is produced in varying amounts by beta cells, but the body is unable to use it effectively. While maturity-onset diabetes is thought to have a greater genetic component than juvenile diabetes (several modes of inheritance may be involved), non-genetic factors also play a strong role. Being overweight usually contributes to its onset. The risk that a SIBLING of an individual with the disorder will develop it is estimated at between 5% and 10%. The risk that a child of an individual with the disorder will develop it is 5% to 10%. Research has also identified a correlation between the number of times a woman is pregnant and an increased risk of developing NIDDM.

This form is usually treated with diet, weight control and exercise. Oral medication or insulin may be required by some individuals.

(There is also a more rare form of maturity-onset diabetes, maturity-onset diabetes of the young [MODY], transmitted as an AUTOSOMAL DOMINANT trait in some families, with onset usually in adolescence or young adulthood.)

These two types serve as an exception to a general rule regarding genetic disorders: Usually, the most severe form of a disorder shows the clearest genetic basis. But in this disorder, the genetics of the more severe juvenile form are less clear than that of the milder maturity-onset type.

### Diabetes in Pregnancy

Diabetes can have a profound impact on pregnancy. Control over the disorder may be complicated by pregnancy, which requires a normalization of blood sugar that may risk frequent hypoglycemia. The risk of a major congenital malformation in an infant of a diabetic mother is estimated at two to three times greater than the general population's. The overall incidence of BIRTH DEFECTS in offspring of insulin-dependent diabetic mothers is estimated to be 6% or higher. Among the malformations are the caudal regression sequence, an otherwise rare malformation combining failure of the bones of the lower spine and thighs to form properly. The kidneys and cardiovascular system may also be affected, and neural tube defects or other anomalies of the central nervous system may occur.

The cause of this teratogenic effect is not understood. However, poor control over the disorder seems to increase the risk of CONGENITAL MALFORMATIONS. It is imperative that pregnancies of diabetic women be carefully monitored.

There is also a condition called gestational diabetes that most commonly appears in pregnancies of overweight women over the age of 35 who have had large babies, were large babies themselves and have a family history of diabetes. While symptoms are mild in the mother, it can produce the same complications for the newborn as other forms of diabetes. Affected infants tend to be large babies with low blood sugar and exhibit respiratory distress, though gestational diabetes does not increase the risk of congenital malformations.

For more information, contact:

Juvenile Diabetes Foundation International
432 Park Avenue South
New York, NY 10016
(212) 889-7575

American Diabetes Association, Inc.
2 Park Avenue
New York, NY 10016
(212) 947-9707
(800) 232-3472

**diaphragmatic hernia**    See EVENTRATION OF THE DIAPHRAGM AND DIAPHRAGMATIC HERNIA.

**diaphragm, eventration of the**    See EVENTRATION OF THE DIAPHRAGM AND DIAPHRAGMATIC HERNIA.

**diastrophic dysplasia**    The name of this form of short-limbed DWARFISM was borrowed from the field of geology in 1960: Diastrophism is the process of the bending of the earth's crust that creates mountains, ocean basins and other features of the planet's surface. In this disorder it refers to the flexion contractures, or permanent bending of the knees, elbows and hips exhibited in some affected individuals. The disorder is variable in its expression.

Like many other forms of short stature caused by defective skeletal development, for many years this disorder was erroneously classified as a form of ACHONDROPLASIA. Many cases of "achondroplasia with CLUBFOOT" are actually diastrophic dwarfism. Additionally, it has been said that this disorder has frequently been erroneously labeled as ARTHROGRYPOSIS in hospital diagnostic files.

At birth, individuals exhibit severe clubfoot (talipes equinovarus) and malformations of the hands, particularly the so-called "hitchhiker's thumb." Fingers are short and broad, and their mobility is reduced. As individuals grow, the face takes on a characteristic appearance, with a narrow nasal root, long, broad philtrum (the groove extending from the bottom of the nose to the upper lip), prominent mouth and square jaw. These features were referred to by the now outdated term "cherub dwarf."

In most cases, cysts of the cartilage of the ears swell soon after birth, resulting in a "cauliflower ear" deformity, though in most cases hearing remains unimpaired.

There is mesomelic limb shortening (shortening of forearm and lower leg). Congenital joint dislocations are common, and individuals have a distorted gait, with a tendency to walk on their toes. The trunk has an extreme swayback appearance (lumbar lordosis) beginning at an early age. The chest is barrel-shaped and there may be lateral curvature of the spine (SCOLIOSIS) as well. These abnormalities of the spinal column may cause severe neurological complications.

Defects of development of the larynx produce a characteristic soft rasping or hoarse voice. Intelligence is normal. The average male adult height is approximately 43 inches.

Diastrophic dysplasia is inherited as an AUTOSOMAL RECESSIVE trait. About one-quarter of affected infants under medical care die due to respiratory difficulties. (A lethal variety of this disorder, also inherited as an autosomal recessive trait, has been reported.)

PRENATAL DIAGNOSIS has been achieved using ULTRASOUND to detect skeletal abnormalities in the fetus.

For more information, contact:

Little People of America, Inc.
P.O. Box 633
San Bruno, CA 94066
(415) 589-0695.

Human Growth Foundation
4720 Montgomery Lane, Suite 909
Bethesda, MD 20814
(301) 656-6904
(301) 656-7540

**diethylstilbestrol, DES**   A synthetic estrogen, a female sex hormone, previously prescribed for women suspected of being at risk for developing complications (such as miscarriage) during pregnancy.

Between 1940 and 1971, approximately two to three million pregnant women were treated with DES, the majority between the years 1946 and 1960. In 1971 the drug was linked to cervical and vaginal CANCER in women (usually 19 to 25 years of age) whose mothers used the drug during pregnancy. These women have been called "DES daughters."

It is estimated that for every 10,000 women exposed during fetal development, approximately 1.4 to 14 develop cervical cancer. A significantly larger proportion (estimated at between 20% and 60%) exhibit other abnormalities of the reproductive system, including structural defects of the cervix, vagina and fallopian tubes. DES daughters are also prone to infertility, miscarriage and premature delivery.

Adverse affects on males whose mothers took DES during pregnancy have not been conclusively documented.

For more information, contact:

DES Action
2845 24th Street
San Francisco, CA 94110
(415) 826-5060

**Di George syndrome**  (thymic alymphoplasia)  CONGENITAL developmental ANOMALY characterized by abnormalities of the immune system and CONGENITAL HEART DEFECTS. The immune system deficiencies are caused by the failure of the thymus gland to develop (see IMMUNE DEFICIENCY DISEASE). In addition, the parathyroid glands, which regulate blood calcium, fail to develop. Named for U.S. pediatrician A.M. Di George (b. 1921), who described it in 1965, it results from an abnormality in the development of the third and fourth pharyngeal pouches of the embryo, from which the aorta forms. Within days of birth, infants may exhibit the grayish or dark purple discoloration of the skin (cyanosis) caused by abnormal amounts of low-hemoglobin blood, due to cardiac abnormalities. Seizures may occur as a result of low calcium. There is FAILURE TO THRIVE, and most die within a month of birth from severe cardiac abnormalities or infections.

In half of the cases, the thymus has completely failed to develop and is underdeveloped in the other half. Once the immune deficiency is identified, infants must be isolated. Those that survive face increased susceptibility to respiratory infections.

In some patients (in particular familial cases) a deletion in the upper portion of the long arm of CHROMOSOME 22 has been found. The offspring of women taking Isotretinoin (ACCUTANE) once a day in the treatment of severe cystic acne, have features that resemble the Di George syndrome. Exposure to alcohol in utero may also cause similar features.

More than half of affected infants share characteristic facial features. The placement of the eyes on the face is uneven; one may be slightly below the other or they may be wide-set (HYPERTELORISM). The eye slits (palpebral fissures) are slanted toward the nose. The nose itself is upturned (anteverted nares), and the groove below the nose that meets the lip (philtrum) is short. The upper and lower lip form a cupid-bow shape. The outer ears (pinnae) may be small, low-set or rotated slightly backward, and malformed.

The incidence is unknown, but it has been found in 3% of children who succumb to congenital heart disease.

**disability development**    See DEVELOPMENTAL DISABILITY.

**discoid lupus erythematosus**    See LUPUS.

**discordance**    The expression of a specific trait in only one member of a pair of TWINS. (See also CONCORDANCE.)

**DNA**    See DEOXYRIBONUCLEIC ACID.

**DNA probes**    Short segments of DEOXYRIBONUCLEIC ACID (DNA) that can be used to identify some genetic abnormalities. The DNA segments are obtained by using RESTRICTION ENZYMES, which chemically cut the DNA at specific points.

A DNA probe is prepared from normal CHROMOSOMES with the normal complement of genes. Each probe is specially labeled with either a radioactive or chemical tag that identifies the DNA gene sequence of the particular segment being used. The probe can then be used as a standard against which the DNA of an individual can be compared.

After obtaining a DNA sample from an individual, often a fetus, the DNA is cut into fragments by use of restriction enzymes and mixed in solution or on a filter with selected DNA probe fragments. Similar fragments from both sets of DNA will stick together while the others wash away. Often, other individuals in the family will also have been tested and a study made of the family's normal genetic makeup. Thus, genetic deviations or abnormalities in the DNA of the individual being tested can be disclosed by a comparison of the family's DNA structure and the segments of the DNA probe that unite with the DNA of the tested person. Where no family study has been possible, DNA probes can be used in some instances where previous research has established that the presence or absence of a particular genetic sequence at a specific location indicates a genetic defect, as in the prenatal diagnosis of SICKLE-CELL ANEMIA, THALASSEMIA and ALPHA 1-ANTITRYPSIN DEFICIENCY.

## Table X
## Empiric Risks* for Down Syndrome Live Birth

| Source | Risk (%) |
|---|---|
| Young mother with previous trisomy 21 (or other trisomy) life birth, miscarriage, or stillbirth | About 1 |
| Occurrence of trisomy 21 in a 2nd- or 3rd-degree relative; maternal age below 35 | Somewhat increased but still less than 1 |
| Rare families with two or more cases of trisomy 21 | Risk markedly increased for 1st-and 2nd-degree relatives |
| Mother with a 21/13, 21/14, or 21/15 translocation | About 15 |
| Father with a 21/13, 21/14, or 21/15 translocation | About 5 |
| Mother with a 21/22 translocation | About 10 |
| Father with a 21/22 translocation | About 12 |
| Either parent with a 21/21 translocation | 100 |
| Decreased levels of maternal serum alpha-fetoprotein | Recent studies indicate increased risk |

*Maternal-age specific risks not included

Reproduced with the permission of the National Genetics Foundation, Inc., from R.B. Berini and E. Kahn (eds.), *Clinical Genetics Handbook* (Orodell, N.J.: Medical Economics Co., Inc., 1987). All rights reserved.

**dolichocephaly**    See CRANIOSYNOSTOSIS.

**dominant**    See AUTOSOMAL DOMINANT.

**Donahue syndrome**    See LEPRECHAUNISM

**Down syndrome**    Characterized by mental deficiency and typical facial features, Down syndrome is the most common identifiable form of MENTAL RETARDATION. It is named for J. Langdon Down (1828-1896), a British physician and early champion of education for the retarded, who in 1886 described a condition he called MONGOLISM in a series of lectures entitled "On some of the mental afflictions of childhood and youth." "Mongolism" referred to the vertical folds of skin obscuring the juncture of the upper and lower eyelids on either side of the nose (epicanthal folds), which, along with the upslanting of the eyes, give individuals an Oriental appearance. However, use of the term mongolism is presently discouraged.

Down syndrome is a CHROMOSOME ABNORMALITY caused by the presence of a third copy of chromosome 21, and the condition is consequently also called trisomy 21. It is the first condition in humans that was found to be caused by a chromosomal abnormality, and was identified as such in 1959 by French pediatrician Jerome Lejeune (though in 1932, Dutch physician P.J. Waardenberg speculated that this could be the cause). The presence of the third chromosome is most often the result of a cell-division error during meiosis, when chromosome pairs normally split in the formation of sperm and egg cells. Thus, the sperm or egg has two chromosome 21s prior to conception, instead of the normal single copy. (In 75% of the cases, the extra chromosome is thought to be in the egg, and in 25% in the sperm.) In approximately 4% of cases, Down syndrome may also result from a translocation, in which extra chromosome 21 material, rather than an entire extra chromosome, is present. Perhaps another 1% of cases are the result of MOSAICISM, a condition in which the error in cell division occurs after the egg has been fertilized, so that some of the individual's cells exhibit the extra chromosome 21, while other cells have only the normal pair. These individuals are generally less severely affected.

Characteristic facial features, in addition to epicanthal folds, include eyes slanted upward away from the nose (mongoloid obliquity), possibly with a speckling at the periphery of the iris (Brushfield spots), and large tongue (MACROGLOSSIA) that often protrudes from an open mouth, making normal speech difficult. Cognitive development HANDICAPS further speech development. (Speech development in infancy is estimated to lag seven months behind unaffected infants.) Other oral abnormalities include fissured lip, delayed eruption or missing teeth and, rarely, CLEFT PALATE. The chin is usually small (micrognathia) and the neck short with extra skin. The outer ears (auricles) tend to be small, and hearing loss is common, with an estimated 75% exhibiting some degree of hearing impairment. Hands are typically short and broad, with a mild incurving (CLINODACTYLY) of the fifth finger. A single crease in the palm (SIMIAN CREASE) is present in about 30% of those with the syndrome. Muscle tone is frequently poor and newborns are often "floppy" (hypotonia).

Congenital cardiac abnormalities are present in about 40% to 50% of affected individuals, and they may lead to death in infancy. They also have 20 times the risk of the general population of developing leukemia (see CANCER). About 12% may have digestive tract problems such as esophageal or intestinal blockages. Ultimately, individuals with Down syndrome develop an Alzheimer's-like dementia, characterized by the development of amyloid plaques in the brain (see ALZHEIMER'S DISEASE) and many succumb to complications by the age of 35. Less than 3% live beyond the age of 50.

The overall incidence is estimated at between one in 650 and one in 1,000 live births. Risks of having an affected infant rise dramatically with maternal age (as they do for all chromosomal abnormalities). Under age 30, the chances of having an affected child are estimated at one in 1,000, while chances are put at one in 35 for women aged 44 and one in 10 at age 49. The reason for the increased risk is unknown but is thought to be due to the female's possessing all her oocytes, or egg cells, at birth. Thus, they may be exposed to environmental agents or deteriorate over time, so that they are more prone to errors when being transformed into eggs at advanced maternal age. There is also increased risk among women who have had a previous child with the syndrome, or those who themselves have Down syndrome (though pregnancy is rare in this condition).

There is a wide variation in the degree of retardation among affected individuals. Until the 1970s, the majority were institutionalized, but new attitudes and educational opportunities are enabling many of them to lead productive and meaningful lives. A little over half have IQs of 30 to 50, classified as moderate retardation, and are capable of achieving some degree of self-sufficiency. Children with Down syndrome tend to be very sociable and loving. A television series about a family with a teen-ager with Down syndrome, "Life Goes On," debuted in 1989.

Prenatal diagnosis is possible with AMNIOCENTESIS and CHORIONIC VILLUS SAMPLING and is recommended for all pregnancies beyond the age of 35. There have been reports of success in suspecting Down syndrome after finding specific abnormalities on ULTRASOUND or by finding low levels of ALPHA-FETOPROTEIN in the blood of pregnant women. The diagnosis is ultimately confirmed through amniocentesis.

For more information, contact:

National Down Syndrome Congress
1800 Dempster Street
Chicago, IL 60068
(312) 823-7550
1-800-232-NDSC

National Down Syndrome Society
141 Fifth Avenue, Suite 75
New York, NY 10010
(212) 460-9330
800-221-4602

Association for Children with Down
Syndrome, Inc.
2616 Martin Avenue

Bellmore, NY 11710
(516) 221-4700

**drug abuse**    A large number of infants are believed to be exposed to illegal drugs in utero due to maternal drug abuse. Surveys of pregnant women in hospitals across the country have found at least 11% of women use illegal drugs during pregnancy, exposing an estimated 375,000 newborns a year to potential damage. This is considered a conservative estimate. The drugs include cocaine, marijuana, heroin, methadone, amphetamines and PCP, and their use appears to transcend social and economic boundaries.

These figures do not include maternal abuse of alcohol, which is considered to be a larger problem. (Abuse of prescription drugs can also cause problems with pregnancy and fetal development.)

Infant damage associated with maternal drug abuse includes prenatal strokes, retarded fetal growth, premature birth, low birthweight, abnormalities of the development of genital, urinary and abdominal organs, and seizures after birth.

Additionally, pregnant drug abusers may have a difficult time receiving help for their dependency; due to liability concerns, some addiction treatment programs will not knowingly treat pregnant women. (See also COCAINE; FETAL ALCOHOL SYNDROME; MARIJUANA; and TERATOGEN.)

For more information, contact:

National Association for Perinatal
    Addiction Research and Education
11 East Hubbard Street
Northwestern University Medical School
Chicago, IL 60611
(312) 329-2512

National Clearinghouse for Alcohol
    & Drug Information
P.O. Box 2345
Rockville, MD 20852
(301) 468-2600

**Dubowitz syndrome**    Infants with this disorder, first described in 1965 by Victor Dubowitz, professor of pediatrics at the Royal Postgraduate Medical School in London, usually have low birth weight, an unusually small head (MICROCEPHALY) and are slightly built. They also have a distinct facial appearance marked by sparse hair, a high sloping forehead, flattening of the ridges above the eyes, drooping upper eyelids (PTOSIS), folds of skin at the inner corners of the eyes (EPICANTHUS) and prominent or low-set ears. As they grow they usually develop an uneven jaw, a high nasal bridge and general facial asymmetry. Some are retarded (generally mildly) and most have a hoarse, high-pitched voice. Behavior problems may be seen.

During the first year of life the infant usually develops a skin rash on the face and limbs (eczema) and may suffer from chronic diarrhea. Affected males may have undescended testes (CRYPTORCHISM) and may have a condition known as HYPOSPADIAS, where the opening of the urethra is located on the underside of the penis.

The basic defect causing this AUTOSOMAL RECESSIVE disorder has not been found. To date there have been approximately 30 cases reported, most occurring within a few families. Surgery may be necessary to correct various abnormalities but the overall prognosis for a normal life span is favorable.

**Duchenne muscular dystrophy**    See MUSCULAR DYSTROPHY.

**ductus arteriosus, patent (PDA)**
See PATENT DUCTUS ARTERIOSUS.

**duodenal atresia or stenosis**    The congenital blockage of the upper segment of the intestine, the duodenum. In those affected, usually the duodenum is constricted (stenosis), rather than completely unconnected (atresia) due to developmental failure. Occurring in an estimated one of every 10,000 births, it is often associated with DOWN SYNDROME; approximately 30% of individuals with this condition have Down syndrome, though the cause of this intestinal blockage is unknown. Most cases are SPORADIC. A little over half of those with this condition under medical care were low birthweight infants. It is often associated with other anomalies. Generally, it is not diagnosed until a few days after birth. If not treated and repaired surgically, death will result, though more than 60% of affected infants survive.

**Dupuytren contracture**    Disorder characterized by progressive flexion deformities of the fingers, particularly the fourth and fifth digits, resulting in permanent bending of the affected fingers. Onset may begin in infancy, though symptoms are most obvious after age 40. Eventually, the hand loses functional ability due to the inability to extend the fingers.

It is named for Guillaume Dupuytren (1775-1835), the preeminent French surgeon of the early 19th century, who first published a report of the disorder in 1833. It exhibits familial aggregation (see FAMILIAL DISEASE) and is thought to be inherited as an AUTOSOMAL DOMINANT disorder with partial sex-limitation; the ratio of affected males to females is six to one. It is often seen in association with PEYRONIE DISEASE.

**dwarfism**    A general term for conditions of short stature. Prior to 1900, classification of dwarfism was rather unrefined, leading to frequent misdiagnosis of various forms and leaving little reliable historical data on incidence or other aspects of the disorders. Classification has improved greatly in recent years due to advanced diagnostic techniques and increased research. The medical profession now recognizes some 200 conditions associated with dwarfism. About half are specific disorders; the remainder represent rare, unidentified conditions that have been seen in one family or individual. ACHONDROPLASIA accounts for approximately half of all cases of dwarfism.

There are more than 500,000 adults below 5 feet in height, and an estimated 500,000 children with growth deficiencies. (Individuals are generally considered dwarfed if their full-grown height is below 4 feet 10 inches [145.4 cm]. Approximately 3% of adult females are estimated to be under 4 feet 11 inches in height, and 3% of adult males under 5 feet 4 inches [160.2 cm].) However, the majority of infants seen by doctors—due to parental concern about growth deficiencies—are merely exhibiting delayed development and will ultimately reach normal adult height.

In the majority of types of dwarfism, life span and intelligence are normal, though some forms are lethal or associated with severe mental impairment.

Dwarfs have been seen in the human population throughout history. They are believed to have been given magical significance in the prehistoric world, and they often occupied unique positions of importance in recorded history. Skeletal remains of achondroplastic dwarfs have been found by archaeologists at prehistoric sites, and figurines and amulets in their shape dating to these same periods have also been found. The pharaohs and their nobles are said to have delighted in having dwarfs in their households, and there are many statues, drawings and records attesting to their special status in Egypt. The Egyptian god Ptah was sometimes depicted as a dwarf, and mummified remains of dwarfs have been found in royal tombs as well as in tombs of dwarfs themselves. They were also invoked in spells involving childbirth and other rituals. Dwarfs continued as court favorites during the Roman Empire; many emperors kept dwarfs, sometimes as trusted advisers. Through the Middle Ages their popularity in royal households remained constant, and they were seen in nearly every court, often fulfilling the role of jester. This practice lingered in Russia and Sweden well into the 19th century.

The term "dwarf" was formerly used to describe short-statured individuals with disproportionate physiques. "Midget" was used to describe a short-statured individual of normal body proportions. (This dwarfing is not actually proportionate, as upper/lower body segment ratios may not be in the normal range.) However, contemporary short-statured individuals regard the term midget as derogatory. The origin of the objection to this term is believed to be due to its circus sideshow associations as well as being a remnant of resentment from a time when proportionate short-statured individuals were perceived by those of abnormal proportions as having fewer social disadvantages. Preferred terminology today includes "dwarfs" and "small," "little" or "short" people.

Proportionate dwarfing (physiologic dwarfing) is usually caused by one of several factors:

*Chromosome Abnormalities*. Missing or abnormal (e.g., rearranged) chromosomes are responsible for some forms of short stature, for example, TURNER SYNDROME.

*Hormone Failure*. There may be disturbances or deficiencies of the pituitary or thyroid glands, which are responsible for regulating normal growth.

*Primary Growth Disturbances*. Some infants do not respond to normal growth factors. This is often the case in certain malformation syndromes. (See PITUITARY DWARFISM SYNDROMES.)

*Secondary Growth Failure*. Growth may be stunted by disease, such as kidney failure, or as a result of fetal exposure to certain TERATOGENS.

*Poor Nutrition*. Chronic malnutrition can result in short stature.

*Inherited Short Stature*. This is the most common form of short stature. If parents are short-statured, their offspring tend to be short-statured as well.

(For information on specific forms of proportionate dwarfing, see also SECKEL SYNDROME, HALLERMANN-STREIFF SYNDROME, PYGMIES, CORNELIA DE LANGE SYNDROME; LEPRECHAUNISM; NOONAN SYNDROME.)

Disproportionate dwarfing is usually the result of defective skeletal development (skeletal dysplasia). There are over 100 recognized dysplasias that result in short stature, and they usually result from an inherited single gene, a metabolic disturbance or an unknown factor.

Disproportionate forms of dwarfism are classified as either short-limb or short-trunk types, depending on whether the limbs or trunk show the most evidence of dwarfing. The short limb type is further classified by the section of the limb most affected. In rhizomelic dwarfing, the sections closest (proximal) to the trunk, the upper arms and thighs, are most shortened. Mesomelia indicates primary involvement of the middle portion of the limbs. Acromelia designates the distal portions, or the extremities of the limbs, the hands and feet. Most cases of disproportionate dwarfing are hereditary, but a significant number are the result of new mutations.

For information on specific forms of disproportionate dwarfism, see also: ACHONDROGENESIS; CAMPTOMELIC DYSPLASIA; DIASTROPHIC DYSPLASIA; METAPHYSEAL CHONDRODYSPLASIA; HYPOCHODROPLASIA; KNIEST DYSPLASIA and PYCNODYSOSTOSIS.

Diagnosis may require multiple specialists, e.g., geneticist, endocrinologist, orthopedist and diagnostic procedures, including X rays, hormone tests, chromosome analysis or other tests.

Treatment is usually multidisciplinary, involving orthodontist, endocrinologist, geneticist, neurologist, physical therapy, often dentist, psychologist and ophthalmologist. Psychosocial and genetic counseling can help answer questions from affected individuals and relatives.

Hormone replacement with growth hormones may be of use in cases of growth hormone deficiency (see PITUITARY DWARFISM SYNDROME) and perhaps in Turner syndrome.

Prenatal diagnosis may be possible for some skeletal dysplasias using ULTRASOUND. Diagnosis is dependent on specific disorder.

For more information, contact:

Little People of America, Inc.
P.O. Box 633
San Bruno, CA 94066
(415) 589-0695

Human Growth Foundation
4720 Montgomery Lane, Suite 909
Bethesda, MD 20814
(301) 656-7540

Parents of Dwarfed Children
11524 Colt Terrace
Silver Spring, MD 20902
(301) 649-3275

**Dyggve-Melchior-Clausen syn-drome**    A rare inherited form of short-trunk DWARFISM. Infants who are born with the syndrome have a short neck, protruding broad chest (PECTUS carinatum) and small head (MICROCEPHALY). Signs of MENTAL RETARDA-TION may develop in the first year of life. As the child learns to walk, a waddling gait becomes noticeable. Other characteristics include short, broad pelvic hip bones (ilia), short fingers, toes and wrists, and pronounced curvature of the lower back (lumbar lordosis). Restricted joint mobility and contractures are seen. It was first described by Danish physicians Holger V. Dyggve, J.C. Melchior and J. Clausen in 1962.

X rays reveal that the spinal column is abnormally shifted toward the front of the body. This may result in damage to the spinal cord. However, there are surgical procedures available to correct bone abnormalities. The disorder resembles the mucopolysaccharidoses but does not involve the same biochemical pathways.

The illness may be inherited as either an AUTOSOMAL RECESSIVE trait or, much more infrequently, an X-LINKED recessive trait. The autosomal recessive form is associated with severe mental retardation and extremely short stature. The rare X- linked recessive type is associated with normal intelligence and less diminution of stature, and appears to be a different disorder. There is no test at present to diagnose the disorder prenatally.

Less than 50 cases of Dyggve-Melchior-Clausen Syndrome have been reported. It may particularly be seen among those of Lebanese background. The life span of affected individuals is difficult to predict, but those with mental retardation generally live into their twenties, while those of normal intelligence live into their forties.

**dysautonomia**    See FAMILIAL DYSAU-TONOMIA.

**dysgenesis**    Defective or abnormal formation of an organ or portion of the body, particularly during embryonic development.

**dyslexia**    A defect in reading and writing unaccompanied by other impairment of intellectual function. The concept of a specific syndrome involving the inability to read evolved in the 19th century, and was articulated in German neurologist A. Kussmaul's description of "word blindness" in 1881. The term *dyslexia* was first used in 1887 by R. Berlin, a professor in Stuttgart, Germany who noted a loss of reading ability among some patients who suffered stroke or trauma.

Dyslexia is thought to be caused by a central nervous system inability to organize graphic symbols. One of the hallmarks of the disorder is the inversion and transposition of letters and numbers when writing or reading, but this is actually not present in the majority of cases. An alternative diagnostic indication is a reading level less than 80% of mathematical level.

While dyslexia likely has numerous origins, familial cases are well-documented. One study of the immediate family of children with dyslexia found that 45% of 75 first-degree relatives examined were considered affected. A hereditary form, transmitted as an AUTOSOMAL DOMINANT trait, with reduced PENETRANCE in females, has been identified. A defective gene has been postulated to be on the short arm of chromosome 15 (see CHROMOSOME).

For more information, contact:

Orton Dyslexia Society
724 York Road
Baltimore, MD 21204
(301) 296-0232
(800) 222-3123

**dysostosis**  A general term for defective bone formation, or ossification, a characteristic of many genetic disorders affecting the skeletal system. However, it is more properly used to describe malformations of individual bones either singly or in combination. This is as opposed to the osteochondrodysplasias, more generalized abnormalities of cartilage or bone growth and development. Examples of dysostoses are CRANIOSYNOSTOSIS, KLIPPEL-FEIL SYNDROME, SPONDYLOTHORACIC DYS-PLASIA, TREACHER-COLLINS SYNDROME and POLYDACTYLY.

**dysplasia**  The abnormal organization of cells into tissues during embryonic development. It involves the process of histogenesis (the origin and development of tissue) and is rarely confined to single organs.

**dysplasia of the nails with hypodontia**
See TOOTH-AND-NAIL SYNDROME.

**dystonia** (torsion dystonia; dystonia musculorum deformans)  Incapacitating neurologic (nerve) disorder that causes repeated and uninterrupted twisting and writhing. It may affect a single muscle, a group of muscles, such as those in the arms, legs or neck, or the muscles of the entire body. In children, the legs, back and arms are most frequently affected, while in adults, manifestations in the face and neck are most common. It is a disorder of movement that does not affect memory, intellect or physical senses.

Early symptoms may be very mild and noticeable only after long exertion, or during times of stress or fatigue. Handwriting may deteriorate after a few lines. There may be foot-cramps, or one foot may drag or tend to pull up after walking or running. The neck may turn involuntarily, especially when tired. There may be tremors and speech difficulties. Dystonic motions may lead to permanent physical deformities by causing tendons to shorten and connective tissue to build up in the muscle.

First described in 1907, the prevalence of the disorder is uncertain, with estimates of between 11 per million and 248 per million of the population, though these estimates may be low due to undiagnosed cases. There is no definitive test for the condition. Diagnosis is based on observation of symptoms and tests of muscles. The cause is unknown, though it is thought to involve the basal ganglia, which lie at the base of the brain and are responsible for controlling movement. Generalized dystonia is thought to be more common in Ashkenazi Jews (those of Eastern European ancestry) and possibly individuals of northern Swedish extraction.

Dystonia occurs in three forms. The two childhood forms, which comprise the majority of cases, are hereditary in nature, one transmitted as an AUTOSOMAL DOMINANT and one as an AUTOSOMAL RECESSIVE trait. (It has been suggested that there may be an X-LINKED form, as well.) A third, primarily adult-onset, acquired, localized form (focal dystonia) may be the result of birth injury, infections, drug reactions, trauma, exposure to heavy metals, carbon monoxide or other environmental influences.

Currently there is no treatment for the disorder, but symptoms can sometimes be controlled by muscle relaxants or by drugs that affect the metabolism of chemicals responsible for transmitting nerve impulses. Early diagnosis and counseling to help deal with the emotional adjustment to the illness are important. Spontaneous remission occurs in 5% to 10% of cases.

Prenatal diagnosis and carrier screening is not possible.

*Autosomal recessive dystonia.* The age of onset is between five and 16 years, usually beginning in the foot or, less often, the hand. Involuntary dystonic movements may progress rapidly to all limbs and torso. The progression slows considerably after adolescence. This form has been thought to be most common among Ashkenazi Jews (those of Eastern European ancestry), with an estimated one in 70 to one in 100 carrying the gene for the disorder. The mode of inheritance of dystonia among Ashkenazi Jews remains controversial. In fact, recent evidence suggests that it may actually be autosomal dominantly inherited with low PENETRANCE.

*Autosomal dominant dystonia.* Symptoms usually emerge in late adolescence or early adulthood, though the age of onset shows a wide range. Symptoms often begin in the torso, and a common feature is the involuntary neck muscle movements (torticollis). Progression, while slow, is continual. A gene for dominant dystonia has been mapped to the long arm of CHROMOSOME 9.

*Focal dystonia.* Though not hereditary, and comprising the minority of cases, these localized dystonias represent some of the most interesting and perplexing movement disorders, and include writer's cramp, blepharospasm (characterized by uncontrolled blinking, which may eventually render an individual unable to see), and oromandibular dystonia, which causes the mouth to pull open or shut tight, creating difficulties of speech and swallowing. Meige's disease, a combination of blepharospasm and oromandibular dystonia, is also called Brueghel's syndrome, because the 16th-century Flemish artist, Peter Brueghel the Elder, painted individuals with this condition.

For more information, contact:

Dystonia Medical Research Foundation
8383 Wilshire Blvd.
Suite 800
Beverly Hills, CA 90211
(213) 852-1630

The Dystonia Foundation
425 Broad Hollow Road
Melville, NY 11747
(516) 249-7799

National Foundation for Jewish Genetic
    Diseases
Suite 1200

609 Fifth Avenue
New York, NY 10017
(212) 753-5155

## dystonia musculorum deformans
See DYSTONIA.

# E

**ear, hairy**   See HAIRY EAR.

**Ebstein anomaly**   A CONGENITAL HEART DEFECT that manifests itself (as do many others) with heart murmurs, congestive heart failure and a bluish or grayish color of the skin (cyanosis) caused by insufficient oxygen. Named for Wilhelm Ebstein (1836-1912), a German physician who described it in 1866, the anomaly consists of the downward displacement of the tricuspid valve (which separates the right atrium and right ventricle), possibly interfering with nerve impulses that control the muscular contractions of the heart, and increasing the risk of sudden cardiac arrest and death.

The extent of the defect is highly variable and may be severe enough to cause fetal or neonatal death. Among those who survive, symptoms include shortness of breath (dyspnea) following exertion, weakness and fatigue, and abnormally rapid heart beat (tachycardia). The heart may appear enlarged upon examination by X ray.

Inheritance is believed to be MULTIFACTORIAL, though AUTOSOMAL RECESSIVE transmission has also been suggested in some cases. Maternal ingestion during pregnancy of lithium, a drug often used to treat MANIC DEPRESSION has been implicated as a cause in some cases.

Incidence is estimated at one in 50,000 in the general population and one in 20,000 of live births. It is thought to account for perhaps one in 200 cases of CONGENITAL HEART DISEASE.

For more information, contact:

Mended Hearts
7320 Greenville Ave.
Dallas, TX 75231
(214) 750-5442

International Bundle Branch Block
   Association
6331 West 83rd St.
Los Angeles, CA 90045-2899
(213) 670-9132

Coronary Club, Inc.
9500 Euclid Avenue
Cleveland, OH 44106
(216) 444-3690

**ectodermal dysplasia (ED)**   A group of rare disorders resulting from abnormal development of the ectoderm, the outer layer of fetal tissue that develops into skin, hair, teeth, nails, sweat glands, glands of the mouth, the nervous system, parts of the eye, the pineal gland and parts of the pituitary and adrenal glands. Any disorder that involves defective development of more than one ectodermal structure is considered to be a form of ED.

Historical data concerning this group of disorders dates back to an account by a Mr. W. Wedderburn, whose description, in 1838, of the "toothless men of Sind," members of a Hindu kindred in the vicinity of Hyderabad, India, was cited by Charles Darwin in *The Variations of Animals and Plants Under Domestication* in 1875.

> I may give an analogous case, communicated to me by Mr. Wedderburn, of a Hindoo family in Scinde, in which ten men, in the course of four generations, were furnished, in both jaws taken together, with only four small and weak incisor teeth and with eight posterior molars. The men thus affected have very little hair on the body, and become bald early in life. They also suffer much during hot weather from excessive dryness of the skin. It is remarkable that no instance has occurred of a daughter becoming affected ... though the daughters in the above family are never

affected, they transmit the tendency to their sons: and no case has occurred of a son transmitting it to his sons. The affection thus appears only in alternate generations, or after long intervals.

The condition was named ectodermal dysplasia by Dr. Ashley A. Weech in 1929, in a report in the *American Journal of Diseases of Children.* A dysplasia refers to any abnormal development. (German F.G. Danz, in 1792, had described two Jewish boys born with no hair and no teeth.)

As the teeth are so often affected, individuals need early and ongoing comprehensive dental care.

Any ectodermal structure may be involved. The skin may be lightly pigmented, thin, delicate and prone to infections or rashes. Scalp and body hair may be thin, sparse or lightly pigmented. Some or all of the teeth may be missing or malformed. Teeth that are present tend to erupt late and may be peg-shaped or pointed. Eyes may have CATARACTS, corneal clouding, nystagmus, strabismus and other ocular defects. There may be a hearing disorder. Some individuals exhibit learning disabilities.

Though there is great variability among the forms of ED, and within individual cases of any given form, ED is often divided into two major types, based on whether or not the individual can sweat normally. In hidrotic EDs, the production of sweat is normal. In hypohidrotic EDs, which tend to be more severe, sweat is greatly reduced or absent.

The increased severity of hypohidrotic EDs is generally the result of the deficiencies of the sweat glands, which render the body unable to regulate internal temperature. Overheating, often to the point of heat exhaustion, may occur, especially in hot weather. Additionally, respiratory infections are common as the protective secretions of the mouth and nose are absent.

Characteristic facial features of this form include flat face around the cheekbones and nose, with a depressed nasal bridge. The forehead is broad, with prominent ridges above the eyes. The lips may protrude, and the eyes may be dry and prone to develop abrasions or cataracts.

Because the ectoderm forms so many structures, ectodermal dysplasias take many different forms. The primary features of some of the more recognized of the over 100 different syndromes are listed below.

*Book syndrome (*AUTOSOMAL DOMINANT. White hair and missing teeth.

*Chands Ed (*AUTOSOMAL RECESSIVE). Curly *H*air, Ankyloblepharon (fused eyelids), Nail *D*ysplasia. Curly hair, defective nails, fused eyelids.

*Christ-Siemens-Touraine syndrome, CST; hypohidrotic ED (*AUTOSOMAL RECESSIVE, X-LINKED recessive). This is the best known of EDs. Decreased sweating, absent or undeveloped eyebrows and eyelashes, sparse hair, small and missing teeth, deficient tears and sensitivity to light (photophobia). Classic CST is an X-linked recessive trait affecting only males, though HETEROZYGOTE females may be missing teeth or have patchy areas of decreased hair (hypotrichosis) or decreased sweating. An autosomal recessive form has a similar phenotype.

*Clouston ED; hidrotic ED* (autosomal dominant). Sparse, dry, blond, and slow-growing hair, defective nails, scanty eyebrows and lashes, defective teeth and nail abnormalities characterize this disorder.

*Ectrodactyly-ED-cleft lip-palate; EEC syndrome* (autosomal dominant). Ectrodactyly (split hands and feet), cleft lip/palate, recurring infections, corneal scarring, tear duct malfunction or anomalies, scant hair, abnormal teeth and nails, no hyperthermia, MENTAL RETARDATION.

*Hay-Wells syndrome* (autosomal dominant). Fused eyelids (ankyloblepharon), hair, nail and skin abnormalities, cleft lip and palate.

*Hypertrichosis lanuginosa* (autosomal dominant). Excessive hair, of extreme degree; often appeared as "sideshow" performers. Descriptions have included "The Dog-Faced Boy" or "The Sacred Hairy Family."

*Hypomelanosis of Ito* (autosomal dominant). Asymmetric, bizarre hypopigmented areas of skin (whorls or lines), ocular defects, abnormal

or missing teeth, hypohydrosis, mental retardation, seizures. Affected individuals may be found to have chromosomal MOSAICISM.

*Incontinentia pigmenti* (X-linked dominant). Absent hair, missing teeth, malformed teeth, marbled pigmentation pattern appearing at birth or during first weeks of life, ocular defects.

For more information, contact:

National Foundation for Ectodermal
    Dysplasia
108 North First Street, Suite 311
Mascoutah, IL 62258
(618) 566-2020

**ectopia cordis**    *Ectopia* refers to the congenital displacement or malposition of an organ or body part. *Cordis* refers to the heart. In this condition, the infant is born with the heart outside of the thoracic cavity. It is generally incompatible with life.

For further information, see CONGENITAL HEART DEFECTS.

**ectrodactyly**    A congenital absence or malformation of the fingers or toes, ranging from partial to complete absence of a finger or toe, which occurs sporadically, to cleft hand or foot deformity (lobster claw deformity) or to absence of all but the fifth finger or toe. Cleft hand and foot deformities are generally characterized by absence of the central finger or toe and clefting into the near portion of the hand or foot, with webbing of the remaining fingers or toes on each side of the cleft. The more severe malformations usually occur in both hands (bilaterally), and foot involvement is frequent.

Several genetically distinct traits appear to be associated with the defect, showing AUTOSOMOL DOMINANT transmission with considerable variability in severity.

Ectrodactyly (as manifested by cleft hand) occurs in approximately one in 55,000 to one in 70,000 newborns. Reconstructive surgery may be helpful in repairing the deformity. Prenatal diagnosis has been accomplished by ULTRASOUND. (See

also ECTRODACTYLY-ECTRODERMAL DYSPLA-
SIA-CLEFTING SYNDROME.)

### ectrodactyly-ectrodermal dysplasia-clefting syndrome (EEC syndrome)

The primary manifestations of this rare syndrome are lobster claw deformity of the
hand (ECTRODACTYLY), abnormalities of
skin and its appendages (ECTODERMAL DYS-
PLASIA) and CLEFT LIP and palate. Other oral
features of the syndrome include absence of
teeth, usually the permanent incisors, decreased formation of enamel, deeply fur-
rowed tongue and dryness of the mouth.

The absence of a tear duct opening may be
associated with increased tearing and inflammation of the eyelids and the tear sac. There
may also be simultaneous inflammation of the
corneas and the mucous membrane covering
the eyeball (which occurs due to dryness) and
sensitivity to light (photophobia).

The scalp hair, eyelashes and eyebrows
may be sparse, and nails may be underdeveloped and brittle. Skin biopsy may reveal absence of sweat glands or irregular clustering
of sweat pores. A child with the syndrome
may have difficulty regulating body temperature due to a decrease in sweating.

ULTRASOUND examination during pregnancy may detect many of these abnormalities. The majority of patients with hand or foot
deformity and cleft lip/palate require surgical
correction of the anomaly. Opening of the tear
duct is essential to prevent chronic inflammation, which can lead to blindness.

Intelligence and life span are rarely affected.

The basic cause of this disorder is unknown.
It appears to be inherited as an AUTOSOMAL
DOMINANT trait with a variable degree of severity of its manifestations among affected
individuals, even within families.

### education

Individuals affected with
some genetic or congenital conditions associated with MENTAL RETARDATION (such as
DOWN SYNDROME) were historically regarded
as largely uneducable. However, new approaches and opportunities for their education reveal a higher degree of learning
ability than previously thought possible.

In the United States, individuals handicapped
by a genetic disease, congenital anomaly or for
any other reason must (by law) have access to
the same educational opportunities as non-handicapped individuals (see HANDICAP). The
1975 Education of the Handicapped Act provides federal financial assistance to states to
ensure that each child with handicap(s) receives a free, appropriate public education.

Institutions receiving this financial assistance must provide educational services that
meet handicapped children's individual needs
as adequately as those services provided for
non-handicapped children. Additionally, it is
required that handicapped and non-handicapped children be educated together, to the
extent possible. Parents and guardians may
review education and placement decisions
made on behalf of their child, and be given due
process to challenge those decisions.

Children with handicap(s) must also have
equal opportunity to participate in extracur-
ricular activities such as counseling, physical education, recreational athletics and
transportation.

These guidelines apply to primary, secondary and postsecondary education.

For more information, contact:

The Center for Handicapped Children and
    Teenagers
2351 Clay Street, Suite 512
San Francisco, CA 94115
(415) 923-3549

The Council for Exceptional Children
1920 Association Drive
Reston, VA 22091
(703) 620-3660

### Edward syndrome (trisomy 18)

A
CHROMOSOME ABNORMALITY in which there

is an extra chromosome 18. Named for English medical geneticist J.H. Edward (b. 1928) who published a description in 1960, it occurs in an estimated one in 7,000 live births, with females being affected three times as often as males. It is characterized by a variety of developmental abnormalities of the chest, hands and feet, joints, skeletal muscles, heart, kidneys and genitals. Fingerprints are also abnormal. The hands, often clenched (with the index finger overlapping the third and the fifth over the fourth), are frequently held next to the head in what has been described as a "pleading" position.

The characteristic face includes an elongated, narrow skull (dolichocephaly; see CRANIOSYNOSTOSIS) with a prominent bulge at the back of the head (prominent occiput). Ocular abnormalities include small eyes (microphthalmia), eye slits (palpebral fissures) that are short, and clouding of the cornea. The mouth is small, as is the chin (micrognathia). The ears are low set and poorly formed. The breast bone (sternum) is characteristically short. The "rocker-bottom" feet have prominent heels.

Infants have low birth weight and fail to thrive. About one-third succumb within the first month of life, half within the first two months, and 90% within one year. Females tend to survive much longer than males (134 days mean survival time vs. 15 for males). Mental and developmental retardation is universal.

For more information, contact:

Support Organization for Trisomy 18, 13
   and Other Related Disorders (S.O.F.T.)
c/o Kris and Hal Holladay
1522 E. Garnet
Mesa, AZ 85204-5957
(801) 882-6635

**EEC syndrome**    See ECTRODACTYLY-ECTODERMAL DYSPLASIA-CLEFTING SYNDROME.

**Ehlers-Danlos syndrome (EDS)**    A group of disorders of the connective tissue, which includes tendons, ligaments, skin, bones, cartilage and the membranes surrounding blood vessels and nerves. These highly variable disorders can be characterized by easily bruised and highly elastic skin that is prone to tear, extreme joint laxity giving the appearance of double-jointedness, and multiple chronic dislocations and broken bones. Premature birth is common in some forms, due to early rupture of the fetal membranes. At birth, there are often scars on the forehead and chin. The ears frequently stick outward. The skin is often described as "velvety," or like chamois. Bruised skin heals with peculiar, "cigarette paper" scars. Normal bumps and bruises can result in serious injury. In some patients most surgery can be undertaken only at great risk, due to fragile tissue and uncontrollable bleeding, and in some forms of the disorder major heart problems, rupture of major blood vessels, aortic aneurysms and internal bleeding can create lethal complications.

The syndrome is named for eminent Danish dermatologist Eduard Ehlers (1863-1937) and French dermatologist Henri A. Danlos (1844-1912), who described various forms of the condition in the early 1900s.

An inherited disorder, at least 13 varieties have been identified, transmitted in AUTOSOMAL DOMINANT, AUTOSOMAL RECESSIVE and X-LINKED forms. The forms vary in their severity. Some are associated with mild symptoms. Others can result in severe disability and death, as described above. Typically, there is little variability among affected family members.

Incidence is estimated at approximately one in 200,000 births, though it may be much higher, since mild NOW is thecases may REMAIN remain undiagnosed. Physicians may regard the continual bone breakage some affected individuals exhibit as attributable to clumsiness.

The basic cause is not known for all types of the disorder. In some forms, defective biosynthesis of collagen appears to play a role. Tissue strength and limited elasticity are associated with normal collagen structures.

There is no accepted method of prenatal diagnosis for all forms of EDS, though theoretically AMNIOCENTESIS and CHORIONIC VILLUS SAMPLING can successfully detect those forms associated with known enzyme defects. (See also CUTIS LAXA.)

For more information, contact:

Ehlers Danlos National Foundation
P.O. Box 1212
Southgate, MI 48195
(313) 282-0180

**Elephant Man**    See NEUROFIBROMATOSIS; PROTEUS SYNDROME.

**elfin faceies with hypercalcemia**    See WILLIAMS SYNDROME.

**elliptocytosis**    See HEREDITARY ELLIPTOCYTOSIS.

**Ellis-van Creveld syndrome**    (chondroectodermal dysplasia)    A rare form of short-limbed DWARFISM. First reported in 1940, it is named for Richard Ellis (1902-1966), professor of pediatrics at the University of Edinburgh, and Simon van Creveld (1894-1971), a pediatrician in Amsterdam and authority on HEMOPHILIA. According to medical folklore, they met on a train while traveling to a medical congress and wrote a description en route of the syndrome that now bears their names.

While approximately 100 cases have been reported, half of them have been in an inbred religious group, the Old Order Amish, living in the vicinity of Lancaster, Pennsylvania.

In addition to short stature, the disorder is characterized by the presence of extra fingers (POLYDACTYLY) and CONGENITAL HEART DEFECTS, most typically atrial septal defect.

At birth, the head and face are normal, but there are frequent dental and oral abnormalities, such as NATAL TEETH, and a pseudocleft of the upper lip referred to as "partial hare lip" or "lip-tie." Dental abnormalities become more prominent with age. Fingernails and toenails are poorly formed. The upper and lower limbs are short, particularly in their middle (mesomelic) sections. The trunk and head size are relatively normal.

The disorder is inherited as an AUTOSOMAL RECESSIVE trait. Approximately half of patients die in early infancy due to cardiorespiratory difficulties. The majority of the survivors have normal intelligence.

For more information, contact:

Little People of America, Inc.
P.O. Box 633
San Bruno, CA 94066
(415) 589-0695

**encephalocele**    The protrusion of brain tissue through a congenital skull defect. The brain pushes out with a bulging sac covered by skin and brain membranes (meninges) and containing cerebrospinal fluid that normally cushions the brain. An encephalocele may form at the lower back of the head (occipital encephalocele), at the rear of the side of the skull (posterior parietal encephalocele) or in the front (anterior encephalocele) on the face.

The most common type is the occipital, which may be associated with an abnormally small head (MICROCEPHALY), with the head flexed backward against the spine. An enlarged head caused by fluid accumulation (HYDROCEPHALUS) is also possible in some cases, especially with the posterior parietal type. An anterior encephalocele appears as a swelling at the base of the nose, which may progress and become associated with hydrocephaly, wide-set eyes (HYPERTELORISM) pulsating bulging eyes (exophthalmos) and difficulties with breathing, vision and feeding.

Mortality can range from 60% when hydrocephaly is present to 100% when there is a combination of massive occipital encephalocele and microcephaly. Treatment can involve surgery to close the skull opening and drain the cerebrospinal fluid from the sac. Among those who survive, about half will have various physical disabilities, including paralysis, BLINDNESS, seizures, retarded growth and defective muscular coordination (ataxia). MENTAL RETARDATION of varying degree can be as high as 40%.

Failure of the skull and bones to close properly, which can be detected at birth, will allow encephalocele formation. The basic genetic defect is not known. Frequency of encephalocele ranges from one in 2,000 to one in 5,000 live births. ULTRASOUND examination and detection of an elevated level of alpha-fetoprotein produced by the fetus is employed in prenatal diagnosis.

Encephaloceles may be components of other syndromes, such as MECKEL SYNDROME and AMNIOTIC BAND SYNDROME. They have been reported in association with teratogenic insults, including maternal rubella (see MEASLES), DIABETES MELLITAS and WARFARIN EMBRYOPATHY.

### enchondromatosis (Ollier disease)

Benign, slow-growing tumors of bone cartilage, resulting in a wide variety of skeletal deformities affecting primarily the long bones of the arms and legs. It includes bowing of bones, enlargement of the finger and toe bones, shortening of the limbs and deviation of the larger forearm bone (ulna) in its connection to the wrist. Bones may fracture easily, and the tumors may become cancerous (chondosarcoma) later in life. Enchondromes may also occur in other disorders.

The disorder is detectable after birth through clinical findings and X-ray examination. The exact cause of this rare disorder is not known, and most cases occur sporadically. Orthopedic procedures may alleviate some of the physical problems associated with this disorder.

### endocrine neoplasias, multiple (MEN)

See MULTIPLE ENDOCRINE NEOPLASIAS (MEN).

### enzyme

An organic catalyst required for a biochemical reaction; though enzymes do not enter into these reactions, they must be present for the reactions to occur. There are hundreds of enzymes in the human body. Composed of complex proteins, they are produced by RIBONUCLEIC ACID (RNA), which is a copy of a segment of DEOXYRIBONUCLEIC ACID (DNA); the DNA holds the master blueprint for the assembly of these enzymes. Genes are themselves segments of DNA. Thus, if there is a change or mutation in a gene, it is a change in the DNA, and this change in the blueprint may result in faulty enzyme assembly. This is the basis of hundreds of hereditary enzyme deficiency diseases. (See also BIOCHEMICAL ASSAYS.)

### epicanthal fold    See EPICANTHUS.

### epicanthus (epicanthal fold)

Taken from the Greek "epi," upon or over, and "kanthos," corner of the eye, this is a fold of skin that covers the inner corner of the eye; commonly seen in Orientals, to a lesser degree among blacks and in a significant percentage of prepubertal whites. The small skin fold, joined to both the upper and lower eyelids, obscures the juncture of the lids. While primarily a benign condition of only cosmetic interest, it is also a frequent feature of many GENETIC DISORDERS, for example DOWN SYNDROME.

There are three major theories about how this condition arises: That it is caused by excessive skin at the base of the nose, poor development of the bridge of the nose or retention of the fetal epicanthal fold, which is normally present in the fetus from the third to sixth month of prenatal life.

Epicanthus is variable in its expression. When present as an isolated characteristic rather than part of a larger syndrome, epicanthus is inherited as an AUTOSOMAL DOMINANT trait. It occurs in males and females with equal frequency. Approximately 70% of Orientals and perhaps 50% of blacks exhibit epicanthus. It occurs in about 20% of white infants at age one, a figure that drops to an estimated 3% by age 12 as the fold of skin gradually disappears. In rare cases where the epicanthus is pronounced it may create vision problems by interfering with the field of view. Cosmetic surgery can remove the obstructing skin. Epicanthus may also make the bridge of the nose appear flat and give the usually mistaken impression that the eyes are misaligned. However, essentially this is a benign condition unless it is part of a larger syndrome.

**epidermolysis bulossa (EB)**   A group of genetic disorders characterized by blistering of the skin and mucosal membranes, ranging in expression from mild to lethal, depending on the specific type of the disorder. (Bullae are large blisters filled with fluids.)

Copious blistering may occur after mild irritation or, in severe forms, without any skin friction, and may also form in the mouth, the gastrointestinal, genitourinary and respiratory tracts.

In severe forms, blistering causes the loss of body fluids, blood and proteins, and may result in dehydration, anemia and growth retardation.

The basic defect that causes the disorders is unknown, and there is no cure. The overall incidence of EB is estimated at one in 50,000 live births, though it has also been estimated that between 25,000 and 50,000 Americans have some form of the disorder. Treatment is aimed at preventing the mechanical traumas that lead to blistering. Relatively important forms of the disorder (which are classified on the basis of whether or not they lead to scarring, on their mode of inheritance and on their microscopic appearance) include:

*Dominant simplex.* This AUTOSOMAL DOMINANT form usually appears soon after birth, or when the infant begins to crawl, and blistering most commonly affects the hands and feet. The severity of the lesions often lessens by puberty.

*Dominant dystrophic.* A childhood form of EB, with onset before the age of one year in 20% of cases. Blistering appears on the ankles, knees, elbows, hands and feet. Oral blistering occurs in about one-fifth of the cases. It is inherited as an AUTOSOMAL DOMINANT trait. Some improvement is common with age. This form has been diagnosed prenatally by a finding of elevated ALPHA-FETOPROTEIN levels in the AMNIOTIC FLUID.

*Recessive dystrophic.* In this AUTOSOMAL RECESSIVE form, blistering begins soon after birth and can occur spontaneously. The eyes, teeth, mouth and esophagus are also commonly involved, in addition to blistering of the skin. Severe scarring occurs as the blisters heal, leading to hand deformities and obstruction of the esophagus. Death often occurs in childhood.

*Recessive lethal (Herlitz type).* Appears at birth, and complications (including excessive bleeding due to rupturing of blisters) cause death by the age of three months. Both of these latter forms have been detected prenatally by obtaining samples of fetal skin via FETOSCOPY for biopsy.

For more information, contact:

The Dystrophic Epidermolysis Bullosa
   Research Assn. of America, Inc.
Kings County Hospital Center
41 Clarkson Ave.
Building E, 6th Fl., Rm. E6101
Brooklyn, NY 11203
(718) 774-8700.

**epilepsy, hereditary**   See   HEREDITARY EPILEPSY.

**epiphyseal dysplasia, multiple**   See
MULTIPLE EPIPHYSEAL DYSPLASIA.

**epispadias**   A malpositioned opening of
the urethra, the duct that carries urine from
the bladder. Similar to but more rare than
HYPOSPADIAS. In this congenital condition,
the urethral opening is located above the
normal position on the penis or vagina
(rather than below it, as in hypospadias).

**EPP**   See PORPHYRIA.

**erythropoietic protoporphyria (EPP)**
See PORPHYRIA.

**essential hypertension**   Chronic elevated blood pressure in the arteries. Found
in 20% or more of any large population
group in the United States, if not brought
under control, hypertension can lead to
stroke, heart disease, kidney disease, vision
disturbances and death. It is twice as common in blacks as in whites.

Between 90% and 95% of hypertension is
classified as "essential" or "primary," and
has no discernible cause. However, it is believed that many of these cases are due to
multifactorial inheritance, that is, the result
of the action of several genes in concert with
environmental agents such as diet, lack of
exercise, smoking and stress. Currently,
there are no accurate figures that allow genetic counseling or estimation of recurrence
risks for relatives of affected individuals.
Estimates of hypertension in children and
adolescents range from 1% to 11%.

Maternal hypertension during pregnancy
is associated with increased health risks
for both the mother and the fetus.

**ethics**   Advances in human genetics
have raised a host of ethical and legal issues.
Efforts to address them lag far behind
science's ability to move the questions from
the realm of speculation to reality.

ABORTION issues have received the most
attention, and extend beyond the question of
a woman's right to abortion or society's
right to limit access to this procedure. For
example, if abortion is acceptable in cases
when prenatal diagnosis discloses the presence of a disorder, what constitutes a disorder severe enough to warrant an abortion?
To what extent should genetic analysis and
abortion be used to "engineer" a family's
offspring, or the population as a whole?

Non-abortion issues now receiving the attention of geneticists, lawmakers, philoso-
phers, private citizens, employers and other
interested parties include the following:

May companies bar fertile women from
jobs where they might be exposed to teratogenic chemicals that can harm unborn children?
(See TERATOGEN; PROTECTIVE EXCLUSION.)
Or, can a fertile woman demand to be transferred from a job, such as working on a VIDEO
DISPLAY TERMINAL (see VDTS) because she
fears the reproductive effects of exposure?
Additionally, with increased knowledge of the
impact of maternal health on pregnancy, what
level of lifestyle or behavior may be required by society in order to protect the
unborn child from maternal neglect?

As genetic analysis becomes more sophisticated, it may be possible to screen individuals not only for potential defects in
offspring, but also for their own predisposition to develop genetically-influenced disorders, such as ALCOHOLISM and CORONARY
ARTERY DISEASE. Thus, concerns have
been expressed that genetic testing may
become an instrument for discrimination
in employment and insurance.

Diagnosis of some disorders, such as
HUNTINGTON'S CHOREA, may require tissue
samples from several family members.
Should family members be required to donate
this material against their wishes?

It has been suggested that a woman who
knows she is at reproductive risk for some genetic conditions may be liable if she fails to tell,
for example, her sister about the risk, and the sister
subsequently gives birth to an affected infant.

Also to be dealt with is the maintenance of severely deformed infants for the harvesting of organs and tissues (see ANENCEPHALY). If it is acceptable for fetal tissue to be used, is it acceptable for a woman to conceive precisely for this purpose? If this is acceptable for humanitarian purposes, such as supplying tissue to a family member who can only be helped this way, is it acceptable strictly for financial compensation?

Following the Supreme Court's lifting of most restrictions on abortion in 1973, the federal government in 1974 created an ethics advisory board for research involving human embryos and fetuses. The board was suspended in 1980. A number of medical schools and other organizations are creating committees and boards to deal with these issues. However, it seems certain that advances in science will continue to far outpace society's ability to answer the questions they raise.

For more information, contact:

The Hastings Center
255 Elm Road
Briarcliff Manor, NY 10510
(914) 762-8500

Kennedy Institute of Ethics
Georgetown University
Washington, DC 20057
(202) 687-6729

**ethnic groups**    All ethnic groups, that is, populations sharing a common genetic and geographic heritage, demonstrate greater incidence of one or more inherited conditions than the incidence displayed by the general population. This increased incidence may be due to the isolated, inbred population, in which a mutant gene is more common, or may simply be due to improved medical record-keeping or research in a given area. Scandinavian populations, for example, are noted for increased incidence of several rare hereditary disorders, and this increase may be due to both of the factors cited above. (See Table XI.)

The first to suggest inbreeding as a factor in higher rates of familial disorders found in population isolates was Joseph Adams in "A Treatise on the Supposed Hereditary Property of Disease," published in 1814.

Among the many disorders historically linked with particular ethnic groups are SICKLE-CELL ANEMIA in blacks, CYSTIC FIBROSIS in whites, THALASSEMIA in populations of Mediterranean ancestry, TAY-SACHS disease in Ashkenazi Jews and ACATALASIA in Japanese. (See also AMISH; JEWISH GENETIC DISEASES and MORMONS.)

**ethnocephaly**    See    HOLOPROSENCEPHALY.

**eugenics**    The science or study of the genetic and prenatal influences that affect expression of certain characteristics in offspring. The term was coined by English scientist Francis Galton (1822-1911) in 1833; he defined it as the improvement of a population by selective breeding of its best specimens. While this had long been practiced by farmers in plants and animals, Galton's concept of applying it to the human population was enthusiastically championed by many, initiating a eugenics movement that would hold sway for the next half century, until its ethical implications and practical problems, as well as Nazi policies and atrocities committed in its name, discredited it.

In the United States and Canada, the movement was responsible for the passage of laws forbidding mentally deficient individuals from having children. These statutes were enforced through compulsory sterilization, and the laws remained on the books in some states and provinces until after World War II. The Cold Spring Harbor Laboratory on Long Island, New York, one of the most respected genetics research centers in the world, was founded as the Eugenics Records Office, and became a center for the promulgation of these policies. Tens of thousands of mentally deficient individuals were sterilized in the United States, mostly

## Table XI
## Ethnicity of Genetic Disease

| Ethnic Group | Genetic Disorders |
| --- | --- |
| Acadian (Nova Scotia) | Niemann-Pick disease, Type D |
| American Indian | Congenital dislocation of hip, gallbladder disease |
| Amish (Pennsylvania) | Cartilage-hair hypoplasia, Ellis-von Creveld syndrome |
| Armenian | Familial mediterranean fever |
| Blacks | Sickle-cell disease, alpha and beta-thalassemia, G6PD deficiency, polydactyly, hypertension |
| Chinese | Alpha-thalassemia, G6PD deficiency |
| Eskimo | Congenital adrenal hyperplasia, methemoglobinemia, pseudocholinesterase deficiency |
| French Canadian (Quebec) | Tyrosinemia, Morquio syndrome, Tay-Sachs disease |
| Finns | Aspartylglucosaminuria, congenital nephrotic syndrome, lysinuric protein intolerance |
| Hutterite | Meckel syndrome, Bowen-Conradi syndrome |
| Irish | Phenylketonuria, neural tube defects |
| Japanese | Acatalasia |
| Jews | |
|   Ashkenazi | Abetalipoproteinemia, Bloom syndrome, Factor XI deficiency, familial dysautonomia, Gaucher disease (Type I), mucolipidosis IV, Niemann-Pick disease (Type A), pentosuria, spongy degeneration of the brain (Canavan disease), Tay-Sachs disease, torsion dystonia. |
|   Sephardic | Ataxia-telangiectasia (Morocco), congenital deafness (Morocco), cystinosis, cystinuria (Libya), familial Mediterranean fever |
|   Oriental | Alpha-thalassemia (Yemen), beta-thalassemia (Kurdistan), G6PD deficiency (Kurdistan, Iran, Iraq), Dubin -Johnson syndrome (Iran), phenylketonuria (Yemen), thrombasthenia of Glanzmann (Iraq) |
| Lebanese | Dyggve-Melchior-Clausen syndrome, juvenile Tay-Sachs disease |
| Mediterranean (Italian, Greek) | Beta-thalassemia, G6PD deficiency, familial Mediterranean fever |
| Mennonites (Old Colony, Canada) | Congenital adrenal hyperplasia, hypophosphatasia, Leigh's disease, Tourette syndrome, diabetes mellitus |
| South African Afrikaaner | Porphyria variegata, Huntington disease |
| SE Asian (Laotian, Thai, Vietnamese) | Alpha and beta-thalassemia |
| Scottish | Cystic fibrosis, phenylketonuria |

Source: Adapted from V.A. McKusick, *Mendelian Inheritance in Man*, 5th ed. (Baltimore: Johns Hopkins, 1978), pp. lix–lxi.

between the 1920s and the 1950s. In Virginia, approximately 8,300 were sterilized between 1924 and 1972, under a state law that was upheld in a landmark Supreme Court decision of 1927. In that ruling, Justice Oliver Wendell Holmes made a now notorious comment: "Three generations of imbeciles are enough."

In Nazi Germany, a system of eugenic health courts was established, and ordered the sterilization of more than half a million people between 1933 and 1940. These individuals were judged to be mentally retarded, psychologically disturbed, physically deformed or suffering from some other illness. Nazi physician Josef Mengele also conducted eugenic breeding experiments using 1,500 pairs of TWINS, both monozygotic and dizygotic (identical and fraternal).

China in 1988 began a program requiring individuals with an IQ of 49 or below to be sterilized if they are married or intend to marry.

**euthanasia, passive**   See PASSIVE EUTHANASIA.

**eventration of the diaphragm and diaphragmatic hernia**   Difficulty in breathing is a hallmark of both of these disorders, abnormalities of the diaphragm, the membrane separating the abdomen from the thoracic (chest) cavity. The lungs are in the thoracic cavity, and the motion of the diaphragm controls breathing.

## Eventration of the Diaphragm

An elevated diaphragm (eventration). This creates problems because the lung may have only minimal room to expand on the affected side. This abnormality may cause the space between the lungs (mediastinum) to shift to the opposite side, which may further impair lung function by compressing the otherwise unaffected lung. This disorder is thought to be due to the failure of a fetus to develop adequate muscle in the diaphragm. Complete congenital absence of muscle in the diaphragm is the most rare form of this disorder, and is incompatible with life.

The condition can also be acquired during delivery (see BIRTH INJURY) due to damage to the nerve controlling the diaphragm muscle and may be either temporary or permanent depending on whether the nerve is merely stretched or irreversibly damaged. Prognosis is excellent if surgery is performed before the infant has deteriorated from chronic oxygen insufficiency, prolonged failure of the lungs to expand (atelectasis) and associated pneumonia.

## Diaphragmatic Hernia

There are two types of diaphragmatic hernias. In posterolateral diaphragmatic hernias, the breathing difficulty is caused by the protrusion of an abdominal organ through the diaphragm into the chest cavity. (Posterolateral refers to the location of the hernia, in back and to the side of the breast bone [sternum].) Infants with this condition may appear bluish at birth. Symptoms progress with this condition as swallowed air distends hollow internal organs and tissues, pushing them into the chest and causing further heart/lung compression. The less developed the lungs are, the earlier the onset of symptoms and the higher the risk of death.

This condition occurs twice as often in males as in females. It is thought to be the result of an imbalance in timing in fetal development. As a result the intestines may migrate into the chest (thoracic) cavity through an abnormal opening in the diaphragm and compress the undeveloped lung buds.

The second type of diaphragmatic hernia, called a retrosternal hernia, may also affect newborns but usually isn't recognized until later in infancy and childhood. (Retrosternal refers to the location of the hernia, directly behind the sternum.) In most cases these extremely rare hernias occur on the right side of the body and seldom are they large enough to cause serious symptoms. It is theorized that this type of hernia occurs due to failure of muscular ingrowth during fetal development, or failure of the diaphragm to fuse properly.

Individuals with diaphragmatic hernias may enjoy a normal life span without disability if the repair is straightforward, lung development is normal and there are no other irregularities.

Inheritance modes for either of these conditions have not yet been determined. Diaphragmatic defects may be identified prenatally by ULTRASOUND examinations.

**exercise**    Moderate physical exercise has not been found to have an adverse impact on fetal health in women with normal pregnancies.

A Brown University study of fetal cardiac response found no impact from exercise, except for a brief period of reduced fetal heartbeat rate following extremely strenuous workouts. However, the American College of Obstetrics and Gynecologists recommends   that pregnant women maintain a pulse rate of no more than 140 beats per minute in exercise, and that they taper off slowly when completing their workouts.

**expressivity**    The degree to which an individual who has inherited the genes for a specific trait exhibits the characteristics of that trait. The term was coined by German neuropathologist Otto Vogt in 1926 (at the same time, he introduced a related term, PENETRANCE). (Vogt was an esteemed clinician of his time; he was summoned to Moscow from Berlin to attend Lenin after his first and second, and ultimately fatal, stroke. Critical of the Nazis as they came to power, Vogt was relegated to working as a stretcher-bearer in

World War II.) Many inherited conditions have a variable degree of expressivity, that is, the characteristics of the condition vary from mild to severe. In others, expressivity has little variation, with all cases exhibiting uniform characteristics and prognoses.

Generally, expressivity in AUTOSOMAL DOMINANT disorders is variable, while the expressivity in AUTOSOMAL RECESSIVE disorders tends to be more uniformly severe.

**exstrophy of bladder**   The protrusion of the bladder through the abdominal wall, caused by the failure of the abdomen to close properly during fetal development. This condition is surgically correctable.

# F

**Fabry disease**   A hereditary ENZYME deficiency. Caused by the deficiency of alpha-galactosidase A, this SYNDROME, seen mostly in males, is characterized by the accumulation of a glycosphingolipid (a derivative of a fat) trihexosyl ceramide, or GL-3, within the cardiovascular-renal system, the skin, eyes and mucous membranes in the mouth. Clusters of dark-red, raised, dot-like lesions of the skin (called angiokeratomas) usually appear during childhood and increase in size and number with age. They often appear in a "bathing suit" distribution, that is, on the buttocks, back, penis, scrotum, inner thighs and around the navel. The accumulation of GL-3 in the walls of small blood vessels leads to kidney disease, heart disease and stroke.

Named for J. Fabry (1860-1930), the German dermatologist who first described it in 1898, an English surgeon and dermatologist, W. Anderson (1842-1900), independently described it that same year.

In childhood affected males experience burning pain in the hands and feet (acroparesthesia). The pain may be triggered by exercise, fatigue, fever, emotional stress or change in temperature or humidity. They often

have diminished ability to sweat. Nausea, vomiting, diarrhea and abdominal or side pain is common. There may also be swelling of the legs due to subcutaneous accumulation of lymph (lymphedema).

Retarded growth and delayed puberty are common. Ocular abnormalities include swelling and distortion of the blood vessels in the conjunctiva and retina. A characteristic "whorl"-like deposit in the cornea is seen. These abnormalities do not interfere with vision. Cardiovascular and renal involvements increase with age.

The disorder exhibits X-LINKED recessive inheritance. Thus it is males who are primarily affected with the disorder. Female CARRIERS, however, often develop angiokeratomas and may have problems with burning pains. Very few have kidney or heart problems. However, the characteristic eye changes are commonly noted. A rough estimate for the frequency of the disorder is one in 40,000 individuals.

In the past those affected by the disorder usually died by the fourth decade, either from kidney failure or cerebrovascular complications. Recent advances in kidney dialysis and transplantation have improved the outlook for affected individuals.

PRENATAL DIAGNOSIS is possible via AMNIOCENTESIS or CHORIONIC VILLUS SAMPLING. At the present time, treatment is symptomatic, but researchers are working toward the possibility of enzyme replacement therapy for this disease.

**facio-scapulo-humeral dystrophy**
See MUSCULAR DYSTROPHY.

**failure to thrive**   A general term for the inability of an infant to gain weight and grow appropriately. It is often seen in infants affected by a variety of CONGENITAL ANOMALIES and congenital or early-onset GENETIC DISORDERS. There are also a myriad of other non-genetic or non-congenital causes.

**fallot, tetralogy of**   See TETRALOGY OF FALLOT.

## familial adenomatous polyposis (FAP)
See CANCER.

## familial cirrhosis
Cirrhosis, a degeneration of the liver due to scarring and replacement with connective tissue, has been observed in multiple siblings in several families with non-affected parents. Familial cirrhosis most likely represents a heterogeneous (that is, of varying causes; see HETEROGENE-ITY) group of disorders, and in some instances nongenetic factors may be responsible for the familial aggregation. (These cases do not include, for example, WILSON'S DISEASE, type IV GLYCOGEN STORAGE DISEASE and GALACTOSEMIA), which are well known causes of familial cirrhosis.)

In India, Indian childhood cirrhosis also affects multiple siblings. Onset usually occurs between six and 18 months of age. Progressive lethargy, jaundice, abdominal swelling and fever develop four to seven months before death.

## familial disease
A disease that occurs in several individuals of the same family with greater frequency than would be dictated by chance. This would obviously include genetic DISORDERS (both single-gene and MUL-TIFACTORIAL) but can also include environmentally-caused diseases, as a family shares a common environment.

The fact that some disorders now known to be genetically influenced often appeared to run in families has been noted since antiquity. For example, Jews recognized that HEMO-PHILIA affected only male members of a family. Among the familial conditions recognized by Hippocrates (ca. 460-ca. 377 B.C.), the father of medicine, were epilepsy (see HEREDI-TARY EPILEPSY), blue eyes and baldness, all of which are now known to be genetically influenced. (See also "INTRODUCTION.")

## familial dysautonomia
(Riley-Day syndrome)   A rare disorder of the autonomic nervous system and sensory system confined almost exclusively to Ashkenazi Jews (of Eastern European ancestry). As a result of defective development of the sensory system, individuals generally cannot feel pain or distinguish between hot and cold, and therefore are prone to injure themselves without realizing it. For example, they are unaware if a bone breaks or if they are being burned. Because of deficits in the autonomic nervous system, they have unstable blood pressure, body temperature (often with unexplained fever) and heart beat. Ingested food or liquid may go into the lungs rather than the gastrointestinal tract, often leading to repeated attacks of pneumonia.

This disorder was first identified in 1949 by U.S. pediatricians C.M. Riley and R.L. Day, and for some time was identified as "Riley-Day SYNDROME," but familial dysautonomia is the current preferred designation. (*Dysautonomia* refers to the disturbed function of the autonomic nervous system.)

Babies born with familial dysautonomia are "FLOPPY INFANTS" with poor muscle tone (hypotonia) and have difficulty feeding because they do not have a normal suck reflex. Perhaps the most distinctive sign is that they cannot produce tears when they cry or when foreign objects get in their eyes. The resulting irritation can create ocular problems and is a serious consequence of the disorder.

Ninety-five percent develop lateral spinal curvature (SCOLIOSIS), often beginning early in life. Other associated features are stunted growth, clumsiness, speech difficulties, drooling and uncontrollable vomiting attacks. There is generally no mental impairment. The tongue of affected individuals lacks taste buds (fungiform papillae), and the resulting flat, smooth appearance of the tongue is useful in establishing the diagnosis.

The disorder is inherited as an AUTOSO-MAL RECESSIVE trait, and about one in 30 to one in 50 Ashkenazi Jews is thought to be a CARRIER of the defective GENE. The incidence among the at-risk population is thought to be one in 10,000 live births, though a recent study in Israel found a higher incidence (one in 3,703). There is no method of detecting carriers or PRENATAL DIAGNOSIS for this disorder. A frequently used diagnostic test involves the injection of histamine into the skin. Affected individuals will not get the characteristic redness (flare) around the injection.

In the past, approximately half of all cases succumbed to respiratory infections or other problems by the age of five, but now 80% are surviving beyond childhood, with many surviving into the adult years. (SEE also INDIFFERENCE TO PAIN.)

For more information, contact:

Dysautonomia Foundation, Inc.
20 East 46th Street, 3rd Floor
New York, NY 10017
(212) 949-6644

Dysautonomia Treatment & Evaluation Center
New York University Medical Center
530 First Avenue, Suite 3A
New York, NY 10016
(212) 340-7225

National Foundation for Jewish Genetic Disease
250 Park Avenue, Suite 1000
New York, NY 10017
(212) 371-1030

**familial Mediterranean fever**   This disorder is characterized by short, recurrent bouts of fever accompanied by pain in the abdomen, chest and/or joints, and a red rash. The attacks have their onset between the ages of five and 15 years, and frequency and duration of the episodes are unpredictable. It is most common in Middle Eastern ethnic groups, Armenians and Sephardic Jews (those who lived in Spain and left during the era of the Inquisitions, settling in various countries bordering the Mediterranean). There have also been reports of clusters of the disorder in individuals of Irish and Italian descent.

While there is no specific treatment, the disorder is not life-threatening, though

AMYLOIDOSIS, an accumulation of amyloid, a starch-like material, may accompany the disorder and damage internal organs. The abdominal symptoms have caused many undiagnosed patients to undergo needless exploratory abdominal surgery.

The disorder is inherited as an AUTOSOMAL RECESSIVE trait. Frequency in some at-risk populations has been estimated as high as one in 2,700, with CARRIER frequency estimated at between approximately one in 25 and one in 50. Colchicine, a medicine used to treat gout, has been used as a treatment.

**familial nephritis**   (Alport syndrome) A hereditary form of kidney failure often associated with DEAFNESS. Symptoms include blood and protein in the urine (hematuria; proteinuria) and elevated blood pressure. Hereditary nephritis is also known as Alport syndrome. In 1927, South African physician A.C. Alport (1880-1959) identified the combination of hematuria and sensorineural deafness (deafness caused by anomalies in the auditory nerves, rather than conductive deafness which is caused by anomalies in physical structures of the hearing organs) as a specific syndrome. The family he described had been the subject of reports dating to 1902. Most cases of familial nephritis represent Alport syndrome, though forms of the disease without deafness have been described. These latter in particular are quite heterogeneous, that is, have a different genetic basis but a common expression with AUTOSOMAL DOMINANT, AUTOSOMAL RECESSIVE and X-LINKED dominant forms described. The hematuria is rarely severe, and the blood in the urine may require microscopic examination for detection. The kidney disease is generally more severe in males, leading to eventual kidney failure and death between the third and fourth decade of life if untreated. Females tend to have a relatively benign course, with no decrease in life expectancy.

In classic Alport disease, in addition to the progressive high frequency sensorineural deafness, there are generally also eye lesions, which may lead to visual deterioration. The kidney has specific changes evident on electron microscopy, and the defect appears to be related to an abnormality of type IV collagen, a component of connective tissue. This disorder is inherited in an X-linked manner, with males exhibiting more severe manifestations than females. The gene responsible appears to be on the middle of the long arm of the X-chromosome.

## familial panhypopituitary dwarfism
See PITUITARY DWARFISM SYNDROMES.

## familial polyposis of the colon (FPC)
See CANCER.

## Fanconi anemia (Fanconi pancytopenia)
Syndrome characterized by multiple CONGENITAL abnormalities, bone marrow failure and CHROMOSOME ABNORMALITIES, and named for Swiss pediatrician Guido Fanconi (1882-1979), who described it in 1927. While the disorder is variable in expression, the manifestations are potentially severe and life threatening.

Infants tend to have LOW BIRTH WEIGHT. The skin often exhibits abnormal pigmentation, consisting of generalized small patches of darkened skin and café au lait spots. The face is asymmetrical, with a small head (MICROCEPHALY), small eyes (microphthalmia), drooping eyelids (PTOSIS) and malformed ears. They may have various abnormalities of the thumb, congenital hip dislocation and deformities of the ribs and vertebrae. There are frequently abnormalities of the genitourinary tract and CONGENITAL HEART DEFECTS. Muscles on the upper trunk and shoulders may be underdeveloped. Some individuals have MENTAL RETARDATION, and DEAFNESS has been reported.

Bone marrow failure develops at approximately seven or eight years of age, and it involves the decreased production of the entire range of blood cells—red cells (resulting in anemia), white cells and platelets—due to abnormalities of the bone marrow, where the blood cells are produced. The decrease in number of blood cells is progressive and often lethal. There is also an increased tendency to develop leukemia and other CANCERS, and the CHROMOSOMES, upon examination, display a propensity for breakage.

The basic defect that causes Fanconi's anemia is unknown. It is inherited as an AUTOSOMAL RECESSIVE trait.

CARRIER screening is not currently possible. However, PRENATAL DIAGNOSIS has been accomplished in at-risk pregnancies by findings of increased chromosome breakage in fetal cells collected via AMNIOCENTESIS.

For more information, contact:

Fanconi's Anemia Support Group
   International
c/o Frohnmayer
2875 Baker Blvd.
Eugene, OR 97403
(503) 421-8453

## Fanconi pancytopenia
See FANCONI ANEMIA.

## Farber lipogranulomatosis
See LIPOGRANULOMATOSIS.

## favism
Common in Sicily and Sardinia and recognized since antiquity, this is a hereditary deficiency of an ENZYME (glucose-6-phosphate dehydrogenase) in red blood cells, resulting in a sensitivity to fava beans (*Vicia fava*), which are staples of the diet in the population at risk. (Fava beans are also the main commercial source of L-dopa, a drug used in the treatment of PARKINSON'S DISEASE.)

It appears that the bean produces a substance that induces the breakdown (hemolysis) of enzyme-deficient red blood cells. Ingestion of as little as one seed of a fava bean, or inhalation of pollen, is enough to precipitate an attack. These episodes are characterized by malaise, headache, dizziness, fever, acute hemolytic ANEMIA, vomiting and diarrhea. Within approximately 24 hours, the skin takes on a yellowish tone (jaundice) and hemoglobin from the destroyed red cells is found in the urine (hemoglobinuria). It may lead to prostration and coma.

The sensitivity apparently diminishes over time, for children are more commonly affected than adults. The condition has been observed even in nursing infants whose mothers ingested the bean.

**fetal alcohol syndrome (FAS)**   Though a link between excessive alcohol consumption during pregnancy and BIRTH DEFECTS has been noted since the time of the ancient Greeks, a specific syndrome of defects associated with fetal exposure to alcohol was identified only in 1973. Designated fetal alcohol syndrome (FAS), it is characterized by INTRA-UTERINE GROWTH RETARDATION, typical facial features, MENTAL RETARDATION, and defects of the central nervous and cardiac systems. It is thought to be one of the most common cause of mental retardation, behind DOWN SYNDROME, FRAGILE X SYNDROME and SPINA BIFIDA. (Some health experts believe it is the number one cause.) The degree of mental retardation varies, with the average IQ between 63 and 68. Affected individuals exhibit poor hand-eye coordination, hyperactivity, trembling and poor attention span.

Characteristic facial features include a small head (MICROCEPHALY) and eyes, folds of the skin that obscure the inner juncture of the eyelids (EPICANTHUS), short, upturned nose (anteverted nares), thin upper lip and underdeveloped philtrum, the groove extending from the middle of the upper lip to the nose. Those affected may also exhibit dental abnormalities in childhood, including upper and lower teeth that fail to meet properly when biting (malocclusion).

Alcohol, a small molecule, easily passes through the placenta and enters the fetal bloodstream. It remains in the FETUS longer than in the adult. Drinking binges further exacerbate risks to fetal development. In addition to direct consequences of alcohol abuse, drinking may cause vitamin and mineral deficiencies in the mother, which may also contribute to fetal malformations.

Most infants with FAS are born to chronic alcoholics. The risks of occasional or moderate drinking (generally considered one or two drinks per day) are unknown, though there is agreement that the more alcohol a pregnant woman drinks, the greater the risk to her fetus. Some organizations, such as the National Institute on Alcohol Abuse and Alcoholism, go as far as to recommend total abstinence during pregnancy.

An estimated one-third of infants born to chronic alcoholic mothers are believed to exhibit some degree of fetal alcohol syndrome. FAS infants are of below average birthweight and at one year of age are typically only 65% of normal length (see LOW BIRTHWEIGHT). Those who don't have the full-blown syndrome, but exhibit some symptoms, are said to have fetal alcohol effects (FAE).

Fetal alcohol syndrome is estimated to occur in approximately one in 700 to one in 2,000 live births. In various studies, FAE has been estimated to occur in from 1.7 per 1,000 live births to 90.1 per 1,000 live births. (See also ALCOHOLISM.)

For more information, contact:

National Center for Education in Maternal
  & Child Health
38th and R Streets, NW
Washington, DC 20057
(202) 625-8400

Fetal Alcohol Syndrome Research Center
C.S. Mott Center
275 East Hancock
Detroit, MI 48201
(313) 577-1485

**fetal aminopterin syndrome**   Aminopterin is a drug prescribed for treatment of CANCER. Taken during the first trimester of pregnancy, it can cause severe abnormalities and fetal death. Fetal exposure after the first trimester may induce a variety of bone deformities and MENTAL RETARDATION. (See also TERATOGENS.)

**fetal face syndrome**   See ROBINOW SYNDROME.

**fetal imaging**    Obtaining an image of the fetus in the uterus. This can be of great help to the physician in determining the gestational age of the fetus and its general condition, as well as aiding in PRENATAL DIAGNOSIS of various disorders. The main techniques for fetal imaging are ULTRASOUND and FETOSCOPY. Fetoscopy carries certain risks and is not frequently employed.

Another method of fetal imaging is by X ray. This is usually done to visualize the fetal skeleton at 17 to 19 weeks. The injection of a special water-soluble contrast dye provides information about the position of the fetus. Since some of the dye is swallowed by the fetus, this procedure also indicates its swallowing ability and the condition of its gastrointestinal tract. Risks are uncertain: There has been speculation that infants exposed to X rays in utero have higher incidence of childhood CANCER.

**fetal surgery**    Surgery performed on an infant prior to birth. Though most BIRTH DEFECTS are best treated after birth, a small and growing number are amenable to treatment prior to delivery. In most instances where surgery is performed, the infant would not survive without surgical intervention. Risk to the health of the mother, and her ability to have future pregnancies, are also considerations in fetal surgery decisions.

Among the conditions that may in some cases be suggested for surgery are HYDROCEPHALUS, herniated diaphragm (see EVENTRATION OF THE DIAPHRAGM AND DIAPHRAGMATIC HERNIA), hydronephrosis, an obstruction of the urinary tract, and multiple pregnancies, in which selected embryos are aborted to improve chances of survival of the remaining ones (see MULTIPLE BIRTHS; ABORTION).

The surgery may be performed through the amniotic sac while the infant is in the womb, or an incision may be made in the abdomen and the fetus partially removed. In the latter operation, the fetus is usually out of the womb for between three and 30 minutes.

It has been discovered that operations on infants before birth leave no scars. Some cosmetic surgeons suggest that facial deformities such as CLEFT LIP, or more serious conditions such as APERT SYNDROME could be successfully treated before birth and heal with no trace.

The first human fetal surgery in the United States was performed in 1981, by Dr. Michael R. Harrison of the University of California at San Francisco, on an infant with hydronephrosis. Hydrocephalus was the first condition successfully treated. Currently, animals are being used to test experimental surgery and to practice surgical techniques for fetal repair of hernias of the diaphragm and SPINA BIFIDA, as well as for transplant techniques for fetal organs and fetal cells.

Non-surgical fetal treatments have been performed, including transfusions, and administration of drugs such as digitalis for heart failure or vitamin B12 for prenatally diagnosed methylmalonic acidemia.

For more information, contact:

International Fetal Medicine and Surgery
  Society
3rd & Parnassus Avenue
San Francisco, CA 94143-0510
(415) 476-4086

**fetal tissue sampling**    Collection of a small amount of tissue from a developing embryo. Fetal tissue samples can currently be obtained by one of several methods: AMNIOCENTESIS, CHORIONIC VILLUS SAMPLING, FETOSCOPY or directly under ultrasound guidance. Amniocentesis will provide tissue samples (essentially fetal skin and bladder cells) suspended in the amniotic fluid; chorionic villus sampling involves suction of tissue from tiny fronds at the edge of the placenta; and fetoscopy allows cutting out of a tiny tissue sample from the fetus itself. Newer techniques allow for direct sampling without the fetoscope under ultrasound guidance. The most common of these is CORDOCENTESIS and involves direct sampling of fetal blood from the umbilical vein. In this technique, also called percutaneous umbilical blood sampling or PUBS, a needle is placed in the vein under ultrasound guidance. Similarly, fetal skin or tissue biopsies can be done by use of a tiny biopsy forceps or needle directed by ultrasound. Risks are involved in all of these procedures, with amniocentesis being the safest and most commonly used technique.

**fetoscopy**   Direct visualization of the fetus, placenta and umbilical cord by the use of a fetoscope, a thin, flexible, fiberoptic tube that can be inserted into the uterus. The field of view and depth of focus is limited, although a 5X magnification is possible.

ULTRASOUND imaging is vitally important in fetoscopy. The position of the fetus, the placenta and the umbilical cord must be determined accurately in advance to avoid injury, and to guide the path of the instruments. Local anesthesia is used, and an incision is made in the mother's abdomen. A thin tube (cannula) containing a sharp, pointed surgical instrument (trocar) is inserted through the incision, piercing the wall of the uterus, and then into the amniotic cavity. Once the cannula is in place, the trocar is withdrawn and the fetoscope with its viewing lens is inserted.

While direct visualization of the fetus can provide valuable information, fetoscopy is primarily used to obtain fetal blood and tissue samples used in PRENATAL DIAGNOSIS. Drawing of blood from the placenta and using a forceps device inserted with the fetoscope to snip a tissue sample from the fetus are extremely delicate operations. They are undertaken only when absolutely necessary for prenatal diagnosis of blood or GENETIC DISORDERS that cannot be more safely obtained through other procedures, such as AMNIOCENTESIS and DNA analysis. Even in skilled hands, fetoscopy carries a 3% to 6% risk of fetal death and miscarriage and a 10% risk of premature birth (see ABORTION, PREMATURITY).

When required, fetoscopy is performed at 17 to 20 weeks of gestation; because of the risk factors involved, it is infrequently used and is undertaken only after careful consideration and consultation between the prospective parents and an obstetrical team. The procedure has been largely replaced by other ultrasound guided techniques. For example, CORDOCENTESIS can be used to obtain fetal blood samples: Under ultrasound guidance a needle can be placed in the umbilical vein to obtain blood without the need to introduce the large-sized fetoscope. The risks of cordocentesis are much lower, about 1%. Similar techniques can be used for other biopsies.

**fetus**   The developing offspring within the uterus. In humans, the developing infant is regarded as a fetus from the third month of pregnancy to birth; prior to the third month it is referred to as an embryo.

**fibrodysplasia ossificans progressiva (FOP)** (myositis ossificans)   The formation of misplaced bony lesions (ossification) in soft tissues, such as connective tissue, skeletal muscle, tendons and ligaments. There are also typical foot and hand malformations associated with FOP: misaligned and shortened big toes, abnormally small thumbs and incurved fifth fingers. Onset usually occurs before age four but may occur as late as puberty. About 30% experience hearing loss, another 30% easy bruisability.

Ossification typically begins in the head, neck, spine or shoulders, and goes on to involve many sites, including the chest, hips, ankles, wrists and, least commonly, hands. Each new lesion is painfully tender and swollen for several weeks until it becomes bony. As ossification continues, the individual finds it increasingly difficult to accomplish tasks unassisted, such as getting out of bed, dressing and bathing. Currently, no surgery or drug therapy affects the course of the disease.

The basic defect that causes FOP, an extremely rare condition, is unknown. It has been suggested, however, that the abnormal cells that eventually become the misplaced (heterotopic) bony lesions develop on the 43rd to 44th day after conception and become spread out at incorrect sites in the body. FOP is inherited as an AUTOSOMAL DOMINANT trait, though most cases have been SPORADIC. There is an increased incidence associated with advanced paternal age.

**fifth disease**    Viral disease, caused by parvovirus 19, that takes its name from being the fifth of six pediatric disorders identified by scientists. The first four were rubella, MEASLES, scarlet fever and Dukes disease, which is a mild form of scarlet fever. The sixth disorder is exanthema subitum, also called roseola infantum.

Maternal infection with fifth disease during pregnancy can cause stillbirth or miscarriage, though the risk is thought to be small. The virus suppresses the fetal bone marrow, causing severe ANEMIA, congestive heart failure and fluid retention. Unlike rubella, there has been little evidence that fifth disease can cause BIRTH DEFECTS; however, this is not clear.

First reported in Europe in 1889, it usually occurs in the spring and winter among children from two to 12 years of age, and its most striking feature is a characteristic rash resembling a slap mark, usually found on the face and occasionally spreading to other parts of the body. Symptoms of fever and rash typically persist for about a week. Infection can be diagnosed via a sophisticated blood test. Some fetuses that have been severely anemic due to maternal infection have been treated with blood transfusions in utero.

**Finnish-type sialuria**    See SALLA DISEASE.

**FLK syndrome**    "FLK" stands for "Funny-Looking Kid," and was a general term for infants affected with various malformation SYNDROMES, particularly those involving multiple facial abnormalities. Considered demeaning and insensitive, it is no longer in use.

**floppy infant**    An infant with poor muscle tone (hypotonia), exhibiting an inability to move limbs or other parts and presenting a limp, floppy appearance. It is common among newborns with many GENETIC DISORDERS and other CONGENITAL ANOMALIES.

**focal dermal hypoplasia**    See GOLTZ SYNDROME.

**focal dystomia**    See DYSTONIA.

**Forbes disease**    See GLYCOGEN STORAGE DISEASE.

**fragile site**    Specific points of the CHROMOSOMES that are prone to break, or at least to appear broken. When the chromosomes are "damaged" in this manner, the chromosomal aberrations that ensue may result in GENETIC DISORDERS. Translocations may occur at these sites, and they may have importance in the genetic changes underlying CANCER. (See also FRAGILE X SYNDROME; CHROMOSOME ABNORMALITIES.)

**fragile X syndrome**    X-LINKED trait, and the second most common identifiable cause of genetic MENTAL RETARDATION after DOWN SYNDROME. It was first identified by geneticist Herbert Lubs, who observed the chromosomal defect responsible for the syndrome in 1969.

Some people have chromosomes that when studied in the laboratory, have a tendency to "break" or "tear." The damage to these aberrant chromosomes typically occurs in particular regions, called FRAGILE SITES. Most of the time these fragile sites are not associated with medical problems, but a pronounced gap in one such region, at the end of the long arm of the X chromosome (referred to by cytogeneticists as

Xq27-Xq28; see CHROMOSOME ABNORMALI-TIES), is associated with fragile X syndrome.

In addition to moderate to severe mental retardation, other characteristics of individuals with fragile X syndrome may include large ears, large testes (macroorchidism), large jaw (prognathism), speech delays, prominent forehead, double- jointedness, autistic symptoms and occasional self-mutilation.

For unexplained reasons, fragile X syndrome does not behave in the typical manner of an X-linked trait. Nearly 20% of fragile X males are silent CARRIERS, who are unaffected by the SYNDROME but can pass the fragile X chromosome to their female offspring. About one-third of female fragile X carriers, who would be expected to be asymptomatic, exhibit some symptoms of the disorder.

Since the late-19th century it has been noted that males institutionalized for mental retardation outnumber females by five to four. The fragile X syndrome and other forms of X-linked mental retardation account for part of the difference.

Fragile X syndrome is estimated to affect one in 2,000 males and to be responsible for 10% of mentally retarded males. It has been described in whites, blacks, Indians, Filipinos, Japanese and Zulus.

PRENATAL DIAGNOSIS is possible through examination of tissue cultures obtained by AMNIOCENTESIS. However, the tissue must be cultured in a medium very low in folic acid. In this environment, the characteristic lesion can be detected by chromosomal analysis.

Folic acid is a form of vitamin B, and there have been attempts to treat fragile X individuals with vitamin B therapy, but the results thus far are generally considered inconclusive.

For more information, contact:

The Fragile X Foundation
P.O. Box 300233
Denver, CO 80203
(303) 861-6630

**Fraser syndrome**   See ABLEPHARIA.

**Freeman-Sheldon syndrome**   See WHISTLING FACE SYNDROME.

**Friedreich's ataxia**   Ataxias are disorders characterized by neuromuscular disturbances resulting in the loss of coordination and balance, and Freidreich's ataxia (FA) is the most common inherited form. It is named for Nikolaus Friedreich, a German neurologist who, in the 1860s, published the first description of a mysterious inherited disease marked by progressive loss of coordination and nerve degeneration.

FA typically begins in the first or second decade of life. Clumsiness is exhibited in the upper or lower extremities, along with a peculiar swaying and irregular movements. As the disease progresses, there is further impairment of limb coordination, gradual loss of sensation in affected limbs, and muscle weakness. Eventually, speech can become affected, making communication difficult. Lateral curvature of the spine (SCOLIOSIS) usually develops, often with disabling results. Foot deformities and heart disease are also frequent features. As many as 40% of affected individuals have DIABETES. Within five years of onset, use of a wheelchair may be required. Complications are often fatal. The mean age of death is 37, though some that have come to medical attention appear to have a normal life expectancy.

While the cause of FA is unknown, neurons that transmit sensory information from the limbs to the spinal cord display degenerative changes.

The incidence is difficult to judge, as many affected individuals may be misdiagnosed. Estimates of the total number of affected individuals in the United States range from approximately 7,500 to 20,000. It is generally inherited in an AUTOSOMAL RECESSIVE manner, though there may be an AUTOSOMAL DOMINANT form.

Recently, the location of the GENE responsible for FA was mapped at CHROMOSOME 9. As a result of this discovery, for the first time, CARRIER detection in members of the immediate family should be possible by GENETIC LINKAGE studies, as well as by PRENATAL DIAGNOSIS in families with one or more affected children.

A number of drugs in development may help alleviate some symptoms of this disorder, but currently there is no cure.

For more information, contact:

Friedreich's Ataxia Group in America, Inc.
P.O. Box 11116
Oakland, CA 94611
(415) 655-0833

Muscular Dystrophy Association
810 Seventh Ave.
New York, NY 10019
(212) 586-0808

**frontometaphyseal dysplasia**    Rare hereditary disorder marked by a peculiar facial appearance, dental abnormalities, multiple joint contractures (see ARTHROGRYPOSIS) and skeletal deformities. The ridges above the eyes (supraorbital ridges) tend to be prominent and the chin pointed and small. Onset of skeletal deformities begins in early childhood. Lifespan and intelligence are normal in most of those affected. It is inherited as an X-LINKED trait with severe manifestations in males and variable but generally more mild manifestations in females.

**fructose intolerance**    (fructose-1-phosphate aldolase deficiency)    Fructose is a sugar present in foods such as fruits, sugar cane, corn syrup, honey and fruit juices. Table sugar or sucrose contains fructose and glucose. Fructose intolerance occurs when the body is unable to metabolize fructose because of the hereditary absence or defi-

ciency of the ENZYME fructose-1-phosphate aldolase. Ingestion of fructose under these conditions results in the blocking of the formation of glucose, a sugar essential as a major source of energy for the body.

In infants born with fructose intolerance, the continued feeding of foods containing fructose will have serious complications, leading to nausea, vomiting, FAILURE TO THRIVE, seizure, caused by an abnormally low level of blood sugar (hypoglycemia), enlarged liver (hepatomegaly), jaundice, excessive fluid in the tissues (edema), abnormal pooling of fluid in the abdominal cavity, malnutrition and wasting, eventual liver failure, dehydration and death. When the disorder is not discovered, infants with fructose intolerance who continue to be fed foods containing fructose often die between two and six months of age.

The disorder can be detected after birth by a fructose tolerance test or a liver biopsy that will disclose the enzyme deficiency. Once the determination is made, all fructose-containing foods must be completely avoided. Full recovery will follow with a normal life span.

This rare disorder is inherited as an AUTOSOMAL RECESSIVE trait. As the gene for the deficient enzyme has been cloned, and several mutations causing the disease identified, DNA-based diagnosis is now possible. This can potentially be used as an alternative to loading tests or liver biopsy for diagnosis, or for carrier detection and prenatal diagnosis in certain families

**fructose-1-phosphate aldolase deficiency**    See FRUCTOSE INTOLERANCE.

**fucosidosis**    Very rare syndrome, identified in well under 100 children and caused by a deficiency of the ENZYME alpha-L-fucosidase, which results in abnormal intracelluar accumulation of fucose, a sugar containing compounds such as glypolipids, lipoproteins, oliogosaccharides and polysaccharides. Three and possibly four forms of fucosidosis have been identified. Children with more severe forms of the disorder (types I and II) do not generally survive beyond six years of age.

In type I, mental and motor development stop at age 10 months, followed by progressive deterioration of the nervous system and muscle weakness, followed in turn by the onset of spasticity and tremor and a loss of awareness of environmental contact—eventually resulting in a state of total unresponsiveness.

Frequently, physical characteristics include thick skin, short head with a prominent forehead, heavy eyebrows, wide-spaced eyes (HYPERTELORISM), flat nose and thick lips. The chest is broad, and lateral curvature of the spine (SCOLIOSIS) may be evident. The heart is often enlarged. Severe enlargement of the liver and spleen are evident (hepatosplenomegaly), giving affected infants an appearance resembling children with Hurler syndrome and other MUCOPOLYSACCHARIDOSES.

Type II is similar to type I, though less severe. Degenerative processes usually begin at age 18 months. Type III manifests itself later than types I and II, perhaps around age three years. Deterioration of mental and motor skills and nervous system is less rapid. Skin lesions may develop, primarily in the pubic area. These lesions are termed angiokeratomas and are dilated blood vessels whose walls are filled with accumulated substances and resemble those seen in FABRY DISEASE. Type IV is similar to type III, except that the skin is thin and dry and no skin lesions are present. Individuals with types III and IV survive longer than those with types I and II, perhaps living into their third decade.

A specific diagnosis may be made by low white blood cell or skin fibroblast activity of alpha-L-fucosidase. PRENATAL DIAGNOSIS may be made by examining fetal cells obtained via AMNIOCENTESIS or CHORIONIC VILLUS SAMPLING.

This disorder displays an AUTOSOMAL RECESSIVE inheritance pattern. There may be a higher frequency in children of Italian descent.

# G

**G syndrome** (Opitz-Frias syndrome; hypertelorism-hypospadias syndrome) The characteristic facial appearance of individuals with G-syndrome includes asymmetric skull, wide-spaced eyes (HYPERTELORISM), flat bridge of the nose, prominent ridge on the side of the skull, slit-like eyelids that are often slanted either slightly upward or downward, a fold of skin that obscures the inner juncture of the eyelids (EPICANTHUS), upturned nose (anteverted nares) and abnormal development of the ear with some degree of backward rotation. Additionally, there are genital and perhaps anal abnormalities in males. Typically, males have HYPOSPADIAS, the malposition of the urethral opening on the underside of the penis. Affected infants have a hoarse or harsh cry.

Frequently the swallowing mechanism is faulty, which may result in choking and coughing. If such a defect is present, alternative methods of feeding are essential to ensure survival. Swallowing capacity improves with time—usually a few months to one year—to the extent that individuals are able to eat a normal diet. Death, when it occurs, generally is due to aspiration or starvation. In mild cases, prognosis for life span and reproductive ability appears normal. About two-thirds of patients may have some mild to moderate MENTAL RETARDATION.

The "G" in G syndrome is taken from the first letter of the last name of the family in which this condition was initially observed. This is a method of naming disorders favored by geneticist Dr. John Opitz, chairman of the department of medical genetics at Shodair hospital in Helena, Montana, who first identified the condition in 1969.

This rare syndrome appears to be an AUTOSOMAL DOMINANT trait that occurs with some male sex limitation (see SEX LIMITED). There is currently no method of PRENATAL DIAGNOSIS.

**galactokinase deficiency**    Symptoms of this enzyme deficiency are CATARACTS in early infancy, associated with an excess of the sugar galactose in the blood (GALACTOSE-MIA). Affected individuals lack the ENZYME galactokinase, which helps metabolize galactose. This disorder is a variant form of galactosemia. The sole clinical significance of this deficiency is that the accumulation of unmetabolized galactose eventually leads to cataracts.

This disorder can be detected at any age by blood and urine tests. Newborns are routinely screened for galactosemia in many states, and depending on what test is used, galactokinase deficiency may be found. A diet that excludes milk, milk products and other sources of galactose prevents cataract formation and can reverse cataracts that have just begun to form. Cataracts can also be removed surgically.

Life span is normal, although cataracts may recur, requiring further surgery.

Galactokinase deficiency is inherited as an AUTOSOMAL RECESSIVE trait. First observed in three Gypsy families, well under 100 individuals with the disorder are known. Its frequency is estimated at one in 100,000 or less.

**galactosemia**    A rare hereditary metabolic disease observed in the newborn that can lead to MENTAL RETARDATION, BLINDNESS and ultimately death. It is caused by the inability to convert galactose (a milk sugar) into glucose (blood sugar), the body's fuel. This inability results from the absence of galactose-1-phosphate uridyl-transferase, the ENZYME responsible for this conversion.

Inherited as an AUTOSOMAL RECESSIVE trait, galactosemia is estimated to occur in approximately one in 20,000 to one in 60,000 live births.

The disease usually appears within the first few days of life, following ingestion of breast milk or formula. Early symptoms include lethargy, feeding difficulties, vomiting, jaundice and an enlarged liver (hepatomegaly). Affected individuals may also exhibit irritability, FAILURE TO THRIVE, diarrhea and severe bacterial infections. Untreated, it may lead to

death. Those who survive, even with prompt treatment, often fail to grow, may be mentally retarded, develop CATARACTS and may suffer liver and kidney damage.

Galactosemia is the most common cause of cataracts in infancy. The elevated level of galactose and other sugars in the blood allows them to be absorbed into the cells of the lens of the eye. There, the sugars absorb water, swelling the eye to the extent that it loses transparency.

Many states have mandatory neonatal screening programs for galactosemia. Diagnosis is made on the basis of blood tests that measure the infant's level of conversion enzyme activity in the blood cells. Affected newborns exhibit no enzyme activity, while CARRIERS have about half the normal activity level. Galactose will also be present in the urine of those affected.

PRENATAL DIAGNOSIS is possible via AMNIOCENTESIS. Though it has been recommended that pregnant women who are known CARRIERS, or whose infants have been diagnosed in utero, should exclude galactose from their diets it is not established that this is effective. Affected individuals may have to eliminate galactose from their diets for their entire lives.

For more information, contact:

The American Liver Foundation
998 Pompton Avenue
Cedar Grove, NJ 07009
(201) 857-2626
(800) 223-0179

The Children's Liver Foundation, Inc.
155 Maplewood Avenue
Maplewood, NJ 07040
(201) 761-1111

**gallbladder anomalies**    This group of ANOMALIES takes many forms. In its most extreme variation, the gallbladder is completely absent (gallbladder agenesis), usually in association with incomplete development of the bile ducts. Another variation is duplication of the gallbladder. Other, very rare variations include: bilobed gallbladder, in which the gallbladder is partially divided (but not separated into two duplicate organs); diverticulum of gallbladder, in which a portion of the gallbladder herniates through a weak spot to form an extra pouch on the outside of an organ; floating gallbladder, in which the membrane (mesentery) that attaches the gallbladder to the body is greatly elongated; and anomalous location or ectopic gallbladder, in which the gallbladder is displaced to the left or the rear or is inside the liver.

The basic defect that causes these conditions is unknown. Normal life span is not affected, and the condition is usually asymptomatic except in circumstances where a floating gallbladder turns, twisting the mesentery, cutting off the organ's blood supply and causing pain, nausea and vomiting.

The genetic basis for the disorders is unknown. CONGENITAL absence of gallbladder occurs in approximately one in 3,300 live births, and duplications of gallbladder in one in 4,000 live births. Other variations are extremely rare. Currently, there is no PRENATAL DIAGNOSTIC method available, though the gallbladder may be visualized by prenatal ULTRASOUND (fetal gallstones have been diagnosed in this way).

**gampsodactyly**   See CLAWFOOT.

**Gardner syndrome**   See colorectal cancer under CANCER.

**gastroschisis**   The failure of the abdominal wall to close completely before birth. As a result, the viscera are exposed at birth and usually protrude through the opening. Typically the opening is small (three to five cm; 1.2-2 in) and to the right of the umbilicus, the point at which the umbilical cord joins the abdomen. The umbilicus is not affected, as contrasted with OMPHALOCELES. The intestines may be abnormally short. In some cases,

the protrusion causes blockage of the intestines or abnormal attachment to other structures.

The cause is not known. The defect is found in about one in 10,000 to one in 15,000 live births. Most cases are SPORADIC, but familial occurrence has been documented in five families.

In contrast with omphalocele, gastroschisis is not associated with an increased incidence of other anomalies.

**Gaucher disease (GD)**   Named for Dr. Philippe C.E. Gaucher, a French physician who first described the disease in 1882, Gaucher disease is an inherited metabolic disorder that leads to the accumulation of a particular lipid, a fatty substance, in internal organs.

GD, like other similar metabolic disorders, is referred to as a STORAGE DISEASE, due to the accumulation, or storage, of material in the body. The accumulation is the result of a deficiency of the ENZYME acid ß-glucosidase, which is necessary to break down a particular lipid, glucosyl ceramide. As it accumulates, the glucosyl ceramide is stored in the scavenger cells of the body, which, taking on a characteristic appearance unique to those affected with this disorder, are called "Gaucher cells." This lipid, which is normally present in only small amounts, accumulates in the spleen, liver and bone marrow and, in some cases, in the lungs. (It accumulates in the central nervous system only in types 2 and 3.)

Gaucher cells in the bone marrow can cause bone and joint pain, fractures and other orthopedic problems. Accumulation in the spleen and liver causes enlargement of these organs and can lead to blood abnormalities such as ANEMIA, easy bruising and impaired blood clotting.

Affected individuals experience pain, frequent nosebleeds, anemia, lack of energy, infections and extremely distended abdomens. At present, therapy for the disease is symptomatic. As the bones weaken, surgery may be required for hip or knee joint replacement. Surgical removal of the enlarged spleen may be necessary to correct the problems related to low blood counts.

Although GD affects all racial and ethnic groups, it is particularly prevalent in Ashkenazi Jews (of Central and Eastern European ancestry) and is the most common genetic disorder among this population: As many as one in 25 are estimated to be CARRIERS of the GENE for this disease.

Inherited as an AUTOSOMAL RECESSIVE disorder, its incidence is estimated to be approximately one in 2,500 live births among Ashkenazi Jews and one in 40,000 live births in the general population. It has been estimated that there are approximately 20,000 affected individuals in the United States.

There are three types of GD, differing in their severity, course and incidence. The three forms are differentiated by the absence or presence and severity of primary neurologic manifestations.

*Type 1—chronic (Non-Neuronopathic) form.* This is by far the most common form, with wide variability in the symptoms and severity. Features may include enlarged spleen and liver (hepatosplenomegaly), low blood count, bleeding episodes, bone deterioration, fractures and, rarely, acute liver complications. There is no mental or neurological involvement.

Symptoms of Type 1 GD usually appear in childhood or early adulthood, but diagnosis may be made as early as the first weeks of life, though some patients are not detected until mid- or late-adulthood. Some who come to medical attention have severe disease in childhood, while others may be completely asymptomatic when diagnosed at 60 or more years of age. The signs may be an enlarged abdomen, blood abnormalities or orthopedic problems. Due to the variability of this disorder, it is difficult to predict its severity in any given individual. There is no classic, predictable disease course.

*Type 2—infantile form.* This type is extremely rare, and shows no predilection for any particular racial or ethnic group. Onset is in infancy, with diagnosis generally made by six months of age. The hallmark of this form is rapid nervous system deterioration, with death by the age of two years.

*Type 3—juvenile form.* This form is very rare, except in a particular region of Sweden, where most cases have been identified. It begins in childhood, with all the manifestations of Type 1 disease but has neurologic disease similar to Type 2, except with a slower progression. Involvement of the brain creates neurological problems, including retardation, seizures and abnormal body and eye movements, leading to death, often by 20 to 30 years of age.

Carrier testing for GD is possible with a blood test to determine the level of the enzyme acid ß-glucosidase. PRENATAL DIAGNOSIS for all forms of GD is possible with CHORIONIC VILLUS SAMPLING or AMNIOCENTESIS.

There is a significant amount of research currently underway on this disorder, as it is considered a model that may help unravel the mysteries of other storage and enzyme deficiency diseases, including specific therapy for these diseases by enzyme or gene replacement strategies. Other storage diseases include TAY-SACHS DISEASE, FABRY DISEASE, MUCOPOLYSACCHARIDOSES and GLYCOGEN STORAGE DISEASE.

For more information, contact:

National Gaucher Foundation
1424 K Street, 4th Floor, NW
Washington, DC 20005
(202) 393-2777

The National Foundation for Jewish
    Genetic Diseases
250 Park Avenue, Suite 1000
New York, NY 10177
(212) 371-1030

Comprehensive Gaucher Disease Clinic
The Center for Jewish Genetic Diseases
The Mount Sinai Medical Center
1 Gustave L. Levy Place
New York, NY 10029
(212) 241-6944

**gene mapping**   The assignment of GENES to specific points on a CHROMOSOME. Knowing the location of genes that cause hereditary disorders is an important tool in the diagnosis, and perhaps the eventual treatment, of these conditions. The first example of gene mapping was accomplished in 1911, when the gene for COLOR BLINDNESS was assigned to the X CHROMOSOME. It was another 50 years before genes could be mapped to autosomes, or non-sex chromosomes, but by the end of the 1980s, approximately 1,700 genes had been mapped.

In the United States, the federally sponsored Genome Project is currently undertaking the mapping of the location of every gene found in the human genetic material, or GENOME.

**genes**   The basic units of hereditary traits. Chemically, they are composed of DEOXYRIBONUCLEIC ACID (DNA), strings of complex, nucleic acid-based "super" molecules. Genetically, they are the determinants of the characteristics that identify living things as individuals and as members of a species. They are passed from generation to generation bundled within CHROMOSOMES, ever replicating and dividing in new combinations.

The term "gene" was introduced in 1909 by Wilhelm Ludwig Johannsen (1857-1927), a pharmacist's apprentice from Copenhagen who went on to become a respected figure in genetics and botany. (He also introduced the term GENOTYPE). He defined a gene as an accounting or calculating unit of heredity. However, the concept of genes had already been accepted, called by names such as "physiological units," "gemmule," "idioplasm," "micellae" and "pangene."

Genes exist in pairs, strung together to form the 23 chromosome pairs found in the nucleus of every somatic, or non-sex, cell. It is estimated that if all this genetic material packed into each cell were unraveled, it would stretch six feet.

Each gene occupies a specific point (locus) on a chromosome, and each gene in a pair is called an ALLELE. Alleles are often dominant or recessive. Dominant genes are so named because their action will dominate or override the influence of a dissimilar allele in the pair. Recessive genes are so named because their action will be recessed or overridden by a dissimilar allele. Individuals who have identical alleles for a given trait, either both dominant or both recessive genes, are said to be HOMOZYGOTES, or homozygous for a given trait. Those who have dissimilar alleles, or genes, one dominant and one recessive, are said to be HETEROZYGOTES, or heterozygous for the trait. (The alleles for blood type, for example, are neither dominant nor recessive, but A, B and O, representing the three major blood types.)

Genes display a great variety. Some control several functions. Others modify the workings of yet a third. Some appear to be master genes regulating the action of several others. Some turn on and off at different ages. And approximately half of the estimated 50,000 to 100,000 gene pairs found in each human cell have, as yet, no discernible function at all. Indeed, the concept of what constitutes a gene (as opposed to merely a small segment of genetic material) is not entirely clear.

Many hereditary disorders are caused by genes that have been damaged or changed. (Damage or aberration in the chromosomes themselves, rather than in single genes, is also responsible for hereditary conditions. See CHROMOSOME ABNORMALITIES.) These changes are called MUTATIONS. Most mutations are harmless, but some have the ability to seriously affect the individual who possesses this mutation, whether acquired from inheritance or, in rare situations, from spontaneous mutation. These gene mutations may be either dominant or recessive. For a recessive condition to appear in an individual, he or she must be homozygous, that is, have two recessive mutant genes. For an individual to have a dominant condition, he or she needs only one gene for the disorder, that is, needs to be a heterozygote for the disorder to manifest itself. Homozygotes for dominant conditions, that is, those with two identical dominant mutant genes, often exhibit extremely severe symptoms of the condition, or die in utero. (See also AUTOSOMAL DOMINANT, AUTOSOMAL RECESSIVE; GENOME; "INTRODUCTION.")

**gene splicing**    See RECOMBINANT DNA.

**genetic code**    The instructions present in the DNA (see DEOXYRIBONUCLEIC ACID) of living cells that control the synthesis of proteins and polypeptides from AMINO ACIDS. These instructions are contained in CODONS, and are present in all viruses, bacteria, plants and animals. Alterations in the genetic code result in genetic variations, which results in all our individual differences as well as in genetic disorders. If one were to have a written printout of an individual's genetic code, including all the genetic material from both parents, using just one letter for each nucleotide (the individual molecules making up the DNA), the printout would fill the pages found in over 25 sets of *The Encyclopaedia Britannica*.

**genetic counseling**    The process of helping parents, prospective parents or others understand genetic information and issues that may have an impact on them and their families.

This counseling may be offered to prospective parents in helping them evaluate risks for hereditary or genetic conditions to their offspring—based on familial history, age, lifestyle or other factors that may influence the health of their offspring—or the counseling may be offered to parents following the birth of an affected individual. Where risks are known or suspected, or a genetic ANOMALY has been discovered during PRENATAL DIAGNOSIS, counseling also involves explaining the options available. However, the goal of the counselor is to allow the parents or prospective parents to make informed decisions on their own, not to tell them what to do, as there is no option that

is either right or wrong; the individuals being counseled must decide what is best for them.

The information that must be explained includes the diagnosis, when a particular condition has been identified in an offspring, the prognosis, or outlook for the future impact of the condition, and available treatment. When the condition is diagnosed prenatally, counseling information also includes information on options such as termination of the pregnancy (see ABORTION) or, in rare cases, FETAL SURGERY. Information about recurrence risks for future pregnancies is also a key component of counseling. The counseling also may involve extensive diagnostic procedures, in an effort to determine the exact cause or nature of a birth defect or other anomalous condition in an affected individual. It can also involve screening individuals from populations known to have an increased risk for some hereditary disorders to determine if they are CARRIERS for the trait, when carrier detection is possible.

Genetic counseling began during the 1950s and 1960s, as advances in genetic research revealed the hereditary basis of a growing number of genetic conditions, and advances in diagnostic techniques, such as AMNIOCENTESIS (which was perfected by the end of the 1960s) allowed the identification of some of these disorders.

Genetic counseling may be offered by family physicians or by specialists trained in genetics. It is recommended for families in which an offspring exhibits BIRTH DEFECTS, MENTAL RETARDATION, developmental delay, short stature or growth disorders, AMBIGUOUS GENITALIA or chronic neurologic or neuromuscular disorders.

It is also recommended in families with a known history of a GENETIC DISORDER, when parents are consanguinous (see CONSANGUINITY), and when maternal age is 35 years or older. (See Tables XII and XIII.)

For more information, contact:

National Society of Genetic Counselors
233 Canterbury Drive

Wallingford, PA 19086
(215) 872-7608

American Society of Human Genetics
9650 Rockville Pike
Bethesda, MD 20814
(301) 571-1825

**genetic disorder**   Any disorder with its origin in a variation of DNA (see DEOXYRIBONUCLEIC ACID), the genetic material in the cell nucleus that controls HEREDITY as well as the production of ENZYMES and other proteins. GENES, and the CHROMOSOMES on which they are found, are constructed from DNA.

Not all genetic disorders are hereditary, that is, passed from parent to offspring through the action of genes, though the majority are. For example, sporadically-occurring chromosomal aberrations passed from parent to offspring, or variations that occur in the chromosomes soon after conception (see CHROMOSOME ABNORMALITIES), can cause disorders that are not hereditary, though they are genetic. Also, genetic disorders are not necessarily CONGENITAL, or apparent at birth (see BIRTH DEFECTS). They may have ages of onset ranging from early infancy to late adulthood.

Genetic disorders fall in three categories: MENDELIAN, or single-gene disorders; chromosomal disorders; and MULTIFACTORIAL disorders. Mendelian disorders result from the action of a single gene or gene pair. They are inherited in dominant and recessive fashion, following laws of inheritance first articulated by Gregor Mendel. More than 4,200 known or suspected single gene disorders have been reported to exist, and are estimated to occur in about 1% of the human population.

Chromosome disorders result from the addition or deletion of genetic material in the cell, or from an abnormal arrangement of the chromosomes. DOWN SYNDROME, for example, is a chromosomal disorder caused by the presence of an extra, third copy of chromosome 21. KLINEFELTER SYNDROME, a rela-

## Table XII
## Indications for Genetic Counseling

- Family history of a known genetic disorder or recurrent pathologic condition
- Birth defects—single anomalies, multiple defect patterns, metabolic disorders
- Mental retardation or developmental delay
- Chronic neurologic or neuromuscular childhood disorders
- Short stature and other growth disorders
- Dysmorphic features
- Ambiguous genitalia or abnormal sexual development
- Carrier status for a genetic disease with increased incidence in specific population groups—sickle-cell, Tay-Sachs, thalassemia
- Infertility, sterility, or fetal wastage
- Exposure to potentially mutagenic or teratogenic agents
- Pregnancy at age 35 or older
- Genetic risks in consanguinity
- Adult-onset disability of genetic origin
- Behavioral disorders of genetic origin
- Cancer, heart disease and other common conditions with a genetic component

Reproduced, with the permission of the National Genetics Foundation, Inc., from R.B. Berini and E. Kahn (eds.), *Clinical Genetics Handbook* (Oradell, N.J.: Medical Economics Co., Inc., 1987). All rights reserved.

tively common chromosomal disorder that occurs only in males, is caused by the presence of an extra X chromosome.

Multifactorial disorders are those caused by the action of several genes in concert with environmental influences. These make up the greatest number of genetic disorders by far, and include CLEFT-LIP or cleft palate, CONGENITAL HEART DEFECTS, NEURAL TUBE DEFECTS (SPINA BIFIDA and ANENCEPHALY), SCHIZOPHRENIA and ESSENTIAL HYPERTENSION.

Genetic disorders are estimated to account for approximately 30% to 50% of all infant hospitalizations. More than 5% of all individuals under the age of 25 are believed to have

## Table XIII
## Sample Prenatal Genetic Screen*

Name _____ Patient #_____ Date #_____

| | | |
|---|---|---|
| 1. Will you be 35 years or older when the baby is due? | Yes_____ | No_____ |
| 2. Have you, the baby's father, or anyone in either of your families ever had any of the following disorders? | Yes_____ | No_____ |
| • Down syndrome (mongolism) | Yes_____ | No_____ |
| • Other chromosomal abnormality | Yes_____ | No_____ |
| • Neural tube defect, ie, spina bifida (meningomyelocele or open spine), anencephaly | Yes_____ | No_____ |
| • Hemophilia | Yes_____ | No_____ |
| • Muscular dystrophy | Yes_____ | No_____ |
| • Cystic fibrosis | Yes_____ | No_____ |

If yes, indicate the relationship of the affected person to you or to the baby's father: _____

| | | |
|---|---|---|
| 3. Do you or the baby's father have a birth defect? | Yes_____ | No_____ |

If yes, who has the defect and what is it? _____

| | | |
|---|---|---|
| 4. In any previous marriages, have you or the baby's father had a child, born dead or alive, with a birth defect not listed in question 2 above? | Yes_____ | No_____ |
| If yes, what was the defect and who had it? | Yes_____ | No_____ |
| 5. Do you or the baby's father have any close relatives with mental retardation? | Yes_____ | No_____ |

If yes, indicate the relationship of the affected person to you or the baby's father: _____

Indicate the cause, if known:_____

| | | |
|---|---|---|
| 6. Do you, the baby's father, or a close relative in either of your families have a birth defect, any familial disorder, or a chromosomal abnormality not listed above? | Yes_____ | No_____ |
| If yes, Indicate the condition and the relationship of the affected person to you or to the baby's father: | Yes_____ | No_____ |
| 7. In any previous marriages, have you or the baby's father had a stillborn child or three or more first-trimester spontaneous pregnancy losses? | Yes_____ | No_____ |
| Have either of you had a chromosomal study? | Yes_____ | No_____ |

If yes, indicate who and the results: _____

| | | |
|---|---|---|
| 8. If you or the baby's father are of Jewish ancestry, have either of you been screened for Tay-Sachs disease? | Yes_____ | No_____ |

If yes, indicate who and the results: _____

| | | |
|---|---|---|
| 9. If you or the baby's father are black, have either of you been screened for sickle cell trait? | Yes_____ | No_____ |

If yes, indicate who and the results: _____

| | | |
|---|---|---|
| 10. If you or the baby's father are of Italian, Greek, or Mediterranean background, have either of you been tested for ß-thalassemia? | Yes_____ | No_____ |

If yes, indicate who and the results: _____

| | | |
|---|---|---|
| 11. If you or the baby's father are of Philippine or Southeast Asian ancestry, have either of you been tested for a-thalassemia? | Yes_____ | No_____ |

If yes, indicate who and the results: _____

| | | |
|---|---|---|
| 12. Excluding iron and vitamins, have you taken any medications or recreational drugs since being pregnant or since your last menstrual period? (include nonprescription drugs.) | Yes_____ | No_____ |

If yes, give name of medication and time taken during pregnancy: _____

*Any patient replying "YES" to questions should be offered appropriate counseling. If the patient declines further counseling or testing this should be noted in the chart. Given that genetics is a field in a state of flux alterations or updates to this form will be required periodically.

Source: American College of Obstetricians and Gynecologists, *ACOG Technical Bulletin*, 108(1987), p. 3.

a genetic disorder, and when late-onset multi-factorial disorders are included, about 60% of all individuals are thought to have genetically-influenced conditions. Genetic influence also appears to play a strong role in premature adult death (below age 50) from all natural causes, including infections and cardiovascular disease. (See also "INTRODUCTION.")

For more information, contact:

March of Dimes Birth Defects Foundation
1275 Mamaroneck Avenue
White Plains, NY 10605
(914) 428-7100

National Organization for RareDisorders,
   Inc. (NORD)
P.O. Box 8923
New Fairfield, CT 06812
(203) 746- 6518

**genetic linkage** The association of genes located near each other on the same CHROMOSOME. As a result of this linkage, these genes are usually inherited together. (Linkage of traits was first seen in studies of coat color in house mice published by A.B. Darbishire in 1904.)

In some single gene disorders, where the specific gene defect is unknown or cannot be disclosed through PRENATAL DIAGNOSIS, the diagnostic information needed may sometimes be obtained through observation of gene linkage; the presence of the second marker gene, which may be perfectly normal, will disclose the presence of the linked defective gene.

An advantage of this technique is that no special knowledge is required as to which specific gene, or what specific defect in a known gene, has caused the problem. If the linkage can be shown, then the diagnosis can be made with some degree of certainty.

The major disadvantage of this technique is that linkage may be different for different families. Thus, many members of the family involved will have to be tested in order to know which genetic marker will work effectively to disclose the linkage. The family study

must be undertaken prior to pregnancy or early in pregnancy, when linkage is to be used for prenatal diagnosis. In many cases, it is not possible to perform such an in-depth family study, and linkage analysis, therefore, will not be completely reliable.

Another potential problem is the possibility that the linkage relationship between the marker gene and the disease gene is altered due to recombination or crossing over. This occurs when the two chromosomes of a chromosome pair join together. When the chromosomes exchange material, if that exchange occurs between the marker and the gene of interest, they will not be inherited together. The frequency of this occurring is related to the distance between the two genes. The closer the two are, the less likely their linkage will be lost. (See also GENETIC MARKERS.)

**genetic markers** Indicators that identify the presence of specific genes or genetic defects. Often, the genetic marker, or marker gene, will identify a DNA segment that indicates the presence of a particular genetic disorder without identifying the actual genetic defect, which may remain unknown; an example is the genetic markers that are used to identify cystic fibrosis and HUNTINGTON'S CHOREA. These markers are signposts linked to the disease gene. The marker gene and the disease gene, located close to each other on the same chromosome, are inherited together.

Some genetic markers involve specific biochemical variations, while other genetic markers depend on the variation among individual chromosomes that occurs when DNA is cut by restriction enzymes.

RESTRICTION ENZYMES and DNA PROBES are often used in establishing genetic markers. DNA fragments produced by restriction enzymes, when mixed in solution with a DNA probe, will result in marking, or identifying, a particular segment of DNA that contains, or is close to, a specific gene.

Identifiable markers for genetic defects have aided in the prenatal diagnosis of disorders that previously could not be diagnosed

## Table XIV
### Incidence of Genetic or Partially Genetic Diseases per 1,000 Live Births

| Disease Category | British Columbia 1967-69 Study | | Present Study (1952-83) Sum of | | UNSCEAR Reports | | |
|---|---|---|---|---|---|---|---|
| | Minimal | Adjusted | Highest Rates | 1966 | 1977[a] | 1982 | 1986 |
| Dominant[b] | 0.6 | 0.8 | 1.4 | 10.0 | 10.0 | 10.0 | 10.0 |
| X linked | 0.3 | 0.4 | 0.5 | ... | ... | ... | ... |
| Recessive | 0.9 | 1.1 | 1.7 | 2.0 | 1.1[c] | 2.5 | 2.5 |
| Chromosomal: | | | | | | | |
|   Numerical | 1.6 | 2.0 | 1.9 | 4.0 | 4.0 | 4.0 | 3.4 |
|   Structural | ... | ... | ... | ... | ... | ... | 0.4 |
| Multifactorial: | | | | | | | |
|   Congenital | 36.0 | 43.0 | 23.1 | 25.0 | 90.0 | 90.0 | 90.0[d] |
|   Other | 16.0 | 47.0 | 23.9 | 15.0 | ... | ... | ... |
| Genetic unknown | ... | ... | 1.2 | ... | ... | ... | ... |
| Total | 55.0 | 94.0 | 53.2 | 56.0 | 105.0 | 107.0 | 106.0 |

[a]The values used in the report of the BEIR committee in 1980 (8) were essentially identical to those in the 1977 UNSCEAR report.
[b]The figures from the UNSCEAR reports include autosomal and X-linked dominants.
[c]The change from 1.1 to 2.5 was made by UNSCEAR to include those disorders whose mutant genes are maintained by heterozygous advantage.
[d]Includes congenital anomalies and other multifactorial disorders.
[e]The sums are not exact owing to rounding.

Source: Patricia A. Baird, "A Population Study of Genetic Disorders in Children and Young Adults," *American Journal of Human Genetics*, 42 (1988):677-693.

before birth. For example, cystic fibrosis could not be diagnosed prenatally until the discovery of a genetic marker closely linked to the gene for this disease. The gene that causes the disease isn't itself identified, but it is closely linked to the marker. If the marker is present, so must the defect in the gene be present. Now, not only can it be diagnosed before birth, but also carriers of this defect can be identified in families with cystic fibrosis, which means that parents who might conceive a child with cystic fibrosis can be made aware of this risk. (See also GENETIC LINKAGE.)

**genetic screening**   Testing groups of individuals to identify defective GENES capable of causing hereditary disorders. Screening is especially useful in populations known to be at increased risk for possessing mutant genes, such as blacks for SICKLE-CELL ANEMIA and Jews for TAY-SACHS DISEASE. In addition, newborn genetic screening programs exist for identifying infants with CONGENITAL disorders whose potentially devastating consequences, if diagnosed early, may be treatable. Examples are PHENYLKETONURIA (PKU) and CONGENITAL HYPOTHYROIDISM. (See Table XIII.)

**genetics**   The scientific study of heredity, the transmission of inherited characteristics from parent to offspring. The term was coined by English zoologist William Bateson, who formally suggested its adoption by the scientific community in 1906. (See also "INTRODUCTION.")

**genodermatosis**   Any genetically-influenced disease of the skin. These include EHLERS-DANLOS SYNDROME, PORPHYRIA, ICHTHYOSIS, EPIDERMOLYSIS BULLOSA, NEUROFIBROMATOSIS, TUBEROUS SCLEROSIS, ECTODERMAL DYSPLASIA, STURGE-WEBER SYNDROME and many others.

**genome**   The entire complement of genetic material found in the CHROMOSOMES. There are an estimated 50,000 to 100,000 GENES in the human genome. The Human Genome Project, a federally-funded effort headed by the National Institutes of Health in Washington, DC, along with the Dept. of Energy, is currently underway to map the entire genome and identify the position of each of these genes, along with their corresponding functions, on the 23 pairs of chromosomes. Nobel laureate James Watson was named the first director of the effort, which has been estimated to require 15 years and approximately $3 billion to complete, involving hundreds of scientists in government, university and private laboratories across the United States.

Currently, approximately 5,000 genes are known and about 1,700 have been identified and located. The entire human haploid genome (that is, the genetic material on one of each pair of chromosomes) is three billion bases of DNA (see DEOXYRIBONUCLEIC ACID). (Each gene is composed of a number of these bases.) Just printing out this sequence, using one letter for each base of DNA, would occupy the equivalent of 13 sets of the Encyclopaedia Britannica. Whether much of this is "junk DNA" or contains unidentified genes is at present purely speculation. Successfully mapping the genome would have tremendous application in the identification and potential treatment of hereditary and GENETIC DISORDERS.

For more information, contact:

The National Center for Human Genome
  Research
Building 1, Room 203
National Institutes of Health
9000 Rockville Pike Blvd.
Bethesda, MD 20892
(301) 496-0844

**genotype**    The genetic makeup of an individual. This is contrasted to the PHENOTYPE, which refers to the physical appearance or characteristics of an individual. An individual will not always have characteristics that reflect his or her genotype. For example, some AUTOSOMAL DOMINANT disorders are not exhibited in all the individuals who possess the GENES for them. The degree to which the characteristics of a specific given gene (also referred to in a more limited sense as a genotype) are exhibited in an individual is referred to as EXPRESSIVITY, and the degree to which a genotype manifests itself in a population is referred to as PENETRANCE.

The term "genotype" was introduced in the early 1900s by Wilhelm Ludwig Johannsen (1857-1927), a pharmacist's apprentice from Copenhagen who went on to achieve considerable renown in the fields of genetics and botany. He also introduced the terms "gene" and "phenotype."

**genu varum**    See BOWLEG.

**German measles–rubella**    See TORCH SYNDROME.

**geroderma osteodysplastica**    See WALT DISNEY DWARFISM.

**giant**    See GIGANTISM.

**gigantism**    Excessive growth or development of any part of the body. Pituitary gigantism results from excessive growth hormone. Cerebral gigantism or SOTOS SYNDROME is a generally SPORADIC disorder of unknown cause resulting in large size, MENTAL RETARDATION and other problems.

Throughout history, there have been well-documented cases of "giants," individuals whose height and size was far above normal. Typically, these conditions are the result of hyperactivity of glands that regulate growth, are not visible at birth, and occur sporadically, the cause remaining unknown.

**Gilbert disease**    Hereditary liver disorder, named for French physician and liver specialist Nicolas A. Gilbert (1858-1927) who first described it in 1901. It is a benign, congenital condition characterized by a fluctuating elevation in serum bilirubin, a yellow pigment excreted by the liver. Bilirubin is produced by the breakdown of hemoglobin from red blood cells and is transported to the liver where it is chemically modified and excreted in the bile.

The onset of the condition usually occurs during the teens or early adulthood. While symptoms are rarely significant, occasionally mild jaundice may appear, and the white of the eye may become yellow. Other than excess serum bilirubin, upon examination, all liver functions are normal. It requires no treatment and will not interfere with a normal lifespan.

The estimated prevalence of Gilbert syndrome is reportedly as high as 3% to 7% of the adult population. Inherited in an AUTOSOMAL DOMINANT fashion, it results from deficient activity of the ENZYME glucuronyl-transferase in the liver.

For more information, contact:

The American Liver Foundation
998 Pompton Avenue
Cedar Grove, NJ 07009
(201) 857-2626
(800) 223-0179

## Gilles de la Tourette syndrome   See
TOURETTE SYNDROME.

## Glanzmann thrombasthenia   See
THROMBASTHENIA OF GLANZMANN AND NAEGELI.

## glaucoma, congenital   See CONGENITAL GLAUCOMA.

## globoid cell leukodystrophy (GLD)
See KRABBE DISEASE.

## glucose-6-phosphate   dehydrogenase deficiency (G6PD)   The most common inherited ENZYME deficiency, it is caused by a variety of MUTATIONS at a single gene locus. At least 150 such variations have been described. Transmitted as an X-LINKED recessive trait, it affects males almost exclusively. This enzyme is produced by a single GENE on the X CHROMOSOME.

The enzyme G6PD is involved in the repair of oxidation damage, which is critical in maintaining the membrane of red blood cells. The disorder is generally asymptomatic, though when triggered it results in episodes of hemolytic ANEMIA, blood disorders caused by the premature destruction of red blood cells. The episodes may be triggered by exposure to certain drugs (e.g., quinine and derivatives), chemicals, infections, or ingestion of fava beans (see FAVISM).

There is a wide variability of severity among the forms of G6PD, depending on the severity of the inherited deficiency. Like SICKLE-CELL ANEMIA and THALASSEMIA, the disorder is common in populations originating in malaria-prone areas of the world, as the deficiency bestows resistance to malaria.

Many newborns of Mediterranean or Oriental ancestry with jaundice (neonatal hyperbilirubinemia) of unknown origin are found to be G6PD-deficient. Overall, G6PD deficiency is estimated to affect 400 million people worldwide. There are several common G6PD variants:

*Type B.* This is the usual form of the enzyme found in whites and in most black individuals. G6PD enzyme activity is normal.

*Type A+.* This variant, occurring in about 20% of black males in the United States, reduces normal G6PD activity by about 10%.

*Type A-.* Found in about 12% of black males in the United States, it results in a reduction of G6PD activity by 10% to 20%. Enzyme activity declines as cells age. If hemolysis occurs, it will affect older cells, leaving young red blood cells with normal enzyme levels, making diagnosis difficult. Hemolysis may occur after drug exposure.

*Type B-.* Two percent to 5% of U.S. males of Mediterranean ancestry have this variant. Enzyme activity is decreased a maximum of 5%, though it may not be decreased at all. Both young and old red blood cells may have reduced G6PD activity.

*G6PD Chinese; G6PD Canton.* These variants are common in Chinese populations and cause a reduction in enzyme activity to only 4% to 25% of normal.

*G6PD Mediterranean.* Found in Greeks, Italians etc. Activity is only 0-5% of normal. Hemolysis is provoked by drugs or favism.

**glutaric aciduria**    Affected individuals exhibit chronic problems with involuntary body movements. There is a wide variety of ceaseless, involuntary, rapid, highly complex, jerky motions or slow, writhing movements that are especially severe in the hands (choreoathetosis). Many of those affected contort themselves, holding one arm and shoulder back with the head drawn back to one side (dystonic posturing). They are usually mentally retarded. Death is sometimes caused by an acute movement disorder episode.

At birth, infants appear normal, but within the first year they exhibit vomiting, diminished muscle tone (hypotonia) and abnormally high acid levels in the blood (acidemia).

Laboratory tests reveal elevated concentrations of glutaric and 3-hydroxy-glutaric acids in urine. Glutaric acid concentrations are also elevated in serum, cerebrospinal fluid, and tissues. Glutaconic acids may occasionally be found in urine. The underlying abnormality is a deficiency of the ENZYME glutaryl CoA dehydrogenase.

Prenatal detection is possible by enzyme assay testing of cultured amniotic cells obtained via AMNIOCENTESIS. At birth, the disorder can be detected by performing enzyme assay tests on white blood cells.

This rare disorder is inherited as an AUTOSOMAL RECESSIVE trait, and the risk of occurrence in the general population is unknown. It is treatable with a special diet and with riboflavin (a B-complex vitamin). Most patients do not survive to childbearing age.

Glutaric aciduria type II is a separate disorder in which not only glutaryl CoA dehydrogenase is deficient but also other enzymes involved in fatty acid metabolism—hence its more appropriate name, multiple acyl CoA dehydrogenase deficiency. It varies in severity from overwhelming metabolic illness with death in the newborn period to milder cases with later onset in childhood with neurologic

abnormalities, low blood sugar, hypotonia and heart abnormalities.

**gluten-induced enteropathy** (celiac disease)    Condition caused by an inability of the small intestine to digest and absorb nutrients, and resulting from a hereditary sensitivity to gluten, a protein compound found in wheat and rye.

Onset is usually in late infancy or early childhood, but may begin in adult life. Symptoms include FAILURE TO THRIVE, passage of loose, pale, bulky, greasy and foul-smelling stools, and irritability. Affected individuals exhibit small stature, deficiencies of vitamin D, folic acid and iron, and increased risk of lymphatic system and gastrointestinal malignancies. There may also be an increased risk for DIABETES MELLITUS, autoimmune thyroiditis and lung diseases.

Both genetic and environmental factors have been implicated in the inheritance of celiac disease; the exact mechanism has not been clearly defined. The condition occurs in about one in 2,000 live births. However, there is a wide variability of incidence among various population groups, reflecting both genetic differences among these groups and differences in consumption of wheat.

With a gluten-free diet, most patients have a normal life span, although an increased risk of malignancy may persist.

**glycogen storage disease (GSD)**    A group of inherited metabolic disorders of the liver and muscle, rendering the body unable to break glycogen down into glucose, the form of sugar it needs to produce energy. As a result, there is an abnormal storage and accumulation of glycogen in tissues, especially the liver or muscle. One of the most common signs is a greatly enlarged liver (hepatomegaly). The other common symptom of some forms is muscle weakness.

Normally, the body stores excess sugar in the liver and muscles in the form of glycogen, a compound containing multiple branching chains of glucose molecules; these are molecules that are "branched" like a tree, rather than organized into a single long chain. Liver ENZYMES convert it back to glucose when the body needs energy. (Enzymes that control this activity are "debranching" enzymes.) The body can survive for days or weeks without eating, due to this conversion process. However, individuals with GSD cannot convert glycogen to glucose. They must be fed every few hours around the clock, so that there is a constant supply of glucose from ingestion. Even with intensive dietary management, some individuals may suffer growth retardation, convulsions caused by low blood sugar, bleeding problems, enlarged liver and abdomen, gout and increased susceptibility to infections. In severe cases, brain damage or early death may occur.

The various manifestations an individual exhibits depend on the specific type of the disease (see below). For example, in the forms affecting muscle, the muscle's ability to break down its stores of glycogen to get "fuel" for muscle contraction is impaired, resulting in fatigue and weakness.

The GSDs are inherited as AUTOSOMAL RECESSIVE traits (except for type IX, which may be either autosomal or X- LINKED recessive). There is a wide variability in the severity of the various types of GSD. However, even in mild forms, individuals may not achieve normal height, and may not be able to compete physically with other children their age.

Treatment generally consists of dietary management; in some forms (e.g., type I) nighttime infusion of glucose directly into the stomach is required, either through a drip tube inserted through the nose, or through creation of a surgical opening into the stomach from the abdomen. Liver transplants have been successful but are generally reserved for the most severe cases.

Perhaps as many as 20 types of GSD have been identified, based on the specific enzyme deficiencies that cause them. Some of the best-known forms are:

*Type I (von Gierke disease)*. Named for German pathologist Edgar O.K. von Gierke

(1877-1945), who described it in 1929, this is the most common and severe form of GSD. Much of the above description relates to this disorder. It is caused by a deficiency of the ENZYME glucose-6-phosphatase. The liver and kidneys are most affected. There may be gross enlargement of the abdomen and kidneys, growth retardation, chronic hunger, fatigue and irritability. Low blood sugar (hypoglycemia) is a major associated problem. Gout and bleeding problems are less common features. In the past, individuals rarely survived into adulthood, but improved treatment makes survival beyond childhood the rule. However, liver tumors (both benign and malignant) may develop.

Type Ib GSD refers to those children whose disease is indistinguishable from those with type I GSD but who have normal levels of glucose-6-phosphatase. In fact, if these enzyme levels are measured in fresh, not frozen, tissue it can be shown to be deficient. These children suffer a severe form of the disease and also suffer abnormalities of their white blood cells, causing recurrent infections.

*Type II (Pompe disease)*. This is generally a severe infantile form first described by Dutch pathologist J.C. Pompe (1901-1945) in 1932. It is due to a defect in alpha-1,4-glucosidase (sometimes called acid maltase).

Type II GSD is actually a lysosomal STORAGE DISEASE and was the first disease to be recognized as such. In the other GSDs the glycogen that accumulates is not stored in the lysosomes, the digestive compartments of the cell, as in this form.

Involvement of organs is generalized, with the heart becoming greatly enlarged. Individuals present a FLOPPY INFANT appearance, with little muscle tone (hypotonia) and severe weakness. The tongue may also be enlarged (MACROGLOSSIA). The average age of death is five months, with survival beyond the first year highly unlikely, due to cardiorespiratory failure.

There is also an early childhood form of the disease characterized by slowly worsening muscle weakness with no heart abnormalities.

It resembles a MUSCULAR DYSTROPHY and causes death before adulthood. An adult form also exists with onset of muscle weakness after the age of 30. These forms exhibit some enzyme activity where the infantile form has none.

*Type III (Forbes disease; Cori disease).* This form is similar to type I, though with milder symptoms. Described by U.S. pediatrician G.B. Forbes in 1953, it is caused by a deficiency of the debranching enzyme in the liver and muscle tissue. The liver and heart and skeletal muscles are primarily affected. Diagnosis is usually based on liver and muscle biopsies. This condition is compatible with normal life expectancy, though individuals may develop muscle disorders as they grow older. Treatment is dietary with only rarely a need for continuous night feeds.

*Type IV (Andersen disease).* In this very rare and severe form, described by U.S. pediatrician and pathologist Dorothy H. Anderson (1901-1963) in 1952, cirrhosis of the liver occurs along with scarring of the affected muscles and heart. It is the result of a defect in the branching enzyme. Death usually occurs before the age of two years.

*Type V (McArdle disease).* Named for British pediatrician B. McArdle (b. 1911), who described it in 1951, this is a mild form of GSD, involving only skeletal muscles. Individuals are essentially normal, though severe muscle cramping occurs during heavy exercise. Muscle fatigue is seen in the teenage years, and progressive weakness in adulthood. Muscle phosphorylase is the enzyme deficient in this form.

*Type VI (Hers disease).* Though extreme enlargement of the liver may accompany this form, it is considered mild. It results from a deficiency of liver phosphorylase. Individuals may exhibit short stature, but they can lead normal lives without requiring any treatment.

*Type VII.* This is considered a mild form, resulting from a deficiency of phosphofructokinase. It resembles type V.

*Type IX.* This form has its onset in childhood, but symptoms may disappear during adolescence. Its primary feature is an enlarged liver, and it is caused by a deficiency of liver phosphorylase kinase. It resembles type VI. It is inherited as an X-LINKED recessive disorder or rarely (only one family, perhaps) as an AUTOSOMAL RECESSIVE disorder.

For more information, contact:

The Association for Glycogen Storage
  Disease
Box 896
Durant, IA 52747
(319) 785-6038

The Children's Liver Foundation
7 Highland Place
Maplewood, NJ 07040
(201) 761-1111

**GM1 gangliosidosis**    A rare GENETIC DISORDER characterized by the accumulation of a ganglioside, a carbohydrate-containing fatty substance, in nerves, spleen, liver, kidneys and other organs. Skeletal deformities are also present. Generally evident at birth, the high level of ganglioside leads to cerebral degeneration, and affected infants rarely survive beyond two years of age. These infants often resemble infants with MUCOPOLY-SACCHARIDOSIS. Milder juvenile-onset and adult forms with primarily neurologic symptoms, without other organ involvement, are also known.

First described in 1964, it is inherited as an AUTOSOMAL RECESSIVE disorder. CARRIER detection and PRENATAL DIAGNOSIS are available by measurement of the ENZYME deficient in this STORAGE DISEASE, beta-galactosidase. (TAY-SACHS DISEASE, a disorder with increased incidence in Ashkenazi Jews, is a different gangliosidosis, with storage of a related substance.)

**Goldenhar syndrome**  (oculo-auricular-vertebral dysplasia; hemifacial microsomia)    Syndrome characterized by varying degrees of facial abnormalities, DEAFNESS and, often, poor development (DYSPLASIA) of the spinal column. Named for French physician M. Goldenhar, who published the first description in 1952, it is highly variable in its expression.

The facial abnormalities are often confined to one side of the face (hemifacial), though in severe cases there may be gross distortion of features involving the entire face. When the features are one-sided, it tends to be right-sided. A frequent abnormality is a lateral cleft on one side of the mouth, which may extend across the cheek. The facial bones and muscles are underdeveloped asymmetrically. The eye on the more affected side of the face may be lower than the other. Abnormalities of the ear are also commonly visible, though they usually are present only in one ear. The ears may be malformed or there may be a missing outer ear or external canal. However, the most characteristic ear abnormality—small appendages or tags of skin adjacent to the ear (preauricular tags)—usually appear on both ears.

The hearing problems resulting from this syndrome tend to be conductive, that is, due to anomalies of the structure of the ear canal or bones involved with hearing, rather than due to sensorineural hearing loss, which results from abnormalities in the nerves that transmit impulses from the ear to the brain. The hearing loss, like the observable abnormalities, tends to be unilateral (affect only one side).

High arched palate, crowded teeth and, in some cases, CLEFT PALATE may also be present. The jawbone may be underdeveloped, as well.

Spinal abnormalities may include SCOLIOSIS, extra vertebrae or poorly developed vertebrae, most often in the neck region. CONGENITAL HEART DEFECTS may also accompany the syndrome. Mild MENTAL RETARDATION has been observed in some cases, but most patients are of normal intelligence.

Oral surgery may correct some of the associated dental problems, and cosmetic surgery may lessen the degree of facial asymmetry or correct the ear malformations.

The basic defect that causes the disorder is unknown. Goldenhar syndrome is estimated to occur in between one in 3,000 and one in 5,000 live births. It affects males more frequently than females by a ratio of three to two. Most cases are observed sporadically within families, although it has been suggested that in a few families there has been either AUTOSOMAL DOMINANT or AUTOSOMAL RECESSIVE inheritance in addition to MULTIFACTORIAL inheritance. Estimated risks of recurrence among SIBLINGS or offspring is about 2%.

PRENATAL DIAGNOSIS may be possible via ULTRASOUND.

Though various combinations of features have been given particular designations in the past (e.g., Goldenhar syndrome vs. hemifacial microsomia) these all seem to be variable gradations in the spectrum of severity of a similar malformation syndrome.

For more information, contact:

National Information Center on Deafness
Gallaudet College
800 Florida Avenue, N.E.
Washington, DC 20002
(202) 651-5000

National Association for the Craniofacially
   Handicapped
P.O. Box 11082
Chattanooga, TN 37401
(615) 266-1632

**Goltz syndrome**  (focal dermal hypoplasia)     Incomplete development (hypoplasia) and other abnormalities of the skin, bones, fingers and eyes. In its most severe form, the SYNDROME is lethal to males *in utero* and greatly reduces fertility in females. It was first described in 1962 by Robert W. Goltz, head of dermatology at the University of Minnesota.

At birth, visible skin lesions include scar-like abnormalities, streaks of excess pigmentation, atrophy and prominent blood vessel markings (telangiectasia). In some cases, there are isolated areas with no skin at all.

Often, there are soft yellow patches of subcutaneous fat along the line of the pelvic bones (iliac crest), groin and backs of the thighs. Benign skin tumors (papillomas) are common on and around the mouth, genitals, rectum, armpits and umbilicus. Hair, if it is present, is sparse and brittle.

Abnormalities of the bone include bone thickening (osteopathia striata), rib anomalies and lateral curvature of the spine (SCOLIOSIS). Fingers are frequently webbed (SYNDACTYLY) and may show other abnormalities as well, including absent or anomalous fingernails.

Eyes are affected most commonly by fissures (COLOBOMA) in the iris and retina, although there may also be "crossed eyes" (STRABISMUS), jerky movements of the eye (nystagmus), obstructed tear ducts, failure of the eyes to develop to normal size (microphthalmia) and absence of one eye.

Other complications of Goltz syndrome include incomplete development of the ears, teeth, genitals, lips, palate and head, growth and MENTAL RETARDATION and DEAFNESS. In rare cases, there may be cardiac and kidney abnormalities.

The basic defect that causes this rare disorder is not known. It is thought to be transmitted as an X-LINKED dominant trait, due to the fact that it affects females much more commonly than males. (Under this hypothesis, a large proportion of affected male FETUSES are spontaneously aborted.) Most cases are new MUTATIONS. There is no known method of PRENATAL DIAGNOSIS.

**goniodysgenesis** Arising from abnormal embryonic development of anterior (front) parts of the eye, this CONGENITAL defect may be inherited as an AUTOSOMAL DOMINANT trait and has a wide variation in expression. The vision of some members of a family may be severely affected while others are affected only slightly. Lifespan and intelligence generally are normal. The defect has been divided into four forms according to severity:

*Posterior embryotoxon.* The mildest form, in which a structure known as the Schwalbe line is displaced forward to resemble a prominent white ring on the border of the cornea. About 15% of the population has this defect in varying degrees.

*Rieger anomaly.* A more serious defect, in which the connective tissue supporting the iris is poorly developed or adheres to the displaced Schwalbe line. (When this ANOMALY accompanies defects such as missing or cone-shaped teeth, the condition is known as RIEGER SYNDROME.) GLAUCOMA and CATARACTS are common.

*Peter anomaly.* Faulty cleavage of embryonic structures results in clouding of the center of the cornea and adhesions of the iris, lens and cornea. Vision can be significantly impaired. Familial forms are most often inherited in an AUTOSOMAL RECESSIVE manner.

*Congenital anterior staphyloma.* Characterized by gross disorganization of the structure between the pupil and the lens (anterior chamber). Severe glaucoma is common.

Goniodysgenesis can be detected at birth. Currently, there is no method of PRENATAL DIAGNOSIS. The defect may be isolated, or any of the forms may be associated with other anomalies or systemic abnormalities.

**Gougerot-Carteaud syndrome** See ACANTHOSIS NIGRACANS.

**gout** Gout has historically been identified as a condition afflicting the upper classes, particularly its obese (see OBESITY) and gluttonous members. It has been called "the disease of kings and king of diseases." Recognized since ancient times, those said to have been afflicted include Alexander the Great, Charlemagne, Isaac Newton, John Milton and Charles Darwin.

Characterized by episodes of extreme pain in the foot (especially the big toe, though the instep, ankle, heel or wrist may also be affected), it is a disorder of purine metabolism causing a buildup of uric acid in the blood, resulting in the accumulation of crystals in joints. While most cases are idiopathic (of unknown origin), some (less than 1%) are known to have a genetic component. These cases are heterogenous, that is, various GENE MUTATIONS all result in the same condition. X-LINKED forms have been identified, and AUTOSOMAL DOMINANT transmission has been suggested for some cases, as has MULTIFACTORIAL inheritance. Evidence has been found that both increased rates of uric acid production and impaired elimination of uric acid by the kidney may be involved. In some families studied in which both parents were affected, age of onset and symptoms in their children were unusually early and severe.

The origins of the cases of the early 18th to mid-19th centuries, which helped establish this disorder's reputation as an affliction of the upper classes, have been the subject of interesting speculation. Some suggest these cases were "saturnine gout," caused by the high levels of lead in the port wine favored by the upper classes of the time. Others suggest that dietary excess in general with increased purine intake was at the root of the disorder. Conversely, a hypothesis has been advanced that the power and influence enjoyed by these upper-class gout sufferers points to the influence of GENETICS, with genes transmitting the metabolic deficiency linked with genes associated with increased intelligence.

**granulomatous disease, chronic**   See IMMUNE DEFICIENCY DISEASE.

**Grebe chondrodysplasia**   A rare form of short-limbed DWARFISM (see CHONDRODYSPLASIA). The arms and legs appear progressively shortened along their length, so that the ends of the arms and legs exhibit greater dwarfing than the sections nearer the trunk. The legs are often more severely affected than the arms. Fingers may be very short, resembling toes, and the toes may be almost non-existent. X-ray examination reveals severe developmental defects of the bones of the arms and legs (long bones). Extra digits may also be seen.

This condition, inherited as an AUTOSOMAL RECESSIVE trait, is observable at birth. STILLBIRTH and neonatal mortality rates (within the first four weeks of birth) are high in this condition, but long-term outlook is favorable for those who survive infancy. Intelligence is normal. Adult height is usually between 39 inches and 41 inches (99.1-104.1 cm). The disorder is named for H. Grebe, the physician who first described affected sisters in 1952.

CARRIERS of the trait, that is, those who possess a single GENE for the disorder, may exhibit mild shortness of the hands and feet.

For more information, contact:

Little People of America
P.O. Box 633
San Bruno, CA 94066
(415) 589-0695

Human Growth Foundation
4720 Montgomery Lane, Suite 909
Bethesda, MD 20814
(301) 656-6904
(301) 656-7540

**grief**   Emotions of grief, sadness and anger are common and healthy responses following the death of an infant affected by a GENETIC DISORDER or BIRTH DEFECT. Grief may be felt as intensely when a baby is lost before birth as when a death occurs in infancy, and a grieving process, and opportunities to express feelings, are important parts of coming to terms with the loss of an infant.

These same emotions often occur when an infant is born with a severe genetic condition or birth defect, and experiencing grief in these situations may be equally important.

For more information, contact:

Compassionate Friends
P.O. Box  3696

Oak Brook, IL 60522-3696
(312) 990-0010

Unite, Inc.
c/o Jeanes Hospital
7600 Central Avenue
Philadelphia, PA 19111
(215) 728-2082

A.M.E.N.D. (Aiding Mothers & Fathers
Experiencing Neonatal Death)
c/o Maureen Connelly
4324 Berrywick Terrace
St. Louis, MO 63128
(314) 487-7582

S.H.A.R.E. (Source of Help in Airing &
Resolving Experiences)
St. Elizabeth's Hospital
211 South Third Street
Belleville, IL 62222
(618) 234-2415

**Griffe des orteils**    See CLAWFOOT.

**GSD**    See GLYCOGEN STORAGE DISEASE.

**G6PD**    See GLUCOSE-6-PHOSPHATE DEHY-
DROGENASE DEFICIENCY.

**Gunther's disease**    See PORPHYRIA.

**gynecomastia, hereditary**    See HEREDI-
TARY GYNECOMASTIA.

**gyrate atrophy**    Hereditary vision disorder
with onset during the first decade of life. The
retina (the inner surface of the back of the eye) and
the choroid (the layer of tissue beneath the retina)
degenerate. (Gyrate, meaning ring-shaped, refers
to the circular pattern of atrophy or degeneration
exhibited by the retina and choroid.) NIGHTBLIND-
NESS is progressive. All those affected are nearsighted (myopia). The visual field becomes
increasingly constricted, leaving only a central
tunnel of vision. Remaining vision deteriorates
after the age of 30.

Inherited as an AUTOSOMAL RECESSIVE trait,
this condition is very rare. It is due to the defi-

ciency of the ENZYME ornithine aminotransferase.

# H

**hairy ear**    Excessive growth of coarse hairs
on the outer ear. This is the only trait (other than
maleness) known to be Y-linked; that is, the
gene for it is located on the Y CHROMOSOME.
(See X-LINKED.) This trait has been observed
in India, Israel and Malta.

**Hallermann-Streiff syndrome**    A
small face, mouth and jaw, large forehead
and small, pinched, beaked nose give rise to
the characteristic birdlike features that identify this disorder. In addition, there is always
proportionate dwarfing, with adult height
rarely exceeding 5 feet (see DWARFISM). It
was described in 1948 by Wilhelm
Hallermann (1909- ), a professor of ophthalmology at Göttingen in West Germany, and in
1950 by Bernardo Streiff (1908- ), professor of
ophthalmology at the University of
Lausanne, Switzerland.

Additional facial abnormalities include
prominent scalp and nose veins, small mouth
and double chin. Eyebrows, lashes and hair
are frequently sparse (hypotrichosis), and the
eyes are invariably smaller than normal
(microphthalmia), with CATARACTS. Although the cataracts may disappear, there is
a high incidence of eventual BLINDNESS.
Whites of the eyes (sclerae) may be blue; other
abnormalities of the eye include absence of
the lens (aphakia), squinting or "crossed" eyes
(STRABISMUS), jerky eye movement (nystagmus), presence of a membrane over the
pupil and secondary glaucoma.

Head and facial bones may be somewhat
smaller than usual or incompletely developed,
and the palate is high and narrow. Teeth may
be absent, incomplete or malformed. Overbite
(malocclusion) is common, as are early severe
cavities (caries). MENTAL RETARDATION has
been reported in about 15% of cases. The genitals
may be small or fail to develop completely.

The basic defect that causes Hallermann-Streiff syndrome is not known, nor has its genetic basis been identified. The condition is rare, and both sexes are affected equally. The greatest threat to life is in early infancy, when feeding difficulties and respiratory problems must be overcome. Surgery may be successful in correcting eye and mouth defects. In adults, the ability to reproduce is severely limited. There is currently no method of PRENATAL DIAGNOSIS available for this disorder.

**hamartoma** A CONGENITAL mass of slowly growing, abnormal tissue. They may appear in organs, blood vessels or other tissue. Hamartomatous tissues are similar to the organ they appear in, but the growth is abnormally organized. Hamartomas can cause complications due to the space they occupy, though they are not malignant.

**handicap** Many individuals who are affected by GENETIC DISORDERS and BIRTH DEFECTS are handicapped as a result of these conditions.

Section 504 of the Rehabilitation Act of 1973 (Public Law 93-112) defines a handicapped individual as

anyone with a physical or mental impairment that substantially impairs or restricts one or more major life activities, such as caring for one's self, performing manual tasks, walking, seeing, hearing, speaking, breathing, learning, and working.

The term physical or mental impairment includes, but is not limited to, speech, hearing, visual and orthopedic impairments, cerebral palsy, epilepsy, muscular dystrophy, multiple sclerosis, cancer, diabetes, heart disease, mental retardation, emotional illness, and specific learning disabilities such as perceptual handicaps, brain injury, dyslexia, minimal brain dysfunction and developmental aphasia.

The goal of the Rehabilitation Act of 1973 was to end discrimination against handicapped individuals in employment, housing and education, and assure their access to programs and facilities receiving government funds. The "American National Standard Specifications for Making Buildings and Facilities Accessible to, and Usable by, the Physically Handicapped" is the code that sets the requirements for accessibility.

Amendments to the Fair Housing Act now require that any new multifamily rental or condominium building with four or more units be accessible to the handicapped.

The 1990 Americans With Disabilities Act extended the protection of the 1973 law, prohibiting discrimination in employment against disabled individuals, even in businesses and institutions that don't receive government funds. The law requires businesses to provide "reasonable accommodations" in their facilities for disabled customers and employees.

For more information, contact:

The Center for Handicapped Children & Teenagers
2351 Clay Street, Suite 512
San Francisco, CA 94115
(415) 923-3549

National Easter Seal Society
2023 West Ogden Avenue
Chicago, IL 60612
(312) 243-8400

March of Dimes Birth Defects Foundation
1275 Mamaroneck Avenue
White Plains, NY 10605
(914) 428-7100

**happy puppet syndrome** (Angelman syndrome) First described by H. Angelman in 1965, this disorder is characterized by severe mental retardation, developmental delays and growth deficiency. It takes its name from an abnormal, puppet-like gait and frequent paroxysms of laughter unconnected to emotions of happiness. These laughing fits are thought to result from a defect in the brain stem. Characteristic facial appearance includes a small, squat skull, decreased ocular pigmentation resulting in pale blue eyes, a large mouth with a large, protruding tongue (macroglossia), and widely spaced teeth.

It has been linked to the deletion of the long arm of one member of the pair of CHROMO-SOME 15s. This deleted section is almost always found on the chromosome inherited from the mother (see IMPRINTING, CHROMO-SOME ABNORMALITIES). There have been at least two reports of affected SIBLINGS, raising the possibility of AUTOSOMAL RECESSIVE inheritance, but the vast majority of cases have been SPORADIC.

**harelip**    A colloquial term for cleft lip. (See also CLEFT LIP, CLEFT PALATE AND ASSO-CIATED CLEFTING CONDITIONS.)

**harlequin fetus** (ichthyosis congenita gravis)    A rare and lethal disorder characterized at birth by thick, hardened plates of skin covering the entire body, cracked along lateral fissures where folds of skin would normally appear.

The first description, recorded in 1750 in the diary of Rev. Oliver Hart, a minister in South Carolina, stands as the definitive one.

On Thursday, April ye 5, 1750, I went to see a most deplorable object of a child, born the night before of one Mary Evans in "Chas" town. It was surprising to all who beheld it, and I scarcely know how to describe it. The skin was dry and hard and seemed to be cracked in many places, somewhat resembling the scales of a fish. The mouth was large and round and open. It had no external nose, but two holes where the nose should have been. The eyes appeared to be lumps of coagulated blood, turned out, about the bigness of a plum, ghastly to behold. It had no external ears, but holes where the ears should be. The hands and feet appeared to be swollen, were cramped up and felt quite hard. The back part of the head was much open. It made a strange kind of noise, very low,

which I cannot describe. It lived about forty-eight hours and was alive when I saw it.

The disorder takes its name from the diamond-shaped sections of cracked skin, which create the appearance of a harlequin's suit.

Inherited as an AUTOSOMAL RECESSIVE trait, the basic cause of the condition is unknown. It is very rare, with approximately 30 cases reported. Most infants die in the first week of life, though the longest surviving infant lived to nine months of age. PRENATAL DIAGNOSIS by fetal skin biopsy has been accomplished.

**Hartnup disease**    Symptoms of this condition, usually detected in newborns, are intermittent and variable, and include rashes on parts of the body exposed to ultraviolet light, psychotic disturbances and impaired kidney and intestinal absorption of certain AMINO ACIDS, in particular tryptophan, an amino acid essential for metabolism. (Rashes from ultraviolet light are more common from February to October.)

Although an exact cause for Hartnup disease is unknown, poor nutrition is thought to precipitate onset of symptoms, which resemble those of niacin, or B-complex, vitamin deficiency (pellagra). Good nutrition and niacin (nicotinic acid) supplements help to alleviate symptoms for most of those affected. Though affected individuals have a normal life expectancy and may remain asymptomatic, without treatment mental deterioration may occur in rare instances.

Hartnup disease is inherited as an AUTOSO-MAL RECESSIVE trait. It is named for the first family identified as having the disorder, and was first described at London's Middlesex Hospital in 1956. It occurs worldwide in approximately one in 14,500 live births but is very rare in North America and other areas where high nutritional standards prevent onset of symptoms.

**heart defects, congenital**    See CON-GENITAL HEART DEFECTS.

**heart-hand syndrome** See HOLT-ORAM SYNDROME.

**hemangioma** A CONGENITAL mass of blood vessels, abnormally large either in number or in degree of dilation. These arteriovenous malformations occur in many SYNDROMES, and may occur as isolated MENDELIAN traits. When located near the skin rather than more internally, they impart a sharply delineated, reddish tone to the skin above. (See also PORT WINE STAIN.)

**hemangioma and thrombocytopenia syndrome** An association of a benign growth (tumor) that results from the proliferation of blood vessels (HEMANGIOMA) with a low number of platelets in the blood (thrombocytopenia). Hemangiomas may occur anywhere in the body but are most frequently noticed in the skin and tissue immediately below the skin, where they appear as reddish patches. The low number of platelets occurs partly as a result of becoming trapped in the tumor. ANEMIA (low blood count) can also occur. There may also be a depletion of fibrinogen, a substance in the blood that aids coagulation.

In this syndrome, a normal hemangioma may suddenly double in size, and purplish spots and patches caused by hemorrhaging appear on the skin. The original size of the hemangioma gives no clue as to possible development of the syndrome. It has been detected in persons ranging in age from newborn to 73 years, affects males and females equally and occurs in one in 500 persons with hemangiomas. (Hemangiomas appear in isolation in approximately one in 12 infants below one year of age.) The mortality rate is approximately 20%, usually due to internal hemorrhaging. The primary means of detection is by platelet count in the laboratory. The cause of the syndrome is unknown.

**hematuria, benign familial** See BENIGN FAMILIAL HEMATURIA.

**hemifacial microsomia** See GOLDENHAR SYNDROME.

**hemihypertrophy** Excessive growth or enlargement occurring on one side, or half (hemi), of the body. There is considerable individual variation both in severity and extent of the disorder. Unilateral, or one-sided enlargement can vary from a single digit or limb, or the face, to involvement of half of the entire body. Usually detected at birth, hemihypertrophy may increase with age, particularly with onset of puberty.

Total hemihypertrophy most often involves the right side of the body. Affected areas exhibit thickening of the skin, excessive glandular secretion, excessive hair growth (hypertrichosis) and extra nipples (polythelia). Additional characteristics may include enlarged bones in the involved area and various skeletal manifestations, including fused fingers (syndactyly), enlarged fingers (macrodactyly) or extra fingers (POLYDACTYLY). Between 20% and 30% of affected individuals have benign tumor-like nodules (HAMARTOMA) and various congenital defects and genitourinary anomalies. MENTAL RETARDATION occurs in about 15%.

Where hemihypertrophy is restricted to the head, there may be enlargement of the tongue (MACROGLOSSIA), lips and palate. There is also usually premature loss of baby teeth and concomitant growth of permanent teeth on the affected side.

Hemihypertrophy may affect portions of both sides of the body. It may be limited to a single system (skeletal, nervous, vascular, muscular) or, more frequently, affect multiple systems. It is also associated with development of cancerous growths (neoplasms), such as WILMS TUMOR or renal anomalies in young children, which can reduce life expectancy.

Treatment for hemihypertrophy consists of surgery to equalize leg lengths and plastic surgery to correct facial enlargement and deformities. Periodic examinations are recommended to detect development of neoplasms.

Hemihypertrophy, which may also be associated with a variety of genetic disorders, appears to occur sporadically in the population, although a few undocumented cases of familial occurrence have been reported. It occurs in approximately one in 15,000 live births. More males than females appear to be affected with total hemihypertrophy. PRENATAL DIAGNOSIS with ULTRASOUND and by viewing of the fetus *in utero* via fetoscopy is theoretically possible if there is sufficient enlargement of affected areas.

**hemochromatosis** Disorder characterized by the body's accumulation of excess iron. It appears to be rather common and greatly under-reported, due to the asymptomatic nature of many cases. Variable symptoms make diagnosis difficult. Onset is usually between the ages of 40 and 60. Women tend to develop the disease later than men, as they normally lose significant amounts of iron during menstruation, pregnancy and lactation. In severe cases the accumulation of iron leads to liver damage, which may eventually result in cirrhosis (see FAMILIAL CIRRHOSIS). Pancreas damage may lead to severe diabetes (see DIABETES MELLITUS). Additionally, there may be endocrine and heart problems, ANEMIA, chronic fatigue and impotence. Abdominal pain is common.

One of the first signs of the disorder is a bronzish tint to the skin. If treated promptly, the condition can be controlled. Treatment usually consists of removing blood, as much as two pints a week, until iron levels reach a normal range.

Inherited as an AUTOSOMAL RECESSIVE trait, studies in Europe, the United States and Australia indicate the frequency of this disorder may be as high as one in 300 to one in 400 people. One in 10 to one in 20 individuals may carry the GENE for the disorder. There is close linkage of the gene for HFE and the HLA locus on CHROMOSOME 6. This may help in diagnosing other family members at risk by determining HLA types within the family.

A blood test can be helpful in diagnosing the disorder by measuring serum iron, total iron binding capacity (TIBC) and ferritin in the blood.

There is also a juvenile form, beginning with abdominal pain in childhood and lack of adolescent sexual development in males (hypogonadatropic hypogonadism), and leading to heart failure between the ages of 20 and 30.

For more information, contact:

American Liver Foundation
998 Pompton Avenue
Cedar Grove, NJ 07009
(201) 857-2626
(800) 223-0179

**hemoglobin** The major component of the red blood cells, which carry oxygen from the lungs to the tissues. There are several normal types of hemoglobin, which is composed of heme, the iron-containing respiratory pigment that gives blood its red color, and globin chains. (Heme is also found in plants, where it gives chlorophyll its green color.) There are six known kinds of globin chains in man, designated alpha, beta, gamma, delta, epsilon and zeta, and the specific combination of globin chains determines the type of hemoglobin. The latter two are found only in embryonic red cells.

Hemoglobin A is the major adult hemoglobin (approximately 92% of adult total hemoglobin). It is composed of two alpha chains and two beta chains. Hemoglobin A2 normally constitutes about 2.5% of the blood and is composed of two alpha and two delta chains. It may be increased in beta THALASSEMIA and be decreased in iron deficiency. Hemoglobin F comprises the bulk of hemoglobin in the newborn, and is composed of two alpha and two gamma chains.

Hemoglobins are large molecules; due to their size, they have a propensity to exhibit a large number of MUTATIONS. More than 300 different types of abnormal hemoglobin have been identified. Many of the hemoglobin abnormalities cause no clinical abnormalities. Others may cause ANEMIA or decreased oxygen transport. Below are some of the more common abnormal hemoglobin conditions (hemoglobinopathies):

*Hemoglobin—Alpha chain abnormalities.* Abnormalities of the alpha chain of globins result in four forms of alpha thalassemia, hemoglobinopathies with an increased incidence in Asian populations.

*Hemoglobin C.* This is an AUTOSOMAL RECESSIVE trait that results in a chronic hemolytic anemia, with symptoms including abdominal pain and an enlarged spleen (splenomegaly). It has an increased incidence in blacks in the United States, with an estimated one in 50 carrying a single gene for the trait and one in 10,000 having the two genes required for expression of hemoglobin C disease. The disorder is sometimes associated with SICKLE-CELL ANEMIA. (See also hemoglobin S-C disease below.) This is a single base substitution in the gene for betaglobin resulting in the substitution of lysine for glutamic acid in the sixth AMINO ACID position in the beta chain. This is the same position of substitution as in sickle-cell anemia, but a different amino acid is substituted.

*Hemoglobin F, hereditary persistence of.* This is not an abnormal hemoglobin. The "F" in hemoglobin F stands for "fetal," and it is the primary type produced by the fetus, due to its superiority in absorbing oxygen from maternal blood. During infancy, the body gradually replaces fetal hemoglobin with adult hemoglobin. However, the tendency for the body to continue producing fetal hemoglobin can be inherited as an AUTOSOMAL DOMINANT trait. It was first observed in blacks and has subsequently been seen in Greeks, Thais and other ethnic groups.

*Hemoglobin H.* This is a form of hemoglobin with only Beta chains and no Alpha chains. It is a form of alpha-thalassemia.

*Hemoglobin M.* This type of hemoglobin is called methemoglobin; it is associated with congenital cyanosis, a bluish or grayish tint of the skin caused by oxygen deficiency. In hemoglobin M disease, the iron in the methemoglobin is unable to combine with oxygen. While there is no effective therapy, it is not life threatening due to the compensating presence of normal hemoglobin.

*Hemoglobin S.* This abnormality causes sickle-cell anemia, which was the first disease discovered to be due to a molecular abnormality of hemoglobin. The hemoglobin S causes red blood cells to collapse and assume a sickle shape. The complications that result from this abnormal shape cause anemia. This is an autosomal recessive trait. Unless genes for hemoglobin S are inherited from both parents, the individual will rarely exhibit clinical manifestations from the characteristic sickling of red blood cells.

*Hemoglobin S-C disease.* If a gene for hemoglobin S (sickle cell) is inherited from one parent, and a gene for hemoglobin C from another, the individual will have Hemoglobin S-C disease (sickle-cell-hemoglobin C disease), a mild form of sickle-cell anemia. Symptoms include blood in the urine (BENIGN FAMILIAL HEMATURIA) and pain in bones, joints, abdomen and chest. Onset is usually in the fourth decade, and the condition is not life threatening.

**hemolytic disease of the newborn**    A condition of the newborn characterized by ANEMIA, jaundice, enlargement of the liver and spleen (hepatosplenomegaly) and generalized swelling caused by excessive fluid in the tissues (edema; in newborns, this is called "hydrops fetalis"). It is caused by transplacental transmission of maternal antibody, usually provoked by incompatibility between maternal and fetal blood types. Incompatibilities of the ABO (blood) system are common but are not severe. Much more grave is Rh incompatibility, which may result in profound anemia in the fetus, sometimes severe enough to cause death in utero.

The Rh factor was first discovered on the surface of mature blood cells (erythrocytes) of the rhesus monkey and subsequently found to be present to a variable degree in humans, as well. Individuals who have this factor are said to be Rh positive (Rh+), and those without it are said to be Rh negative (Rh-). An Rh negative mother who is carrying an Rh positive fetus may develop antibodies against the Rh factor (sensitization)—for example, as a result of fetal red cells entering the maternal circulation at the time of delivery. Rh sensitization is prevented by the administration of anti-Rh antibodies to Rh- mothers at the time of delivery to "block" the sensitization process if any fetal Rh+ cells enter the mother's circulation. Unless sensitization is blocked, these antibodies can cross the placenta in a future pregnancy and enter fetal circulation, where they may destroy the red blood cells of an Rh+ fetus.

Close monitoring of the pregnancy can minimize the consequences of this incompatibility. This involves prenatal testing, fetal transfusions and expert obstetrical care.

**hemophilia**   Any of several disorders of the blood clotting process that greatly prolong coagulation time. Coagulation, or clotting, is the body's mechanism to halt bleeding; it involves at least 14 sequential steps, each requiring a specific plasma protein or "factor" normally found in the blood. In hemophilia, one of the factors required for the clotting sequence is deficient or absent.

The condition known as hemophilia has been recognized for thousands of years. In ancient Egypt, women whose eldest child bled to death from a minor wound were forbidden to have more children. By A.D. 400, the Jews knew hemophilia to be an inherited disease, and male babies were permitted to go uncircumcised if they had two brothers who bled to death at circumcision.

In the 19th and 20th centuries hemophilia was common in European royal families. Queen Victoria was a CARRIER, possibly the result of a new mutation inherited from her father or mother; she married her cousin, Prince Albert of Saxe-Coburg and passed the gene to several of her descendants, including Czarevich Alexis, son of Czar Nicholas II and the Czarina Alexandra. Alexandra turned to Rasputin to help cope with her son's disorder, ultimately ceding power to him, which may have helped precipitate the Russian Revolution.

In the United States, the first report of familial incidence was a 1792 newspaper account, and the transmission from unaffected mothers to sons was described in 1803.

The two most common forms of hemophilia are hemophilia A and hemophilia B. Hemophilia A and B have similar symptoms and were not recognized as separate disorders until 1952.

Both hemophilia A and B are X-LINKED recessive genetic diseases. While females carry the trait, they very rarely exhibit any symptoms of the disorder.

Hemophilia A (classic hemophilia), is caused by the deficiency of antihemophilic factor, or AHF, which is most commonly called factor VIII. Hemophilia B (also called Christmas disease, for the name of the family the disorder was first observed in) is caused by the deficiency of PTC (plasma thromboplastin component), or factor IX. Hemophilia A is four times as common, with an estimated incidence of one in 10,000 males, while hemophilia B is estimated to occur in one in 40,000 males. Approximately one woman in 5,000 is a carrier for hemophilia A, and one in 20,000 is a carrier of hemophilia B.

Hemophilia C is the least common and least severe form of hemophilia. It is caused by the deficiency of factor XI (PTA, plasma thromboplastin antecedent) and is seen with greatest frequency in individuals of Ashkenazi Jewish background. In contrast to hemophilia A and B it is inherited as an AUTOSOMAL RECESSIVE disorder. It often manifests itself as bleeding after a dental extraction or with heavy menstrual bleeding.

Hemophilia is typically divided into three classes: severe, moderate and mild, based on the level of clotting factor in the blood. In severe hemophilia, there is less than 1% of normal clotting factor. The degree of severity tends to be consistent from generation to generation.

Contrary to popular understanding, minor cuts and wounds do not present a threat to hemophiliacs. Rather, the gravest danger comes from spontaneous bleeding that may occur in joints and muscles. This is most prone to occur during years of rapid growth, typically between the ages of five and 15 years. Repeated spontaneous bleeding in joints may cause arthritis, and adjacent muscles often become weakened. Pressure on nerves caused by the accumulation of blood may result in pain, numbness and temporary inability to move the affected area. In the past, this often led to permanent crippling disability by adulthood. The development of purified clotting factors in the 1970s, isolated from donated blood, significantly improved the long-term outlook for hemophiliacs. Severe hemophiliacs required transfusions of clotting factors as frequently as once a week.

However, transfusions of clotting factor, which may contain blood products from as many as 1,000 blood donors, created another major health problem for hemophiliacs. Prior to 1984, the clotting factor was not screened for the AIDS virus, and as a result it is estimated that half of all hemophiliacs have become infected with the virus. Yet evidence indicates that, for unknown reasons, HIV-positive hemophiliacs (those who harbor the AIDS virus) do not develop symptoms of AIDS as frequently as HIV-positive individuals from other high risk groups.

Female carriers generally have lower clotting factor levels than non-carriers, facilitating carrier detection. Tests for factor VIII clotting activity can identify carriers of hemophilia A with 90% accuracy. DNA (see DEOXYRYBONUCLEIC ACID) analysis using gene probes can also be used to identify carriers of hemophilia A and B, but it requires that several family members be studied. In some families, not enough information is available to be useful.

PRENATAL DIAGNOSIS of hemophilia is possible. The first step is to determine the gender of the FETUS via AMNIOCENTESIS or CHORIONIC VILLUS SAMPLING. Hemophilia can usually be detected in a male fetus through fetal blood sampling, or with DNA analysis of fetal tissue. (See also VON WILLEBRAND DISEASE.)

For more information, contact:

The National Hemophilia Foundation
The Soho Building
110 Greene St. #406
New York, NY 10012
(212) 219-8180

**hemorrhagic disease of the newborn**
Condition characterized by bleeding (hemorrhaging) in the newborn. Bleeding may be localized (frequently intestinal) or diffuse. It is caused by an inadequate supply of vitamin K-dependent coagulation factors: II, VII, IX and X (components of the blood involved in coagulation). This is usually due to depletion of coagulation factors derived from the mother during pregnancy and the delay in establishment of bacterial flora of the intestine that produce vitamin K. Maternal ingestion of drugs (e.g., dilatin or coumadin) may also cause it. The condition can be treated with vitamin K. Routine administration of vitamin K to infants at birth is now a standard part of neonatal care to prevent this disorder.

**hepatitis**   A viral disease that may result in inflammation of the liver and destruction of the liver cells, potentially leading to fatal scarring (cirrhosis) of the liver. It occurs in three recognized forms: hepatitis A, hepatitis B (HBV) and a more recently identified hepatitis C, which appears to be the most common. Of most concern during pregnancy is HBV.

Hepatitis B, often transmitted by contaminated needles, sexual contact or contact with contaminated blood, can be transmitted to a developing fetus by an infected mother. However, only an estimated 5% are infected in the womb; the majority are infected during birth. Without treatment, an estimated 90% of infected infants will be chronic carriers of the virus, perhaps showing no signs of the disease but capable of transmitting it to others. They also have a greatly increased risk of developing cirrhosis (see FAMILIAL CIRRHOSIS) and liver CANCER. An estimated 16,500 infants are born annually to infected women, and 3,500 become chronic carriers. Approximately 25% will ultimately die of liver cancer or cirrhosis. Maternal infection has also been associated with increased rates of miscarriage (See ABORTION), LOW BIRTH WEIGHT and premature delivery (see PREMATURITY).

It is thought that one-tenth of one per cent of all Americans are chronic carriers of HBV, and the U.S. Centers for Disease Control has recommended that all pregnant women be tested for it. Vaccination with hepatitis B immune globulin soon after birth can prevent 85% to 90% of infected infants from becoming chronic carriers.

Hepatitis A is usually transmitted by contact with fecal material from an infected individual. Maternal infection during pregnancy is not associated with birth defects, though if contracted during the last two weeks of pregnancy, the infant may be born with the infection.

Hepatitis C, transmitted through sexual contact and by transfusions of contaminated blood, is believed to affect 3% to 7% of the U.S. population. An estimated 150,000 Americans are infected annually, with half of them developing chronic hepatitis C. The virus that causes this disorder was not identified until the late 1980s; prior to that time there was no way to test for it, and cases were described simply as non A and non B hepatitis. Diagnosis of hepatitis C is possible by blood test. Research has also indicated that a drug, alpha interferon, can control the infection and prevent liver destruction in this form of hepatitis.

**hepatolenticular degeneration**   See WILSON DISEASE.

**hereditary angiodema**   See HEREDITARY ANGIONEUROTIC EDEMA.

**hereditary   angioneurotic   edema (HANE)**   (hereditary angiodema) Affected individuals exhibit episodes of localized edema (an abnormal accumulation of fluid in body tissues), which can occur under the skin on the face, neck, lips, hands and feet. This causes swelling that is usually not painful, inflammatory or itchy.

Edema of a more serious nature can occur in the mucous membranes of the throat, stomach and intestines, accompanied by abdominal pain and vomiting. Unnecessary abdominal surgery has been performed in situations where the attending physician was not aware of the presence of this disorder, resulting in improper diagnosis of abdominal symptoms.

The greatest danger in this disorder is the occurrence of edema in the throat (larynx). Swelling of the laryngeal mucosa can obstruct the airway to the lungs, and has caused death in 10% to 30% of such cases. A tracheotomy, an incision in the throat to allow insertion of a tube that will permit breathing, is sometimes required.

The disorder can be detected in infancy. While present throughout life, symptoms are generally more severe in adolescence and tend to subside after 50 years of age.

Although first described and named medically in 1882, this disorder and its hereditary nature may have been noted earlier. It has been suggested that American author Nathaniel Hawthorne refers to this disorder in *The House of the Seven Gables*, published in 1851. The book describes members of a family who gurgled when excited and who sometimes died because of this, after a curse to choke on their own blood was placed on an ancestor. Hawthorne recognized that this was a hereditary disease and not a prophetic curse by noting that "this mode of death has been an idiosyncrasy with this family, for generations past … Old Maule's prophecy was probably founded on a knowledge of this physical predisposition."

Episodes of this disorder are recurrent and last from six hours to three days. There appears to be no precipitating event, although they are sometimes associated with menstruation, temperature extremes, physical trauma or emotional distress. The frequency of attacks of this disorder and the degree of disruption of daily living activities varies considerably. Some individuals may have only one episode in a lifetime, while others will experience frequent episodes with abdominal pain or the need for repeated tracheotomies.

The basic cause of the disorder is the deficiency of an inhibitor to the activity of the ENZYME C1 esterase, which is believed to increase the permeability of blood vessels, bringing on the edema.

Inherited as an AUTOSOMAL DOMINANT trait, the disorder has been observed in a large number of ethnic groups, including those originating in Northern Europe, the Mediterranean area and Africa.

Periods of remission can be prolonged by therapy with the androgen danazol. it is an anabolic steroid with little masculizing activity, which increases levels of C1 esterase inhibitor.

**hereditary anonychia** (absent [finger/toe] nails)　The primary characteristic of this CONGENITAL disorder is a partial or complete absence of nails on fingers or toes and various abnormalities of the nails and finger or toe bones. Abnormalities may include underdeveloped nail beds (the portion of the fingers or toes normally covered by nails), or furrowing, thickening or thinning of the outermost layer or horny skin (nail plate) at the nail site. Flattening and spreading out (spatulation) of the bones at the ends of the fingers or toes, or shortening of the finger, toe or hand bones may be seen in some cases.

This rare disorder occurs in both AUTOSOMAL DOMINANT and AUTOSOMAL RECESSIVE forms. It is detectable at birth or may develop at a later age. Life span and intelligence are normal.

Abnormalities of the nails may also be seen as part of malformation syndromes, such as the ECTODERMAL DYSPLASIAS.

**hereditary benign chorea**　An early onset, non-progressive form of chorea (involuntary movements), marked by involuntary twitching of the muscles of the limbs and face. Mental function remains normal. It appears to be inherited as an AUTOSOMAL DOMINANT trait.

Corticosteroids given to an affected individual to control his non-associated asthma attacks have been found, coincidentally, to reduce the frequency and amplitude of the chorea.

It is important to distinguish this benign disorder from the more debilitating HUNTINGTON'S CHOREA.

**hereditary coproporphyria**　See PORPHYRIA.

**hereditary disease**　A disease or abnormal condition that results from the influence of aberrant genes inherited from the mother or father. Hereditary diseases may be transmitted as AUTOSOMAL DOMINANT, AUTOSOMAL RECESSIVE, X-LINKED or polygenic or MULTIFACTORIAL traits. This represents a vast number of disorders. More than 4,300 conditions have been linked to single-gene (autosomal dominant, autosomal recessive, X-linked) defects alone. the number of multifactorial disorders is thought to be much greater.

The fact that some disorders now identified as hereditary tend to run in families has been noted since antiquity. (See also GENETIC DISORDERS; FAMILIAL DISEASE.)

**hereditary elliptocytosis**　A benign hereditary condition in which the red blood cells are oval or elliptical, instead of exhibiting their normal round shape. In the general population, it is estimated to occur in one in 2,000 live births. However, it is extraordinarily frequent in Dyacks (aborigines of Sarawak) and other aboriginal groups in Malaysia and Melanesia, where the incidence is reported to approach 40% of the population. it has been suggested that, like the other red cell disorders, such as hemoglobinopathies (e.g., SICKLE-CELL ANEMIA and THALASSEMIA), elliptocytosis may bestow an increased resistance to malarial parasites. It is inherited as an AUTOSOMAL DOMINANT trait.

**hereditary epilepsy**    Any of numerous brain function disorders, characterized by recurrent seizure attacks with sudden onset. (It is also the most common neurological condition complicating pregnancy.) Seizures occur when normal electrical signals between brain cells temporarily increase or otherwise act abnormally. One percent to 2% of the general population is estimated to have some form of epilepsy, and more males than females are affected. About 5% of the population will have a single seizure at some time in their life.

Eighty percent of epilepsy cases are idiopathic; no cause can be determined. In the other 20%, the epilepsy is secondary to an identifiable cause, often an underlying hereditary defect. Epilepsy or seizures is associated with over 130 genetic conditions. Two relatively common single-gene disorders that often cause seizures are TUBEROUS SCLEROSIS and NEUROFIBROMATOSIS. Even when the cause of an individual's epilepsy is not identifiable, genetic factors undoubtedly influence predisposition to develop seizures. Trauma, infection and tumor are examples of environmental causes of seizures, which may still involve genetic predispositions.

Indications that an individual's epilepsy is genetically influenced include a family history of seizures or the presence of additional abnormalities, such as mental retardation, metabolic disturbance, skin lesions, neurologic problems (including certain specific electroencephalographic abnormalities) and peculiar physical characteristics or anomalies.

In the ancient world, epilepsy was considered a divine affliction, and those affected were thought to be touched by the gods. However, Hippocrates (ca. 460-ca. 377 B.C.), the father of medicine, speculated that this, and other diseases, were actually hereditary: "But this disease seems to me to be no more divine than others … Its origin is hereditary like that of other disease … What is to hinder it from happening that where the father and mother were subject to this disease, certain of their offspring should be affected also?"

Considering all causes of epilepsy, a child with one epileptic parent is five times more likely than a child with non-epileptic parents to develop the condition. The risk is generally highest if the affected parent is the mother. Sons are slightly more likely than daughters to develop epilepsy, no matter which parent is affected. If one of a pair of twins develops epilepsy, the risk of a fraternal twin developing it is 5% to 20%, and 40% to 90% for an identical twin.

Various anticonvulsant drugs or tranquilizers may prevent or reduce the severity of seizures in many forms of epilepsy. (However, some ANTICONVULSANTS may cause BIRTH DEFECTS if taken during pregnancy. In GENETIC COUNSELING of those with epilepsy, the possible teratogenic effects of anticonvulsant drugs are usually more important than the possibility of transmitting the tendency to have seizures to offspring.)

The more common forms of epilepsy include:

*Grand mal epileptic seizures (convulsive seizures; generalized tonic clonic seizures).* This is the most common form of epilepsy. A grand mal seizure often begins with a hoarse cry, leading to unconsciousness, body stiffening and jerking movements. If seizures begin before four years of age, there is a 7.5% chance that siblings or offspring will develop epilepsy before they are 20. If the age of onset is between four and 15 years, the risk drops to 4.3%.

*Petit mal (absence) epileptic seizures.* A petit mal seizure lasts only a few seconds, occurs mostly in children and usually looks like daydreaming or blank staring, though it may be accompanied by blinking or chewing movements, turning of the head or waving of the arms.

Offspring and siblings of a petit mal epileptic have, in general, a 2% to 5% chance of developing the condition, though the risk may be as high as 10% for the daughter of an epileptic mother. Petit mal epilepsy is most likely polygenically inherited, with greater heritability in females.

*Infantile spasms (hypsarrhythmic EEG pattern).* These occur in infancy and childhood; in general, 5% of affected children have a family history of the condition. Some cases are idiopathic, and polygenic factors are the likely culprit; in these the general recurrence rate for siblings is 5% to 10%. Others are associated with genetic syndromes, such as PHENYLKETONURIA and TUBEROUS SCLEROSIS, and there is an X-LINKED form as well. It has been reported that 25% of infants with infantile spasms develop tuberous sclerosis.

*Myoclonic photosensitive epilepsy.* Here, a neurologic hypersensitivity to flashes of light is dominantly inherited. In a small proportion of people with this abnormal EEG pattern, exposure to such light induces seizures. When seizures are present, they appear to be highly inheritable.

For more information, contact:

Epilepsy Foundation of America
4351 Garden City Drive
Landover, MD 20785
(301) 459-3700

Epilepsy Society, Inc.
Ramapo Medical Prof. Bldg.
222 Route 59
Suffern, NY 10901
(914) 357-3490
(914) 294-6185

**hereditary essential tremor**    Familial disease, characterized by late-onset tremors and found to be quite common in certain parts of Sweden and Finland. Onset is usually between the ages of 40 and 50, though it may appear in adolescence, early adulthood or, in exceptional cases, at birth. The tremors begin symmetrically in the hands and arms, and may progress to the facial muscles and tongue, and may cause speech difficulties (dysarthria). The trunk and legs are sometimes involved, and the gait may become rigid and stiff.

Tremors occur at the frequency of three to 12 per second, and are usually exacerbated by fatigue and emotion and relieved by alcohol. The tremor is stationary for long periods following initial appearance of the disorder, but there is further progression in late life. Though progression of the disorder may cease, remission is rare.

Inherited as an autosomal dominant trait, it is estimated that in Sweden one in 10,000

individuals carry the gene for the disorder. However, in one parish the gene frequency is estimated to be as high as one in 22. A study of 210 affected individuals found that all but two could trace their ancestry back to four couples. In Finland, the disorder has been estimated to affect the remarkably high percentage of more than 55% of all persons over 40.

**hereditary gynecomastia**    The enlargement of the breasts in males. As a genetic condition gynecomastia with onset at puberty is associated with AMBIGUOUS GENITALIA, PSEUDOHERMAPHRODITISM, ADRENOGENITAL SYNDROMES, KLINEFELTER SYNDROME and other abnormalities of sexual differentiation. Familial cases have been reported in which gynecomastia is the only abnormality exhibited, and AUTOSOMAL DOMINANT, AUTOSOMAL RECESSIVE and X-LINKED transmission have all been proposed as the method of inheritance. As an isolated occurrence it is quite common among male adolescents; reportedly as many as 40% exhibit mild, benign, transitory gynecomastia during puberty.

**hereditary hemorrhagic telangiectasia**    See    OSLER-WEBER-RENDU SYNDROME.

**hereditary motor and sensory neuropathy**    See CHARCOT-MARIE-TOOTH DISEASE.

**hereditary progressive arthroophthalmopathy**    See    STICKLER SYNDROME.

**heredity**    The genetic transmission of characteristics from parent to offspring. The fact that there are conditions that appear to be passed from parent to offspring has been noted since antiquity. For example, Hippocrates (ca. 460-ca. 377 B.C.), the father of medicine, identified epilepsy, baldness and blue eyes as among hereditary conditions.

These characteristics may be inherited as single GENE traits (that is, AUTOSOMAL DOMINANT, AUTOSOMAL RECESSIVE or X-LINKED dominant or recessive), POLYGENIC (caused by the action of several genes) or MULTIFACTORIAL traits (caused by several genes in concert with environmental influences). Thousands of disorders in humans are hereditary; more than 2,200 different single-gene disorders alone have been confirmed, and more than 2,100 other suspected single-gene disorders have been reported. The number of multifactorial disorders is thought to be much greater. (See also FAMILIAL DISEASE; HEREDITARY DISEASE; MENDELIAN; "INTRODUCTION".)

**Hermansky-Pudlak albinism**    See ALBINISM.

**hermaphrodite**    (hermaphroditism) An individual with the reproductive organs of both male and female. The concept of dual sexuality in one individual is common to many primal myths. Use of the term "hermaphrodite" dates to at least 300 B.C.; it is most likely taken from the son of Hermes and Aphrodite, Hermaphrodite. According to the Roman poet Ovid, he was a normal youth whose being was united with that of a water nymph, thus becoming both male and female. However, it has also been suggested that the term may refer to *hermes*, road markers and stone boundary columns that were dedicated to Hermes, god of the road, which were originally topped with the head of Hermes but were occasionally crowned with the head of Aphrodite.

Throughout the Hellenistic-Roman period, hermaphrodites were depicted on gems, vases and mural paintings, and references to hermaphrodites can be found in the works of the Greek and Roman historians Herodotus and Pliny. The first medical writings attempting to detail actual case histories appeared in the 16th century. However, until late in the Middle Ages, human hermaphrodites were considered monsters.

In affected individuals ovaries and testicles are both present, and the external genitalia and internal reproductive structures are highly variable in form. There may be both ovarian and testicular tissue on one side and either an ovary or a testis on the other; or ovaries and testes may be on both sides (bilateral).

Affected individuals have often been diagnosed in early infancy as the result of efforts to determine their sex in cases of AMBIGUOUS GENITALIA. Diagnosis is made by a variety of methods, including physical examination, endocrine studies, karyotyping and a variety of imaging techniques involving the genitals and reproductive system.

More than half have a 46XX karyotype, that of a normal female, and most of the remainder 46XY, that of a normal male. Thus, chromosomally the hermaphrodite's gender is definitive. However, a very small percentage have both 46XX and 46XY cells lines, and thus are both male and female chromosomally (see CHROMOSOMES; CHROMOSOME ABNORMALITY).

The cause of hermaphroditism is unknown. It has its genesis after the fourth week of pregnancy, when gonadal sex is established. (Prior to that time, though chromosomal sex of an embryo is determined, tissues that form the genitals and reproductive system remain sexually undifferentiated.)

An estimated 80% of hermaphrodites are capable, with surgical and hormonal therapy, of becoming fertile females, and giving birth. However, there are no reports of hermaphrodites raised as males ever siring children. In the past, most hermaphrodites were raised as males. It may be preferable to raise them as females due to the increased chance of reproductive viability. Additionally, because malignancies may develop in abnormal testicular tissue, these abnormal testes should be removed.

True hermaphroditism is rare in humans; little more than 525 cases have been documented. Much more common are conditions of ambiguous genitalia in which individuals appear to be of indeterminate gender, due to lack of development of external genitalia, such as PSEUDOHERMAPHRODITISM, a form of ambiguous genitalia with the presence of only a single type of gonadal tissue.

**Herpes simplex**   See TORCH SYNDROME.

**Hers disease**   See GLYCOGEN STORAGE DISEASE.

**heterochromia irides**   Asymmetry of pigmentation of the irides (eyes of separate colors). It is seen most frequently in WAARDENBURG SYNDROME and in PIEBALD SKIN TRAIT. It may also result from damage to autonomic nerves (cervical branches of the sympathetic nerves) as a result of birth injury. Cervical sympathetics are automatic nerves that govern pupil size, sweating and other functions. When these nerves are damaged, the iris may lose color.

Whether this condition ever occurs as an inherited condition independent of any other syndrome is not clear, though it has been suggested that it occurs in isolated cases as an AUTOSOMAL DOMINANT trait.

**heterogeneity** (heterogeneous)   T h e ability of a single (or very similar) condition(s) to be caused by a variety of genetic or non-genetic causes. Many inheritable disorders, MENDELIAN as well as MULTIFACTORIAL and POLYGENIC, are heterogeneous.

**heterozygote**   An individual with different ALLELES or unlike GENES in a gene pair that controls a given characteristic. In the past, this generally indicated that an individual possessed one dominant and one recessive gene for a given characteristic, but the concept of heterozygosity has become more complex as geneticists have learned that there may be numerous forms (or ALLELES) of a recessive gene. Individuals who are heterozygotes for AUTOSOMAL RECESSIVE traits, and women who are heterozygotes for X-LINKED recessive traits, are often termed CARRIERS.

**high scapula**   See SPRENGEL DEFORMITY.

**hip, congenital dislocation of**   See CONGENITAL DISLOCATION OF THE HIP.

**Hirschsprung disease** (colon aganglionosis)   A congenital dilation of the colon, which prevents feces from passing into the rectum and being excreted, causing constipation, vomiting, dehydration and FAILURE TO THRIVE. Surgical removal of the affected portion of the colon results in immediate recovery in 50% of those treated. Without treatment, in those severely affected the condition may result in death. (An estimated 20% of those affected die in infancy.) It results from the absence of the nerve cells (myenteric ganglia) in the colon that normally propel the movement of feces in the intestine.

Incidence is estimated at one in 8,000 live births, and males are more commonly affected than females by a ratio of approximately three to one. Named for Danish pediatrician H. Hirschsprung (1830-1916), who published a description in 1888, it is believed to be inherited as a MULTIFACTORIAL trait, though no clear method of hereditary transmission has been identified. An increased incidence of Hirschsprung disease has been noted among infants with DOWN SYNDROME. Most often the disorder is a SPORADIC occurrence.

**hirsutism**   Excessive hair growth, typically at puberty and especially in females. The hair may appear on the face, chest, abdomen or extremities. Other secondary sex characteristics remain normal. The cause is unknown, though familial cases have been noted.

**histidinemia**   Histidine is a basic AMINO ACID found in many proteins and, metabolized by the body; it is essential for optimal growth in infants. A deficiency of the ENZYME histidase, normally found in the liver and the thick outer layer of the skin (stratum corneum), results in a failure to metabolize histidine and produces an excess of histidine in the blood and urine of those affected. This defect leads to the condition known as histidinemia. For some years it was believed that this resulted in emotional and behavioral problems, speech impairment, scholastic failure and mild to moderate MENTAL RETARDATION. However, it has become apparent that in the vast majority of cases histidinemia is a harmless biochemical abnormality. In only a small proportion of those with the enzyme deficiency (some believe less than 1%) does it cause significant neurologic dysfunction.

Inherited as an AUTOSOMAL RECESSIVE enzyme defect, histidinemia can be detected in the first week of life by a blood test for histidine or by a test for histidase activity in the stratum corneum.

This defect occurs in approximately one in every 12,000 live births, a frequency approximating that of PHENYLKETONURIA.

In some states, the law has required testing of all newborns for histidinemia. Because of the question of whether histidinemia is really a "disease," the benefit of this screening is controversial.

**HLA**   See HUMAN LEUKOCYTE ANTIGEN.

**holoprosencephaly**   A group of facial malformations caused by defective development of the embryonic forebrain. Essentially, the forebrain fails to divide, or divide properly, into cerebral hemispheres. The type of holoprosencephaly exhibited is determined by the severity of this defective development.

In the most severe form, CYCLOPIA , there is a single eye-globe in the middle of the face and often congenital absence of the nose (arhinia), though there is usually a malformed nose-like structure with no connection to the postnasal space.

In ethmocephaly, another form of holoprosencephaly, there are two closely set eyes (hypotelorism) associated with absence of the nose, though, again, proboscis formation occurs.

Cebocephaly, a third form, is characterized by hypotelorism and a single nostril nose with a blind ending.

Other less severe forms have varying degrees of hypotelorism and abnormalities of the nose (e.g., a flat, boneless nose) and upper lip (e.g., clefts).

Holoprosencephalic infants often have small heads (MICROCEPHALY), and their pregnancies are frequently abnormal, often with excess AMNIOTIC FLUID (polyhydramnios). About 25% require cesarean section delivery.

Holoprosencephaly is estimated to occur in one in 15,000 births. This condition is often seen in CHROMOSOMAL ABNORMALITIES, particularly trisomy 13, 18p-, 13q and triploidy. It may also be seen in syndromes such as the MECKEL SYNDROME. Among spontaneous ABORTIONS, the rate of holoprosencephaly may be as high as one in 250. It is believed to be inherited as an AUTOSOMAL RECESSIVE characteristic in some cases, since there have been many instances of affected SIBLINGS, though there may be a mild AUTOSOMAL DOMINANT form as well. Most often, however, the defect is an isolated occurrence.

Those with the most severe forms of holoprosencephaly do not survive infancy. Infants with milder forms often survive into childhood, though they exhibit moderate to severe MENTAL RETARDATION.

PRENATAL DIAGNOSIS, especially in severe cases, may be accomplished with ULTRASOUND.

**Holt-Oram syndrome** (heart-hand syndrome)   Disorder characterized by defects in the thumbs, hands, arms and heart; first described in 1960 by Mary Holt and Samuel Oram, both cardiologists at Kings College Hospital in London.

The thumb may be absent or partially developed. It may also be finger-like, with three phalanx bones (triphalangeal) rather than the normal two, rendering it nonopposable. In the most severe cases, abnormal bones in the wrist (carpal bones) may further reduce rotation of the thumb as well as the wrist. The arms may be shortened, with the hand attached directly to the shoulder (PHOCOMELIA). The lower limbs are normal.

Atrial septal defect is the most common CONGENITAL HEART DEFECT seen among individuals with Holt-Oram syndrome. In addition, a duct that normally occurs only in the FETUS may decrease the amount of blood circulating in the lungs (PATENT DUCTUS ARTERIOSUS). Ventricular septal defect, transposition of the great vessels, and mitral valve prolapse may also occur.

In most cases both heart defects and upper limb abnormalities occur, although occasionally one may be seen without the other. The degree of the malformations varies among individuals with the syndrome, even within families with multiple affected individuals.

The syndrome is detectable in infancy, with upper extremity abnormalities usually visible at birth. Life span depends on the severity of defects. Surgery can correct some of the heart and skeletal defects. Intelligence is normal.

The basic defect in this rare disorder is unknown. It is inherited as an AUTOSOMAL DOMINANT trait. Prenatal ULTRASOUND and FETOSCOPY may detect the syndrome if the abnormalities are severe.

**homocystinuria**   Disorder that manifests itself in skeletal abnormalities, such as knock knees (genu valgum), high foot arch (pes cavus), either a ridged or a funnel-shaped chest (pectus carinatum or excavatum) and SCOLIOSIS. The abnormalities may be detected visually or by X rays. Restricted mobility of joints and osteoporosis, which leads to fracture, are common. The individuals have a tall, thin appearance, with long, thin extremities and digits resembling those of MARFAN SYNDROME.

Clotting (thrombosis) in blood vessels leading to the heart, lungs, brain and kidneys is also common and may cause death at any time from infancy. Some individuals may have flushed cheeks (malar flush). One-half to two-thirds are mentally retarded.

Most affected individuals who live past age 10 develop a displacement of the lens of the eye (ectopia lentis). This can lead to complications such as progressive near-sightedness, detached retina and glaucoma.

Affected individuals lack the enzyme cystathionine ß-synthase. This results in a buildup of toxic compounds that is assumed to cause the physical symptoms.

Homocystinuria can be detected within two to four days of birth by urine or blood tests. In about half of cases, treatment with vitamin B6 (pyridoxine)  started in infancy prevents all signs of the disorder. In other cases a low-methionine diet can minimize skeletal malformations and ocular changes, and prevent MENTAL RETARDATION and thrombosis.

The disorder is rare, with incidence below one per 100,000 in the general population, but slightly more prevalent in Ireland and among persons of Irish descent. It is inherited as an AUTOSOMAL RECESSIVE trait. Individuals may live past age 50, but the potential for thrombosis greatly reduces life expectancy.

Other rare, variant forms of the disease result from defects in vitamin B12 and folic acid metabolism.

**homozygous; homozygosity**   Having identical ALLELES or identical corresponding GENES for a given trait.

**horseshoe kidney**   A CONGENITAL abnormality in which both kidneys are united at their lower ends, creating a horseshoe-shaped mass rather than two individual kidneys. It occurs in an estimated 1 in 400 live births. Recurrence in families is rare. It is also seen in CHROMOSOME ABNORMALITIES; e.g., 20% of infants with trisomy 18 have horseshoe kidney. It is often entirely asymptomatic, but may lead to obstruction of urinary flow, and therefore to stones, infection or pain. Horseshoe kidney is generally detected by X ray or ULTRASOUND.

**human leukocyte antigen (HLA)** (major histocompatibility complex)   A GENETIC MARKER used in determining the compatibility of tissue for organ transplants. The major histocompatibility complex in humans is found on the short arm of chromosome 6 and is the location (loci) of a number of GENES that play a role in immunological response. The designation for this area on the CHROMOSOME is HLA (human leukocyte antigen).

If an individual is to receive an organ transplant, it is possible to test the compatibility of their HLA type with that of the potential donor. Complications associated with organ rejection will be minimized if the donor's HLA is compatible with the recipient's.

Certain HLA types are associated with a susceptibility to develop a number of diseases. Thus HLA genes appear to be one of the inherited "susceptibility factors" underlying the MULTIFACTORIAL inheritance of a number of common disorders and responsible for the familial incidence of these diseases. The best known example of an association of HLA type with disease susceptibility is the association of ANKYLOSING SPONDYLITIS with HLA B27. Other disorders that are associated with specific HLA types include PSORIASIS, juvenile-onset DIABETES MELLITUS, Graves disease, MYASTHENIA GRAVIS, celine disease and RHEUMATOID ARTHRITIS. Other diseases are closely linked to the HLA gene, and thus HLA types can be used as a marker for the presence of the disease gene. Such is the case for HEMOCHROMATOSIS and congenital adrenal hyperplasia (21-hydroxylase deficiency). HLA types are also used as markers for paternity testing. (See also ADRENOGENITAL SYNDROMES.)

**humeroradial synostosis**  The fusion of two bones of the arm (the humerus of the upper arm and the radius of the forearm) rendering the arm unable to bend at the elbow, or severely limiting its motion at the joint. The basic cause is unknown.

Other abnormalities have been associated with this condition in a few cases, and humeroradial synostosis may also be associated with a number of distinct syndromes. In isolation, this rare condition may be inherited as either an AUTOSOMAL DOMINANT or AUTO-SOMAL RECESSIVE trait. In most cases, the prognosis for a normal life span is favorable, depending on the degree of severity of associated abnormalities.

**humpback, hunchback**  An abnormal curvature of the spine that gives the back the appearance of having a lump or protuberance. Medically, this condition is referred to as kyphosis. A deformity associated with many CONGENITAL and hereditary disorders affecting the skeletal system, it is perhaps best known as the affliction of Quasimodo, the fictional character in Victor Hugo's novel *Notre Dame de Paris* (1831). The condition often occurs in combination with SCOLIOSIS, an abnormal lateral (sideways) curvature of the spine. When the two are seen together, it is referred to as kyphoscoliosis.

**hunchback**  See HUMPBACK.

**Hunter syndrome**  See MUCOPOLY-SACCHARIDOSIS.

**Huntington's chorea** (Huntington's disease; HD)  A progressive disorder of the central nervous system characterized by the development of bizarre, uncontrollable movements (chorea) of the arms, legs, torso and facial muscles, intellectual impairment and severe mental disturbances. Its arrival in the New World can be traced to the 17th century, and manifestations of the disorder may have been responsible for charges made against some men and women of consorting with the devil and of being witches.

In 1630, three men whose families had been persecuted for witchcraft immigrated to America. These men and their descendants had repeated problems with legal authorities, and several were executed for witchcraft. One of the three men subsequently settled in East Hampton, Long Island, in New York, and his progeny were notorious locally for a strange and frightening disease.

While growing up, George Huntington (1850-1916) visited patients from this family, accompanied by his father and grandfather, who were general practitioners. In 1872, after graduating from medical school, he published his first and only paper, "On Chorea," in which he described the disorder that now bears his name.

Approximately 25,000 individuals have been confirmed as having HD, and 125,000 are thought to be at risk for developing the disorder. Most cases in the United States can be traced to these three original settlers, though it is seen in other ethnic groups as well. Cases in South Africa have been traced to Dutch immigrants who settled there in 1658, and in Venezuela to a German sailor who arrived about 1860. An extensive kindred near Venezuela's Lake Maracaibo has been well-documented. It is one-third as prevalent among blacks and very rare in Japanese.

The cause of HD is unknown, though the brains of affected individuals exhibit characteristic deterioration. An area that is important in motor control, the caudate nucleus, is severely shrunken, and spiny neurons, cells that carry impulses within the brain, are destroyed. A neurotoxin, quinolinic acid, normally present in the brain, is found in abnormal concentrations in the affected areas of the brain.

Onset is usually between the ages of 35 and 45, though it has appeared in children as young as two years of age and in adults as old as 80. In these unusual cases, differentation from other neurologic diseases is imperative. Initial symptoms include irritability, clumsiness, depression and forgetfulness. Mood, personality change and uncontrollable movements may precede correct diagnosis by a decade. (Folksinger Woody Guthrie, who was affected, was first thought to be an alcoholic, and later a schizophrenic, before he was properly diagnosed.)

Progressive deterioration of the central nervous system leads to slurred speech, grimacing, compulsive clenching and unclenching of fists and flailing of arms and legs. Ultimately, those affected succumb to pneumonia, heart failure or other complications 15 to 20 years after onset.

HD is inherited as an AUTOSOMAL DOMINANT disorder, with an incidence estimated at between from 4 and 10 per 100,000 births. Age of onset and the rate of progression may be influenced by the gender of the parent from whom the disorder was inherited. When paternally inherited, the most common form of HD begins an average of three years earlier than when maternally inherited. For example, juvenile and adolescent forms are almost always paternally inherited. Late onset cases (age 50 or later) are twice as likely to be maternally inherited. New MUTATIONS are very rare, accounting for perhaps only 0.1% of cases.

There is no cure, though drugs may alleviate some of the associated movement disorders. Antidepressants and counseling may be required; due to the severe mental depression that often accompanies the disorder, by some estimates as many as 25% of those affected are though to attempt suicide.

Generally, those who are at risk or those who are affected have had children before they learn whether they have inherited the condition and are capable of transmitting it to their offspring. A GENETIC MARKER, or a chromosomal signpost that indicates the presence of the HD gene, was discovered on chromosome 4 in 1983, and presymptomatic diagnosis of some individuals with HD, and PRENATAL DIAGNOSIS for HD within some large families, is now possible. Tests require blood or tissue samples from several relatives. Testing is considered 99% accurate and is being done on a limited basis. Those tested undergo additional psychological counseling due to the potentially devastating nature of the results. However, surveys among those at risk and response to the currently available procedure indicates there may not be an overwhelming demand for diagnosis among at-risk individuals. GENETIC COUNSELING for HD is among the most difficult counseling problems.

For more information, contact:

The Huntington's Disease Society of
America, Inc.

140 West 22nd Street, 6th floor
New York, NY 10011
(212) 242-1968

Hereditary Disease Foundation
606 Wilshire Boulevard, Suite 504
Santa Monica, CA 90401
(213) 458-4183

**Huntington's disease**    See HUNT-
INGTON'S CHOREA.

**Hurler syndrome**    See MUCOPOLY-
SACCHARIDOSIS (type I).

**Hutchinson-Gilford progeria syn-
drome**    See PROGERIA.

**hydrocephalus**    An abnormal increase of
cerebrospinal fluid (CSF) within the cranial
cavity, along with the expansion of the ventricles of the brain, enlargement of the skull and
atrophy of the brain. It may result in physical
incapacity, mental retardation, blindness and
death. The term is taken from the Greek words
*hydros* (fluid) and *cephalus* (head).

Within the brain are four fluid-filled cavities called ventricles. There are two lateral
ventricles (one in the center of each cerebral
hemisphere) and smaller third and fourth ventricles (one atop the other in the middle of the
brain, between the lateral ventricles). The ventricles are connected, or "communicate,"
through passageways that lead from the lateral
ventricles into the third and fourth ventricles,
and finally into the spinal column. Small,
flower-like tufts within the ventricles, called
the choroid plexus, produce CSF at a rate of
approximately 350 to 500 cc. every day. (Most
is produced in the larger lateral ventricles.)
After circulating around the brain and spinal
cord, the CSF is reabsorbed into the blood. In
almost all cases, hydrocephalus is caused by a
blockage somewhere in this CSF circulatory
system. The body does not reduce CSF production, and the increase in cranial pressure
caused by the buildup creates serious medical
problems.

If upon examination there is no apparent
blockage, and it appears that fluid is free to
circulate throughout the ventricles, the hydrocephalus is referred to as "communicating."
(That is, the ventricles remain in communication.) However, if blockage is observed within
the CSF circulatory system, the hydrocephalus is said to be "noncommunicating."

The signs of the condition are an enlarged
head (macrocephaly), usually appearing first
as a bulge of the anterior fontanelle, the soft
spot on the forward top portion of the infant's
head. Cranial sutures (the gaps or seams between the skull bones) may be widely separated, the scalp may appear to be stretched and
glistening and scalp veins distended. In severe
cases, the eyes may appear to deviate downward ("sunsetting") due to pressure on the
optic nerve. Vomiting, irritability, lethargy
and seizures are other symptoms.

In those born with the condition, the head
may appear large from birth. When the condition develops before the bones of the skull have
fused, the head will grow larger as the pressure
builds. There will be less swelling, but more
intracranial pressure, when the skull bones have
fused in approximately six to 12 months.

The condition is estimated to occur in one in
500 births. Seventy-five percent to 95% of cases
have their origin in fetal development, the remainder develop hydrocephalus as a result of
complications arising from other conditions.

Hydrocephalus can occur as an isolated
condition, as part of a SYNDROME, or in association with other defects. An X-LINKED recessive form accounts for a significant proportion
of male cases. It accounts for perhaps one-
quarter of all hydrocephalus in males that
result from a narrowing of the communication
between the third and fourth ventricles. Hydrocephalus may also result from in-
traventricular hemorrhages in premature
babies. The blood clot that forms after the
bleeding may block CSF circulation or
reabsorption.

Many children with hydrocephalus may
have developmental delays, disorders of muscle tone and movement, feeding and speech

difficulties, perceptual motor disturbances or sensory disorders. Occasionally there are ocular problems, as well.

In about 30% of cases, an enlarged head is evident at birth. The majority of the remaining cases are diagnosed within the first few months of life, when a disproportionate increase in the size of the head becomes observable. Fifty percent of the cases are identified within the first four months of life and 80% within the first year.

The condition can be confirmed through CT scans of the brain and by measuring CSF pressure within the brain. Prenatal diagnosis of the condition is sometimes possible using ULTRASOUND to detect an enlarged head. A positive finding may require delivery via CESAREAN SECTION due to the increased size of the cranium.

The primary method of treatment is surgical implantation of a shunt, a tube that drains excess CSF from the ventricle of the brain. It typically runs under the skin along the scalp and neck and empties into the abdominal or peritoneal cavity, where it is absorbed into the body. Due to this procedure, affected individuals with proper diagnosis and treatment can live normal life spans relatively uncomplicated by the condition. Successful shunting operations have even been performed on hydrocephalic fetuses in utero, but such operations remain experimental and the role of this procedure is unclear.

As an isolated condition, the prognosis is least favorable when hydrocephalus is present at birth. Almost half of the cases of true congenital hydrocephaly are STILLBORN. One-quarter die soon after birth, only 5% survive. Among the survivors, less than half have normal IQs, with the rest exhibiting mild to severe MENTAL RETARDATION.

Some infants with CONGENITAL hydrocephalus will also have additional abnormalities within the brain and other malformations that affect the brain or other organs of the body. These may be relatively harmless, such as CLEFT LIP and cleft palate, or may have serious consequences, such as heart disease and obstruction of the bowel. In addition, 80% of infants with SPINA BIFIDA may have hydrocephalus as a further complication.

For more information, contact:

The National Hydrocephalus Foundation
Route 1, River Road
Box 210 A
Joliet, IL 60436
(815) 467-6548

Hydrocephalus Parent Support Group
225 Dickinson Street, H-893
San Diego, CA 92103
(619) 726-0507

Guardians of Hydrocephalus Research
  Foundation
2618 Avenue Z
Brooklyn, NY 11235
(718) 854-4443

**hymen, imperforate**   See   IMPERFORATE HYMEN.

**hyperammonemia, congenital**   See UREA CYCLE DEFECTS.

**hypercholesterolemia**   See   CORONARY ARTERY DISEASE.

**hyperglycinemia, nonketotic**   See NONKETOTIC HYPERGLYCINEMIA.

**hyperimmunoglobulin E**   See   JOB SYNDROME.

**hypermobility**   The ability to move joints beyond their normal range of extension; in colloquial language "double-jointedness." It is noted in disorders of the skeletal and connective tissues such as MARFAN SYNDROME and EHLERS-DANLOS SYNDROME. Benign hypermobility syndrome is an AUTOSOMAL DOMINANT disorder with hypermobility of the joints, which may dislocate, but with no skin involvement, as is seen in the Ehlers-Danlos syndrome.

**hyperphosphatasia** Also known as juvenile Paget disease, this is a HEREDITARY DISEASE characterized by numerous skeletal malformations. They include easily fractured bones, bowed legs, short neck, an unusually prominent sternum or chest (pectus carinatum), abnormal curvature of the spine (kyphoscoliosis), an enlarged head and enlarged and pronounced brow (frontal bossing).

During the first year of life, infants exhibit fever and painful and swollen extremities, and between the ages of two and three years develop an enlarged head, often experiencing headaches and vision and hearing loss. Affected individuals frequently have numerous bone fractures, though they heal normally. Growth is affected, but not seriously diminished. Activities such as running, walking or jumping are impaired due to muscle weakness; a movement such as extending the arm from the elbow is often impossible.

Laboratory tests reveal elevated serum acid and serum alkaline phosphatase levels with normal calcium and phosphorus levels. Elevated levels of the amino acid hydroxyproline are found in connective tissue.

The basic defect of this AUTOSOMAL RECESSIVE disorder is not understood. Bones remain weak since fibrous bone never strengthens or becomes compact as they normally would.

**hypertelorism** An abnormally wide distance between the eyes. CONGENITAL ocular hypertelorism is very common in many GENETIC DISORDERS. As an isolated condition, familial cases have been noted, though the mode of inheritance is unclear.

**hypertelorism-hypospadias syndrome** See G SYNDROME.

**hypertension, essential** See ESSENTIAL HYPERTENSION.

**hyperthermia of anesthesia** See MALIGNANT HYPERTHERMIA.

**hypertriglyceridemia** See CORONARY ARTERY DISEASE.

**hypochondroplasia** A form of DWARFISM caused by defective skeletal development (chondrodystrophy). Though it is a distinct disorder, for many years after it was first described in 1913 it was considered a form of ACHONDROPLASIA. (Though it resembles achondroplasia, its features are milder, especially in the hands and spine as well as in the lack of craniofacial involvement.) The degree of height reduction and disproportion of the physique is variable.

Birthweight may be low (see LOW BIRTH WEIGHT). The head appears normal, though the forehead may be prominent. Short stature may not be recognized for two to six years. Mildly affected individuals may remain undiagnosed. The body is thick and stocky with a relatively long trunk and short limbs. The elbows may not fully extend. The hands and feet are short and broad. Bowleggedness (genu varum, see BOWLEG) is sometimes present but often disappears with age. The abdomen may protrude slightly, and individuals may exhibit a swayback appearance (lumbar lordosis). As adults, individuals may experience pain in joints and lower back. Approximately 10% exhibit mild MENTAL RETARDATION. Lifespan is normal. Average height ranges from 51 inches to 57 inches (130 cm to 145 cm).

It is inherited as an AUTOSOMAL DOMINANT trait; while familial incidence is well-documented, most cases appear to be SPORADIC, resulting from new MUTATION, in some cases related to advanced paternal age. The defect that causes the skeletal maldevelopment is unknown. It is estimated to occur approximately one-twelfth as frequently as achondroplasia.

PRENATAL DIAGNOSIS may be possible in at-risk pregnancies based on ULTRASOUND findings of characteristic fetal skeletal deficiencies, and has been accomplished. However, because of the great variability of this condition it may not always be possible.

For more information, contact:

Little People of America, Inc.
P.O. Box 633
San Bruno, CA 94066
(415) 589-0695

Human Growth Foundation
4720 Montgomery Lane, Suite 909
Bethesda, MD 20814
(301) 656-6904
(301) 656-7540

**hypogammaglobulenemia**   See IM-
MUNE DEFICIENCY DISEASE.

**hypophosphatasia**   A HEREDITARY DIS-
EASE resulting in an abnormal balance of bone
calcium and phosphate, causing the bone tissue
to inadequately calcify or not calcify at all. It
occurs in infantile-, childhood- and adult-onset
forms. Depending on the severity of the disorder, effects range from intrauterine death to
modest handicaps in childhood and adulthood.

The infantile form is the most severe. It is
characterized by short, bowed limbs, soft and
beaded ribs, deformed and enlarged joints,
and poor skull formation. Seizures, vomiting
and a high-pitched cry are common. Affected
infants are often stillborn or die early due to
respiratory problems. Some, however, spontaneously improve.

The childhood form is generally milder.
Symptoms may appear after six months of age
and include premature skull bone closure
(craniosynostosis), growth retardation, narrow chest, enlarged wrists, knees and ankles
and bowed legs caused by RICKETS. Additional features are premature loss of baby teeth
and a weakened immune system. Calcification of the kidney and an excess of calcium
in the blood (hypercalcemia) may accompany these symptoms.

The adult form is the mildest and appears
as a reduction or thinning of bone mass (osteoporosis) and occasional bone fractures.

Infantile and childhood forms of
hypophosphatasia are AUTOSOMAL RECES-
SIVE traits, while the adult form is an AUTOSO-

MAL DOMINANT. Occurrence is rare: Approximately 200 cases have been identified. The
frequency of the lethal form is estimated to be
about one per 100,000 live births.

PRENATAL DIAGNOSIS may be achieved by
finding extremely reduced alkaline phosphatase activity (similar to that seen in the blood
of affected individuals) in fetal cells obtained
via AMNIOCENTESIS or CHORIONIC VILLUS
SAMPLING. Prenatal ULTRASOUND has also
been used to diagnose severe infantile cases
before birth.

**hypophosphatemia** (X-linked hypophosphatemia; X-linked vitamin D-resis-
tant rickets)   Condition characterized by
an abnormally low concentration of phosphate in the blood, and detectable by laboratory testing at birth; it results from defective
reabsorption of phosphate by the kidneys. In
addition to the loss of phosphate through the
kidneys, the body does not respond to dietary
levels of vitamin D. Lacking these substances,
bones become soft and easily deformed (RICK-
ETS) as an affected child grows. Other symptoms, which may progress with age, include
slow growth, short stature, dental abnormalities, spinal and skull deformities and joint limitations.

Inherited as an X-LINKED dominant trait, it is
estimated to occur in approximately one in
200,000 live births. It is partially responsive to
early, continual treatment with oral phosphate
and vitamin D supplementation. There is evidence that the location for this defective gene is
on the short arm (p) of the X CHROMOSOME.

**hypoplastic congenital anemia**   See
ANEMIA.

**hypospadias**   Developmental defect of
the urinary tract readily recognizable in the
male at birth. The urethral opening, which is
normally at the tip of the penis, is instead
located on the underside of the penis. Also,
there is a thin, deficient amount of foreskin on
the upper surface of the penis. In approximately
half of those affected, the penis also curves downward due to a fibrous band (chordee) that, com-

bined with the urethral opening on the underside, forces the child to urinate in the direction of his feet rather than in the normal forward direction. If not corrected, chordee can cause painful erection later in life, with an inability to perform sexual intercourse and normal impregnation.

The location of the misplaced opening may be at the juncture of the head and shaft of the penis (60%); along the shaft (15%); at the point where the shaft joins the scrotum (20%); or in the perineum, the area between the scrotum and the anus (5%).

Complications of hypospadias can involve a narrowing (stenosis) of the urethral opening, disease resulting from this obstruction of the urinary tract (obstructive uropathy) and, ultimately, potential kidney failure.

Hypospadias is estimated to occur once in every 186 live births. The exact cause is unknown. It is primarily a male disorder, although a rare misplacement of the urethral opening inside the female vagina occurs about once for every 10,000 cases of male hypospadias.

Corrective surgery is almost always successful, and there is no shortening of the normal life span. Elective circumcision should not be done since the foreskin is used in the corrective surgery, which for psychological reasons is generally done prior to the age of 15 months.

It is the result of MULTIFACTORIAL inheritance in most cases. The risk of a second male being born with hypospadias has been estimated to be about 12%. This increases to 26% in those cases where the father also was born with hypospadias.

**hypothyroidism, congenital**    See CONGENITAL HYPOTHYROIDISM.

---

# I

**I-cell disease**    See MUCOLIPIDOSIS.

**ichthyosis**    Any of several specific hereditary or congenital skin disorders. Its name is taken from the Greek *ichthys*, for fish, and *osis*, for

condition, because the skin of affected individuals, due to its dry, scaly appearance, is sometimes described as resembling fish skin. Ichthyosis occurs in AUTOSOMAL DOMINANT, AUTOSOMAL RECESSIVE and X-LINKED forms. Severity ranges from mild, easily treated cosmetic problems to severe, lethal conditions.

*Ichthyosis vulgaris.* Inherited as an autosomal dominant disorder. Onset occurs in infancy or later, with symptoms of mild scaling seen mainly on the extremities, particularly the palms and soles. Incidence is estimated at approximately one in 300 individuals. A significant proportion of those with dominant forms of ichthyosis who are under medical attention also have asthma, eczema or hayfever.

*Ichthyosis congenita.* This autosomal recessive form may result in death in the first months of life due to complications from severe skin lesions. However, individuals may heal completely or exhibit mild ichthyosis for the remainder of their lives. (See HARLEQUIN FETUS.)

*Lamellar ichthyosis.* Affected infants may be covered with a smooth layer of skin, which is shed in two to three weeks after birth, often leaving the body covered with thick scales, which may persist or disappear spontaneously in early infancy. Inherited as an autosomal recessive trait, this rare disorder is estimated to occur in one in 3,000,000 births.

*X-linked ichthyosis.* As the name implies, this is an X-linked disorder, seen only in males and associated with a deficiency of the enzyme steroid sulfatase. It is similar to ichthyosis vulgaris, though it presents a more striking "fish-skin" appearance. It affects an estimated one in 6,000 males.

**IDDM**    See DIABETES MELLITUS.

**imaging, fetal**    See FETAL IMAGING.

**immotile cilia syndrome**    See KARTAGENER SYNDROME.

**immune deficiency diseases**    Those diseases that result in a breakdown of the immune system, the mechanism by which the body defends itself against viral and bacterial infection, parasitic disease, fungi and other microorganisms. The immune system is also responsible for allergic reactions, for rejecting transplanted organs and perhaps even for the prevention of the development of CANCER.

Immune disorders that result from defects within the immune system itself are called "primary" immunodeficiency diseases. ("Secondary" refers to disorders due to outside influences, such as AIDS.) Many primary immune deficiency diseases are genetically determined, and there is great variability in their severity and incidence. Over 70 of these disorders have been described, excluding a number of unusual variants in which only a few cases have been described.

The immune system operates by first recognizing foreign substances (antigens) and then reacting to them. A variety of different cell types and proteins are responsible for this activity. The major components of the system are B-lymphocytes, T- lymphocytes, phagocytes, immunoglobulins and complement.

When stimulated by antigens, B-lymphocytes mature into plasma cells, which then produce antibodies, specialized serum protein molecules that attack specific antigens. The antibody proteins are called immunoglobulins or gammaglobulins. There are five major classes of these antibodies: immunoglobulins G (IgG), A (IgA), M (IgM), E (IgE) and D (IgD), each with its own special role in attacking antigens.

T-lymphocytes directly attack virus, fungi or transplanted tissue, and also act as regulators of the immune system. They develop in the bone marrow and migrate to the thymus gland, where they mature. ("T" stands for "Thymus.") Each T-lymphocyte reacts with a specific antigen, just as each antibody molecule does. Additionally, T-lymphocytes fall into three categories: "killer" T-lymphocytes actually destroy antigens; "helper" T-lymphocytes assist the killer T- lymphocytes and also help B-lymphocytes produce antibodies; and "suppressor" T-lymphocytes stop the activity of the helper T-lymphocytes. Without them, the immune system would continue reacting

to antigens even after an infection had been destroyed.

Phagocytes ingest and kill microorganisms, and there are various types of these cells: All are either white blood cells or derived from them.

Complement is a group of serum proteins that assist in immune responses, from attracting phagocyte cells to the site of an infection, to coating microorganisms so they are more easily ingested by phagocytic cells.

A defect or deficiency in any one of these systems, or any part thereof, will result in an immune deficiency disease, making an individual more prone to infection.

*Agammaglobulinemia (XLA; X-linked agammaglobulinemia; Bruton's agammaglobulinemia; congenital agammaglobulinemia).* This was the first identified immune deficiency disease, described by Dr. Ogden Bruton at Walter Reed Hospital in 1952.

Inherited as an X-LINKED recessive trait, it is caused by a deficiency or absence of immunoglobulins and results from the failure of B-lymphocytes to mature.

Affected individuals are prone to infections of the mucous membranes, such as the sinuses (sinusitis), respiratory tract (pneumonia in the lungs and bronchitis in the bronchial tubes), eyes (conjunctivitis), nose (rhinitis) and ears (otitis), and the gastrointestinal tract (gastroenteritis). Any of these infections may penetrate the mucous membrane and involve the blood stream or internal organs.

Individuals with this disorder are most prone to bacterial infection, from pneumococcus, streptococcus and staphylococcus, and to common viruses that cause diarrhea and respiratory infections such as colds and flus. In those affected, live vaccines can also cause the disease for which the vaccine is designed to protect against.

The presence of this disorder can be confirmed by testing of immunoglobulins in the blood. The levels will be abnormally low or absent in affected individuals. The test is difficult in infants under the age of six months, since they typically have low levels of these serum proteins. Other tests can establish the effectiveness of those immunoglobulins that are present.

At present, there is no cure for this disorder. Treatment consists of transfusions of gammaglobulins culled from blood donations. Chronic or recurring infections may still occur, requiring laboratory identification of the specific microorganism causing the infection, in order to design a more specific antibiotic therapy.

Most affected individuals can lead relatively normal lives. CARRIER females have normal levels of immunoglobulins, but there has been much recent research that may allow carrier detection in families with this disease.

*Selective IgA Deficiency.* This is the most common of the immunodeficiency diseases, with an incidence estimated as high as one in every 400 people. It is also one of the milder forms; there is a wide variability in expression, and many affected individuals are asymptomatic and thus are not aware of their condition.

In this disorder immunoglobulin A (IgA) may be deficient or absent. The disorder appears to be MULTIFACTORIAL. Some cases are familial and reports of both dominant and recessive inheritance have been published. Other cases appear to be acquired. The most common features of this condition are recurrent or chronic infections and allergies. Food allergies and asthma can occur with selective IgA deficiency.

An additional complication in this disorder is the development of autoimmune diseases, in which the immune system manufactures antibodies that attack the body's own tissues. Examples of autoimmune disease associated with this disorder are RHEUMATOID ARTHRITIS and systemic LUPUS erythematosus.

It is not possible to replace IgA in affected individuals. Gammaglobulin (such as administered for agammaglobulinemia) contains no IgA. Furthermore, if IgA is totally absent, introduction into the body (for example, by receiving blood transfusions) could trigger a massive allergic reaction, characterized by

low blood pressure, difficulty breathing and collapse, as the immune system reacts to what it considers a foreign substance.

Long-term antibiotic therapy may be required in treating this disorder. The long term outlook is dependent on the severity of the individual case and its attendant complications, but generally the outlook is excellent.

*Common variable immunodeficiency (hypogammaglobulinemia).* This disorder is characterized by frequent and unusual infections. They may first occur any time between infancy and the third or fourth decade of life.

It is relatively common and is caused by a variable deficiency of immunoglobulins, hence the name. There may be a deficiency in IgG by itself, or IgG and IgA, or IgG, IgA and IgM. Some patients have few or non-functioning B-lymphocytes, others lack helper T-lymphocytes, and another group has an excess of suppressor T-lymphocytes. The severity of this condition is also highly variable.

The cause is unknown, and while genetic factors appear to be involved, its inheritance pattern does not fit well-defined MENDELIAN patterns in all cases.

Infections typically affect the ears, sinuses, nose, bronchi and lungs. Repeated, severe infections may cause permanent damage to the bronchial tubes (bronchiectasis) or chronic lung disease. Gastrointestinal complaints are also frequent, and may be caused by giardia lamblia, an intestinal parasite.

Both infections of the joint as well as painful joint inflammations (polyarthritis) may develop. Other autoimmune responses may also occur. For example, the body may destroy its own blood cells.

Immunoglobulin replacement can improve this condition and help control infection, though in some cases long-term treatment with a broad array of antibiotics may be required.

*Severe combined immunodeficiency (SCID).* This is the most serious of the primary immunodeficiency diseases. Infections begin in the first few months of life, and they are typically severe and complicated. (The so-called "BUBBLE BOY" had this disorder.)

Most cases of SCID are inherited. Both AUTOSOMAL RECESSIVE and X-LINKED forms have been described.

The three primary causes of SCID are absent or poorly functioning T-helper cells, absent or poorly functioning thymus gland and the absence or defective functioning of cells in the bone marrow that manufacture T- and B-lymphocytes. The reasons for these absences or deficiencies are unknown.

There is also an ENZYME deficiency form of SCID (ADA deficiency, adenosine deaminase deficiency) that allows metabolic poisons to build up in the lymphocytes, slowly poisoning the cells. ADA accounts for approximately half the cases of autosomal recessive SCID, and PRENATAL DIAGNOSIS is possible via CHORIONIC VILLUS SAMPLING. This disorder is a leading candidate for the first human gene therapy trials; normal copies of the defective gene have been cloned, and they would be transplanted into the bone marrow of affected individuals.

Among the most dangerous infectious agents for those with SCID are chicken pox virus (VARICELLA), cytomegalovirus (CMV), herpes simplex virus and MEASLES virus. Fungal, or yeast infections, are also very difficult to treat. Oral thrush (candida), a white fungus, is a common feature, as is diarrhea. The skin may become infected with the same fungus that causes oral thrush.

Tests to establish the diagnosis include lymphocyte counts in a blood smear, and tests to examine the effectiveness of those lymphocytes present. Usually, there is a decreased level of all classes of immunoglobulins.

Children with SCID typically endure repeated hospitalization and must be isolated from children outside the family. Usually they cannot be taken to public places, and contact with relatives should be limited. Siblings exposed to chicken pox or other infectious agents may also present a potential source of infection. In some cases, they cannot absorb food normally, possibly requiring continuous intravenous feeding.

Gammaglobulin replacement therapy can be of some benefit. The most successful therapy is bone marrow transplantation. Bone marrow cells from a normal matched donor, once transplanted, can manufacture the immune system products missing in the SCID individual. The recipient of the first such transplant for SCID, performed in 1968, is still alive and well as of this writing. The success rate after the first 100 of these operations was judged to be approximately 65%.

Without successful bone marrow transplantation, individuals are at constant risk of severe and fatal infection. Prenatal diagnosis has been accomplished by fetal blood sampling and assay of lymphocyte populations.

*Chronic granulomatous disease (CGD).* This form of immune deficiency is characterized by the inability of phagocytes to destroy certain microorganisms. While the phagocytic cells ("scavenger cells") can ingest the microorganisms normally, abnormal metabolism within the cell prevents them from killing the bacteria and fungi once ingested. The rest of the individual's immune system functions normally.

The infections often result in the formation of granulomas, or localized, swollen collections of infected tissue. These may block the intestine or urinary tract and require surgical treatment. The skin, lungs, lymph nodes, liver or bones are most frequently involved. Pneumonia is a recurrent problem.

CGD can be inherited as either an AUTOSOMAL RECESSIVE characteristic or more commonly through X-LINKED recessive transmission. Affected males outnumber affected females by a ratio of four to one.

The disease is usually recognized during infancy. Approximately 80% of those affected have unusually frequent or severe infections during the first year of life. Diagnosis is made by analyzing the function of phagocytic cells.

After identifying the chromosomal location of the X-linked CGD GENE, this gene has been cloned and characterized. This has allowed understanding of the underlying defect in the disorder and has permitted prenatal diagnosis of the condition.

Continuous treatment with oral antibiotics is often recommended. Early treatment of infections is extremely important. Affected individuals are also generally advised to swim only in well-chlorinated pools, since organisms found in other waters may cause infections. They are also advised to refrain from smoking marijuana, since the bacteria aspergillus is found in most samples and can cause lung infections in CGD patients. Dusty conditions, especially caused by spoiled or moldy grass and hay, should also be avoided. CGD occurs in an estimated one in 1,000,000 live births.

The overall incidence of immunodeficiency (excluding IgA deficiency) is estimated to be about one in 10,000 with approximately 400 new cases annually in the United States.

Other immune deficiency disorders include DI GEORGE SYNDROME and ATAXIA-TELANGIECTASIA.

For more information, contact:

Immune Deficiency Foundation
P.O. Box 586
Columbia, MD 21045
(301) 461-3127

**imparidigitate** Having an uneven number of digits (fingers or toes).

**imperforate anus** A large group of anorectal malformations caused by a defect in the development of the tail end (terminus) of the embryo's hindgut, which forms the intestines and other organs of the lower abdomen. Conditions in this category include an external bowel opening that is: (1) in the normal position but too small to function properly (anal stenosis); (2) in an unusual position (ectopic), such as the perineum or scrotum in males, the vulva, vestibule or vagina in females; or (3) not visible at all on examination. Most newborns in the two latter groups will show signs of intestinal blockage within 24 hours because the contents of their bowels at birth cannot be evacuated. Infants with anal stenosis usually develop constipation within days or weeks of birth.

About half of all cases of imperforate anus are accompanied by other abnormalities as well. The majority of associated problems are in the lower spine (lumbosacral malformations) or genito-urinary system; other anomalies may occur in the trachea or esophagus or in the central nervous, cardiovascular or gastrointestinal systems (see VATER ASSOCIATION). These other anomalies account for over 90% of all deaths associated with imperforate anus, which has an overall mortality rate of 10% to 30% in reported cases.

Imperforate anus is seen in approximately one of every 5,000 live births, and males are 50% more likely than females to be affected (three to two ratio). Diagnosis in both sexes is usually made within days of birth. The majority of all cases are SPORADIC, but an AUTOSOMAL RECESSIVE inheritance has been strongly suggested in some families with more than one affected child.

Treatment is usually surgical, with the immediate aim of relieving colon pressure. Enlargement of the external opening is all that is needed for correcting anal stenosis. When the external opening is in the perineum, scrotum, vulva or vestibule, however, plastic surgery to reposition the opening is required. If the external opening is in the vulva or lacking altogether, the newborn usually receives a colostomy until after the first year, when plastic surgery is performed to create an external opening in the appropriate location (anorectal reconstruction).

**imperforate hymen** The central portion of the hymen (which covers the vaginal opening) in this structural flaw fails to develop its normal opening. The external genitalia, vagina, cervix, uterus, fallopian tubes and ovaries are not affected. While it may be detected at birth through investigation of possible causes of accumulation of fluid in the vagina, it usually goes unnoticed until puberty when menstrual flow is blocked and accumulates. The hymen may bulge.

The incidence is believed to be low. Although it was reported that three sisters in one family were affected, heritable tendencies have not been frequently observed. The condition is not necessarily CONGENITAL; some cases may develop as the result of inflammation. It has no effect on fertility.

**imprinting**  A gender-specific molecular process of GENE modification that may activate an otherwise dormant gene. This process is now thought to play a role in the development of several inherited disorders, and may prove to be a significant refinement of Mendel's laws of inheritance. According to MENDELIAN theory, genes inherited from each parent are equal in their influence, and will be expressed or masked depending on whether each is dominant or recessive and on the allele (the form of the gene inherited from the other parent) each is paired with. However, according to preliminary theories of imprinting, in some disorders the gender of the parent from whom the gene is inherited may also determine whether or not a gene will be expressed. In practice, this means an aberrant gene inherited from the father may usually result in a specific disorder, while the same gene, inherited from the mother, will lie dormant.

For example, among those who develop WILMS TUMOR, a childhood cancer, some individuals exhibit a deletion of material on one of their two chromosome 11s (see CHROMOSOME ABNORMALITIES). This damaged chromosome is almost always maternally inherited, that is, passed down from the mother. This suggests that the maternal genes play some role in suppressing tumor development, and that loss of this suppressor function results in the development of Wilms tumor. Absence of the suppressor function is apparently not compensated for by genes on the chromosome 11 inherited from the father.

As another example, both the PRADER-WILLI SYNDROME and the HAPPY PUPPET SYNDROME (Angleman syndrome), two very different disorders, are associated with deletions of the same area of the long arm of chromosome 15. In almost all cases of the Prader-Willi syndrome the chromosome 15 exhibiting this deletion is inherited from the father, while in happy puppet syndrome the damaged chromosome 15 is almost always inherited from the mother. It thus appears that it is essential to have both maternally derived and paternally derived copies of at least some portions of some chromosomes.

An understanding of imprinting may help explain heritability and statistical aspects of inherited disorders that previously appeared to mock the laws of Mendel. Other disorders in which imprinting has been suggested as playing a role include FRAGILE X SYNDROME, RETINOBLASTOMA, several forms of tumors including CANCERs of the breast, colon and lung, and HUNTINGTON'S CHOREA.

**index case**  See PROBAND.

**indifference to pain**  (congenital analgesis)  The first case of this rare hereditary disease is believed to have been reported in 1932, seen in an individual who made a living with a human pincushion act. Though affected individuals can distinguish between feelings of sharpness and dullness, heat and cold, they do not experience feelings of pain. Otherwise, they are neurologically normal. Repeated fractures are common, with deformities often resulting. Some exhibit self-destructive behavior, such as biting the tip of the tongue. Indifference to pain is also a feature of FAMILIAL DYSAUTONOMIA. As an isolated anomaly, it is transmitted as an AUTOSOMAL RECESSIVE trait.

**infantile autism**  A potentially severely incapacitating and pervasive developmental disorder, characterized by unresponsive behavior and bizarre movements of speech, typically appearing during the first 30 months of life. The classic form was described by U.S. child psychiatrist Dr. Leo Kanner in 1943; he noted that in most cases behavior was abnormal from early infancy.

Clinical diagnostic criteria include quantitative impairment in social interaction, in communication, language and symbolic (imaginative) development, and a markedly restricted repertoire of activities or interests. There is slow development or lack of physical, social and learning skills, abnormal interpersonal communication and relations, immature rhythms of speech, poor comprehension of ideas and inappropriate use of words. Senses of sight, hearing, touch, pain, balance, smell and taste may also be abnormal. Individuals may exhibit inappropriate laughing or giggling, repeat phrases said by others (echolalia), have crying tantrums for no observable reason, act as though deaf, resist change in routine, engage in sustained odd play, develop inappropriate attachment to objects, indicate needs by gesture and fail to establish eye contact with others.

It is thought that in the past some affected infants, unwanted by parents, were abandoned in the wilds and later found and called "wild children" or "wolf children." One of the best documented cases was the "Wild Boy of Aveyron," a 12-year-old found wandering in the woods near Aveyron, France, in 1795. He did not speak and related poorly to humans. Modern examination of medical records of the case has led to the conclusion that he was most likely an autistic child. The case was dramatized in the film *L'Enfant Sauvage* by French director Francois Truffaut. A fictional portrait of an autistic adult, portrayed by Dustin Hoffman, was presented in the 1988 Academy-Award-winning film *Rain Man*.

While many autistic children demonstrate skills in music, mathematics or use of spatial concepts (such as assembling jigsaw puzzles), they usually exhibit MENTAL RETARDATION. Sixty per cent have IQ scores below 50; 20% score between 50 and 70; 20% score greater

than 70. However, they may display a wide variability in performance on tests at different times.

Autism is believed to result from several causes, including untreated PHENYLKETONURIA, rubella (see TORCH SYNDROME), chemical exposure in pregnancy, as well as hereditary predisposition leading to disorders of brain development and central nervous system damage. Contrary to earlier theories, it is not caused by improper or cold, detached parenting. One theory of the behavioral aspects of the disorder is that the autistic individual's brain is abnormally susceptible or vulnerable to overstimulation, and that withdrawal from the outer world is an attempt to limit stimulation. The repetitive actions they often engage in may have a calming effect on the cerebral cortex, and their abhorrence of change in routine can also be explained in this context. There is no cure, though symptoms may change or diminish over time. However, 75% function in the retarded range throughout life.

Classic autism has been estimated to occur between one per 2,000 and one per 5,000 live births. A survey that included almost every family in Utah, published in 1989, found a rate of four per 10,000 live births. it is four times more common in males than in females, although females appear to be more severely affected and have a poorer prognosis. Most cases are SPORADIC. However, the Utah survey, the most extensive conducted to its date, found recurrence rates far above the 2% previously accepted. In families with an autistic girl, researchers led by Edward R. Ritivo of the University of California found recurrence risk, or the possibility of a subsequent child being affected, of 14.5%; in families with an autistic boy, recurrence risk was 7%. In families with two affected infants, the figure rose to 35%. Speech delay is common in sibships containing autistic children.

Autistic features are also found in FRAGILE X, LESCH-NYHAN and RETT SYNDROMES.

There is no precise medical test for autism. Diagnosis is often made within the first two years of life, based on clinical observations and parental reports of the child's behavior. Computerized X rays—CT scans—may reveal abnormalities in the ventricles of the brain in autistic children. The most favorable prognostic indicators are an IQ greater than 70 and speech present before the age of five years.

Treatment generally consists of special education programs, counseling and use of behavior modification and medication to control or decrease specific symptoms. In cases of autism identified as resulting from metabolic abnormalities, control of diet may be helpful in mitigating the symptoms. Prenatal detection of this disorder has not been achieved.

For more information, contact:

Autism Society of America
Suite #1017
1234 Massachusetts Ave., N.W.
Washington, DC 20005
(202) 783-0125

**infantile lactic acidosis** See CONGENITAL INFANTILE LACTIC ACIDOSIS.

**infantile osteopetrosis** Brittle, abnormally dense bones that fracture easily characterize this CONGENITAL condition. In fact, fractures may occur during delivery as well as throughout the child's life. Though the fractures tend to heal satisfactorily, deformities frequently develop during childhood. During the first year of life the head becomes enlarged and square in shape with a prominent forehead. Hearing and vision grow progressively worse; ocular abnormalities may include drooping eyelids (PTOSIS), crossed eyes (STRABISMUS) and CATARACTS. Teeth may develop abnormally and are prone to decay. On X rays, bones of the hand may have a "bone in bone" appearance, and ribs appear flared.

Other complications may include severe ANEMIA and enlargement of the spleen, liver and lymph nodes. There is a predisposition to bone and marrow infection (osteomyelitis).

While growth and developmental retardation are common in affected children, intelligence is usually normal.

A diagnosis of osteopetrosis can be made in the third trimester with X rays and possibly could be made earlier with ULTRASOUND. The basic defect of this relatively rare condition, which is inherited as an AUTOSOMAL RECESSIVE trait, is unknown. CARRIERS cannot be detected. It occurs with unusual frequency in Costa Rica, and there and elsewhere it seems to strike offspring of blood relatives (see CONSANGUINITY). The condition occurs with equal frequency in males and females.

The prognosis for children with infantile osteopetrosis is poor. Anemia or a secondary infection often causes death in infancy or early childhood. Bone marrow transplants, however, have been successful for a few patients.

There is also an essentially benign AUTOSOMAL DOMINANT form of the condition. It has a later onset and has only the bony features without the other associated features. Height is normal but osteomyelitis is more common.

**infantile subacute necrotizing encephalopathy of Leigh** Unusual eye movements beginning in infancy or early childhood, generally occurring in association with an infection, are usually the first signs of this rare inherited condition. Bearing the name of English neuropathologist D. Leigh, who published the first description in 1951, symptoms are variable from case to case but may include abnormal eye movements, sluggish pupils, degeneration of the optic nerve, tremors, weakness, numbness and unsteady gait. The irregular eye movements may stabilize or improve slightly when the infection clears but worsen with a second infection. In older children and adolescents the disease may be chronic and unremitting. Stress may also trigger episodes and cause periodic problems with walking. There may also be symptoms involving regulation of the heart, respiration, salivation and swallowing, and signs of cerebellar degeneration. Though complete remissions have been reported in some cases, generally there is a progressive loss of neurologic functions, ultimately resulting in death.

The condition is believed to be inherited as an AUTOSOMAL RECESSIVE trait. Increasing evidence suggests that the biochemical defect involves the pyruvate decarboxylation system, a membrane-bound complex within the cell that produces enzyme-cofactors, substances required by many ENZYMES to function. Blood levels of lactate and pyruvate are increased. The mechanism that produces the brain pathology remains unknown but may be related to the unusually high concentration of lactic acid in the body fluid and tissues (acidosis).

**infertility**    The inability to conceive children. It may be caused by a variety of conditions in otherwise healthy men and women. It is also a feature common to many genetic conditions that affect sexual development or differentiation. (See also KLINEFELTER SYNDROME, TURNER SYNDROME, ABORTION, ADRENOGENITAL SYNDROMES, CHROMOSOME ABNORMALITIES, CRYPTORCHISM, AMBIGUOUS GENITALIA.)

**inguinal hernia**    A hernia is the protrusion of an organ through the wall of a cavity that usually contains it. In this common CONGENITAL developmental defect, a portion of the intestine protrudes through the abdominal wall, and into the inguinal canal, part of the genitourinary system, where it can interfere with urination, development of reproductive organs and cause discomfort. Seen predominantly in males (approximately 90% of those brought to medical attention), it affects as many as one in 100 children. In males the intestine may push into the scrotal sac, blocking the testis from descending. Though it may be corrected surgically, in severe cases intestinal blockage may occur, resulting in intestinal perforation, shock and complications that may lead to death if not treated.

It is caused by the failure of an embryonic structure, the processus vaginalis, to close during fetal development. The hernia is usually either on both sides (bilateral) or, if on one side, most commonly on the right. The condition may be diagnosed from early infancy to early childhood. Symptoms may include an accumulation of fluid (hydrocele) in the groin area, which can be felt during physical examination as a solid mass. Affected infants may exhibit signs of discomfort and distress.

Approximately half of those under medical attention for TESTICULAR FEMINIZATION SYNDROME have inguinal hernias. The cause of the developmental defect is unknown, and various modes of inheritance are suspected of being involved. Inguinal hernias may also be seen as part of other SYNDROMES, particularly those involving connective tissue, such as MARFAN SYNDROME.

**insulin-dependent   diabetes   mellitus (IDDM)**    See DIABETES MELLITUS.

**intestinal atresia or stenosis**    Blockage (atresia) or narrowing (stenosis) of segments of the small intestine. Atresia is more common than stenosis. Characteristic sites of occurrence are the jejunum, the long segment of the small intestine leading from the stomach and duodenum, and the ileum, the long segment leading from the jejunum to the large intestine. In a small percentage of cases, atresia is found in both segments.

Symptoms of atresia—vomiting, constipation and swelling of the abdomen—are evident at birth or within the first week of life. Symptoms of stenosis—diarrhea or constipation—tend to occur later in infancy or may be delayed until childhood or even adulthood. X-ray studies can locate the specific sites.

Intestinal atresia and stenosis are always considered as secondary to other fetal disease processes. The immediate cause of both may be impairment of the blood supply to the membranous sac that contains the abdominal organs (mesentery). Other associated anomalies may also be present.

The defect is found in approximately one in 330 live births in the United States. The risk of recurrence in other siblings or offspring can be high in cases in which atresia in a newborn is associated with another defect characterized by thickening of the contents of the intestine (meconium ileus), as is seen in CYSTIC FIBROSIS. The risk of recurrence in other forms of atresia is low. Except in cases associated with other disorders, (e.g., cystic fibrosis), affected persons have a normal life span. (See also DUDONEAL ATRESIA.)

**intrauterine growth retardation (IUGR)** Growth retardation observable at birth. An estimated 3% to 7% of markedly small babies are classified under this broad category.

A baby born at term (the normal 40 week gestation period) and weighing under 5.5 pounds (2.5 kg) is said to be "small for gestational age," or SGA (as opposed to AGA—"appropriate for gestational age"). Among SGA infants are those with IUGR. Premature infants may or may not exhibit IUGR. Some infants, though born extremely prematurely, nonetheless have a normal weight for their gestational age (see LOW BIRTH WEIGHT, PREMATURITY).

Babies with IUGR have an increased risk during the newborn period of developing hypoglycemia (low blood sugar), hypocalcemia (low blood calcium) and polycythemia (thick blood due to a high number of red blood cells). They are also at increased risk for developing birth asphyxia due to lack of oxygen, infections and hypothermia (low body temperature). There is an increased frequency of congenital anomalies and a three- to 10-time increase in prenatal mortality. Long-term effects may include learning, behavior and neurologic problems.

Ninety percent of cases of IUGR are idiopathic, that is, the cause is unknown. However, several maternal, fetal and environmental factors are associated with the condition: Mothers who are themselves small tend to have smaller babies; first babies are generally smaller than subsequent babies; maternal nutrition can affect the infant's size at birth, as can maternal illnesses and infections. Also associated with an increased incidence

of IUGR are: multiple gestation, that is, carrying more than one fetus; toxemia; abnormalities of the uterus or placenta; maternal use of drugs and especially tobacco; or living at high altitudes during pregnancy. CHROMOSOME ABNORMALITIES and various genetic SYNDROMES and DYSPLASIAS may also cause IUGR.

Some affected infants grow to normal size, while others remain below average throughout their lives. Generally, "catch up" growth, if it occurs, occurs during the first year of life. In some infants, head size and, presumably, brain growth have been relatively spared.

For more information, contact:

Human Growth Foundation
4720 Montgomery Lane, Suite 909
Bethesda, MD 20814
(301) 656-6904
(301) 656-7540

**in utero** Within the womb, or uterus.

**isolated HGH deficiency** See PITUITARY DWARFISM.

**isotretinoin** See ACCUTANE.

**isovaleric acidemia** See SWEATY FEET SYNDROME.

**Ivemark syndrome** See ASPLENIA SYNDROME.

# J

**Jansen-type metaphyseal chondrodysplasia** See METAPHYSEAL CHONDRODYSPLASIA.

**Jansky-Bielschowsky disease** See BATTEN DISEASE.

**Jarcho-Levin syndrome**    See SPON-
DYLOTHORACIC DYSPLASIA.

**jaw winking syndrome** (Marcus Gunn
syndrome)    Curious phenomenon consisting of a drooping (PTOSIS) single eyelid which
opens to a higher level than the non-drooping
eyelid when the mouth opens. If the mouth is
held open, the drooping recurs. If the jaw is
moved to the side of the drooping lid, the
ptosis increases. If the jaw is moved to the
other side, the drooping decreases. Affected
individuals also open their mouths whenever
they look up. Its secondary designation bears
the name of Scottish ophthalmologist R. Marcus Gunn (1850-1909), who described it in
1883.

The drooping eyelid occurs more frequently on the left than the right, and though
many variations have been observed, this phenomenon is rarely observed in both eyes (bilaterally).

This benign condition is detectable soon
after birth, because it is most noticeable during
sucking. The basic cause is unknown. In some
families it exhibits an irregular AUTOSOMAL
DOMINANT inheritance pattern, but this leaves
the origin of many cases unknown. The condition often grows less noticeable with age.

**Jervell and Lange-Nielsen syndrome**
(cardioauditory syndrome; deafness and
functional heart disease)    Irregularities
of heart rhythm, as a result of cardiac electrical
conduction disturbances (which appear on
electrocardiogram examinations as a prolonged Q-T interval), in association with profound congenital DEAFNESS, particularly at
higher frequencies. It is named for Norwegian
physicians A.J. Jervell and F. Lange-Nielsen,
who described it in 1957.

The deafness is sensorineural, that is, involves the sensory nerves. The inner ear exhibits evidence of widespread degeneration of
these nerves. While there may be some hearing of low tones, it is insufficient for normal
learning of speech, and special education is
necessary.

The conduction abnormalities cause heart
arrhythmias that result in fainting spells.
Fainting may begin in infancy or childhood
and is often brought on by physical exertion
or nervousness. The severity and frequency of
attacks are highly variable. They range from
mild spells to loss of consciousness for five to
10 minutes, with temporary disorientation following recovery. Intervals between episodes
range from months or years between attacks
to several a day. If this syndrome is not identified as the cause, the fainting may be mistaken for epilepsy or hysterical episodes.

Transmitted as an AUTOSOMAL RECESSIVE
trait, it has been estimated to have an incidence of between 1.6 and six per million live
births. It has been suggested that carriers of a
single GENE may exhibit mild cardiac abnormalities upon electrocardiogram examination.

Until recently, the cardiac complications
caused death in half the affected individuals
by the age of 15, and survival beyond the age
of 21 was rare. The introduction of proptrano-
lol, a drug that controls characteristic cardiac
rhythmic abnormalities, has reduced mortality
from the disorder to less than 6%.

For more information, contact:

National Information Center on Deafness
Gallaudet College
800 Florida Avenue, N.E.
Washington, DC 20002
(202) 651-5000

American Society for Deaf Children
814 Thayer Avenue
Silver Spring, MD 20910
(301) 585-5400

**Jeune syndrome** (asphyxiating thoracic
dysplasia)    Rare CONGENITAL SYN-
DROME, named for French pediatrician M.
Jeune, who described it in 1954; it is characterized by a narrow, immobile chest (thorax)
and short arms and legs. In general, the long
bones of the arms and legs are short and stubby
and their ends irregular. The cartilage at the

ends of hand and foot bones, the portion of the bone referred to as the epiphysis, is sometimes cone-shaped, and there may be extra fingers and toes (POLYDACTYLY). The ribs have an abnormally short and stubby appearance, and the lungs are often incompletely developed (hypoplastic).

Although this disorder is usually identified at birth by physical appearance and X-ray studies of the chest and pelvis, it may not be detected until weeks or months later when an upper respiratory infection causes acute respiratory distress. Narrowness and immobility of the thorax lead to rapid shallow breathing and cyanosis due to reduced oxygen in the blood. The condition is often rapidly fatal.

Transmitted as an AUTOSOMAL RECESSIVE trait, the basic defect that causes this disorder is unknown. It occurs in two forms, one that results in death within a few months of birth and a second, less fatal form characterized by later kidney disease. There is no method of PRENATAL DIAGNOSIS, although ULTRASOUND may be able to detect anatomic alterations characteristic of this disorder.

**Jewish genetic disease**    Any one of several hereditary disorders that have a significantly increased prevalence among Ashkenazi Jews, those of Eastern European ancestry (as distinguished from Sephardic Jews, those from the Mediterranean area, and Oriental Jews, from Asia). More than 90% of Jews in the United States and Europe are Ashkenazim, as are 45% of Jews in Israel.

The disorders include: BLOOM SYNDROME; FAMILIAL DYSAUTONOMIA; GAUCHER DISEASE; MUCOLIPIDOSIS; NIEMANN-PICK DISEASE; and TAY-SACHS DISEASE.

For more information, contact:

The National Foundation for Jewish
  Genetic Diseases
250 Park Avenue, Suite 1000
New York, NY 10017
(212) 371-1030

**Job syndrome**    (hyperimmunoglobulin E)    According to the book of Job in the Bible (Job 2:7), "Satan … smote Job with sore boils from the sole of his foot unto his crown." Based on this description, in 1966 British Dr. S.D. Davis gave the name "Job syndrome" to a condition affecting two unrelated girls with lifelong histories of bacterial abscesses of skin (boils) and other organs, with little local inflammatory reaction. Since then, there have been several additional reports of this condition.

Other frequent sites of infection, in addition to the skin, are the middle and external ear, sinuses, gums and lungs. Most commonly, the bacterium involved in the recurrent infections is staphylococcus aureus.

Inherited as an AUTOSOMAL RECESSIVE trait, characteristics of this syndrome also include coarse facial features, chronic eczema and elevated levels of immunoglobulin E. There also may be decreased movement of white blood cells to sites of infection (defective chemotaxis).

**Joseph disease**    See AZOREAN DISEASE.

**Jumping Frenchmen of Maine**    Curious condition characterized by an exaggerated startle reflex. It was first studied by Dr. G.M. Beard in 1878, who noted a familial link (see FAMILIAL DISEASE) and reported his observations to the American Neurological Association. He found that some French Canadian lumbermen from the Moosehead Lake region of Maine would respond abnormally to sudden sensory input. A sharp, unexpected sound or touch provoked a sometimes violent cry or movement in response (hence, the "jumping" appellation). Additionally, affected individuals would comply with quick, sudden commands, even if inappropriate. For example, if told to strike another person, they would do so without hesitation, even, according to Beard's

1880 account published in *Popular Science Monthly* "if it was his mother and he had an axe in his hand." Often, they echoed the words of the command. If addressed quickly in a language foreign to them, some would repeat the phrase. A tendency to blurt out whatever is being thought at the time of the stimulus has also been described.

This condition is now known to affect people of almost any nationality and geographic location. Transmitted as an AUTOSOMAL RECESSIVE characteristic, it manifests itself in childhood and lasts throughout life. The basic cause is unknown and there is no effective therapy.

**juvenile diabetes**    See DIABETES MELLITUS.

**juvenile Paget disease**    See HYPERPHOSPHATASIA.K

---

# K

---

**Kabuki make-up syndrome**    Congenital MENTAL RETARDATION syndrome, first described in Japan in 1981. It takes its name from the peculiar facial appearance of affected individuals, particularly the elongated opening for the eyes between the eyelids (palpebral fissures), with the "eversion" (turning inside out) of the outer, or lateral third of the lower eyelids, which resembles the make-up of the actors of Kabuki, a traditional Japanese theatrical form.

Other facial features include a broad, depressed nasal tip, large, prominent earlobes and arched eyebrows. There is also recurrent inflammation of the middle ear in infancy. Skeletal features include dwarfing (see DWARFISM), SCOLIOSIS and a short fifth finger. Abnormalities of the vertebrae, hands and hip joints are observable in X rays.

This rare disorder seems to be most prevalent in Japan. It has been estimated that its prevalence among Japanese newborns is one in 32,000. The cause is unknown. All the patients identified to date have been SPORADIC with no other cases in the family. The findings to date are compatible with an AUTOSOMAL DOMINANT trait in which each affected individual represents a new MUTATION.

**Kartagener syndrome**    (immotile cilia syndrome)    The cilia—small hairline projections of some cells—do not move normally or at all in those affected by this syndrome, due to the cilia's defective structure. Respiratory system effects of the cilia's immotility include thick mucoid nasal secretions, swelling of multiple nasal sinuses, recurrent respiratory infections, mouth breathing due to nasal polyps, and chronic bronchitis. These occur during an affected child's first year, in most cases. Chronic middle ear inflammation may result in some hearing loss, and coughing may become chronic.

Thick mucus blocks the sinuses, eustachian tubes and lobes of the lung, predisposing these areas to infection. It also has been noted that in some affected individuals mucus collects because they have little or no means to remove it from the tracheobronchial tract; the cilia normally responsible for this locomotion are impaired.

Other complications of Kartagener syndrome may include a partial or complete reversal of organ positions (situs inversus) (including a lower right, rather than left, testicle). The heart may be on the right side rather than the left (dextrocardia). Cardiac anomalies may also be present, and their severity tends to be related to the degree of situs inversus. Adult males may be sterile, due to immotile sperm. Semi-sterility in females has been observed.

Kartagener syndrome is inherited as an AU-TOSOMAL RECESSIVE trait by about one in every 50,000 Americans. Life expectancy is essentially normal, though respiratory problems, if severe, can limit rigorous physical activity. About 30% of patients undergo lung surgery. Antibiotic therapy is almost constantly required. Especially in infants, aerosols, postural drainage and decongestants are needed several times daily to assist breathing.

**karyotype**    An individual's CHROMO-SOMES, particularly when seen reproduced in a microphotograph and displayed in a standardized format, with the chromosome pairs arranged by size. The karyotype can reveal CHROMOSOME ABNORMALITIES responsible for several genetic anomalies, such as DOWN SYNDROME and KLINEFELTER SYNDROME.

**King syndrome**    See    MALIGNANT HYPERTHERMIA.

**kinky hair disease**    See MENKES SYN-DROME.

**kleeblattschadel anomaly** (cloverleaf skull)    A severe form of CRANIOSYNOSTO-SIS, a group of disorders characterized by premature closure of the gaps (sutures) between the skull bones, causing the skull to grow in aberrant directions. In this form, the skull bones fuse during fetal development, causing distorted growth that gives the head a cloverleaf appearance: a high, peaked forehead, with prominent bulges on both sides of the head. Those severely affected are typically stillborn or die in early infancy, while those who survive exhibit severe MENTAL RETARDATION due to central nervous system complications arising from intracranial pressure.

The cause of this rare condition is unknown, and it generally occurs sporadically. It may occur as an isolated malformation or as part of another condition (e.g., as a severe form of a craniosynostosis SYNDROME or other skeletal DYSPLASIA, such as thanatophoric DWARFISM).

For other forms of craniosynostosis, see APERT SYNDROME; CARPENTER SYNDROME; CROUZON DISEASE; and PFEIFFER SYNDROME.

**Klinefelter syndrome**    A genetic endocrine disorder that affects approximately one in 500 live-born males, characterized by the lack of normal sexual development, infertility and psychological adjustment problems. It bears the name of H.F. Klinefelter (b. 1912), a U.S. physician who observed several of the patients he first described (in 1942) while a Fellow at Harvard University under Dr. Fuller Albright, whose name is associated with several hereditary disorders.

The SYNDROME is caused by a CHROMO-SOMAL ABNORMALITY, in which individuals have an extra X CHROMOSOME (XXY, instead of the normal XY male chromosomal complement, or KARYOTYPE). Approximately 10% of affected males have a mixture of cells with both normal and abnormal chromosome complements, a condition referred to as MOSA-ICISM. Klinefelter syndrome is probably the most common single cause of deficient sexual development and infertility found in humans.

The penis and scrotum are well differentiated, and the condition may remain unrecognized until puberty, at which time incomplete masculinization or development of some female characteristics, such as enlarged breasts (GYNECOMASTIA, seen in an estimated 50%) brings them to medical attention. At puberty there is decreased androgen (a male sex hormone) production. Infertility is complete. Body and pubic hair are sparse. The testes remain abnormally small. Legs are long in proportion to arms and trunk, and individuals tend to be about 2.5 inches (6.4 cm) above average height. Muscles fail to develop fully and the voice may remain high-pitched. Fat distribution about the body may give them a somewhat feminine physique. Individuals rarely develop acne.

As compared with normal males, individuals with this syndrome have a slightly greater incidence of physical disorders, including cardiac, hearing and dental anomalies, as well as a variety of psychological problems including social maladjustment, emotional disturbances, alcoholism and reportedly are at increased risk of incarceration. About 15% have below average intelligence. (One percent of all males with IQs of 90 or below are estimated to have Klinefelter syndrome.) Those of normal intelligence often have learning disabilities and may be passive and poorly motivated.

Life span appears normal, though breast tissue in affected men has a risk for developing CANCER 20 times greater than males in the general population.

Affected individuals are reported to account for approximately one in 75 to one in 25 of all cases of male infertility, one in 100 males in institutions for the mentally retarded, and one in 169 males in psychiatric facilities.

Counseling and hormonal therapy can decrease the effects of the disorder. PRENATAL DIAGNOSIS is possible by chromosomal analysis of fetal cells gathered via AMNIOCENTESIS or CHORIONIC VILLUS SAMPLING.

**Klippel-Feil syndrome** Massive congenital fusion of neck vertebrae is the outstanding feature of this disorder, named for French neurologists Maurice Klippel (1858-1942), head of the department of medicine at the Hospital Tenon in Paris, and Andre Feil, his intern, who first described it in 1912. This developmental defect is associated with a variety of anomalies, which can include a short neck with the child's head appearing to sit directly on the trunk, limited head movement, a very low hairline at the back of the head, low-set ears, crossed eyes, DEAFNESS, CLEFT PALATE, elevation of the shoulder blades (SPRENGEL DEFORMITY), flaring shoulder and back (trapezius) muscles, spinal deformation

(SCOLIOSIS), CONGENITAL HEART DEFECTS and undeveloped kidneys.

Neurologic defects may also develop, and include involuntary muscle contractions (spasticity), brisker than normal reflex reactions (hyperreflexia) and paralysis of one side of the body (hemiplegia), of the lower portion of the body and both legs (paraplegia) or of all four extremities and the trunk (quadriplegia). Affected individuals may also exhibit an involuntary movement of one part of the body simultaneous with voluntary or reflexive movement of another part (synkinesis).

It has been estimated that this disorder occurs about once per every 35,000 individuals, with over 65% of severe cases occurring in females. The exact cause is unknown, though it has been suggested that faulty development of spinal segments along the neural tube in the embryo is a determining factor. Currently, there is no method for PRENATAL DIAGNOSIS of this disorder.

**Klippel-Trenaunay-Weber syndrome** Deformities of the limbs and digits are the most notable characteristics of this SYNDROME. Typically, one limb or one side of the body is predominantly affected. The deformities of the extremities, which can usually be seen at birth, include enlargement (hypertrophy), benign tumors composed of masses of blood vessels (HEMANGIOMAS) on and beneath the skin, swollen and twisted veins (varicosities) and, occasionally, abnormal communication between an artery and vein (arteriovenous fistula). Extra, missing, malformed or webbed digits may be part of the syndrome, as may hemangiomas of the intestinal or urinary tracts, lymph tumors on the skin and general nonspecific enlargement of internal organs. Usually, but not always, the hypertrophied area has a hemangioma or other visible vascular (blood vessel) abnormality. In the unusual case, the vascular abnormality will most often affect another limb or, less frequently, the buttocks, lower back, flank or side of the chest.

Involvement of the head and face is rare; when it occurs, it is most frequently in the form of a PORT WINE STAIN. Facial involvement in this syndrome may be associated with MENTAL RETARDATION.

Most affected individuals have a reasonably favorable prognosis, though ulcers and chronic skin problems are not uncommon. Surgery may be necessary to remove a severely disproportionate digit, to amputate a limb if the vascular abnormality has been severe enough to cause clotting difficulties or to correct an ateriovenous fistula.

The condition was first described in 1900. It is named for Maurice Klippel (1858-1942), Paul Trenaunay (born 1875), who was Klippel's junior colleague in Paris when the first case was described, and Frederick Parkes Weber (1863-1962), an eminent London physician who described numerous genetic syndromes and who further delineated this condition in 1907 and 1918.

The basic defect that causes Klippel-Trenaunay-Weber syndrome is unknown. Almost all cases have occurred sporadically. PRENATAL DIAGNOSIS is possible with ULTRASOUND.

For more information, contact:

National Congenital Port Wine Stain
  Foundation
123 E. 63rd Street
New York, NY 10021
(212) 755-3820

**Kniest dysplasia**   A rare form of disproportionate DWARFISM. At birth the limbs appear disproportionately small, but the disproportion reverses as growth occurs, with the trunk appearing stunted as a result of spinal curvature (SCOLIOSIS). The long bones of the leg grow short and bowed. Characteristic facial appearance includes a flat "dish-face" countenance with a wide nasal bridge, large eyes and broad mouth. About half of the cases have CLEFT PALATE.

There may be developmental delays in walking and speech, but intelligence is usually normal. Recurrent respiratory distress in infancy is common. A swayback (lumbar lordosis) of the spine develops, as well as spinal curvature (kyphoscoliosis). The joints of the knees, elbows and hands are enlarged and prominent, and show a limited range of motion. Permanent bending of the joints (flexion contractures) occurs. Degenerative arthritis may leave affected individuals incapacitated by late childhood. Severe nearsightedness (myopia) may lead to retinal detachment. Frequent middle ear infections and loss of hearing are also common. Inherited as an AUTOSOMAL DOMINANT trait, lifespan is unaffected.

For more information, contact:

Little People of America, Inc.
P.O. Box 633
San Bruno, CA 94066
(415) 589-0695

Human Growth Foundation
4720 Montgomery Lane, Suite 909
Bethesda, MD 20814
(301) 656-6904
(301) 656-7540

**koala bear syndrome**   See CHONDRODYSPLASIA PUNCTATA, rhizomelic type.

**Krabbe disease** (globoid cell leukodystrophy; GLD)   A rapidly progressive, fatal form of infantile LEUKODYSTROPHY. Onset is usually between the ages of three and six months, with irritability and hypersensitivity to external stimuli, feeding difficulties and sometimes stiffness of the limbs. Infants frequently cry without apparent cause. It quickly progresses to severe mental and motor deterioration, loss of muscle tone (hypotonia), seizures, BLINDNESS and DEAFNESS. There is no treatment. Death usually occurs before three years of age.

The disorder was first described in 1916 by Danish neurologist K.H. Krabbe (1885-1961), who observed the condition in two siblings and noted the familial connection (see FAMILIAL DISEASE). Additionally, he described the globoid cells in the white matter of the brain that are considered the hallmark of the disorder. Globoid cells are large, irregular histiocytic (scavenger) cells that often contain multiple nuclei. The spinal fluid protein is elevated and nerve conduction velocities reduced.

The underlying cause is a deficiency of galactocerebroside ß-galactosidase, a lysosomal ENZYME that normally breaks down galactocerebroside, the main lipid component of myelin, into ceramide (a fat) and galactose (a sugar). (Myelin is the substance in the white matter that protects the axons, nerve fibers that transmit impulses in the nervous system.) As a result, galactocerebroside and its derivatives are thought to accumulate in cells of the brain, destroying the cells that produce myelin.

Inherited as an AUTOSOMAL RECESSIVE trait, Krabbe disease is a very rare disorder, though its incidence is unknown. There is a report of high frequency in Israel in an isolate of Druze, a religious group founded in Egypt in the 11th century. Diagnosis is made either on the basis of abnormal ENZYME activity consistent with the disorder, or on the finding of globoid cells in brain biopsies following death. CARRIER detection is possible on the basis of deficient enzyme activity. PRENATAL DIAGNOSIS is possible by enzyme assay of cultured fetal cells obtained via AMNIOCENTESIS or CHORIONIC VILLUS SAMPLING.

This disorder has been reported in several mammalian species, and the "twitcher" mouse as well as a canine form are serving as a model for studies of the condition.

For more information, contact:

United Leukodystrophy Foundation, Inc.
2304 Highland Drive
Sycamore, IL 60178
(815) 895-3211

**KUF's disease**    See BATTEN DISEASE.

**Kugelberg-Welander disease**    See SPINAL MUSCULAR ATROPHY.

**kyphosis**    See HUMPBACK.

# L

**lactic acidosis, congenital infantile**
See CONGENITAL INFANTILE LACTIC ACIDOSIS.

**lactose intolerance**    The inability to digest lactose, a complex sugar found in milk, due to a deficiency of the ENZYME lactase, which triggers the breakdown of lactose into the more digestible simple sugars, glucose and galactose. Without such a breakdown, lactose is retained in the gut, resulting in bacterial fermentations and the influx of water into the intestine via osmosis.

After ingesting dairy products, individuals with this syndrome will experience symptoms ranging from bloating and abdominal cramps to severe diarrhea with frothy, sour-smelling stools. In milk-fed infants born with lactose intolerance, diarrhea can be followed by dehydration, malnutrition and even death if correct diagnosis is not made. Early detection by lactose loading test and, more importantly, by assay of intestinal enzyme through biopsy, followed by replacement of milk with a lactose-free preparation, can facilitate a normal life expectancy.

CONGENITAL lactose intolerance appears to be rare, but an adult-onset form can develop later in life, due perhaps to a gradual reduction in lactase production with aging. The exact risk of adult-onset lactose intolerance is unknown. However, more than 50% of American blacks are reported to suffer from this disorder. It is less life-threatening than the congenital form, possibly due to larger body size and less dependence on milk as an important dietary element.

Congenital lactose intolerance is believed to be inherited as an AUTOSOMAL RECESSIVE trait, whereas the adult-onset form is probably an AUTOSOMAL DOMINANT trait. However, the mode of inheritance in either case has not been definitely ascertained.

**Langer-Giedion syndrome**    Named for L.O. Langer and A. Giedion, who described it in 1974, this syndrome exhibits characteristic facial features recognizable at birth, including a bulbous nose, thin lips, sparse scalp hair, thick tented nostrils, large protruding ears with thickened edges, a small head (mild MICROCEPHALY) and a small lower jaw (micrognathia). During infancy, loose skin will produce excess skin folds about the neck, but this disappears as the child grows older.

Other characteristics apparent as the child develops include abnormal curvature of the spine (SCOLIOSIS), thin ribs, uneven limb growth, excess joint looseness that permits an abnormal range of joint movement (HYPERMOBILITY), loss of muscle tone (hypotonia), wing-shaped shoulder blades, hearing difficulties, a fusion of two or more toes or fingers (SYNDACTYLY), abnormally short fingers with one or more permanently bent to the side (clinobrachydactyly), short stature, cone-shaped ends (epiphyses) of finger and toe bones rather than normally rounded ends, causing tapering of the digits, and many bony outgrowths on bone surfaces (multiple cartilaginous exostoses) that may require surgery. Also, many small areas of skin discoloration will be present on the upper trunk, legs, neck, scalp and face, some of which will be flat and smooth and others raised and solid (cutaneous maculopapular nevi).

Mild to moderate MENTAL RETARDATION is common to all affected individuals, with a marked delay in ability to speak. Upper respiratory tract infections are common in infancy but diminish as the child grows. The disorder

shares many features with the TRICHORHINOPHALANGEAL SYNDROME.

This syndrome is rare, and the basic defect and mode of transmission is unknown. Most cases are SPORADIC. In a large percentage of cases a chromosome deletion has been found involving a segment of the long arm of chromosome 8 (see CHROMOSOME ABNORMALITIES).

**Langer-Saldino type achondrogenesis**
See ACHONDROGENESIS.

**Laron-type pituitary dwarfism**    See PITUITARY DWARFISM.

**Larsen syndrome**    Named for Loren J. Larsen, chairman emeritus of the orthopedic surgery department at the Shriner's Hospital for Crippled Children in San Francisco, who first described it in 1950. This disorder is characterized by CONGENITAL joint dislocations involving the elbows, wrists, hips and knees, flat facial features with a depressed nasal bridge, wide-set eyes (HYPERTELORISM) and a prominent forehead. Other abnormalities include partial dislocation of the shoulders, spatulate thumbs, short hand bones, short nails, cylindrical nontapering fingers and clubfeet. Complications may involve respiratory difficulties in infancy, CONGENITAL HEART DEFECTS and CLEFT PALATE.

Both AUTOSOMAL DOMINANT and AUTOSOMAL RECESSIVE forms of this disorder have been identified. It may be diagnosed at birth by physical and X-ray examination.

Prevalence of the disorder is not known, and there has been inadequate long-term data to provide a definitive prognosis. It appears, however, that the prognosis can be relatively good with aggressive orthopedic management.

**laryngomalacia**    The most common CONGENITAL abnormality of the voicebox (larynx), this condition makes breathing noisy and difficult for affected infants. The pyramid-shaped cartilage structures at the back of the larynx (arytenoids) and the cartilage flap that covers the entrance to the larynx (epiglottis) during swallowing are spongy and flutter excessively. An abnormal high-pitched breathing sound on inhaling (stridor) and a bluish tint of the skin due to lack of oxygen (cyanosis), especially during feeding, result. The stridor increases when the infant sleeps or cries vigorously.

Laryngomalacia can be detected one to six months after birth with direct examination of the larynx. The symptoms usually subside gradually after the age of 18 months. To assist the infant's breathing, feeding must be frequently interrupted, and the position of least obstruction must be maintained. In severe cases, there may be a failure to gain weight, and a tracheotomy may be required.

The cause of laryngomalacia is unknown, though it is more common in males. It is not generally considered to be genetic, though families have been reported in which AUTOSOMAL DOMINANT inheritance has been suggested. Life span and intelligence are not affected.

## Laurence-Moon-Biedl Syndrome
See BARDET-BIEDL SYNDROME.

**LCAT deficiency**   See LECITHIN: CHOLESTEROL ACYL TRANSFERASE.

**lead**   Fetal exposure to high levels of lead during pregnancy may result in stunted growth and MENTAL RETARDATION. However, the effects of exposure to low levels of lead during pregnancy are uncertain.

In the 1800s, women in the lead industry were frequently exposed to high levels of lead and frequently became sterile or had miscarriages. Currently, fetal lead poisoning is rare, though lead found in old house paint and in polluted soil or water may damage infants who ingest it. (See also TERATOGEN.)

**learning disability**   See MENTAL RETARDATION; DYSLEXIA; HANDICAP; EDUCATION.

**Leber optic atrophy**   First described by German ophthalmologist Theodore von Leber (1840–1917) in 1871, this rare hereditary disorder causes a sudden and rapidly progressive loss of central vision, the area of clearest acute vision in the eyes. The optic nerve atrophies (deteriorates), wasting away until central vision is destroyed.

It affects mostly males (85%) in their late teens to mid-20s, but has been reported in individuals from five to 65 years of age. It usually appears in both eyes (bilaterally) and headaches may accompany the onset of visual loss.

The genetic cause of this disorder is unusual. It breaks all rules of MENDELIAN inheritance. All studies indicate that transmission is through females with no documentation of it being passed on by males. It has now been shown that this is because the disorder results from a mutation in mitochondrial DNA. An individual inherits all of his or her mitochondria from his or her mother, hence this unusual inheritance pattern. Mitochondria are organelles within the cells that contain their own DNA, distinct from DNA in the nucleus.

**Leber's amaurosis congenita**   Congenital retinal disease, named for German ophthalmologist T. von Leber (1840–1917), who first published a description in 1869. It causes moderate to severe BLINDNESS in infants due to a degeneration of the retina. (The term *amaurosis* means complete loss of vision, especially when it occurs for no apparent reason.) Signs of poor vision are usually evident in the first few months of life, although they can appear anytime during the first year and sometimes beyond that.

Infants may rub or poke at their eyes, sometimes vigorously enough to cause the eyeball to retract into the socket (enophthalmos).

Initial eye examination may disclose crossed eyes (STRABISMUS), constant and involuntary back-and-forth eye movements (pendular nystagmus), cataracts or an absent or minimal reaction of the pupils to stimulation by light (pupillary reflex), in addition to retinal abnormalities.

Associated neurological disorders can include MENTAL RETARDATION, epilepsy, DEAFNESS, loss of muscle tone (muscular hypotonia) and an abnormal increase in cerebrospinal fluid (CSF), causing enlargement of the head (HYDROCEPHALY).

Two forms of the disease, which is a congenital form of RETINITIS PIGMENTOSA, are known: stationary and progressive. Those affected with the stationary form can retain fair vision. However, most common is the more severe, progressive form, which results in eventual blindness. A normal life span is possible, except in the cases where neurological disorders are severe enough to cause early death. The progressive form may often be associated with other problems such as skeletal or kidney abnormalities. For example, children with ZELLWEGER SYNDROME may exhibit this ophthalmologic abnormality.

The basic cause of this disorder is unknown. As an isolated defect, it is inherited as an AUTOSOMAL RECESSIVE trait and occurs in approximately one in 33,000 live births. In cases where it occurs as part of a specific syndrome, it may have a different inheritance pattern.

**lecithin: cholesterol acyl transferase (LCAT) deficiency**    Deficiency believed to prevent the body from maintaining the normal balance between cholesterol and other cholesterol compounds called esters, resulting in an excess of fats in the blood (hyperlipidemia), a decrease in the red blood cell count (ANEMIA), some abnormal red blood cells (target cells) and excess protein in the urine (proteinuria). Opacity of the cornea is also seen with LCAT deficiency. All affected individuals have very low or absent levels of LCAT ENZYME in their blood plasma.

The deficiency, first recognized in 1966 and described in only seven families, causes progressive kidney failure and possibly accelerates the depositing of fats on the artery walls (atherosclerosis). Dietary fat restriction is necessary. The disease's progression may be prevented by frequent transfusions of plasma with normal levels of LCAT. Renal dialysis is available in the event of kidney failure.

No method of CARRIER detection for this rare deficiency, which affects less than one in 100,000 people, is known. In a region in western Norway about one in 25 individuals may be carriers of this gene, but few cases have been seen elsewhere. It is inherited as an AUTOSOMAL RECESSIVE trait, and is probably detectable at birth by plasma enzyme determination.

**leopard syndrome**    See MULTIPLE LENTIGINES SYNDROME.

**leprechaunism (Donahue syndrome)**
First described by W.L. Donahue in 1954, this rare disorder, evident at birth, is characterized by striking facial and physical features. The face has been described as "grotesque" and "elfin-like." The nasal bridge is flat, nostrils flared. The lips are thick and large, the eyes prominent and the ears low-set. Infants may have excessive facial hair (hirsutism). The features are quite coarse, not cute as the leprechaun label might suggest.

Excessive skin folds, lack of subcutaneous tissue, and low birthweight give infants an emaciated appearance. The striking physical appearance is usually sufficient for diagnosis. Insulin levels may be very high.

Breast enlargement is common in males and females, as are penile and clitoral enlargement. The hands and feet are also large.

Leprechaunism is inherited as an AUTOSOMAL RECESSIVE trait. To date, approximately 30 well-documented cases have been reported. The basic cause of the disorder is due to a defect on the cellular surface receptor for insulin. Though PRENATAL DIAGNOSIS has not been achieved, it may be possible. Affected infants exhibit severe motor and MENTAL RE-TARDATION and progressive wasting. All have died between the ages of six months and one year.

**Lesch-Nyhan disease**   Syndrome, seen only in males, characterized by bizarre, self-destructive behavior and severe motor and MENTAL RETARDATION. Unless affected individuals are physically restrained, they will engage in acts of self-mutilation, which may result in the tips of their fingers being chewed off and almost total detruction of the lips. (The lower lip is more frequently severely damaged.) However, the sensation of pain remains undiminished, and affected individuals are usually more comfortable when restrained.

At birth, infants appear normal and develop without incident for the first six to eight months of life. However, increased irritability may be noticed by three months of age. Gradually, motor control deteriorates. Infants become unable to sit or support their heads. Prominent spastic movements develop. Mental retardation is noted. Hand restraints become required to control self-destructive behavior, and sometimes selected baby (deciduous) teeth must be extracted to stop lip biting. (Lip biting decreases with age.)

The disorder was first described by M. Lesch (b. 1939) and W.L. Nyhan (b. 1926) of Johns Hopkins University in 1964. However, a pre-Incan ceramic figure excavated near Lima, Peru, is thought to display a representation of the characteristic self-mutilation of the lips and nose seen in this condition. Dr. Nyhan brought attention to this figure in a 1972 article in *Hospital Practice*.

Lesch-Nyhan syndrome is caused by the almost total absence of an ENZYME essential for the control of uric acid production (hypoxanthine guanine phosphoribosyltransferase). This is the first condition identified in which a specific biochemical abnormality can be associated with a specific pattern of aberrant behavior. While excessive uric acid produc-tion can be controlled with drugs, there is no decrease in self-mutilation or improvement in mental function. Death usually occurs during the teens or the 20s, primarily as a result of infection or kidney failure. Individuals with milder forms of deficiency of this enzyme exhibit elevated uric acid levels, GOUT, kidney stones and kidney failure.

Inherited as an X-LINKED trait, it is estimated to occur in one in 100,000 live births. CARRIER testing is available, and PRENATAL DIAGNOSIS is possible by the finding of reduced enzyme activity in fetal cells collected via AMNIOCENTESIS or CHORIONIC VILLUS SAMPLING.

**leukemia**   See CANCER.

**leukodystrophy**   Genetically determined, progressive disorders of the nervous system affecting the brain and spinal cord. The term is taken from the Greek *leuko*, for white, referring to the white matter of the nervous system, and *dystrophy*, meaning disordered (*dys*) growth (*trophy*).

The white matter of the nervous system contains a complex chemical substance called myelin. Composed of at least 10 lipids, complex fatty substances, the myelin forms a sheath that insulates the axon, a strand of nerve fiber that conducts nerve impulses. The nervous system contains billions of axons. The leukodystrophies destroy the myelin sheath, and sometimes the nerve cell (neuron) itself may be affected. This interferes with the conduction of electrical impulses, resulting in loss of function of the nervous system.

Each form of leukodystrophy affects one of the lipids that make up this myelin sheath, or destroys the axon itself. Most have their onset in infancy or childhood. First symptoms are often a loss of muscle tone (hypotonia), irritability, spasticity and weakness. There is a steady decline in mental function, motor activity and vision. The condition progressively worsens, impairing mental and physical abilities and resulting in death.

There is at present no recognized effective therapy, though there is ongoing research into the usefulness of bone marrow transplants in some patients.

Most of the conditions, while affecting all populations, are quite rare. Most are inherited as AUTOSOMAL RECESSIVE traits, though some forms are X-LINKED.

For information on specific forms of leukodystrophies, see ADRENOLEUKO-DYSTROPHY, ALEXANDER DISEASE, CANAVAN DISEASE, KRABBE DISEASE, METACHROMATIC LEUKODYSTROPHY, PELIZAEUS-MERZBACHER SYNDROME and REFSUM DISEASE.

For more information contact:

United Leukodystrophy Foundation, Inc.
2304 Highland Drive
Sycamore, IL 60178
(815) 895-3211

**limb-girdle dystrophy**    See MUSCU-LAR DYSTROPHY.

**linkage, genetic**    See GENETIC LINK-AGE.

**lipogranulomatosis** (Farber lipogran-ulomatosis)    A rare storage disorder char-acterized by progressive and rapid physical and mental debilitation, resulting in death. Well under 100 cases have been diagnosed, with the majority succumbing by two years of age. (However, one patient survived to at least 17 years of age.) Its secondary eponymic des-ignation is taken from U.S. pediatrician S. Farber who first described the condition at the Mayo Clinic in 1952.

In infants, lumpy masses over the wrists and ankles (and other pressure-bearing areas) occur within the first few months of life. Signs of central nervous system disease are also evident. Other symptoms include hoarseness, noisy breathing, slowed development and chronic FAILURE TO THRIVE. Severe painful joint swelling and restriction of movement is progressive, and there is gradual cerebral fail-ure. Recurrent pulmonary infections are also common. In delayed-onset cases joint swell-ing is detected at age two or three years.

Inherited as an AUTOSOMAL RECESSIVE trait the SYNDROME is the result of an inborn error of metabolism, caused by a deficiency of the ENZYME acid ceramidase, with the result being the accumulation of the fat, ceramide. There is no treatment available.

**lip pits or mounds**    Small pits or open-ings on the exposed surface of the lips. These appear either in the angles at the juncture of the upper and lower lips (commissural lip pits) or adjacent to the midline of the lower lip (paramedian lip pits). Pits of the upper lip are very rare.

Paramedian lip pits frequently are associ-ated with CLEFT LIP or palate, fusion of the eyelids or development of wing-like skin folds (pterygium) located behind the knees.

Lip pits are evident at birth. No treatment is prescribed for the commissural variety. Paramedian lip pits and pits of the upper lip may require surgery. Intelligence and life span are unimpaired.

The cause of this SYNDROME is unknown. Lip pits affect both sexes with equal fre-quency, and familial occurrences of com-misssural and paramedian lip pits suggest AUTOSOMAL DOMINANT transmission. Pits of the upper lip probably are of nongenetic ori-gin.

The van der Woude syndrome of lip pits and cleft lip or palate is an important autoso-mal dominant cause of facial clefts. Because of variable expressivity, the parents may have only lip pits but their offspring may have cleft lip or palate. Thus, in all cases of clefts, the child and parents should be examined to look for lip pits.

Commissural lip pits are reported to occur in approximately one in 80 to one in 500 whites, about one in 50 American blacks and approximately one in 110 Native Americans.

**lissencephaly syndrome**    (Miller-Dieker syndrome)    Lissencephaly means "smooth brain," that is, a brain without convolutions (gyri). Infants affected with this rare developmental anomaly exhibit an abnormally small head (MICROCEPHALY), small mandible, bizarre facial appearance, FAILURE TO THRIVE and retarded motor development. It is invariably fatal, either in infancy or early childhood. It is caused by subtle deletions of the short arm of chromosome 17 (see CHROMOSOME ABNORMALITIES). Where these deletions have not been detectable by standard chromosome analysis, molecular studies have demonstrated small deletions and loss of genetic material. Formerly considered an AUTOSOMAL RECESSIVE disorder, it is now known that most familial cases result from chromosomal rearrangements. PRENATAL DIAGNOSIS is possible using cytogenetic or molecular studies. Lissencephaly may also be a feature of other syndromes.

**Little's disease**    See CEREBRAL PALSY.

**live birth**    A birth in which the infant exhibits signs of life, such as heartbeat, respiration or movement of voluntary muscle. In some countries, infants who die within 24 hours of delivery are not considered to be live births, a distinction that may have considerable impact on birth and neonatal mortality statistics.

**localized absence of skin**    Individuals with this rare disorder are born with skinless patches, usually limited to areas of the scalp. These patches have the appearance of ulcers, sometimes covered by a thin membrane. Usually, the affected area develops a scab that heals itself within a few weeks, leaving only a fine, depressed hairless scar. If the defective patch is large, skin grafts may be necessary. Such incomplete development of an organ, in this case the skin, is referred to as aplasia.

In more severe forms of this disorderer, the underlying skull, the covering of the brain (meninges), and brain may be included in the defect, and the trunk and limbs, particularly the lower legs, may be affected. In extremely rare cases, the syndrome is associated with CLEFT LIP or palate, extra fingers or toes (POLYDACTYLY), eye abnormalities, tumors of the blood vessels (HEMANGIOMAS), SPINA BIFIDA with MENTAL RETARDATION, CONGENITAL HEART DEFECTS and CHROMOSOME ABNORMALITIES.

A few hundred cases have been reported. There is some suggestion that it is inherited as an AUTOSOMAL DOMINANT trait, although some cases appear to be AUTOSOMAL RECESSIVE. Prognosis is favorable, except in those few cases with associated complications.

**Lou Gehrig's disease**    See AMYOTROPHIC LATERAL SCLEROSIS (ALS).

**Louis-Bar syndrome**    See ATAXIA-TELANGIECTASIA.

**low birth weight**    Weight of 2,500 grams, or 5.5 pounds or less, at birth. Approximately 5.7% of white and 13% of non-white liveborn infants in the United States are low birth weight, as are more than two-thirds of 45,000 infants who die each year in the United States (see Table XV). Low birthweight babies have at least five times the mortality rate of babies weighing 6.5 to 9.5 pounds, considered normal birth weight. Low birth weight infants are also more likely to suffer from long-term developmental disabilities than infants of normal weight.

Low birth weight is usually associated with PREMATURITY (birth before the 37th week of pregnancy; normal gestation is 40 weeks), but it can also be seen in full-term infants who exhibit fetal growth retardation. (All infants, whether born prematurely or at full term, can be classified as either "small for gestational age" [SGA] or "appropriate for gestational age" [AGA].) Lack of adequate development of their organ systems leaves low birth weight infants vulnerable to a host of health problems. There are different problems associated

### Table XV
### Percent of Babies Born at Low Birthweight, Selected Countries, 1982

| Rank | Country | Percent | Rank | Country | Percent* |
|------|---------|---------|------|---------|----------|
| 1 | Norway | 3.8 | 14 | Canada | 6.0 |
| 2 | Sweden | 4.0 | 14 | Denmark | 6.0 |
| 2 | Netherlands | 4.0 | 16 | German Democratic Republic | 6.2 |
| 4 | Finland | 4.1 | 17 | Italy | 6.7 |
| 5 | Ireland | 4.7 | 18 | U.S. (Total) | 6.9 |
| 6 | Switzerland | 5.2 | 19 | United Kingdom | 7.0 |
| 6 | France | 5.2 | 20 | Hong Kong | 8.0 |
| 6 | Japan | 5.2 | 21 | Costa Rica | 8.5 |
| 9 | Germany, Federal Republic | 5.5 | 22 | Chile | 9.0 |
| 10 | Belgium | 5.6 | 23 | Korea, Republic of | 9.2 |
| 10 | Austria | 5.6 | 24 | Colombia | 10.0 |
| 12 | *U.S. (White)* | 5.7 | 25 | Hungary | 11.8 |
| 13 | Greece | 5.9 | 26 | *U.S. (Black)* | 12.6 |

Source: *A Briefing Book on the Status of American Children, 1988* (Washington, D.C.: Children's Defense Fund, n.d.).

with premature infants when compared to SGA ones.

RESPIRATORY DISTRESS SYNDROME, an insufficiency of lung function, is one of the most common and acute problems associated with prematurity, accounting for 25,000 deaths a year in the United States.

Low body temperature causes additional problems. Instead of using energy from food for growth, low birth weight infants use it to maintain body warmth. Hypoglycemia, low levels of sugar in the blood, is frequently seen in these infants, and if untreated can lead to MENTAL RETARDATION and severe brain damage. Jaundice of the newborn is another common disorder. RETINOPATHY OF PREMATURITY may result in blindness.

Certain maternal factors are associated with increased incidence of low birth weight. Teenage mothers are more likely to have low birthweight infants. Twenty-five percent are born to teenagers, with the risk for a low birth weight infant greatest for those under 16. Women who have previously given birth to low birth weight infants are also at increased risk, as are those who will give birth to twins or any multiple birth.

Maternal health can also have a profound impact on birth weight. Maternal genetic disorders, DIABETES MELLITUS, high blood pressure, kidney and respiratory problems, have all been associated with low birth weight infants. Poor maternal nutrition also has been shown to have a potential negative impact on the infant's size at birth. Folic acid deficiency, which results from an insufficient amount of meats and leafy vegetables in the diet, can lead to megaloblastic ANEMIA of pregnancy, and may cause miscarriage.

Alcohol, cigarettes and drugs also appear to contribute to a birth weight that is considerably below that of infants in comparable groups who do not use these substances (see TERATOGENS).

Currently, the percentage of infants born with low birth weight is increasing, rising 2.4% between 1985 and 1987. (The percentage dropped 9% from 1975 to 1985.) The rate of infants born weighing less than 3 pounds, 4 ounces, considered very low birth weight, increased 6.8% between 1975 and 1987. Very low birth weight infants have at least 90 times the mortality rate of babies with normal birth weights.

**Lowe syndrome**　Named for U.S. pediatrician Charles U. Lowe, senior member of a group that in 1952 described three male children with the condition, this disorder is also called the "oculo-cerebro-renal syndrome," due to the three major organ systems involved (eye, brain and kidney).

Inherited as an X-LINKED trait, it appears almost exclusively in males, though a very small number of affected females have been reported. This may be due to a second mode of inheritance or a coincident CHROMOSOME ABNORMALITY, or may be like the situation for other X-linked disorders where females show a wide spectrum of variability of involvement. It occurs in all races, though most reported cases have been of white or Asian ancestry. The incidence is unknown, with estimates on the number of affected individuals worldwide ranging between a few hundred and a few thousand. As of the mid-1980s, at least 150 cases had been reported in the medical literature.

At birth, affected individuals tend to have high, prominent foreheads, sparse hair and protruding ears. Undescended testicles are common. They often have a high palate and small mouth, which may result in extensive dental problems.

The ocular abnormalities include CATARACTS, GLAUCOMA, corneal degeneration and crossed eyes (STRABISMUS). Any one of these may cause significant visual disability. Cataracts, a clouding of the lens, are present at birth or may appear in the neonatal period. Unless surgically treated soon after birth, the infant will not have the visual stimulation necessary to fully develop useful vision. Glaucoma develops in about half of affected individuals, causing pressure within the eye to increase to the point that it damages the optic nerve, and may lead to total blindness. Scar tissue (keloid) may form on the cornea, the clear covering on the front of the eye, often causing progressive blindness.

Abnormalities in the central nervous system associated with this disorder include MENTAL RETARDATION, typically in the mild to moderate range, with some individuals exhibiting severe retardation. Some have seizures and serious behavioral problems, such as intense temper tantrums, hyperactivity and mild self-abuse. These abnormalities may be the result of abnormal brain development during fetal life.

Poor muscle tone (hypotonia) is another feature in most affected infants, resulting in a FLOPPY INFANT appearance. Poor head control and sucking reflex may cause feeding problems in infancy. Typically, motor development is significantly delayed.

Kidney abnormalities may not be present at birth, but are usually apparent by one year of age. The kidney is unable to reabsorb phosphate, potassium, AMINO ACIDS and other important substances from the blood, leading to a "wasting" of these substances. This can create serious metabolic problems.

Soft or broken bones and RICKETS are another common finding. Almost all affected individuals exhibit short stature. They are also prone to respiratory infections and constipation due to poor muscle tone. Joint swelling and arthritis may develop during teenage years.

The basic cause of this disorder is unknown. Diagnosis is made on the basis of the presence of the characteristic features of the disorder. Female CARRIERS may have cataracts, which may aid in GENETIC COUNSELING. Recently, the Lowe syndrome GENE was found to be closely linked with DNA markers on the long arm of the X-chromosome, which allow for carrier detection and PRENATAL DIAGNOSIS in at-risk families. The main cause of death in infancy is chronic renal insufficiency. Deaths at all ages have been reported from kidney failure, dehydration and pneumonia. With no complications, affected individuals live into their 20s and 30s.

For more information, contact:

Lowe's Syndrome Association
222 Lincoln Street
West Lafayette, IN 47906
(317) 743-3634

**lung cancer**   See CANCER.

**lupus**  (lupus erythematosus, LE; discoid lupus erythematosus; systemic lupus erythematosus, SLE)   A widespread disorder that can affect either the skin (discoid lupus erythematosus) or multiple internal organ systems (systemic lupus erythematosus, SLE). Its prevalence (it is more common than MULTIPLE SCLEROSIS, MUSCULAR DYSTROPHY, leukemia and CYSTIC FIBROSIS) and the difficulty of diagnosing the more serious internal form due to the extreme variability of symptoms, make it a major health problem. While found in all races and ethnic groups, it primarily affects women of childbearing years, though it can appear at any age.

Lupus is an autoimmune disease, that is, a disorder in which the immune system attacks the body's own tissue (see IMMUNE DEFICIENCY DISEASE). The exact cause is unknown, though it is thought to result from a combination of genetic, viral and environmental influences. Genetic factors appear important as indicated by twin studies that show 60% CONCORDANCE in identical twins and the fact that familial aggregation of the disorder has been clearly demonstrated (see FAMILIAL DISEASE). Many relatives of affected individuals have abnormal proteins in their blood, though they may not have symptoms of the disorder. There is a 12.8% incidence of SLE among first-degree relatives (parents, SIBLINGS, children) of patients with this disorder. In addition, there is accumulating evidence that specific HLA types (HLA-D2 or -D3, see HUMAN LEUKOCYTE ANTIGEN) are more common in patients with SLE than in the general population. The incidence is higher among American blacks than among American whites (three to four times higher), and certain North American Indian tribes (Sioux, Crow, Arapahoe) have an even greater predisposition. The female hormone estrogen may also play a role, as indicated by the preponderance of pre-menopausal female cases. (Ten percent of the cases are caused by adverse reactions to drugs.)

The first record of this disorder was probably made by Hippocrates in the fourth century B.C.; he described a disease characterized by the erosion and scarring of facial skin. Many centuries later the condition was given the name *lupus*, Latin for "wolf." There is dis-

agreement over whether the name derives from the resemblance of the facial lesions to the bite of a wolf, or because the characteristic butterfly-patterned red rash across the bridge of the nose and cheeks resembles the markings on the face of a wolf. The word erythematosus (from the Greek word *erythema*, meaning redness or flush) was added in the 1840s to distinguish this condition from other skin disorders. (At the time, physicians confused the condition with a form of tuberculosis, due to the rash's resemblance to tubercular lesions.) At the turn of the century, Canadian physician Sir William Osler added the word "systemic" to distinguish the form that involves internal organs from the form confined to the skin.

Ninety percent of patients are women, with half developing symptoms between the ages of 15 and 30. Lupus is estimated to occur in one in 400 to one in 500 women, affecting between 500,000 and one million Americans. Over 50,000 new cases are diagnosed, and 6,000 deaths are attributed to the disorder annually in the United States. Some suspect the disorder is even more prevalent, with many mild cases never coming to the attention of the medical community.

The symptoms can appear in any part of the body, though the most commonly involved areas are the skin, joints, blood, heart, lungs and kidneys.

*Discoid LE.* This mild form is generally confined to the skin and is characterized by a disc-shaped or butterfly-patterned rash that appears on the face. Raised, scaly red areas may also occur on the scalp, ears, chest and arms. Only about 2% to 5% of affected individuals exhibit internal symptoms of lupus, as well, though as many as 50% experience joint ache and fatigue. Seventy percent of patients with the disorder are women, with symptoms usually appearing between the ages of 20 and 40. Discoid lupus is diagnosed relatively easily by the characteristic skin rash.

Discoid lupus can be treated with corticosteroids, natural or synthetic hormones that can suppress inflammation. Antimalarial drugs may be prescribed for cases that don't respond to corticosteroids.

*Systemic lupus erythematosus (SLE).* The baffling nature of this disorder has much to do with the extreme variability of expression. No two individuals display the same symptoms, and the symptoms often mimic other disorders, including RHEUMATOID ARTHRITIS, dementia, stroke, psychosis, epilepsy, kidney disease, ALLERGY and hypochondria. Its severity is also highly variable, ranging from mild to life-threatening. The writer Flannery O'Connor succumbed to complications of SLE, and four weeks before her death wrote: "The wolf, I'm afraid, is inside tearing up the place. I've been in the hospital 50 days already this year."

The facial lesion that characterizes the discoid form is observed in only 5% of newly diagnosed SLE patients. It may begin, like rheumatoid arthritis, with swelling of joints of the hands, feet, ankles or wrists. (Lupus is classified as a chronic inflammatory rheumatic disease of the connective tissue, in the same family as rheumatoid arthritis.) Additional symptoms may include fever, skin rashes, chest pain, extreme fatigue, loss of appetite, weight loss, sores in the mouth or vagina, increased susceptibility to infection and hair loss. Some affected individuals display RAYNAUD DISEASE, painfully cold fingers and toes caused by spasms of the small blood vessels resulting from cold or intense emotions. Sjorgren's syndrome, a dryness of the mucous membranes throughout the body, is exhibited in some cases.

The disease may begin in any of several organ systems and spread to others. The membranes surrounding the heart, lungs or abdominal organs may become inflamed. The gastrointestinal tract may be involved. In the cardiovascular system, SLE may mimic rheumatic heart disease or an arterial clot. Nerve damage may affect sensations and movement. Brain involvement may be misdiagnosed as a mental disturbance. In severe cases it may attack the kidney and cause kidney failure, a common cause of death among those who succumb to the disorder.

The diagnosis is based on medical history, physical examination and laboratory tests. The most reliable test involves screening for high levels of proteins called antinuclear antibodies (ANA) in the blood, which may indicate a problem in the immune system. However, due to the variability of symptoms, individuals suspected of having the disorder may be required to undergo a wide variety of diagnostic procedures.

While there is no cure, many symptoms can be treated and managed with corticosteroids and antimalarial drugs, in addition to aspirin, nonsteroidal anti-inflammatory and immunosuppressive drugs.

Though it is a lifelong condition, the symptoms appear and disappear unpredictably. Some have no recurrence after the initial symptoms disappear. During periods of remission, flare-ups of symptoms can be triggered by insufficient rest, overwork, stress, irregular living habits and discontinuance of medication prescribed to control symptoms. About 40% of affected individuals are sensitive to ultraviolet radiation and must protect themselves from exposure to sunlight. Allergy-producing substances in hair colorings and cosmetics may also trigger reactions. In the mid-1970s, 80% of patients did not survive five years after diagnosis. Now, due to improved therapy, 80% to 95% of affected individuals live at least 10 years after diagnosis.

Currently there is no method of PRENATAL DIAGNOSIS. Many affected women who become pregnant will not experience any complications due to the disorder, though a slight worsening of their condition may occur. However, these women face an above-average risk of spontaneous ABORTIONS and STILLBIRTHS. This may be due to the presence of lupus anticoagulant, an acquired inhibitor of blood coagulation that circulates in the blood of patients with SLE. This is not associated with bleeding but paradoxically with excessive clotting. The presence of the anticoagulant is associated with pregnancy loss. In addition, the offspring of mothers with SLE are at risk for developing CONGENITAL heart block, a potentially life-threatening disturbance of cardiac rhythm. In this condition, the conduction of the electrical stimulus to cardiac contraction is delayed. So striking is the association between SLE and congenital heart block that it is recommended that all infants born to mothers with SLE be evaluated for heart block and conversely that mothers of all infants with heart block should be evaluated for evidence of lupus. Similarly, investigation for lupus anticoagulant has become a part of the evaluation of all couples with recurrent pregnancy loss.

For more information, contact:

Lupus Foundation of America, Inc.
1717 Massachusetts Ave., N.W., Suite 203
Washington, DC 20036
(202) 328-4550

The American Lupus Society
23751 Madison Street
Torrance, CA 90505
(213) 373-1335

The SLE Foundation of America
149 Madison Avenue
New York, NY 10016
(212) 685-4118

**lupus erythematosus, LE**   See LUPUS.

**Lyme disease**   Though named for the town of Lyme, Connecticut, where it was first recognized by a team of Yale University medical researchers in 1975, this tick-borne bacterial infection occurs in many parts of the world. Symptoms include red, ring-like rashes, arthritis-like joint pain and swelling, and flu-like episodes. Untreated, it may damage the heart, brain, central nervous system and liver.

Lyme disease contracted during pregnancy has been associated with spontaneous ABORTION, CONGENITAL HEART DEFECTS, BLINDNESS and delayed development. Additionally,

at least two infants have been born with Lyme disease, apparently contracted from the mother in utero.

While a dearth of data prevents definitive conclusions about the potential teratogenic nature of the disease, pediatricians with experience with the infection recommend that pregnant women who develop any signs of Lyme disease seek immediate medical attention.

# M

**McArdle disease**   See   GLYCOGEN STORAGE DISEASE.

**McCune-Albright syndrome**   Condition of skin and skeletal abnormalities first described in 1936 and 1937 by Donovan James McCune (1902–1976), a pediatrician at Columbia University in New York, and Fuller Albright (1900–1969), an endocrinologist at the Massachusetts General Hospital (Albright's name is attached to several skeletal disorders).

Irregularly shaped, coffee-colored splotches (café au lait spots) are observed on the forehead, neck, back and buttocks. Skeletal lesions are found throughout the long bones, especially the lower limbs, replacing bone tissue with sharp, gritty, glass-like splinters (fibrous dysplasia). These result in pain, leg fractures, a limping, waddling gait, leg length discrepancies and a characteristic bowing or "hockey-stick" deformity. Bowing of the legs may appear as early as the first year of age, and nearly always prior to age 10. Multiple fractures may result in partial or complete disability. Rib fractures predispose some patients to pneumonia. Bony lesions of the skull and facial skeleton can cause bone overgrowth of facial passages, and may result in BLINDNESS or DEAFNESS. There may be protrusion of an eye associated with visual disturbances and enlarged distorted jaw and facial asymmetry in approximately 25% of the cases.

Accelerated skeletal growth in childhood produces adults of short stature. PRECOCIOUS PUBERTY is common in females, less frequent in males. Onset of menstruation (menarche) may occur as early as three months of age, but more often between one and five years. Development of breasts and secondary sexual characteristics follows, appearing between five and 10 years of age. Overactive thyroid glands are seen in 20% of these cases.

The cause of this syndrome is unknown. Reported cases have been SPORADIC and may be detected at birth by the characteristic pigmented skin blotches, or later by sexual precocity or bone deformities. Life span may be normal except where there is extensive bone degradation. Bone deformities are treated by orthopedic surgery. The drug medroxyprogesterone is used to control sexual precocity.

**Machado-Joseph disease**    See AZO-
REAN DISEASE.

**McKusick-type metaphyseal chondro-
dysplasia**    See METAPHYSEAL CHON-
DRODYSPLASIA.

**macroglossia**    An abnormally large tongue. This condition is common in DOWN SYNDROME and many other genetic syndromes.

**madarosis**    A very rare CONGENITAL condition characterized by underdeveloped eyelashes. Typically those who are completely lacking eyelashes are also missing eyebrows and scalp hair.

The cause of this disorder, which involves incomplete formation of hair follicles, observable with a microscope, has not yet been determined. The pattern of inheritance is uncertain, though in a few families it appears to be an AUTOSOMAL DOMINANT trait.

**Madelung deformity**    A CONGENITAL deformity of the wrist resulting in pain and limited motion of the wrist and elbow. It is named for German physician Otto W. Madelung (1846–1926) who described it in 1878. Females are more frequently affected than males by a ratio of four to one. Inherited as an AUTOSOMAL DOMINANT trait, it is caused by the overgrowth of the ulna, one of the two bones of the forearm. Madelung deformity is also seen in individuals with the autosomal dominant disorder dyschondrosteosis. (Individuals possessing two copies of the dominant dyschondrosteosis gene, that is, HOMOZY-GOTES for this gene, have a disorder named mesomelic DWARFISM, type Langer.

**major histocompatibility complex**
See HUMAN LEUKOCYTE ANTIGEN.

**male pattern baldness**    Though not a disease or disorder, affected males have often sought a cure for this condition, characterized by the gradual loss of hair on the head. Severe early baldness is believed to be inherited as an AUTOSOMAL DOMINANT trait with expression only in males. However, women may also be affected if they inherit two copies of the GENE, that is, if they are homozygotes for the baldness gene. It is said to affect at least 50% of white men and 25% of white women. Blacks are less frequently affected, and baldness is relatively rare among Native Americans and Orientals.

In 15% of affected white men, the condition progresses until only a fringe of scalp hair remains. Women are rarely as severely affected, and the condition's appearance is usually different than that in men.

That baldness tends to run in families has been noted since the time of the Greeks, a link noted by Hippocrates (ca. 460–ca. 377 B.C.), the father of medicine. Specific patterns of balding can often be seen through successive generations, suggesting the operation of a single major gene. The descendants of President John Adams are a well-known example among geneticists of an inherited pattern of baldness.

Treatment has traditionally consisted of the use of hairpieces and wigs to cover the bald areas. More recently, hair transplants and treatment with the drug minoxidil have helped alleviate the condition in some men. Minoxidil is a drug developed for the treatment of high blood pressure. Excessive hair growth (hypertrichosis) was noted as a side effect. This "side effect" has been capitalized upon and now the drug is more often prescribed for this than for its primary use. (See also ALOPECIA.)

For more information, contact:

Bald-Headed Men of America
3819 Bridges St.
Morehead City, NC 28857
(919) 726-1855

H.A.I.R., Inc.
Help Alopecia International Research
P.O. Box 691487
Los Angeles, CA 90069
(213) 851- 5138

National Alopecia Areata Foundation
P.O. Box 5027
Mill Valley, CA 94941
(415)383-3444

**malformation**   See ANOMALY.

**malignant hyperthermia (MH)**   (hyperthermia of anesthesia; King syndrome) Disorder that can cause death during or soon after surgery due to an at-risk individual's reaction to any of several commonly used general anesthetics. The administration of anesthesia triggers a chain reaction in those affected beginning with increased metabolic rate and muscle rigidity. The body temperature may be elevated as high as, reportedly, 110° Fahrenheit or more (hyperthermia). Death results from cardiac arrest, brain damage, renal shutdown or internal hemorrhaging. Those who survive an episode may exhibit impaired function of the brain, kidneys or other major organs.

The disorder was first described by Drs. Michael Denborough and Roger Lovell in 1960 in Australia. At the time, the mortality rate of those who had MH attacks in surgery was 80%. Since 1979, the drug dantrolene has been used as an antidote, reversing the course of these attacks, and mortality rate is now estimated at perhaps 10%.

MH occurs by itself, as an isolated entity, and has also been found in association with a number of other neuromuscular diseases, including MYOTONIC DYSTROPHY and myotonia congenita. The tendency to develop MH, as an isolated entity, is generally inherited as an AUTOSOMAL DOMINANT trait, though in some families (rarely) it appears to be an AUTOSOMAL RECESSIVE or MULTIFACTORIAL trait. It is estimated that as many as one in 200 people may carry the defective GENE that triggers these episodes. They may undergo surgery several times successfully without exhibiting any symptoms of the condition.

The disorder has been identified in almost all Western countries, as well as Japan, Australia and New Zealand. In the United States, it most commonly affects whites of Northern European ancestry. Attacks occur most frequently in older children and young adults.

Some physical characteristics appear to be common in families susceptible to MH. They include a history of unexplained high fevers, unusual muscle weakness, spinal deformities, a history of muscle cramps and an inability to exercise in high heat.

Pigs have a similar disorder that is triggered by periods of stress, and there have been suggestions, though unproven, that in some individuals at risk for MH, episodes can also be triggered by intense stress or by exercise. It has also been suggested that there may be a link between MH and heat stroke.

Susceptibility for MH may be detected via a muscle biopsy with studies of muscle contraction after pharmacologic stimulation. However, these studies require removal of a significant amount of muscle tissue by an invasive procedure, are highly specialized, and are available at only about 10 centers across the United States—and do not reliably detect 100% of individuals at risk for developing MH. Thus, because of the potential catastrophic consequences, anyone with a first-degree relative (parents, offspring, SIBLINGS) who exhibited symptoms of MH during surgery must be considered at risk.

At-risk individuals undergoing surgery can be anesthetized with alternative agents, with special care taken to monitor them during and after the operation.

For more information, contact:

Malignant Hyperthermia Association of the
 United States
P.O. Box 3231
Darien, CT 06820
(203) 655-3007

**mandibulo-facial dyostosis**    See
TREACHER COLLINS SYNDROME.

**manic depression** (manic    depressive psychosis; affective disorders)    An episodic psychological disturbance that manifests a tendency toward depression alternating with occasional periods of energized alertness, grandiosity and other signs of mania. It is called a bipolar disorder, indicating the presence of mania and depression or mania alone, as opposed to unipolar, which refers to depression alone. A familial aggregation and strong genetic predisposition to these disorders has long been recognized, both medically and popularly, as has been noted in the lyrics to a Memphis Slim song:

My Mama had them
Her mama had them
Now I've got them, too
Folks, you've got to inherit the blues

The mode of inheritance in most genetically-determined cases is unknown. One form seen in an AMISH family with a history of manic depression appears to be an AUTOSOMAL DOMINANT form. A 1987 report suggested the aberrant GENE was found on the tip of the short arm of chromosome 11. However, research published subsequently cast doubts on this assertion. A Jewish family in Israel has been suggested to have an X-LINKED form, with the mutant gene found on the X CHROMOSOME. Other groups and affected individuals may have yet different forms. (Two million in the United States are thought to be affected.)

Recurrence risks for near-relatives tend to be highly variable, even more so than for SCHIZOPHRENIA. First-degree relatives (parent, child, sibling) of an affected individual have about a 7% risk of having a bipolar disorder and an equal risk for a unipolar disorder. (Unipolar disorders also appear to have a genetic component, though less strong than bipolar disturbances.) Female first-degree relatives are from one and a half to two times as frequently affected as males. The risks approximately double if both a parent and sibling are affected.

Antidepressant drugs can alleviate some symptoms. From 10% to 20% of those under medical care are reported to commit suicide.

The cause of bipolar disorders is unknown, but one theory holds that it may involve abnormalities in the transport of sodium and lithium in the brain. Thirty percent of affected individuals under medical supervision have such an abnormality in their blood cells; their affected relatives show similar signs, while unaffected relatives have no such transport defect. About 1% of the general population will develop a major bipolar disorder within their lifetime; as many as 5% may develop a milder unipolar depressive psychosis.

**manic depressive psychosis**    See
MANIC DEPRESSION.

**mannosidosis**    A hereditary deficiency of the ENZYME alpha-mannosidase, this metabolic disorder results in accumulations of mannose-rich compounds in body cells and organs.

After the first few years of life, there is a progressive coarsening of facial features, marked by a high forehead, prominent jaw bone, low flat nose, short neck, large tongue (MACROGLOSSIA), enlarged hands, feet and ears. DEAFNESS is common, as is delayed motor development. Growth is retarded and speech is delayed. MENTAL RETARDATION is characteristic, with IQs generally in the 50 to 70 range.

Other symptoms include spoke-shaped opacities in the lenses of the eyes, mild muscle weaknesses, spleen and liver enlargement (hepatosplenomegaly), HUMPBACK (kyphosis), demineralization of the long bones (osteoporosis) and umbilical or INGUINAL HERNIAS.

The SYNDROME is inherited as an AUTOSOMAL RECESSIVE trait, and there appears to be some concentration among Scandinavians. There also is a juvenile-adult-onset form of the disorder. Symptoms range from the mild to the more severe depending upon the form of the condition that is inherited. Diagnosis of mannosidosis is based on reduced levels of the enzyme alpha-mannosidase in blood constituents.

CARRIER detection is not simple but PRENATAL DIAGNOSIS is possible through finding reduced enzyme levels in cultured AMNIOTIC FLUID (or chorionic villus) cells. Prognosis depends upon the form of the disease. The early- onset form may be fatal in early childhood.

An animal model exists among cattle. A similar neurodegenerative disease due to a deficiency of beta-mannosidase has been described in goats and recently several cases have been found in humans.

**maple syrup urine disease**    An infant-onset metabolic disorder resulting in deterioration of the nervous system. First described in 1954, it is named for the urine's characteristic maple syrup odor. Untreated, death usually occurs before the age of one year.

Inherited as an AUTOSOMAL RECESSIVE trait, it is caused by defective metabolism of the AMINO ACIDS leucine, isoleucine and valine. Initial symptoms, evident soon after birth, include vomiting, lethargy, feeding problems and poor muscle tone (hypotonia). As the condition progresses, mental and physical retardation commonly result. It can be managed by a controlled diet that excludes foods with the amino acids that cannot be metabolized. However, this dietary management is difficult and must be initiated within 10 days of birth.

Maple syrup urine disease is estimated to occur in one in 200,000 live births. However, among conservative Mennonites, a religious isolate in eastern Pennsylvania, frequency has been estimated as high as one in 176 live births. Prenatal diagnosis is possible by enzyme assay of cultured fetal cells gathered via AMNIOCENTESIS.

For more information, contact:

Families with Maple Syrup Urine Disease
24806 SR 119
Goshen, IN 46526
(219) 862-2992

**Marcus Gunn syndrome**    See JAW WINKING SYNDROME.

**Marfan syndrome**    A genetic disorder of the connective tissue that primarily affects the skeletal, ocular and cardiovascular systems.

The condition takes its name from Bernard-Jean Antonin Marfan (1858–1942), a founder of French pediatrics who in 1896 described it in a five-year-old girl with poor muscle development and abnormal spinal curvature, whose limbs, fingers and toes were long and thin.

In the skeletal system, the most distinguishing characteristic is excessive height with long extremities, including fingers and toes. Defects in the cardiovascular system, which become more threatening with age, are the major health consideration.

The biochemical basis for the disorder is unknown, and presently there is no way of making a definitive diagnosis of Marfan syndrome. Identifying affected individuals is accomplished by testing suspected cases for signature indicators of the disorder, as well as ascertaining family history. It is inherited as an AUTOSOMAL DOMINANT trait, and is believed to affect one in 10,000 individuals, making it more prevalent than CYSTIC FIBROSIS and HEMOPHILIA. Twenty-five percent of the cases are the result of new mutation, and, as with many other dominant disorders, the rate of mutation appears to be linked to increased paternal age. Non-affected parents have an estimated one in 40,000 to one in 50,000 chance of giving birth to an infant with Marfan caused by a new mutation.

There is a great variability in expression of this condition. Even within families with more than one affected member the severity and specific features displayed can vary tremendously. Most of the characteristic features become more pronounced with age, making diagnosis generally easier at older ages.

Many Americans first became aware of the syndrome following the death of Olympic star Flo Hyman in 1986. At the age of 31, she collapsed and died of a ruptured aortic aneurysm during a volleyball tournament in Japan. She had never been diagnosed as having the disorder. Almost a decade earlier, collegiate basketball player Chris Patton died from the same manifestation of Marfan during a pickup basketball game. Although the prognosis for this condition has improved dramatically in recent years due to new therapies, the difficulty in recognizing the disorder, and its often sudden, fatal consequences has led Dr. Reed Pyeritz of Johns Hopkins Medical Institutions in Baltimore, Maryland, to say, "Often the first person to make the diagnosis of Marfan is the coroner."

Medical historians question whether the violinist Niccolo Paganini, noted as having exceptionally long fingers (a hallmark of the disorder), may have had Marfan syndrome. Additional attention has been focused on Abraham Lincoln, with some citing his excessive height and lean frame as evidence that he had Marfan and was likely to have died unnaturally early, even if spared an assassin's bullet. However, more recent historical examination notes that his hands were well-proportioned, he had no spinal curvature or chest deformity, and he was exceptionally muscular, none of which is typical for individuals with Marfan syndrome. Additionally, he was farsighted, which is extremely rare in the disorder.

Bones and ligaments are affected in many different ways. In addition to excessive height, arms and legs are often disproportionately long (dolichostenomelia), as are the fingers (ARACHNODACTYLY). The arms, when fully extended, may have a span considerably greater than body height. The joints may have the ability to bend beyond their usual limit (HYPERMOBILITY). This can cause clumsiness and precipitate repeated dislocations. Feet are usually flat. Spinal curvature (SCOLIOSIS) is common and may be severe. It can develop rapidly and may require surgical intervention. The breast bone may protrude (pigeon breast, *pectus carinatum*) or be indented (funnel chest, *pectus excavatum*).

The face, like the rest of the body, may be long and narrow, with a highly arched palate and crowding of teeth caused by a narrow jaw. There are a number of associated ocular abnormalities, as well. The most common is myopia, or nearsightedness. The lens may be dislocated (that is, off center). Since this anomaly is observed in few other disorders, it is an important clue in diagnosing the syndrome. Retinal detachment may occur, requiring affected individuals to refrain from recreational activities that may subject them to blows to the head, which could precipitate detachment.

The cardiovascular characteristics, perhaps the most consistent features, are also the most serious. Most common is mitral valve prolapse. This occurs when the mitral valves, which separate the chambers of the heart, like the joints, are "floppy" and don't effectively cover the opening. The condition is found in 75% to 85% of cases. Complications of mitral valve prolapse can include abnormalities of heart rhythm (arrhythmia), infection of the valve (endocarditis) and, rarely, sudden death.

The aorta, the artery that carries all the oxygenated blood pumped from the heart, is the area most seriously affected. The wall of the aorta may become seriously weakened, even to the point where the vessel may suddenly rupture with fatal consequences. (The bulging area caused by the weakened tissue is termed an aneurysm.) Furthermore, the dilation of the aorta that over time precedes this rupture may allow blood to flow back into the heart and can ultimately cause heart failure.

New surgical procedures for replacing this damaged section of the aorta are greatly increasing life expectancy among those who exhibit serious cardiac problems. Beta blockers, drugs that lower blood pressure, are also often prescribed to reduce the risk of ruptured aneurysms.

Cardiovascular abnormalities can be detected with an echocardiogram, a test that uses high frequency sound waves (ULTRASOUND) to create a sonar scan of the heart.

Women with Marfan must be carefully monitored during pregnancy, due to the extra strain this places on their hearts. In addition, vigorous exercise and competitive sports should be avoided.

Currently there is no accepted method of effective PRENATAL DIAGNOSIS for this disorder, though sonography has been used in at-risk pregnancies; in at least one, abnormally long limbs were detected.

For more information, contact:

National Marfan Foundation
382 Main Street
Port Washington, NY 11050
(516) 883-8712

Johns Hopkins Medical Institutions
Division of Medical Genetics
Baltimore, MD 21205
(301) 955-3122

**marijuana**    Previously labeled as a suspected TERATOGEN, its effects on fetal development are unclear. Studies have been contradictory, and statistical data on incidence of birth defects in marijuana users surveyed is hard to interpret due to the presence of other potential contributing factors, such as cigarette smoking, alcohol use and maternal health. Women who smoked marijuana have been reported to have had prolonged, difficult or unexpectedly fast labor. In some studies LOW BIRTH WEIGHT and PREMATURITY were associated with marijuana, while in others they were not. Infants born to marijuana users have been reported to have tremors and altered visual response in the first few days after birth, but these abnormalities have disappeared within a month.

The impact of paternal use of marijuana on levels or viability of sperm is also unclear.

**Markers, genetic**    See GENETIC MARKERS.

**Maroteaux-Lamy syndrome**    See MUCOPOLYSACCHARIDOSIS.

**maturity-onset diabetes**    See DIABETES MELLITUS.

**measles (rubeola)**    A viral infection that, if contracted during pregnancy, can cause PREMATURITY, LOW BIRTH WEIGHT or miscarriage (see ABORTION). However, it has not been linked to BIRTH DEFECTS. If infection occurs near delivery date, the infant may be born with measles, with severity of symptoms ranging from mild to fatal.

Measles, also called rubeola, should be distinguished from rubella (German measles), a viral infection that can cause birth defects if contracted during pregnancy. (See also TERATOGEN, TORCH SYNDROME).

**Meckel syndrome** (Gruber syndrome) Invariably fatal syndrome characterized by multiple, severe physical abnormalities. The head is small (MICROCEPHALY) and the skull often has an opening at the back, or hernation, through which brain tissue protrudes (occipital ENCEPHALOCELE). The forehead is sloped, and the eyes may be small or completely absent (microphthalmia; anophthalmia). Other anomalies include CLEFT PALATE, extra fingers or toes (POLYDACTYLY), polycystic kidneys and incomplete development of the genitalia. The abdomen and lower trunk may be swollen due to enlargement of the kidneys and liver, and may in some cases make delivery difficult. CLUBFOOT is common, as are other anomalies of the limbs. Infants are either stillborn or die soon after birth.

It is named for Johann Friedrich Meckel, who first described it in 1822. It is often referred to as Gruber or Meckel-Gruber syndrome for Dr. D.G. Gruber, who described it in 1934.

This rare condition is inherited as an AUTOSOMAL RECESSIVE trait. PRENATAL DIAGNOSIS is possible by ULTRASOUND with identification of either the encephalocele, enlarged cystic kidneys or polydactyly. An elevated alphafetoprotein level may also be seen in many cases with encephalocele.

**median cleft face syndrome** A CONGENITAL developmental abnormality characterized by wide-spaced eyes (HYPERTELORISM) and a CLEFT that creates some degree of a vertical separation in the middle of the face. The skull itself may also be fissured. The severity of the median clefting ranges from broadening of the nasal tip to complete separation of the nose or nose and lip into two parts. Clefting of the palate also may be evident in severe cases. Other less common physical features include abnormally small eyeballs (microphthalmia), benign cysts located on the globe of the eye, fissures of the upper eyelid, CATARACTS, ear abnormalities, deformities of the fingers, and undescended testes. Approximately 20% of affected indi-

viduals may exhibit mild MENTAL RETARDATION.

The basic cause of this rare syndrome is unknown, and most cases occur sporadically. Corrective and reconstructive surgery may repair some clefts. Life span is unaffected, and psychosocial therapy may help affected individuals adjust to their appearance.

**Mediterranean anemia** See THALASSEMIA.

**Mediterranean fever, familial** See FAMILIAL MEDITERRANEAN FEVER.

**Melanoma** See CANCER.

**Mendel, Gregor** See MENDELIAN.

**Mendelian** Genetic traits that follow patterns of inheritance described by Austrian monk Gregor Johann Mendel (1822–1884). He was the first to deduce correctly the basic principles of heredity. Mendelian traits are also called "single GENE" or "monogenic" traits, because they are controlled by the action of a single gene or gene pair. More than 4,300 human disorders are known or suspected to be inherited as Mendelian traits, encompassing AUTOSOMAL DOMINANT, AUTOSOMAL RECESSIVE and X-LINKED dominant and X-linked recessive conditions. Overall incidence of Mendelian disorders in the human population is about 1%. Many non-anomalous characteristics that make up human variation are also inherited in Mendelian fashion. (Non-Mendelian traits are inherited in POLYGENIC, caused by the action of several genes, or MULTIFACTORIAL, caused by the action of several genes in concert with environmental influence, fashion.)

A monk in Brünn (now Brno), in Moravia (now a part of Czechoslovakia), Mendel, who had studied physics and mathematics, noticed that garden pea plants had varying traits. For example, some unripe pods were yellow, others green; some varieties were tall, others were dwarfed. The position of the flowers, whether clustered at the top, or distributed along the stem, also varied, as did the physical appearance of the peas themselves, being either smooth or wrinkled. In 1856 he began experiments in which he cross-bred pea plants, with the goal of studying the hereditary transmission of these and other characteristics and the statistical relation of the subsequently-appearing traits. Based on his observations, he hypothesized that each trait in the offspring is controlled by only two factors, one from the male and one from the female, and that these traits were either dominant or recessive: A dominant trait would override the influence of its complementary hereditary factor; the influence of a recessive trait would recede when paired with a dominant one. (See Table XVI.)

He presented his finding to the Natural History Society of Brünn, which published them in 1859, and was also in communication with Karl von Näegeli, one of the most respected botanists of the day. However, the importance of his work went unrecognized until 1900, when three researchers independently rediscovered his findings. (See also Introduction, "The History of Genetics.")

**meningocele**   A skin-covered, sac-like protrusion of the membranes (meninges) covering the brain or the spinal cord. It is one defect in the spectrum of NEURAL TUBE DEFECTS. Its origin is POLYGENIC (caused by several different genes), and it occurs in approximately one out of 20,000 live births, equally distributed between males and females.

In spinal meningocele, the neural material from the spinal cord does not extend into the sac, although there is usually an opening in the spine (SPINA BIFIDA), which requires surgical correction. In general, there is no paralysis or sensory loss with either cranial or spinal meningocele. It can occur in isolation or as part of another syndrome.

Meningocele can be repaired surgically. With repair during the first year of life, the prognosis is favorable.

**Menkes syndrome**   (kinky hair disease)
A hereditary inability to absorb and use copper is the hallmark of this syndrome, first described by U.S. pediatrician/neurologist J.H. Menkes in 1962. Affected infants appear normal at birth, but near the end of the first year of life begin to show signs of drowsiness, increased difficulty with feeding, poor visual development and a tendency to have an abnormally low body temperature (hypothermia). By the age of three months, muscle spasms and seizures are evident.

As the disorder progresses, there is a marked FAILURE TO THRIVE, severe MENTAL RETARDATION and a deficient physical growth. The scalp hair is characteristically short, sparse, twisted and unruly. Eyebrow hair is whitish and lacks color. Other symptoms include an abnormally small head (MICROCEPHALY) with a short, broad nose, full cheeks, small lower jaw (micrognathia) and a lack of facial expression. Loss of muscle tone (hypotonia) and a depressed sternum, or breast bone (pectus excavatum), are also characteristic. X-ray examination may disclose bone spurs on the long bones of the arms and legs and flaring of rib ends.

Degeneration of the central nervous system results in increased reflex reaction (hyperreflexia), muscle contractions and stiff, awkward movements (spasticity), and paralysis affecting all four limbs (quadriparesis).

Transmitted as an X-LINKED recessive trait, this rare disorder occurs only in males and has been estimated to occur once in every 35,000 to 40,000 live births, with only about 50 reported cases. Death within the first or second year of life occurred in 90% of those initially identified. Some CARRIERS of the trait have been identified through examination of the scalp hair. Prenatal diagnosis research has also shown elevated levels of copper in AMNIOTIC FLUID in case of this disorder.

Carrier testing is difficult but PRENATAL DIAGNOSIS has been accomplished by studies of copper uptake in fetal cells obtained by AMNIOCENTESIS or CHORIONIC VILLUS SAMPLING.

**Table XVI**
**Modes of Mendelian Inheritance, Related Sex Ratios and Risks of Recurrence**

| Code | Mode of transmission | Sex ratio | Risk of recurrence for | |
|------|---------------------|-----------|------------------------|--|
| AR | Autosomal recessive | M1:F1 | Patient's sib: | 1 in 4 (25%) for each offspring to be affected |
| | | | Patient's child: | Not increased unless mate is carrier or homozygote |
| AD | Autosomal dominant | M1:F1 | Patient's sib: | If parent is affected 1 in 2 (50%) for each offspring to be affected; otherwise not increased |
| | | | Patient's child: | 1 in 2 |
| AD-85%± penetrance | Autosomal dominant with about 85% penetrance | M1:F1 | Patient's sib: | If parent is affected <1 in 2 (<50%) for each offspring to be affected; otherwise not increased |
| | | | Patient's child: | <1 in 2 |
| AD-60%± penetrance | Autosomal dominant with about 60% penetrance | M1:F1 | Patient's sib: | If parent is affected 1 in 3 (30%) for each offspring to be affected, 1 in 2 for inheriting mutant gene; otherwise not increased |
| | | | Patient's child: | 1 in 3 (30%) for each offspring to be affected, 1 in 2 for inheriting mutant gene |
| X-linked R | X-linked recessive (rare) | M1:F0 | Patient's sib: | If mother is a carrier 1 in 2 (50%) for each brother to be affected and 1 in 2 (50%) for each sister to be a carrier |
| | | | Patient's child: | 1 in 1 (100%) for carrier daughters; not increased for sons unless wife is a carrier |
| X-linked D | X-linked dominant (rare) | M1:F2 | Patient's sib: | If affected parent is female 1 in 2 (50%) for each sib to be affected. If affected parent is male 1 in 1 (100%) for each sister to be affected; not increased for brothers |
| | | | Patient's child: | If patient is female 1 in 2 (50%) for each offspring to be affected; if patient is male 1 in 1 (100%) for daughters, not increased for sons |

Source: Daniel Bergsma (ed.), *Birth Defects Compendium*, 2nd ed. (New York: A.R. Liss, 1979).

**mental retardation** Impairments of learning, social adjustment and maturation, characterized by below-average intellectual function and behavioral development. A major health problem, it handicaps more infants than any other childhood disorder; an estimated 150,000 infants a year are born with, or will later be diagnosed as having, mental retardation, and it is thought to affect between 1% and 3% of the general population.

Mental retardation can result from genetic abnormalities, exposure to environmental agents, prematurity, intrauterine or birth trauma, or a combination of these and other factors. However, in the majority of those affected (estimates of 40% to 80%), the cause cannot be determined.

As a genetic condition, mental retardation can be inherited as an AUTOSOMAL DOMINANT, AUTOSOMAL RECESSIVE, X-LINKED, POLYGENIC or MULTIFACTORIAL trait, or as a result of CHROMOSOME ABNORMALITIES. Approximately 12% to 25% of those affected are thought to have single-gene (autosomal dominant, autosomal recessive or X-linked) forms. It is also a feature of approximately 200 CON-GENITAL conditions. Other genetic disorders (for example, PHENYLKETONURIA, CONGENI-TAL HYPOTHYROIDISM, GALACTOSEMIA) can result in mental retardation if undetected and untreated following birth.

Studies in mental institutions indicate mental retardation of unknown origin occurs in multiple siblings in a considerable number of cases, and these may be due to rare recessive disorders. It has also been estimated that about a third of normal persons carry a recessive gene for a low-grade mental defect.

Though there are no precise means of measuring the extent of mental retardation, those with IQs below 70 are considered to be retarded, and their retardation is classified in one of four categories: mild, moderate, severe or profound. Ninety percent of affected children are in the mild range, with IQs in the range of 52 to 67. They are educable and may learn to function independently as adults, though they require special education. Mild retardation may be difficult to diagnose; since infants develop at different rates, diagnosis in these cases is often delayed until two to three years of age. Those in the moderate range (IQs of 36 to 51) may attain some degree of independence as adults and also require special education. In the severe range (IQs of 20 to 35) affected individuals can learn minimal conversation and self-care skills, though they require supervision throughout life; institutionalization may be necessary. Those with profound retardation (IQ below 20) may acquire only minimal self-care skills and toilet training. Language development is usually minimal, and total supervision is required. One percent of newborn infants are severely to profoundly retarded. However, many of them succumb to associated conditions, so that by seven years of age, only an estimated 0.3% to 0.4% of the population have IQs below 50.

Mild or moderate retardation is usually multifactorial in cause, that is, caused by the action of several genes in concert with envi-ronmental influences, while severe cases are more likely to be due to genetic defects alone; at least one-third of severely retarded individuals are believed to have genetic abnormalities. Perhaps half of the remainder are genetically influenced.

The risk of recurrence in family members—and the possibility of PRENATAL DETECTION—is dependent on the form of mental retardation. However, mild retardation is much more likely to be seen in multiple family members than severe retardation.

Among the more well-known conditions or syndromes with which mental retardation is associated are CRANIOSYNOSTOSIS, DOWN SYNDROME, FRAGILE X SYNDROME, PHENYL-KETONURIA, fetal exposure to rubella (see TORCH SYNDROME) and alcohol (see ALCO-HOLISM; FETAL ALCOHOL SYNDROME), AMINO ACID disorders, and STORAGE DISEASES. (See also EDUCATION; HANDICAP; listings under DOWN SYNDROME.)

For more information, contact:

Mental Retardation Association of
   America
211 East 3rd South, Suite 212
Salt Lake City, UT 84111
(801) 328-1575

Association for Retarded Citizens
2501 Avenue J
Arlington, TX 76006
(817) 840-0204

**mesomelic dwarfism**   See MESOMELIC DYSPLASIA.

**mesomelic dysplasia**   (mesomelic dwarfism)   A group of conditions of short-limbed DWARFISM characterized by shortening of the mesomelic or middle portion of the limbs. Several forms are recognized, differentiated by the clinical and, more importantly, radiographic (observable by X-ray) differences.

*Langer type.* This form is named for radiologist L.O. Langer, who described it in 1967. It is characterized by severe shortening of the forearms and lower legs and malformations of the wrist. The elbows may not extend fully. Intelligence and lifespan are normal. Adult height is about 51 inches (129.5 cm). Inherited as an AUTOSOMAL RECESSIVE trait, individuals carrying a single copy of the GENE appear to have dyschondrosteosis—a short forearm with bowing at the radius, often with dislocation or limitation of movement at the elbow or wrist. It is those with two copies of the gene (HOMOZYGOTES) who have significant dwarfism.

*Nievergelt type.* Described by German physician K. Nievergelt in 1944, the forearms and lower legs are shortened and deformed from a mild to a severe degree. Dimpling of the skin on the forearms and lower legs may result from bony protruberances of the limbs. Motion of elbows and fingers may be limited. Intelligence and lifespan are normal. Adult height has been generally between 53 inches and 58 inches (134.6–147.3 cm) in the very few reported cases. It appears to be an AUTOSOMAL DOMINANT trait.

*Reinhardt-Pfeiffer type.* Described by German physicians K. Reinhardt and R.A. Pfeiffer in 1967, this is a moderate form of mesomelic short-stature, and has been described in only one family, inherited as an AUTOSOMAL DOMINANT trait. The lower legs are most affected, and the skeletal deformities may be progressive. Adult height was between 59 inches and 67 inches (149.9–170.2 cm), and intelligence and lifespan normal.

*Werner type.* Described in 1915 in Germany by gynecologist P. Werner, this form is characterized by extreme shortening of the lower leg, extra fingers or toes (POLYDACTYLY) and absence of thumbs. Bones of the ankles are also deformed. Forearms are normal, but the wrist bones may be deformed, and wrist movement may be limited.

Intelligence is normal, as is lifespan. Inherited as an AUTOSOMAL DOMINANT trait, the severity of the condition is highly variable.

For more information, contact:

Little People of America, Inc.
P.O. Box 633
San Bruno, CA 94066
(415) 589-0695

Human Growth Foundation
4720 Montgomery Lane, Suite 909
Bethesda, MD 20814
(301) 656-6904
(301) 656-7540

## metachromatic leukodystrophy (MLD)

Form of LEUKODYSTROPHY, a group of degenerative, progressive disorders of the nervous system. It takes its name "metachromatic" from the coloration of affected white matter cells after they are chemically stained during laboratory analysis; components of the same tissue take on various shades or colors, all differing from the color of the dye they are stained with.

The disorder is caused by the absence of the ENZYME arylsulfatase A (ASA), which normally breaks down sulfatides, a component of myelin, the protective sheath that covers the axons, nerve fibers that transmit electrical impulses. The sulfatides would normally be broken down into cerebrosides. The consequent accumulation of sulfatides in the brain, peripheral nerve, kidney, liver and gall bladder causes the breakdown of myelin, though the reason for this destruction is unclear.

MLD occurs in three forms: late infantile, with symptoms appearing between about 14 months and two years of age; juvenile, with onset between the ages of four years and 16 years of age; adult, with onset after the age of 16.

In the late infantile form, first described in 1933, symptoms begin with poor muscle tone (hypotonia), unsteady gait, speech abnormalities and arresting of mental development. The disorder is progressive, with ultimate loss of voluntary muscle control (apraxia), inability to communicate (aphasia), dementia and BLINDNESS. Death usually occurs between the ages of three and six years. There is no generally recognized treatment, though successful treatment with bone marrow transplatation is being explored. The potential of this treatment is not yet clear.

The other two forms display wide variability of expression, though they are also progressive and lead to death. In the adult form, initial symptoms have usually been psychiatric, leading to a diagnosis of SCHIZOPHRENIA. Disorders of movement and posture appear later. Until recently, most adult cases were diagnosed after death, though biochemical screening for indicative levels of enzyme activity now allows more timely detection. This method has found unsuspected cases among individuals institutionalized for mental disorders. Other diagnostic methods include CAT (computerized axial tomography) scanning, analysis of cerebrospinal fluid (CSF), and findings of low arylsulfatase A in tissue and white blood cells.

(In another disorder, multiple sulfatase deficiency, the enzyme ASA is decreased as are many other sulfatases, resulting in a syndrome of MLD characterized by MUCO-POLYSACCHARIDOSIS, ICHTHYOSIS and DEAF-NESS.)

MLD is inherited as an AUTOSOMAL RE-CESSIVE trait. Incidence has been estimated at between one in 40,000 and one in 50,000 live births in the general population. CAR-RIER detection is possible, but difficult. PRE-NATAL DIAGNOSIS is possible in at-risk pregnancies.

For more information, contact:

United Luekodystrophy Foundation, Inc.
2304 Highland Drive
Sycamore, IL 60178
(815) 895-3211

**metaphyseal chondrodysplasia**    Term describing several forms of short-limbed DWARFISM. *Metaphyseal* refers to the area of the bones involved, the metaphyses, which are the growth areas near the ends of the bones. *Dysplasia* refers to defective development, and *chondro* to cartilage. The defective development of the cartilage causes characteristic abnormal flaring of the metaphyses observable in X rays. The bones of the arms and legs (long bones) show the most evidence of the abnormality. Several varieties have been identified. The Schmid type is relatively common, the McKusick type well-known but uncommon and the remainder rare. Immunologic and endocrine abnormalities are important aspects of several forms.

*McKusick type (cartilage-hair hypoplasia.* This disorder was first observed in the Old Order AMISH, a religious community in the area of Lancaster, Pennsylvania, where it is relatively common. It is also relatively common in Finns in Finland and is seen in other groups. The McKusick referred to is Dr. Victor McKusick, a well-known geneticist at Johns Hopkins University in Baltimore, Maryland.

Body length is reduced but weight is normal at birth. The elbows have somewhat limited extension and ankles are deformed. As infants age, a single leg may bow inward or outward. Hands and feet are short and pudgy, and the fingers and toes show extreme flexibility of motion. By nine to 12 months of age, X rays can detect the characteristic abnormalities.

The hair is light and sparse, and a distinctive feature is the small width of the hair shafts when examined microscopically. Immunity is deficient and individuals affected are prone to infections, particularly during infancy and early childhood. Individuals have an increased susceptibility to chicken pox and other infections caused by the VARICELLA-ZOSTER virus, due to a defect of the cellular immune system, and may be left with deep pocked scars. The infection may be severe and lethal.

It is inherited as an AUTOSOMAL RECESSIVE trait. Adult height is usually between 41 inches and 57 inches (104.1–144.8 cm).

*Schmid type.*    First described in 1949, this

disorder is variable in its expression, with females being less severely affected than males. Increased paternal age has been associated with SPORADIC cases resulting from new MUTATIONS.

The dwarfing and short-limbed disproportion are usually seen by 18 months to 24 months of age. The first sign is a BOWLEGedness, and is usually noted when infants begin walking. As they age, the bowing increases, producing a waddling gait and contributing to degenerative arthritis in the hips.

The abnormalities of the metaphyses of the bones revealed in X rays are variable, from mild to gross. They appear to heal with bedrest, but reappear when weight is placed on them.

It is inherited as an AUTOSOMAL DOMINANT trait. Average adult height is 51 inches to 63 inches (129.5–160 cm).

*Jansen type.* Named after the Dutch orthopedist and founder of that specialty in his country, this is a very rare form, inherited as an AUTOSOMAL DOMINANT trait. Permanent bending of joints (flexion contractures) is severe. Patients are severely dwarfed and disabled. Asymptomatic hyperglycemia is seen but its association is not understood. About 10 cases have been reported. Adult height averages about 47 inches (119 cm.). Lifespan is normal.

*Metaphyseal chondrodysplasia with thymolymphopenia.* "Thymolymphopenia" refers to an involvement of the thymus and lymph glands that is characteristic of this form. As a result of this involvement, the condition is lethal, with affected infants exhibiting severe combined immunodeficiency disease (see IMMUNE DEFICIENCY DISEASES).

The short-limb condition is present at birth, along with evidence of ECTODERMAL DYSPLASIA, and often with skin disorders, including CUTIS LAXA, lack of scalp hair and scaly skin. Infants exhibit FAILURE TO THRIVE and are prone to bacterial, fungal and viral infections, which lead to death in infancy.

The condition is rare and is transmitted as an AUTOSOMAL RECESSIVE trait.

For more information, contact:

Little People of America, Inc.
P.O. Box 633
San Bruno, CA 94066
(415) 589-0695

Human Growth Foundation
4720 Montgomery Lane, Suite 909
Bethesda, MD 20814
(301) 656-6904
(301) 656-7540

**metatropic dysplasia**     (metatropic dwarfism)     Metatropic, from the Greek *metatropis*, meaning changing pattern, refers to the reversal of the proportions of the dwarfing (see DWARFISM) observed in affected individuals. Cases of the disorder are believed to have been first described in 1892 in Germany.

At birth, infants appear to have relatively short limbs and a relatively long, thin trunk. Craniofacial appearance is normal. Body length is usually normal during the neonatal period, but in late infancy, the spine begins to exhibit backward and lateral curvature (kyphoscoliosis), resulting in a short-trunk dwarfism. The kyphoscoliosis usually becomes severely incapacitating.

The limbs continue to exhibit dwarfing, and the bones of the arms and legs have a "barbell" shape upon X-ray examination. Additionally, the coccyx (the lower end of the spinal column) may be unusually long, resulting in what appears to be an almost tail-like appendage.

Generally inherited as an AUTOSOMAL RECESSIVE trait, metatropic dysplasia is relatively rare. While many affected individuals die in infancy, survival into the third decade of life is common, with height generally between 45 inches and 47 inches (114.3–119.4 cm). PRENATAL DIAGNOSIS is theoretically possible by findings of abnormal limb length via ULTRASOUND, but the dwarfism is usually diagnosed at birth. A less severe AU-TOSOMAL DOMINANT form is also known.

For more information, contact:

Little People of America, Inc.
P.O. Box 633
San Bruno, CA 94066
(415) 589-0695

Human Growth Foundation
4720 Montgomery Lane, Suite 909
Bethesda, MD 20814
(301) 656-6904
(301) 656-7540

**methylmalonic acidemia**   A group of disorders characterized by the inability to metabolize methylmalonic acid or by a defect in the metabolism of vitamin B12. The blood and urine exhibit an excessive level of the AMINO ACID glycine (hyperglycinemia), with an accompanying high level of ketones (ketoacidosis), which are substances normally processed by the liver from fats in food. Low blood sugar (hypoglycemia) is common. Methylmalonic acid, which is not normally found in the blood or urine, will also be detected. Also, an abnormally small number of circulating white cells in the blood (neutropenia) and a decrease in the number of blood platelets (thrombocytopenia) will be evident.

Repeated episodes of ketoacidosis may produce mental confusion, breathing difficulties, nausea, vomiting, dehydration and, if untreated, coma followed by death. MENTAL RETARDATION and marked growth retardation have been observed in those who survive the high rate of death in early infancy. Convulsions and fungus infections may also develop.

Inherited as AUTOSOMAL RECESSIVE traits, the incidence is about one in 50,000 live births. There is no current method of identification of CARRIERS. PRENATAL DIAGNOSIS possible by testing for the presence of methylmalonic acid in the mother's urine or in the AMNIOTIC FLUID, as well as by detection of the ENZYME defects in fetal cells.

Treatment is complex, including dietary management, often vitamin B12 supplements and possibly other agents such as carnitine.

**Michelin tire baby syndrome**   First described and named in 1985, the syndrome was reported in two families. The first individual brought to medical attention was a three-year-old girl with deep skin folds on the back and on the arms and legs, reminiscent of the appearance of the "Michelin Tire Man" used in advertisements for the Michelin Tire Company. Some adult relatives had skin creases on wrists and forearms that apparently were remnants of similar skin folds in infancy. It is believed to be inherited as an AUTOSOMAL DOMINANT trait.

One researcher has suggested that this congenital anomaly has existed throughout human history; German pediatrician Hans-Rudolf Wiedemann, founder of the Society for Anthropology and Human Genetics, has called attention to a sculpture on a bronze door of the cathedral of Hildesheim in northwestern Germany, which depicts Eve nursing her infant son who appears to have features of this syndrome.

**microcephaly**   A small head, often with a receding forehead and large ears and nose; it is usually an associated feature of other disorders, rarely occurring in isolation, though infants with true hereditary microcephaly, an AUTOSOMAL RECESSIVE disorder, have only head and facial abnormalities as physical symptoms.

Microcephaly is sometimes visibly obvious in newborns by the characteristic forehead, flattened back of the head, and small or closed fontanels, the "soft spots" between the skull bones. It is most often diagnosed by measuring the infant's head circumference, though it may be diagnosed prenatally via ULTRA-SOUND.

Physical growth is generally retarded and children learn to walk more slowly than their normal counterparts. There is a delay in speech and mental development. Some patients experience seizures and spasticity and may exhibit cross eye (STRABISMUS). Personality and mood are variable and may vacillate to extremes. Nearly 90% suffer from some form of prenatal brain damage. However, it is important to note that not all individuals with microcephaly will be retarded and have neurologic abnormalities; some are entirely normal.

This defect may be caused by a number of factors: GENETICS, CHROMOSOME DISORDERS, environment and factors of unknown origin. Environmental causes include prenatal radiation, infections (including rubella and toxoplasmosis) and drugs or agents (TERATOGENS), such as alcohol. Women with PHENYLKETONURIA (PKU) also give birth to microcephalic children. A number of multiple anomaly SYNDROMES have microcephaly as a feature.

Microcephaly may be inherited, but the GENE is considered extremely rare. In the general population, microcephaly due to genetic factors occurs in one in 30,000 to 50,000 live births, and in one per 10,000 births due to the other mentioned causes. In some population isolates, frequency may be as high as one in 2,000 births.

True hereditary microcephalics live an average-length life span, yet some die early due to other congenital defects or infectious diseases.

**middle-ear infections**    Among the most common illnesses in children. Middle-ear infections occur when bacteria in the nose and throat migrate to the inner ear, causing irritation, inflammation and a buildup of fluid behind the eardrum. The condition, also termed otitis media, is painful and may be accompanied by temporary hearing loss.

Several studies indicate that the tendency to develop middle-ear infections is inherited, and the infections are more common among white or Native American than among black or Hispanic children. About 10% of white children in one genetic study of the condition were affected. Susceptibility to otitis media

thus appears to be MULTIFACTORIAL, with some genetic disposition.

The infections can be easily treated with antibiotics. However, if left untreated, the buildup of fluid pressure can break the eardrum. Long-term problems with hearing and speech may result.

(Children are more prone to middle-ear infections than adults because their relatively short and horizontal eustachian tubes facilitate the migration of bacteria from the nose and throat to the ear.)

**midget**    Historically, this term has been used to describe short-statured individuals with normal body proportions, as opposed to "dwarfs," disproportionate short-statured individuals. (Actually, the body may not be proportionate, as upper/lower body segment ratios are not always in the truly normal range.)

The term midget is currently considered derogatory by short-statured individuals and its use is discouraged. The origin of the objection to this term is believed to be due to its circus-sideshow association and also to be a remnant of resentment from a time when proportionate short-statured individuals were perceived by those of abnormal proportions as having fewer social disadvantages. Preferred terminology includes "dwarf," and "small," "little" or "short" people.

Proportionate short stature may be caused by CHROMOSOME ABNORMALITIES, hormone failure, primary growth disturbances, secondary growth failure, poor nutrition and inherited short stature.

For more information on proportionate short stature, see DWARFISM and PITUITARY DWARFISM SYNDROMES.

**Miescher's syndrome**    See ACANTHOSIS NIGRACANS.

**migraine headaches**    Headaches accompanied by nausea and vomiting, often preceded by sensory disturbances, most commonly of a visual aura, such as a blind spot or twinkling lights. Migraines affect 5% to 10% of the population, and demonstrate an undoubted familial aggregation (see FAMILIAL DISEASES). In a study of 500 individuals who sought medical help for the condition, more than 90% had one parent who was similarly affected. Among offspring of two affected individuals, more than 80% were affected. Among offspring of one affected parent, more than 60% also had migraines, as opposed to less than 4% of the offspring of unaffected parents. Though it has been suggested that the tendency to develop these headaches is inherited as an AUTOSOMAL DOMINANT disorder, it is difficult to be sure that a single GENE is responsible for this common condition.

**Miller-Dieker syndrome**   See LISSEN-CEPHALY SYNDROME.

**Minimata disease**   CONGENITAL mercury poisoning seen in the town of Minimata in southern Japan. Affected infants were among the offspring of pregnant women who ate fish from Minimata Bay, seafood that had high levels of mercury from industrial wastes discharged into the bay. Between 1953, when it was first observed, and 1971, 134 cases were reported.

The mercury caused central nervous system disorders, resulting in death in an estimated 38% of affected infants and brain damage in more than 25% of the survivors. Affected infants had small heads (MICROCEPHALY) and severe brain damage manifest as CEREBRAL PALSY. A similar epidemic occurred in Niigata, Japan, in 1964.

**miryachit**   A "jumping disorder" reported in Siberia (in the present Soviet Union) in the late 19th century, characterized by an exaggerated startle response, similar to JUMPING FRENCHMEN OF MAINE.

Miryachit, which means "to act foolishly," was characterized by extreme imitative behavior.

**miscarriage**   See ABORTION.

**mitral valve prolapse**   See CONGENITAL HEART DEFECTS.

**Moebius syndrome** (congenital facial diplegia)   Form of congenital facial paralysis first described by Dr. P.J. Moebius in 1888. It is caused by the abnormalities in the sixth and seventh cranial nerves or the portions of the brain from which they derive. CLUBFOOT (talipes equinovarus) and permanently bent fingers (flexion contractures; see CAMPTODACTYLY and ARTHROGRYPOSIS) have been associated with some cases.

It is most commonly a sporadic occurrence though in some cases it is believed to be inherited as an AUTOSOMAL DOMINANT trait.

More external cranial nerve involvement or MENTAL RETARDATION is seen in about 15% of cases, and the syndrome may be associated with other non-neurologic defects as well.

**Mohr syndrome**   See ORAL-FACIAL-DIGITAL SYNDROME.

**mongolian spots**   Blue-gray areas of discolored skin seen on the lower back, thighs and sometimes shoulders of the newborn. These spots are benign and gradually fade. They are estimated to occur on 80% of non-white and 10% of white infants.

**mongolism**   An archaic term previously used to describe individuals with DOWN SYNDROME, or trisomy 21, a congenital form of MENTAL RETARDATION. (See also CHROMOSOME ABNORMALITIES.) Its name was taken from the characteristic appearance of the eyes in this disorder: The eye slits (palpebral fissures) slant upward, away from the nose (mongoloid obliquity) and a small excess of skin adjacent to the nose obscures the juncture of the bottom and top eyelids. This is called an EPICANTHAL FOLD. Both mongoloid obliquity and epicanthal folds, while associated with numerous birth defects and inherited congenital syndromes in Western populations, are normal in Asians, hence the appellation.

**monilethrix**   A defect of the hair shaft characterized by beaded and brittle hair. (The beaded appearance is observable under a microscope.) It usually appears by the second month of life and may result in ALOPECIA, the loss of scalp hair. The degree of hair loss among affected individuals is variable and may fluctuate over time. While there is no effective treatment, one affected individual reportedly responded to endocrine therapy.

   Monilethrix is inherited as an AUTOSOMAL DOMINANT trait and has been studied extensively in several families. Some researchers suggest an AUTOSOMAL RECESSIVE variety may exist as well.

**monosodium glutamate sensitivity**
See CHINESE RESTAURANT SYNDROME.

**monosomy**   See CHROMOSOME ABNORMALITIES.

**Mormon**   There are approximately one million Mormons in the religious community centered in the Salt Lake City, Utah, area. Most are descended from 20,000 pioneers who came to the area little more than a century ago. They tend to have large, extended families (some numbering in the thousands) and, due to church teachings, keep detailed records of their ancestors and ancestry. These provide perhaps the most extensive PEDIGREES available to genetic researchers. A computerized data base of these genealogical records has been created,

as well. For these reasons, some Mormon families have been extensively studied by geneticists seeking data on the heritability of diseases, particularly cancers of the colon, breast and lung, and melanoma.

**Morquio syndrome**   See MUCOPOLYSACCHARIDOSIS.

**mosaicism**   The condition in which some of an individual's cells have a normal KARYOTYPE, or complement of CHROMOSOMES, while other cells exhibit a CHROMOSOME ABNORMALITY. Thus the individual has cells of two or more different chromosomal constitutions. This condition exists when an abnormality in chromosomal division occurs soon after conception. Subsequently, this aberration is exhibited in those cells descended from this first chromosomally aberrant cell, while the remainder are normal. Among the conditions in which mosaicism is sometimes seen is DOWN SYNDROME.

   In females, in any one cell, only one X CHROMOSOME (of the two) is active, and the other is inactivated. This process of X-inactivation is random, and either X chromosome (paternal or maternal) may be "switched off" in each individual cell. This process occurs early in embryonic life and thus all females are in a sense mosaics since they have two populations of cells: one population with the maternal X active, one with the paternal X active. Therefore females are mosaic with respect to most X-LINKED GENES.

**mucolipidosis (ML)**   A group of rare hereditary ENZYME deficiency diseases. In each of these, the deficiency of a single enzyme causes various chemical substances to accumulate in cells throughout the body, resulting in progressive damage that ranges from problems in the joints leading to decreased mobility, to severe mental and physical retardation with complications in all organ systems. Because the disorder involves the accumulation or "storage" of these compounds, it is one of a group of disorders called STORAGE DISEASES. However, what is stored is not actually a lipid in many cases, and therefore some authorities have proposed changing the named mucolipidosis to oligosaccharidosis.

(See MUCOPOLYSACCHARIDOSIS for a discussion of a group of storage diseases that share many of the features of ML; other disorders often grouped with the mucolipidoses are FUCOSIDOSIS, MANNOSIDOSIS and ASPARTYLGLUCOSAMINURIA.)

The combined incidence of the various forms of ML is estimated at one in 25,000 live births. There are four recognized types of this condition, all transmitted as AUTOSOMAL RECESSIVE traits. PRENATAL DIAGNOSIS is possible with AMNIOCENTESIS and CHORIONIC VILLUS SAMPLING.

*Mucolipidosis I–sialidosis.* A disorder resulting from the deficiency of the ENZYME neuraminidase, producing neurologic abnormalities (see NEURAMINIDASE DEFICIENCY).

*Mucolipidosis II–I-cell disease.* Characterized by the early onset of severe psychomotor retardation, short stature, CLUB FEET, CONGENITAL DISLOCATION OF THE HIP and restricted joint mobility, the face has a typical coarse appearance with thick hair, a high narrow forehead, heavy eyelashes, depressed nasal bridge, upturned nose (anteverted nares), and low-set ears. The upper lip is thick, and the gums are very markedly enlarged. The teeth rarely erupt. The hands and feet are stubby, and the wrists widened.

Repeated respiratory infections are common during the first year of life, along with failure to thrive and lack of psychomotor development. Death usually occurs before the age of six years. Less than 50 cases have been reported. The fundamental defect is in an enzyme that "targets" many other enzymes to the lysosomes (the "digestive" organelles of the cell). Thus all these secondary enzymes' activities are deficient within the lysosome, allowing the molecules that these enzymes should have digested to accumulate. This ac-

cumulation has a characteristic appearance termed "I-cell," for inclusion cell.

*Mucolipidosis III—pseudo-Hurler polydystrophy.* First described in 1966, and characterized by growth retardation and progressive stiffening of the joints, this is essentially a milder form of I-cell disease. Joint stiffness (unaccompanied by pain or swelling) begins by two to four years of age, primarily affecting the hands and shoulders. Clawhands, the extreme permanent bending of the joints at the ends of the fingers, become apparent by age six.

The facial features are broad and coarse, the neck short. During formative years, the joints of the hips and elbows become affected. Carpal tunnel syndrome, a soreness and weakness of the thumb, may develop. The skin becomes tight and hardened. The corneas of the eyes show progressive clouding. As the mobility of the joints decreases, individuals may be unable to raise their arms above their heads. At eight to 10 years, they are usually below the third percentile in height for their age. Joint stiffness stabilizes around the time of puberty.

Additional common findings include mild MENTAL RETARDATION, CONGENITAL HEART DEFECTS and enlargement of the liver and spleen (hepatosplenomegaly).

By adulthood, joint stiffness results in a considerable HANDICAP. Surgery can often correct the carpal tunnel syndrome. The progressive destruction of the hip joints, which may be apparent by the late teens, is the most disabling aspect of the disorder.

As in ML II (I-cell disease), there is a deficiency or abnormality of glycoprotein N-acetylglucosaminylphosphotransferase activity. In ML III the defect is partial, while in ML II it is complete.

*Mucolipidosis IV.* First described in 1974, the features, which manifest during the first year of life, are profound mental and motor retardation and visual impairment. Individuals' motor development never progresses beyond the age of 15 months. None can walk unsupported. Many cannot sit up without being supported. None can control utensils with their fingers. Language abilities also never progress beyond this developmental age. Some may verbalize five to 10 words, but most are completely uncommunicative. Corneal clouding is evident.

There are no abnormalities of the skeleton or internal organs, and there has been speculation that many cases may remain undiagnosed. The condition can be confirmed by electron microscopic examination of cells, which reveal the abnormal storage organelles (specialized areas within the cells) that typify the disorder. It may be more common in Ashkenazi Jews than in the general population. The prognosis and lifespan of individuals is unknown, though patients have survived into their mid-20s.

For more information, contact:

Mucolipidosis IV Foundation
6 Concord Drive
Monsey, NY 10952
(914) 425-0639
(718) 434-5067

National MPS Society, Inc.
17 Kraemer St.
Hicksville, NY 11801
(516) 931-6338

## mucopolysaccharidosis (MPS)   A

group of STORAGE DISEASES; because of an ENZYME deficiency specific to each type, mucopolysaccharides are not properly metabolized, and therefore accumulate or are "stored" within the cells. This accumulation typically results in multiple problems, including severe skeletal deformities and MENTAL RETARDATION.

Mucopolysaccharides are components of various kinds of connective tissue, and include dermatan sulfate, an important constituent of skin and blood vessels, and heparan sulfate, typically found in the walls of blood vessels. Excess mucopolysaccharides leak from their storage sites into the urine and form the basis of several commmon screening tests for the disorder.

At least six basic types (most encompassing several sub-types) have been identified. All are inherited as AUTOSOMAL RECESSIVE traits, except for Hunter syndrome (MPS II), which is inherited as an X-LINKED recessive trait and is seen only in males. Overall incidence of MPS is estimated at one in 25,000 live births.

### Types of MPS

| | |
|---|---|
| MPS I– | Hurler syndrome |
| | Scheie syndrome |
| | Hurler/Scheie syndrome |
| MPS II– | Hunter syndrome, mild |
| | Hunter syndrome, severe |
| MPS III– | Sanfilippo-A |
| | Sanfilippo-B |
| | Sanfilippo-C |
| | Sanfilippo-D |
| MPS IV– | Morquio-A |
| | Morquio-B |
| MPS V– | Vacant—formerly Scheie syndrome |
| MPS VI– | Maroteaux-Lamy, classic severe |
| | Maroteaux-Lamy, intermediate |
| | Maroteaux-Lamy, mild |
| MPS VII– | Sly |

Below are descriptions of the more prevalent forms of MPS.

*Hurler syndrome (MPS I).* The classic features of this disorder are growth failure after infancy, mental retardation, HUMPBACK and short, broad bones, especially in the hands, which lead to stiffness and limitation in movement of the joints. It is named for German pediatrician Gertrud Hurler (1889–1965), who described the condition in 1919.

Decelerated physical and mental growth becomes apparent during the latter part of the first year. Growth usually stops by two years of age. The face develops coarse features, including prominent forehead, thick earlobes, full lips and broad, low nasal bridge. Corneal clouding is present. The nostrils are upturned (anteverted nares), and a continual runny nose is common. The mouth is usually held open, especially after the age of three years. There is a protruding abdomen, deformity of the chest, shortness of the spine and enlargement of the liver and spleen (hepatosplenomegaly). Mental retardation becomes more severe with age. Death usually occurs by age 10 due to pneumonia or heart failure. It is caused by the deficiency of the enzyme alpha-L-iduronidase.

PRENATAL DIAGNOSIS may be made based on studies of enzyme activity in cultured fetal cells obtained by AMNIOCENTESIS or CHORIONIC VILLUS SAMPLING.

*Scheie syndrome (MPS I-S).* This form is characterized by moderately short stature, clouding of the corneas, and joint limitations leading to clawed hand. Intelligence is normal. No major abnormalities are seen in infancy until the appearance of progressive corneal clouding, which leads to decreased vision by the third or fourth decade. It is named for Harold Scheie, professor of ophthalmology at the University of Pennsylvania, who described it in 1962.

Patients tend to have moderately short, stocky and muscular physiques, with a short neck and broad, short hands. The same mucopolysaccharides accumulate as in Hurler SYNDROME and the same enzyme, alpha-L-iduronidase, is deficient. Therefore, the precise gene MUTATION must be different in the two disorders.

*Hunter syndrome (MPS II).* This syndrome, which has a mild and a severe form, has the symptoms of a less severe form of Hurler syndrome (MPS I), with onset typically between the ages of two and four years. It is named for Charles Hunter (1873–1955), a prominent physician in Winnipeg, Canada, who described it in 1917, calling it "gargoylism." During his military service in London in World War I, Hunter presented two brothers with the condition at the Royal Academy of Medicine. He intended the term gargoylism to describe the coarse facial features of affected individuals and to suggest the appearance of gargoyles decorating the architecture of churches such as Notre Dame cathedral. (It came to be used to describe other mucopolysaccharidoses as well.) However, similar features are common to many genetic conditions. Considered demeaning and insensitive, the term "gargoylism" is no longer used.

Characteristic facial appearance includes a flat nose with wide nostrils and depressed nasal bridge, thick lips, tongue and gum. Individuals often have excessive hair (hypertrichosis) and low hairlines. Breathing is noisy, accompanied by runny nose. The liver and spleen are enlarged. Mental deficiency often becomes apparent at approximately age five or six years. Deterioration is typically progressive after age five or six. In severe cases, physical activity decreases, speech is reduced, there is difficulty ingesting solid food and weight decreases. Respiratory infections may become more severe and frequent, and may cause death. Cardiac complications may also lead to death.

In the severe form, death usually occurs between the ages of five and 14 years, though survival to age 60 has been reported in the more mild form.

Female CARRIERS can be detected by enzyme assay, and prenatal diagnosis is possible.

*Sanfilippo syndrome (MPS III).* First recognized in 1963, this appears to be the most common form of MPS, manifest primarily as a neurologic disease. It bears the name of U.S. pediatrician Sylvester J. Sanfilippo, who described it in 1963. Growth is normal or accelerated for one to three years, followed by slow growth. Joint mobility is only mildly restricted in the elbows and knees. The face develops coarse features, including moderate enlargement of the head, sunken nasal bridge, heavy eyebrows and eyelashes, thick lips and abundant, coarse scalp hair. Behavioral problems include restlessness, aggressiveness, diminished attention span and sleep disturbances. These behavioral problems are often what bring individuals to the attention of physicians. Mental development slows and then deteriorates by 18 months to three years of age. Eventually individuals regress to a vegetative state.

Individuals may die during adolescence due to pneumonia, though one-third may survive into their thirties. Prenatal diagnosis is available through enzyme assay. There are, however, four types of this syndrome, each with different ENZYME deficiencies. The exact form of the disease must be determined in each family for accurate diagnostic testing.

*Morquio syndrome (MPS IV).* First described in 1929 by Luis Morquio (1867–1935), professor of pediatrics in Montevideo, Uruguay, this form of MPS is marked by growth failure and progressive spinal deformity. It is essentially a skeletal DYSPLASIA. The first symptoms, flaring of the rib cage, frequent upper respiratory tract infections, hernias and growth deficiency, become apparent by 19 months to two years of age. The facial features become coarse, with broad mouth, widely spaced teeth and upturned nose (anteverted nares). The neck is very short, and the head appears to rest directly on the shoulders. Abnormalities of the bones of the spine in the neck can lead to injury to the spinal cord. The extremities appear disproportionately long, as the trunk is shortened due to involvement of the bones of the spine. Individuals exhibit a semicrouching stance with "knock knees." Corneal clouding occurs after age 10, and progressive deafness during adolescence. Adult height rarely exceeds 39 inches (about 1 m.). Intelligence is usually normal.

Prenatal diagnosis is available by studying cultured fetal tissue for enzyme activity. Though respiratory insufficiency or cardiac complications may result in death in adolescence, longer survival has been reported.

*Maroteaux-Lamy syndrome (MPS VI).* This syndrome was originally described in 1963 by Pierre Maroteaux, the director of the National Center of Scientific Research at the Hopital des Enfants Malades in Paris, and Maurice Lamy (1895–1975), the first professor of medical genetics at the University of Paris. Development is usually normal until approximately age six, when small stature and spinal deformities are noted. The chest is deformed with a prominent sternum, and the face exhibits coarse features common to MPS: large head, thick eyebrows and scalp hair, flat nasal bridge and upturned nose (anteverted nares), full cheeks and lips. In the more severe form, there is rapid progression to disability with short stature, marked facial and skeletal abnormalities, severely impaired vision and hearing, and prominent cardiac defects. While intelligence is normal, impaired vision and hearing, restricted mobility and psychological adjustment problems may impede the individual's abilities.

Individuals with the mild form have normal lifespans. In the severe form, most succumb to cardiorespiratory problems by the end of the second decade. Bone marrow transplantation has been utilized as an attempt to treat this disorder (as well as some of the other forms of MPS), and the potential benefits of this therapy are currently under intensive investigation.

Prenatal diagnosis is possible by assaying enzyme activity in fetal cells collected by amniocentesis or chorionic villus sampling.

*Sly (MPS VII).* Described in 1973 by U.S. pediatrician and genetics professor William S. Sly, this is a more recently identified form. Symptoms are often visible at birth or appear within the first year of life and include growth retardation, joint contractures and spinal malformations. The characteristic coarse face, short stature and developmental retardation are also present, and there appears to be variability of severity of the symptoms among patients, as with the other forms of MPS. Because few cases have been described, long-term prognosis is unknown.

Prenatal diagnosis is possible by analysis of fetal cells, as with other forms of MPS.

For more information contact:

National MPS Society, Inc.
17 Kraemer Street
Hicksville, NY 11801
(516) 931-6338

**multifactorial** A general term for disorders that have their origins in the effects of one or more GENES, environmental influences or

## TABLE XVII
### Frequencies of the Most Common Multifactorial Disorders Found In a Survey Conducted in British Columbia, Canada

| Multifactorial Condition | 1952–63 | | 1964–73 | | 1974–83 | | Total | |
|---|---|---|---|---|---|---|---|---|
| | N | Rate[a] | N | Rate[a] | N | Rate[a] | N | Rate[a] |
| Diabetes mellitus | 526 | 1,202.3 | 382 | 1,108.3 | 103 | 265.7 | 1,011 | 864.2 |
| Schizophrenic psychoses | 181 | 413.7 | 1 | 2.9 | 0 | 0.0 | 182 | 155.6 |
| Affective psychoses | 10 | 22.9 | 0 | 0.0 | 0 | 0.0 | 10 | 8.5 |
| Borderline mental retardation | 314 | 717.7 | 63 | 182.8 | 1 | 2.6 | 378 | 323. |
| Mild mental retardation | 181 | 413.7 | 37 | 107.4 | 5 | 12.9 | 223 | 190.6 |
| Epilepsy | 807 | 1,844.6 | 502 | 1,456.5 | 228 | 588.1 | 1,537 | 1,313.8 |
| Strabismus | 924 | 2,112.0 | 3,566 | 10,346.3 | 1,450 | 3,740.0 | 5,940 | 5,077.5 |
| Asthma | 124 | 283.4 | 53 | 153.8 | 71 | 183.1 | 248 | 212.0 |
| Inguinal hernia | 0 | 0.0 | 196 | 568.7 | 1,997 | 5,150.8 | 2,193 | 1,874.6 |
| Eczema | 37 | 84.6 | 4 | 11.6 | 3 | 7.7 | 44 | 37.6 |
| Anencephaly | 58 | 132.6 | 45 | 130.6 | 50 | 129.0 | 153 | 130.8 |
| Spina bifida | 214 | 489.1 | 117 | 339.5 | 67 | 172.8 | 398 | 340.2 |
| Encephalocele | 5 | 11.4 | 7 | 20.3 | 8 | 20.6 | 20 | 17.1 |
| Congenital hydrocephalus | 48 | 109.7 | 99 | 287.2 | 76 | 196.0 | 223 | 190.6 |
| Congenital anomalies of heart and circulatory system | 1,177 | 2,690.3 | 1,699 | 4,929.4 | 1,734 | 4,472.5 | 4,610 | 3,940.6 |
| Cleft palate and cleft lip | 468 | 1,069.7 | 445 | 1,291.1 | 431 | 1,111.7 | 1,344 | 1,148.8 |
| Congenital hypertrophic pyloric stenosis | 23 | 52.6 | 805 | 2,335.6 | 909 | 2,344.6 | 1,737 | 1,484.8 |
| Hirschsprung disease, etc. | 9 | 20.6 | 60 | 174.1 | 43 | 110.9 | 112 | 95.7 |
| Hypospadias and epispadias | 102 | 233.1 | 558 | 1,619.0 | 620 | 1,599.2 | 1,280 | 1,094.1 |
| Clubfoot | 679 | 1,552.0 | 1,433 | 4,157.7 | 1,967 | 5,073.4 | 4,079 | 3,486.7 |
| Congenital dislocation of hip | 197 | 450.3 | 878 | 2,547.4 | 1,322 | 3,409.8 | 2,397 | 2,048.9 |
| Congenital dislocatable hip | 0 | 0.0 | 12 | 34.8 | 622 | 1,604.3 | 634 | 541.9 |
| Total | 6,084 | 13,906.2 | 10,962 | 31,804.8 | 11,707 | 30,195.6 | 28,753 | 24,577.9 |

[a]Per 1 million live births.

Source: Patricia A. Baird, "A Population Study of Genetic Disorders in Children and Young Adults," *American Journal of Human Genetics*, 42(1988), pp. 677-693.

unknown factors acting in combination. (Though the term POLYGENIC is used interchangeably with multifactorial by some, polygenic properly refers to a disorder resulting from the action of two or more genes.) Multifactorial disorders often appear in familial clusters, though they do not conform to dominant or recessive patterns of heredity. They are the most common and least understood of genetic disorders; little is known regarding their exact cause. (See Table XVII.)

Multifactorial disorders include CLEFT LIP or cleft palate, CONGENITAL HEART DEFECTS, NEURAL TUBE DEFECTS (SPINA BIFIDA and ANENCEPHALY), SCHIZOPHRENIA and ESSENTIAL HYPERTENSION.

Risks of recurrence in a given family in which one member has a multifactorial disorder are low, generally estimated in the realm of 3%. Some multifactorial disorders are more common in one gender. In these gender-linked multifactorial disorders, risks for recurrence increase when the affected family member is of the sex in which the condition is typically less common. Recurrence risks also increase if multiple family members are affected or if the problem is more severe in the affected individual (e.g., bilateral cleft lip vs. unilat-

eral). (See also AUTOSOMAL DOMINANT, AU-
TOSOMAL RECESSIVE, MENDELIAN.)

## multiple acyl COA dehydrogenase
See GLUTARIC ACIDURIA.

## multiple births
Giving birth to more than one child from a single pregnancy. Multiple births are associated with increased risks for miscarriage (see ABORTION), as well as greater risks for maternal and infant health and survival. BIRTH DEFECTS and LOW BIRTH WEIGHT are more common in multiple births, as well.

Multiple births have long been the object of interest and speculation. In his *History of Animals*, Aristotle wrote that five was the maximum of infants a woman was capable of producing in a single pregnancy (quintuplets). However, reports of women giving birth to six (sextuplets) and seven (septuplets) infants have been somewhat common from Aristotle's time to the present. Yet no valid reports of such a birth were recorded until 1888, when the birth of septuplets was documented in Italy (and promptly criticized for contradictiong Aristotle's teachings). In 1938 *Look* magazine reported finding a family of septuplets born in 1866, four of whom reached adulthood.

Multiple births, and their associated problems, have become more common as more women use fertility drugs in an effort to conceive. (By 1990, an estimated 20,000 women in the United States annually took fertility drugs; see CLOMIPHENE CITRATE.) These drugs may result in pregnancies in which as many as nine embryos begin to develop at one time. In these situations, intervention may attempt selectively to abort all but one or two of the developing embryos as none would otherwise survive to term. (See also TWINS.)

## multiple endocrine neoplasias (MEN)
Genetically influenced CANCERS of the endocrine glands. These rare conditions are classified into MEN I, II and III based on the site and characteristics of the tumors.

In MEN I, individuals may develop neoplasms or tumors that may appear in more than one gland, including the parathyroids (90%), pancreas (80%), pituitary (65%), adrenal cortex (35%) and thyroid glands (20%). By interfering with the hormonal secretion of these glands, the cancers may produce abnormalities in the bones, kidneys and mucous membranes, enlargement of extremities, headaches and visual disturbances. Predisposition to develop these cancers is inherited as an AUTOSOMAL DOMINANT trait. The tumors usually develop between the age of 10 and 60.

Individuals with MEN II typically have specific cancers of the thyroid (medullay carcinoma) affecting the cells that produce calcitonin (a hormone important in calcium metabolism), as well as overdevelopment of the parathyroid gland and tumors of the adrenal medulla or related nerve tissue (pheochromocytoma). Predisposition is inherited as an AUTOSOMAL DOMINANT trait. Onset may be anytime from early childhood to 60 years. The GENE for this disorder appears to be located on CHROMOSOME 10.

MEN III is also believed to be inherited as an AUTOSOMAL DOMINANT disorder. Affected individuals often exhibit striking, small tumors (neuromas) of mucous tissues, appearing on the lips, tongue, gum, palate, nose and conjunctivae of the eyes. These tumors are usually evident by the age of eight years, and those affected typically have weak and thin physiques with severe muscular wasting and abnormal spinal curvature. They also often have medullay carcinoma of the thyroid or pheochromocytoma like those with MEN II. Onset is from early childhood to age 40.

The tumors may become malignant in all forms of MEN, though early detection increases chances for survival. MEN are believed to result from errors in the development of the neural crest, the embryonic structure from which nerve tissue develops. PRENATAL DIAGNOSIS is currently not available, though linkage analysis (see GENETIC LINKAGE) may in the future prove useful. However, due to hormone imbalances caused by these disorders, sensitive hormone assays make early diagnosis possible.

It is recommended that first-degree relatives (parents, siblings, offspring) of affected individuals undergo annual examinations.

## multiple epiphyseal dysplasia   A

group of skeletal disorders affecting bone formation and resulting in DWARFISM. The epiphysis is a secondary bone-forming (ossification) center in the bones of infants, separated from the parent bone by cartilage. Normally, as skeletal growth proceeds, the epiphysis joins with the parent bone. In this group of disorders, the ossification of the epiphyses of the bones of the arms and legs is abnormal, resulting in mild shortening.

Generally, this form of dwarfism remains unrecognized until the ages of five to 10 years, when short stature begins to become apparent. The dwarfing is of the short-limbed variety, with trunk size remaining normal. The hands, and particularly the thumbs, may appear short and stubby. Affected individuals may exhibit a waddling gait, difficulty in running or climbing stairs, and experience pain and stiffness in the limbs and joints, particularly of the lower limbs. Degenerative arthritis of the hips is common in older individuals under medical care. Physical activities may be limited in those severely affected. Intelligence and lifespan are normal.

The various forms of multiple epiphyseal dysplasia may be inherited as AUTOSOMAL DOMINANT or AUTOSOMAL RECESSIVE traits, though most are dominant.

For more information, contact:

Little People of America, Inc.
P.O. Box 633
San Bruno, CA 94066
(415) 589-0695

Human Growth Foundation
4720 Montgomery Lane, Suite 909
Bethesda, MD 20814
(301) 656-6904
(301) 656-7540

## multiple lentigines syndrome   (LEOP-

ARD syndrome)   LEOPARD syndrome, the secondary name of this condition, refers to the many freckles (lentigines) covering the face and body in 80% of cases, and it is also an acronym for the features of this disorder. (Lentigines differ from freckles in that they are darker, present at birth and not related to exposure to the sun.) LEOPARD stands for *l*entigines, *E*CG abnormalities, *o*cular hypertelorism, *p*ulmonic stenosis, *a*bnormalities of genitalia, *r*etardation of growth, and *d*eafness. In addition, half of all affected infants display winged shoulder-blades, and 35% show some degree of thick, webbed folds of skin from jawbone to mid- shoulder (pterigium coli).

About 95% of affected infants show electrocardiographic (ECG) changes indicating abnormalities in the transfer of heart impulses from one chamber to another (interventricular conduction). Equally common is abnormal narrowing of the heart valve leading to the blood vessel carrying blood to the lungs (pulmonary stenosis). Growth is retarded in 90% of cases, and 75% have very wide-set eyes (HYPERTELORISM).

About half of all affected males also have genital abnormalities such as failure of one or both testicles to descend (CRYPTORCHISM) or a urethral opening on the underside of the penis (HYPOSPADIAS). DEAFNESS due to a lesion in the ear's cochlea occurs in about 35%.

Less common findings include triangular face with prominent forehead (bossing), drooping eyelids (PTOSIS) and other cardiac anomalies such as enlarged heart (hypertrophic cardiomyopathy), abnormal aortic valve (aortic valvular dysplasia) and a hole in the septum, which normally separates the heart's two atria (atrial septal defect).

LEOPARD syndrome is usually detected by age four or five, when lentigines become abundant, though some affected infants never develop lentigines. Detection is easy in cases with the characteristic lentigines, but even those without them can be screened with a detailed examination for accompanying symptoms. Life expectancy is usually not affected, nor is intelligence, unless hampered by deafness or severe pulmonary stenosis. Surgical correction of cryptorchism and cardiac lesions may be necessary in some cases.

Inherited as an AUTOSOMAL DOMINANT trait, the prevalance of this variable disorder is uncertain. Over 70 cases have been reported.

**multiple pterygium syndrome**    Pterygia are fibrous malformations exhibiting with a webbed appearance. In this disorder webbed folds of skin (pterygia) of the neck and armpit, inner part of the elbow, back of the knee and inner surface of the leg are evident at birth. Other defects associated with this disorder include rocker bottom feet, deformed joints, webbed fingers (syndactyly), small penis and scrotum and undescended testicles in males (cryptorchism), and underdeveloped external genitalia in females. Affected individuals may also exhibit folds of skin at the inner corner of the eyes (EPICANTHUS), downward slanting at the outer corners of the eyelids and mouth, low hairline on the back of the neck, and crouched stance. Skeletal deformities include fusion of neck vertebrae and curvature of the spine. Adults are seldom taller than 4.5 feet.

A severe, lethal form of the disorder exists. It is a distinct genetic entity, also an AUTOSOMAL RECESSIVE trait that leads to STILLBIRTH or death in the immediate newborn period due to lack of development of the lungs. Many other pterygium SYNDROMES also exist.

**multiple sclerosis (MS)**    An autoimmune disorder that causes the immune system to attack myelin, the material that forms the protective sheaths surrounding nerve fibers. Mostly seen in females, onset is usually between the ages of 20 and 40 years. Variable symptoms and severity, and the episodic nature of attacks, make diagnosis difficult. Characteristic signs include blurring of vision, slurring of speech, muscle weakness, loss of balance, depression and frequently euphoria. Estimates of the number of those affected have been put as high as 250,000 in the United States (about one in 1,000 individuals).

Though first-degree relatives (parent, SIBLING, offspring) have been estimated to have a risk 15 times that of the general population's for developing MS, the genetic link is nonetheless weak, and the disorder follows no known pattern of inheritance. Even identical twins have only a 50% chance or less of both exhibiting the disorder if one of the pair has it. (However, there may be rare forms that are genetically caused.)

But while the disorder is not hereditary, susceptibility to develop MS appears to have a genetic component. Susceptibility has been linked to a number of different GENES or gene groups. Some of these genes or gene clusters are part of the HLA complex (see HUMAN LEUKOCYTE ANTIGEN), which plays an important role in regulating the immune system, and others are also linked to immune system functioning. Virus infections are also thought to contribute to the eventual onset of MS.

For more information, contact:

National Multiple Sclerosis Society
205 East 42nd Street
New York, NY 10017
(212) 986-3240

**muscular dystrophy**    A group of hereditary disorders characterized by progressive muscle weakness and wasting. The disease process causes healthy muscle cells to be replaced by fat and connective tissue. Muscular dystrophies may be transmitted as AUTOSOMAL DOMINANT, AUTOSOMAL RECESSIVE or X-LINKED traits, depending upon the particular form of the disease. New MUTATIONS can also be responsible for some cases.

*Duchenne muscular dystrophy (DMD).* Named for Guillaume B.A. Duchenne (1806–1875), a French neurologist who first described the disorder in 1861, this is the most common and severe form of muscular dystrophy. It is transmitted as an X-LINKED trait, though approximately one-third of new cases are thought to be the result of a new mutation. Incidence of DMD is estimated to be one in 3,000 to one in 4,000 male births, and there are about 15,000 DMD patients in the United States at any given time.

Symptoms of the disease become manifest between the ages of two and five years, and they include waddling or walking on toes, stumbling, difficulty in running, climbing stairs or getting up from the floor. The wasting of muscles usually begins in the lower trunk and calves, and eventually affects all the major muscle groups. It is sometimes called pseudohypertrophic muscular dystrophy because the enlargement of the calf muscle that is characteristic of this disease is caused not by increased muscle tissue but by the accumulation of fat and connective tissue in the degenerating muscle fibers.

Progression of the disease is rapid. Walking becomes difficult, and skeletal contractures and muscle atrophy follow. Individuals generally require use of a wheelchair by adolescence. About one-third of patients exhibit MENTAL RETARDATION, and death due to respiratory failure occurs before the age of 30 years in most cases.

Currently, the options for treatment are limited. Physical therapy can delay muscle atrophy and deformities. Orthopedic devices can help maintain mobility. Surgery to lengthen contracted tendons is sometimes performed, and medication can help relieve muscle stiffness.

In 1986 scientists identified the defective GENE that causes DMD, located on the short arm of the X CHROMOSOME, and in 1987 they isolated the protein the normal gene produces. The protein has been named "dystrophin," and it is absent in the cells of those with DMD. In 1989 scientists successfully corrected a similar deficiency in mice unable to produce dystrophin by injecting immature muscle cells (myoblasts) into their tissue. Subsequently the mice were able to produce dystrophin. This research may ultimately provide avenues for treating DMD.

Prior to the identification of the defective gene, the primary screening test for DMD CARRIERS and individuals was the presence of highly elevated serum levels of creatine phosphokinase (CK). This test can identify 60% to 70% of CARRIER females. About 5% of carriers have some muscle weakness.

Now RECOMBINANT DNA techniques using the DMD gene have been used in PRENATAL DIAGNOSIS of DMD, as well as for carrier testing in families with individuals affected with DMD, but large scale population screening is not yet available.

*Becker's muscular dystrophy.* Similar in mode of transmission to DMD, it manifests itself later in life and progression is much less severe. It is one-tenth as common as DMD. The protein dystrophin is present in muscle cells of Becker's muscular dystrophy patients, but at levels far below those in unaffected individuals. Becker and DMD result from different mutations in the same gene.

*Facio-scapulo-humeral dystrophy.* This AUTOSOMAL DOMINANT form of muscular dystrophy is very rare, but because of its mode of inheritance it can appear in nearly every generation among families with the disorder. Expression in families is highly variable; some individuals suffer no disability while others experience early incapacitation.

The dystrophy begins in muscles of the face (facio), shoulder (scapulo) and upper arms (humeral). Symptoms usually become evident in the teens, though they may appear at any time from infancy to middle age. There is facial weakness, such as difficulty in closing eyes, whistling and puckering lips. Progression is usually slow, though it may be rapid in some cases. Eventually trunk and leg muscles become involved, and individuals may be unable to walk.

Family studies are usually necessary to identify all affected individuals and establish the risks of recurrence.

*Limb-girdle dystrophy.* This dystrophy is generally inherited as an AUTOSOMAL RECESSIVE trait. The symptoms, weakness in the shoulder or pelvis area, can begin to appear anytime from childhood through early adulthood.

The course of the disease is unpredictable. Progression tends to be slow, particularly if the disease begins in the shoulder, rather than pelvic area. Incapacitation occurs after 20 years or more. By middle age most individuals are unable to walk. Life expectancy is slightly diminished.

Carrier testing and prenatal diagnosis are currently not available for limb-girdle muscular dystrophy.

*Myotonic dystrophy.*   See MYOTONIC DYS-TROPHY.

For more information, contact:

Muscular Dystrophy Association
810 Seventh Avenue
New York, NY 10019
(212) 586-0808

**mutagen**   Any substance capable of causing a genetic MUTATION. Many medicines, chemicals and physical agents such as ionizing radiation, cancer chemotherapeutic agents, and ultraviolet light have this mutagenic ability. (See also TERATOGEN.)

**mutation**   Any inheritable change or alteration in genetic material. Genetic disorders have their origin in mutations that have typically been passed down through generations. However, a proportion of affected individuals may be the result of a new mutation that occurred either in the sperm or egg of one parent or in the embryo. In some dominant genetic disorders that result in death in infancy, all affected individuals are the result of new mutations. Mutations can also occur in the cells of the body after birth (somatic mutation) and may result in tumors.

The discovery that mutations could be artificially induced by exposure to heavy doses of X-rays, reported by Hermann J. Muller (1890–1967) in 1927, was a major advance in genetic research. Muller, then at the University of Texas, was awarded the Nobel prize in 1946 for his work. (See also RADIATION; TE-RATOGEN; "INTRODUCTION.")

**myasthenia gravis (MG)**   Translated from its Greek and Latin derivation, *myasthenia gravis* means "grave muscle weakness," and is characterized by weakness and loss of control over voluntary muscles, most often those responsible for eye movements and eyelids, chewing, swallowing, coughing and facial expression. Muscle control over breathing and the movement of arms and legs may also be affected.

Most cases of MG are not inherited but some show a familial aggregation (2% to 5% of cases) (see FAMILIAL DISEASES), and many of these are believed to be inherited as an AUTOSOMAL RECESSIVE trait, as they most often involve siblings, though they may not always conform to a simple MENDELIAN transmission pattern.

The familial form usually affects young children or adolescents and onset in adulthood is rare. The muscle weakness is static or only slowly progressive. Most frequently, onset of symptoms occurs in the first year of life, and it responds well to treatment with anti-cholinesterase drugs. The anti-cholinesterase drugs prolong the action of acetylcholine in impulse transmission at the motor end plate (where the nerve transmits the impulse to the muscle), by blocking the action of cholinesterase, which ordinarily stops it. Cases with onset between the age of two and 20 years resemble adult MG. (The adult form is the result of an autoimmune disorder that causes the body to destroy receptors between nerve endings and muscles that normally allow control over movement.)

There is also a familial infantile form of MG, "transient myasthenia gravis of the newborn." This form is caused by passive transfer of antibodies associated with the autoimmune disorder of adult MG to the fetus from a myasthenic mother. It occurs in 10% to 15% of babies born to MG mothers and is characterized by respiratory and feeding difficulties in the neonatal period. There is usually total remission after a few weeks, but it can be life threatening if untreated during this time.

For more information, contact:

Myasthenia Gravis Foundation
53 W. Jackson Boulevard
Chicago, IL 60604
(312) 427-6252

**myopia**    Commonly known as nearsightedness, this condition occurs when the eyeball is elongated so that the focal point of parallel light rays lies in front of, rather than on, the retina. It appears to have many possible genetic causes; individual families have shown all the major types of MENDELIAN inheritance. There also appears to be an association between such factors as PREMATURITY, administration of oxygen after birth or maternal disease in pregnancy, and the incidence of myopia. A positive family history alerts parents to watch for mannerisms of nearsightedness, such as squinting. The actual diagnosis is usually made by age three.

On average, visual acuity among those affected ranges between 20/50 and 20/60. However, with corrective lenses, visual acuity may be correctable to 20/30 or better.

It is not unusual to also have a misalignment of the optic axis (STRABISMUS) associated with this condition.

It has been suggested that children with myopia tend to have, on average, higher IQs than those without it, but this has not been convincingly demonstrated.

CONGENITAL myopia is a relatively rare disorder, affecting males and females equally. With corrective lenses prescribed as early as possible, the prognosis is favorable, since most cases of myopia do not deteriorate with age; it is rarely progressive.

There are some specific SYNDROMES with myopia (such as X-LINKED recessive syndrome of myopia and nightblindness) and it may be a part of other disorders (e.g., MAR-

FAN SYNDROME). For the child of an individual with an isolated case of severe myopia, a risk of 4% to 5% for similar severe eye problems has been suggested.

**myositis ossificans**    See FIBRODYSPLASIA OSSIFICANS PROGRESSIVA.

**myotonic dystrophy**    (Steinert disease)    A combination of progressive weakening of the muscles (dystrophy) and muscle spasms or rigidity, with difficulty relaxing a contracted muscle (myotonia). It may also be associated with mild to severe MENTAL RETARDATION, CATARACTS, diminished endocrine function, including atrophy of the gonads, and decreased functioning of the pituitary, thyroid, adrenal cortex or pancreatic islets (the latter leading to a mild form of DIABETES MELLITUS). Among the affected muscles is the heart, leading to cardiac irregularities and often death due to heart failure. The disease is highly variable in the expression of manifestations among different individuals.

It appears to have three possible types, based on age of onset; during infancy, from early childhood to age 20, and after age 20. The average age of detection is in the second decade of life, but there are potentially recognizable symptoms early on—reduced fetal movements in pregnancy, poor sucking reflexes and muscle rigidity in infancy, drooping facial muscles and a characteristic sunkenness at the temples (temporal atrophy).

The condition is progressive, leading to incapacitation, mental deterioration and ultimately death, often by age 50 to 60. Symptomatic relief can be provided for the associated muscle weakness through physical therapy and orthopedic measures.

Inherited as an AUTOSOMAL DOMINANT trait, approximately one-third of the cases may be the result of a new MUTATION. In the infant-onset form, STILLBIRTH and infant mortality rates are high.

The GENE for myotonic dystrophy has been mapped to CHROMOSOME 19. Where appropriate family members are available to document linkage to markers on chromosome 19, PRENATAL DIAGNOSIS is possible.

# N

**Naegeli syndrome** Rare hereditary syndrome, first described by Swiss hematologist O. Naegeli (1871–1938) in 1927. It is a form of ECTODERMAL DYSPLASIA, a group of disorders characterized by abnormalities of the skin, teeth, hair and nails. (These form from embryonic ectodermal tissues during fetal development.) The soles of the feet and the palms of the hands appear thickened (plantar and palmar hypodrosis and hyperkeratosis). Affected individuals are unable to sweat normally and are especially sensitive to heat. Yellow spotting of the tooth enamel is another manifestation.

Inherited as an AUTOSOMAL DOMINANT trait, the basic defect that causes this disorder is unknown. Life span and intelligence are normal.

**nail-patella syndrome** As the name indicates, this disorder primarily affects the nails (fingernails more frequently than toenails) and the kneecaps (patellae). The deformities are apparent at birth. The nails are markedly reduced in size, often with the half toward the inner arm missing, and sometimes the white "moons" at the base of the nails are triangular. Thumbnails are most involved; changes progressively diminish from the index to the pinky finger. If the patellae are present at all, they are underdeveloped and likely to be dislocated.

Other findings associated with nail-patella syndrome are fingers bent sideways (CLINODACTYLY), elbow joints that cannot be fully extended, SCOLIOSIS, underdeveloped shoulder blades, drooping eyelids (PTOSIS),

CATARACTS and, in about 30% of affected individuals, kidney disorders. These renal complications (including kidney failure) are the only ones that may shorten the life span of an individual with this syndrome. Affected individuals must be repeatedly tested to assure early diagnosis and treatment of any renal disease. (About 8% of affected individuals who come to medical attention succumb to renal disease.)

Nail-patella syndrome is an AUTOSOMAL DOMINANT trait with variable EXPRESSIVITY. The basic defect that causes this rare syndrome is unknown, though the responsible GENE has been located on CHROMOSOME 9. It is linked to the gene for ABO blood group. PRENATAL DIAGNOSIS may be possible using linkage studies or ULTRASOUND.

**narcolepsy** (narcoleptic syndrome) A sleep disorder characterized by disabling daytime drowsiness, low alertness, loss of muscle tone (cataplexy), hallucinations, sleep paralysis and disrupted nighttime sleep. Daytime sleepiness occurs so suddenly and with such overwhelming power that some affected individuals refer to it as a sleep attack, with some experiencing several such episodes a day. Periods of sleep following these attacks generally last from a few seconds to 30 minutes, but may last several hours.

Familial narcolepsy was recognized as early as 1877, when an affected mother and son were described, but it was not until 1926 that the disorder was delineated as a specific entity (see FAMILIAL DISEASE).

The disorder seems to be caused by an imbalance in the brain's sleep/wake cycle. Rapid eye movement (REM) sleep and dreaming may occur when the individual is awake, often resulting in intense, vivid hallucinations, sometimes accompanied by frightening auditory, visual and tactile sensations. Occasionally they are difficult to distinguish from reality. Sleep paralysis, the momentary inability to move when waking up or falling asleep, may accompany these hallucinations.

Narcolepsy is a lifelong condition. There is no known cure and no confirmed reports of lasting remission. Symptoms usually become noticeable between the ages of 10 and 30. Subtle at first, they become increasingly severe over the years. The sleep attacks may become profoundly disabling, seriously disrupting social and professional lives. While narcolepsy by itself does not lower life expectancy, affected individuals must be careful to control symptoms while driving or engaging in other potentially dangerous activities.

Drug therapies can help control symptoms. Stimulants can stave off sleep attacks, and depressants are often prescribed to control cataplexy and hallucinations. Naps throughout the day may counter excessive sleepiness.

About half of all narcoleptics have cataplexy. Cataplectic attacks may be triggered by humor (hearing, or especially telling, a joke), competition (playing cards), excitement (viewing or participating in sports) and stress (asking for a pay raise). Individuals may abruptly lose muscle control and collapse into sleep. Attempts to control attacks by avoiding these feelings may restrict the individual's emotional development.

For more information, contact:

American Narcolepsy Association, Inc.
P.O. Box 1187
San Carlos, CA 94070
(415) 591-7979

Association of Sleep Disorders Centers
Stanford University Medical Center
Stanford, CA 94305

**natal teeth**    About one in 3,000 liveborn infants have teeth at birth, a condition believed to be inherited as an AUTOSOMAL DOMINANT trait. Historical figures who are reported to have been born with erupted teeth include Zoroaster, Hannibal, Richard III of England, Richelieu, Mazarin, Mirabeau and Broca. King Louis XIV of France was said to have been "a considerable vexation to his wet-nurses" as a result of this condition.

Natal teeth are also associated with genetic SYNDROMES, including ELLIS-VAN CREVELD SYNDROME and HALLERMAN-STREIFF SYNDROME.

**nephritis, familial**    See FAMILIAL NEPHRITIS.

**nephrosis, congenital**    See CONGENITAL NEPHROSIS.

**neural tube defects (NTD)**    Term describing a variety of CONGENITAL defects of the spine or skull resulting from failure of the neural tube to close, or close completely, an ANOMALY that has its genesis in the fourth week of pregnancy. The neural tube is a region on the back portion of an embryo from which the brain and spinal cord develop. As the embryo grows, the top of the neural tube becomes the brain, and the bottom the spinal cord. When the neural "tube fails to close properly, tissue associated with the brain or spinal cord remains exposed or incompletely protected, resulting in potentially severe developmental disabilities and infant death. Corrective surgery and physical therapy can help alleviate associated physical problems in some cases.

NTDs comprise the most frequent malformations of the central nervous system. The form and severity of an NTD depends on the location and the extent of the defect. They include SPINA BIFIDA (failure of the spinal cord to close), ANENCEPHALY (the failure of the cranium and brain to form or form completely) and ENCEPHALOCELE (protrusion of the brain through the skull, usually in the back of the head). Some NTDs are not open, and while the nerve tissue is incompletely shielded, the defect is covered by skin.

NTDs are caused by the action of several genes either alone (POLYGENIC) or in concert with environmental factors (MULTIFACTORIAL). They may also be part of single GENE disorders (e.g., encephalocele in MECKEL SYN-DROME), or caused by CHROMOSOME ABNOR-MALITIES (e.g., trisomy 18) or teratogenic exposure (e.g., spina bifida caused by valproic acid). There is also an increase in NTDs among offspring of diabetic women (DIABE-TES MELLITUS).

Neural tube defects occur in approximately one to two of every 1,000 live births in the United States, but the true rate of occurrence may be higher, as perhaps half of anencephalics are thought to be spontaneously aborted. Geography is also associated with variations in risk. In Wales and Ireland almost 1% of all newborns have NTDs. In the United States, incidence decreases from North to South and East to West. In New York the rate is approximately two per 1,000 live births, and in Los Angeles it is one per 1,000. NTDs are more common in whites than in other racial groups, and more common in first born children. Affected females outnumber males by a ratio of between two to one and three to two. A woman who has had an infant with an NTD has a risk of recurrence estimated at between 1% and 5%, which rises to 4% to 9% after having two affected infants. (See Table XIX.)

PRENATAL DIAGNOSIS of open NTDs is possible via findings of increased ALPHA-FETOPROTEIN levels found in AMNIOTIC FLUID collected with AMNIOCENTESIS. They may also be seen in utero with ULTRASOUND in some cases. Screening for NTDs is possible in low-risk pregnancies via measuring alpha-fetoprotein levels in maternal blood. A role of VITAMIN supplementation before conception and during early pregnancy in preventing NTDs has been proposed but remains unproven at the present time. It is the subject of several ongoing investigations.

**neuraminidase deficiency**   (sialidosis)   A group of rare hereditary deficiencies of an ENZYME responsible for the metabolism of some polysaccharides, sugar molecules found as components of larger complex molecules, leading to the accumulation of abnormal amounts of polysaccharides in the tissues. There are at least three forms. In one form, onset is in childhood or early adulthood, characterized by seizure-like muscle spasms and progressive loss of vision. A CHERRY-RED SPOT is present on the retina of the eye. Intelligence remains normal. In another form individuals may also have coarse facial features, bony abnormalities, enlarged livers and clouding of the cornea suggestive of MUCOPOLYSACCHARIDOSIS. In a third form the kidney is also involved. The disorder is inherited as an AUTOSOMAL RECESSIVE trait. Definitive diagnosis is based on deficiency of the enzyme alpha-neuraminidase.

**neurodermatosis**   See PHAKOMATOSIS.

**neurofibromatosis (NF) (von Recklinghausen disease)**   One of the most common inherited disorders, with an incidence from one in 2,500 to one in 3,300 births, this potentially disfiguring condition affects an estimated 100,000 Americans. However, there is a great variability of expression and it has been estimated that as many as 95% of cases go unrecognized. In most cases, "café au lait" spots, irregularly shaped, coffee-colored splotches on the skin are the only symptom. Freckling about the armpits is another manifestation.

The disease derives its name from the thousands of neurofibromas, or tumorous growths, that disfigure severely affected individuals. Additionally, these tumors may be found in connective tissue, brain and spinal cord, eye, liver, stomach, bladder, kidney, larynx and intestine. Internal tumors can damage nerves and cause paralysis or blindness. In 3% to 15% of the cases, the tumors turn malignant. Learning disability is exhibited in 40% of the cases, and 2% to 5% are mentally retarded.

It is inherited as an AUTOSOMAL DOMINANT trait, with 50% of cases thought to be the result of new MUTATION. It is also referred to as von Recklinghausen disease and von Recklinghausen neurofibromatosis for Ger-

## Table XVIII
### Neural Tube Defects in the United States
### (approx. 6,000/year)

|  |  | Prognosis | |
| Type (Degree) | Incidence/ 1,000 Births | Neonatal Death (%) | Long-term Disability (%) |
| --- | --- | --- | --- |
| Anencephaly | 0.6-0.8 | 100 | 0 |
| Spina bifida. (open) | 0.5.-0.8 | 33 | 65[*] |
| Spina bifida (closed) | 0.1-0.14 | 7 | 10[*] |
| Total | 1.2-1.7 | 60 | 60[*] |

## Title XIX
### Relative Risks of Occurrence of Neural
### Tube Defects in the United States

| Family History | Risk (Incidence/ 1,000 Births) |
| --- | --- |
| No family history of NTD | 1 |
| Positive family history | |
| Maternal | 10 |
| Paternal | 5 |
| One-parent with NTD | 30 |
| One prior infant with NTD | 20 |
| Two prior infants with NTD | 60 |

[*]Disability has been reported to include lower limb paralysis, sensory loss, chronic bladder or bowel problems, club foot, scoliosis, meningitis, hydrocephalus and mental retardation.

Source: American College of Obstetricians and Gynecologists, *ACOG Technical Bulletin*, 99 (1986), p.1.

man pathologist F.D. von Recklinghausen (1833–1910), who published the first description in 1882.

There is currently no method of PRENATAL DIAGNOSIS or identification of afflicted individuals who are asymptomatic. The site of the defective GENE that causes NF has been located close to the center of CHROMOSOME 17, and this may soon help in identification and treatment of the disorder.

A more severe form, bilateral acoustic neurofibromatosis (also called central NF and NF-2), occurs in one in 50,000 births, and causes multiple tumors of the cranial and spinal nerves. This often results in DEAFNESS, balance disorders and paralysis, requiring multiple surgeries in adolescence or early adulthood. The site of the defective gene that causes this form of NF has been located on chromosome 22.

This disorder came to greater public attention as a result of the popularity of the eponymous Broadway play and movie about Joseph Merrick, the grossly deformed 19th-century Englishman who was exhibited in a freak show as "The Elephant Man."

In an interesting twist, some geneticists now postulate that the Elephant Man didn't suffer from neurofibromatosis at all, but rather from PROTEUS SYNDROME, a greatly disfiguring disease first described in 1976. They note that Merrick's skin and bone deformities (which included a head with a three-foot circumference) were too severe to be caused by neurofibromatosis. Additionally, Dr. Frederick Treves, Merrick's benefactor, never described neurofibromas in his case write-ups of the Elephant Man.

For more information, contact:

National Neurofibromatosis Foundation
141 Fifth Avenue
Suite 7-S
New York, NY 10010
(212) 469-8980
Outside New York: 800-323-7938

## neuronal ceroid lipofuscinosis (NCL)
See BATTEN DISEASE.

## nevoid basal cell carcinoma syndrome    (basal cell nevus syndrome)
Syndrome, present in about one of every 200 patients with basal cell carcinoma (a skin

tumor), characterized by eruptions of the skin and anomalies of the ocular, skeletal, central nervous and endocrine systems.

At birth, ocular defects may include a deformity of the eyelid (dystopia canthorium), abnormally wide spacing between the eyes (HYPERTELORISM) and congenital BLINDNESS. Numerous skeletal problems may also be present at birth, including anomalies of the ribs, spine, feet and digits.

In childhood, multiple jaw cysts begin to appear, followed by multiple basal cell carcinomas. These early skin lesions start out as brownish, dome-shaped papules (raised skin areas) on the upper body. Later they may ulcerate. Adult patients develop a characteristic broad facial appearance due to slightly protruding jaw, swelling around the forehead, sunken eyes and a broadening of the nose.

The prognosis for affected individuals is generally favorable, but is dependent on the location, number and severity of the tumors that characterize the syndrome.

PRENATAL DIAGNOSIS is not yet available, and the basic defect that causes this AUTOSOMAL DOMINANT disorder is not known. About 40% of cases are new MUTATIONS.

**nevus**    CONGENITAL discolorations or anomalous pigmentation of a well-defined area of the skin. Referred to as birthmarks and moles, they appear in various forms, some of which are hereditary.

Pigmented moles have long been observed to show a familial aggregation and are now known to be inherited as an AUTOSOMAL DOMINANT trait. Multiple pigmented moles are also a feature of one chromosomal aberration, TURNER SYNDROME. Multiple pigmented lesions may be seen in a variety of many other disorders such as NEUROFIBROMATOSIS (café au lait spots) or LEOPARD syndrome. (See also PORT WINE STAIN.)

**Niemann-Pick disease**    A group of disorders characterized by the accumulation

of a phosphorus-containing lipid compound, sphingomyelin, in the lysosomes, which are the small digestive structures within cells. This accumulation in the cells of the central nervous system, liver and spleen leads to cell death, and in most cases has fatal consequences. The disorders are classified as STORAGE DISEASES, because they involve the abnormal accumulation or storage of material in the cells.

Four major subtypes (A, B, C and D) have been identified. Type A occurs primarily in infants of Ashkenazi Jews (those of Eastern European ancestry), though it affects all ethnic groups. It was first described by Albert Niemann, a German pediatrician, in 1914. The features of the disorder were more fully detailed by the German physician Ludwig Pick in the 1920s, and the disorder now carries their names.

The primary metabolic defect in the first two forms (A and B) is thought to be the deficient function of the ENZYME sphingomyelinase, which normally helps metabolize the phospholipid, sphingomyelin. The accumulation of lipids in the cells causes them to have a large, pale, "foamy" appearance. These "Niemann-Pick cells," which can be found in the bone marrow, liver, spleen, lymph nodes and lungs, are helpful in diagnosing the condition. The defect in types C and D appears to involve the processing of cholesterol and only secondarily results in any sphingomyelin accumulation.

All forms are inherited as AUTOSOMAL RECESSIVE traits.

*Type A.*    This form is severe and rapidly progressive. The first signs, such as difficulty in feeding and failure to achieve normal developmental milestones, are usually noticed by four to six months of age. The spleen and liver become markedly enlarged (hepatosplenomegaly). About 50% of patients exhibit the retinal abnormality (CHERRY-RED SPOT) characteristic of TAY-SACHS DISEASE. As they age, infants lose control of motor function and mental capacity deteriorates. Infants take on an emaciated appearance with distended abdomens. The skin may have a brownish-yellow discoloration. Recurrent respiratory infections cause severe debilitation, and death usually occurs by three years of age.

The disorder is estimated to occur in one in 25,000 to one in 30,000 infants of Ashkenazic Jewish ancestry. One in 85 to one in 100 Ashkenazi Jews is thought to be a CARRIER of the trait.

*Type B.* In this rare form, which affects all ethnic groups, there is no mental or neurological involvement. Onset is in childhood, and other symptoms are consistent with type A, including presence of Niemann-Pick cells, severe enlargement of the liver and spleen and recurrent infections. There is also lung involvement in this form. Patients have reached adulthood without significant disease-related complications. Life span is generally normal.

*Type C.* This rare form, which occurs in all ethnic groups, exhibits both neurological deterioration and organ involvement. The age of onset is highly variable and may be between one and two years of age or in adulthood, though it most commonly appears later in childhood. There is progressive loss of mental and motor skills. Liver and spleen are enlarged and Niemann-Pick cells are present. Gait abnormalities and ataxia, muscle weakness and seizures occur as the disease progresses. Death usually occurs between the ages of five and 15 years.

*Type D.* Resembles type C but is confined to individuals living in a coastal area of southwestern Nova Scotia with a common ancestor of French (Acadian) extraction. (An adult-onset type E—including patients with disease resembling type C but with onset in adulthood—has also been suggested.) A new classification has been proposed that divides cases into those that are primarily sphingomyelinase-deficient and those that aren't, and subdivides these two types by severity/age of onset (e.g., acute vs. chronic).

PRENATAL DIAGNOSIS of A and B subtypes is possible by observing deficient sphingomyelinase activity in cultured cells gathered through AMNIOCENTESIS. Prenatal diagnosis, previously unreliable in type C, should now be more reliable by specifically measuring cholesterol esterification in fetal-derived-cells.

For more information, contact:

National Foundation for Jewish Genetic Disease, Inc.
250 Park Avenue, Suite 1000
New York, NY 10177
(212) 682-5550

The National Tay-Sachs & Allied Diseases Association
92 Washington Avenue
Cedarhurst, NY 11516
(516) 569-4300

**nightblindness**   The absence or deficiency of vision in the dark, caused by the absence or deficiency of visual purple, a pigment normally found in the retina of the eye and necessary for seeing in reduced lighting. Nightblindness is usually inherited as an AUTOSOMAL DOMINANT trait, when occurring as an isolated non-progressive disorder.

A study of a French family well-known for the condition was published in 1838. Their lineage was traced to Jean Nougaret, a butcher from Provence who settled in a small village near Montpellier in the south of France and who was the common ancestor of everyone in the district with nightblindness. A study of his genealogy found 629 persons, 86 of whom had nightblindness.

There is also a variety commonly found in Japan, named Oguchi disease, for Japanese ophthalmologist Chuta Oguchi (1875–1945). Inherited as an AUTOSOMAL RECESSIVE trait, it is rare in the United States.

It is also a feature of other ophthalmalogic conditions, especially retinal degenerations, such as RETINITIS PIGMENTOSA.

**nonketotic hyperglycinemia**   Glycine is an AMINO ACID found in many animal and plant proteins. A hereditary CONGENITAL defect in the ability of the body to metabolize glycine results in nonketotic hyperglycinemia, a condition in which there is excess glycine in the blood. This is to be distinguished from hyperglycinemia associated with increased ketone levels in the blood, a nonspecific feature of a number of organic acidurias such as PROPIONIC ACIDEMIA. In nonketotic hyperglycinemia, ketones are not elevated; it is a specific disorder of glycine breakdown.

This disorder is characterized by severe convulsions and MENTAL RETARDATION. Within the first few days of life, the affected infant will display lethargic behavior. Convulsions may appear from three days to six weeks after birth. Other complications may include irritability, marked muscular tension (hypertonia), increased reflex reactions (hyperreflexia), an abnormally small head (MICROCEPHALY) and abnormal cavity formation in the brain (PORENCEPHALY).

The exact genetic defect causing this disorder is not known in all cases, although it is known to be inherited as an AUTOSOMAL RECESSIVE trait. A blood test a few days after birth that shows an excess of glycine aids in the detection and diagnosis of this disorder. Glycine levels may be elevated in the urine and also in the cerebro-spinal fluid.

Hyperglycinemia is very rare, and the prognosis for those affected is generally grave, with most dying in infancy. An atypical late-onset form also exists. At present, there is no method for identifying CARRIERS of this disorder and no successful treatment that will allow normal development.

**Noonan syndrome**    Named for J.A. Noonan who described it in 1963, this syndrome is characterized by short stature, ovarian or testicular dysfunction, MENTAL RETARDATION and lesions of the heart or great vessels (blood vessels found primarily on the right side of the heart).

The first report in medical literature of an individual now thought to have Noonan syndrome was published in 1883 by O. Kobolinski. Facial features include wide-set (HYPERTELORISM), downward slanting eyes; skin folds obscuring the inner juncture of the eyelids (EPICANTHUS); flat nasal bridge; upper and lower teeth that fail to meet properly (dental malocclusion); low-set ears with abnormal ear folds that may rotate backward; and short or webbed neck. In addition, the hair in white patients may be light in color and coarse in texture, and is often curly or kinky and extends low on the neck. Abnormalities of the shape of the chest, such as pigeon breast (PECTUS CARINATUM) or funnel chest (pectus excavatum), are common in addition to other skeletal abnormalities. In males the testes may fail to descend (cryptorchism). The appearance of affected individuals is often similar to that of TURNER SYNDROME, though, unlike that syndrome (seen exclusively in females), either gender may be affected.

The severity of the Noonan syndrome is variable. Prognosis for life span, growth and reproductive ability depends on the severity of the specific abnormalities. Therapy may include surgery to correct cardiovascular defects or undescended testes. Hormonal substitution has been used in treating some individuals.

Noonan syndrome usually occurs sporadically, and the basic defect involved is unknown; however, reports demonstrate frequent familial distribution, which may be compatible with AUTOSOMAL DOMINANT inheritance. Prevalence of the disorder may be as high as one in 1,000 and appears to occur with equal frequency in both genders. (See also CONGENITAL HEART DEFECTS.)

**Norrie disease**    Characterized by total blindness in both eyes at birth, this rare X-LINKED hereditary condition occurs only in males. Eyeballs may be abnormally small (microphthalmia), and a gray or gray-yellow mass of tissue is visible behind the lens. This "tumor" must be differentiated from RETINO-BLASTOMA. Often the pupil is dilated and does not react to light. The iris may be poorly developed. At first the lens may be clear, but CATARACTS may form. Eyeballs shrink by the age of 10. Most affected persons are also mentally retarded and frequently suffer severe DEAFNESS as they grow older.

There is close GENETIC LINKAGE of the disorder with certain marker GENES on the X CHROMOSOME, making CARRIER identification and PRENATAL DIAGNOSIS possible in some cases.

**nucleoside phosphorylase deficiency**
An extremely rare immunodeficiency disease. Only about 10 patients have been identified and described. It involves a deficiency of the ENZYME nucleoside phosphorylase and is inherited as an AUTOSOMAL RECESSIVE trait.

Patients with this condition show absent to severely depressed T-cell immunity, while maintaining normal B-cell immunity. However, B-cell immunity deteriorates with age, and patients increasingly suffer from infection, rarely surviving to the age of 10. Immunization with attenuated live viral vaccines, such as measles, can prove fatal.

The enzyme abnormality is demonstrable at birth, though the immunologic function may at first seem normal. There is a possibility that diagnosis could be made in utero by studying enzyme activity in fetal cells. At present, there is no known way to replace the missing enzyme and no effective treatment. (See also IMMUNE DEFICIENCY DISEASE.)

# O

**obesity**   The condition of being 20% or more above ideal body weight. Research has found that some people inherit a strong tendency to become obese. Statistics in the Danish Adoption Register indicate a strong correlation between the weight class of adopted individuals and the body-mass index of their biologic parents, without any similar correlation between adoptees and their adoptive parents.

In some animals, an abnormally low level of the protein adipsin, which is made in fat cells and secreted directly into the bloodstream, has been found to play a role in obesity, possibly influencing appetite or metabolism. It has been theorized that abnormally low levels of adipsin, perhaps an inherited deficiency, may cause hereditary obesity in humans, as well.

**obesity-hypoventilation syndrome**
See PICKWICKIAN SYNDROME.

**occipital horn syndrome**   See CUTIS LAXA.

**ocular albinism**   See ALBINISM.

**oculo-auricular-vertebral dysplasia**
See GOLDENHAR SYNDROME.

**oculo-cerebro-renal syndrome**  See LOWE SYNDROME.

**oculocutaneous albinism**   See ALBINISM.

**OFD syndrome**   See ORAL-FACIAL-DIGITAL SYNDROME.

**Oguchi disease**   See NIGHTBLINDNESS.

**olivopontocerebellar atrophy (OPCA)**
A rare group of disorders characterized by a wasting of portions of the brain: the cerebellum, which lies below the larger cerebrum and behind the spinal column and controls muscular coordination and equilibrium; the pons cerebelli, a bridge-like structure of the brain stem connecting with the medulla oblongata (the enlarged portion of the spinal column at the base of the brain), and the olivary body, which lies on the medulla oblongata. In one system of classification these disorders are broken up into six types, classified according to the mode of inheritance and the nature of the resulting neuromuscular impairment. Others simply consider these disorders to be

among the group of adult-onset ataxias (disorders of coordination) with other associated features. Most forms are AUTOSOMAL DOMINANT while in others AUTOSOMAL RECESSIVE inheritance is seen.

Symptoms usually begin to appear when the affected person is about 30 years old, but they may appear as early as childhood (in some forms) or as late as the 50s or 60s in others. Beginning with a slowly developing unsteadiness of gait, the impairment eventually involves all the limbs. An affected person experiences a slowly progressive loss of muscular coordination (ataxia). Control is lost over muscles used in speaking (dysarthria). Tremors and involuntary movements follow. Muscles may be rigid. In some forms of the disease there may be sensory impairment, mental deterioration, paralysis of eye movement or retinal degeneration with loss of vision. No biochemical abnormalities are known. Affected persons may die of pneumonia or other debilitating disease in their fourth to seventh decade of life. (See also AZOREAN DISEASE; FRIEDREICH'S ATAXIA.)

**omphalocele**    In this CONGENITAL condition, defective embryonic development results in a hole in the abdominal wall, ranging in size from one cm (approximately 3/8 inch) to a massive area covering almost the entire abdomen. Portions of the intestinal tract, covered by a saclike membrane that is either skin or an extension of the inside of the abdominal wall (peritoneum), protrude through the hole at the base of the umbilical cord. Depending on the size of the defect, the contents of the sac range from a small loop of bowel to the entire intestinal tract, including stomach, liver and spleen. The sac may rupture during delivery.

Because elements of the intestinal tract are abnormally positioned, they may not function properly or the blood supply to them may be diminished. The intestine often is rotated and may require corrective surgery. The genitourinary system, cardiovascular system, and rarely the central nervous system may also be

affected. The defect may be seen with CHROMOSOME ABNORMALITIES or as part of the BECKWITH-WIEDEMANN SYNDROME.

The greatest threats to life from omphalocele are infection of the peritoneum and starvation because the intestine is nonfunctional. However, most mortality in individuals with omphalocele is due to associated ANOMALIES. Surgical correction is highly successful and is usually undertaken as soon after birth as possible. If the omphalocele is very large, the abdominal cavity may be too small to contain the viscera; in this case, the protrusion is covered by a pouch of synthetic material and returned to the abdominal cavity in stages as the cavity increases in size.

Although the basic defect that causes omphalocele has not been identified, it is known to occur in approximately one in 6,000 live births and to affect males more frequently than females by the ratio of three to two. ULTRASOUND may detect the presence of omphalocele.

**oncogene**    GENES that appear to play a role in the development of CANCER, perhaps by orchestrating uncontrolled cell growth. First isolated in the 1980s, approximately 50 oncogenes had been identified by the end of the decade. A number of anti-oncogenes have also been identified, which appear to inhibit the development of cancer. It is thought that several cumulative changes must occur before cancer develops. Among the changes, oncogenes must be activated and anti-oncogenes must be deactivated. Two or more oncogenes of different classes may also be required to cooperate before malignant cell growth is triggered.

It is likely that the action of oncogenes and anti-oncogenes underlies most if not all cancers, and it is only how these are triggered that differs from situation to situation. Viruses and other environmental agents are thought to play a part in activating oncogenes. Chromosomal rearrangements may also be involved: Oncogenes are located at the sites of chromosome rearrangements seen in various cancers, such as the Philadelphia chromosome observed in many leukemia patients.

Drs. J. Michael Bishop and Herald E. Varmus of the University of California shared a 1989 Nobel prize for their pioneering work in developing the oncogene hypothesis.

**Opitz-Frias syndrome**   See G SYNDROME.

**oral-facial-digital syndrome**   (OFD syndrome)   A heterogenous (of varying origins) group of disorders with two well-recognized variants, which, though they may be distinguished from one another, are often confused:

*OFD I.*   An X-LINKED dominant disorder, limited to females and lethal in males. It has distinct oral, facial and digital ANOMALIES. Affected individuals have a small, short (partial) midline CLEFT in the lip with bands of fibrous tissue that connect the cheeks and lip to the gums and often cleft the tongue. In addition to cleft palate and a thin nose with a broad nasal root, the position where the upper and lower eyelid meet near the nose (canthi) may be displaced. The skin may be dry and there is thinning of the hair (ALOPECIA) in over half the patients. White nodular cysts of the sebaceous glands and hair follicles (milia) are seen on the face. Central nervous system defects are common (approximately 20%) and MENTAL RETARDATION is seen in over half of those brought to medical attention. Asymmetric shortening of the digits with or without webbing of the digits (SYNDACTYLY), or extra digits (POLYDACTYLY), which may be unilateral or bilaterally asymmetric, may be seen. One-third of patients die in infancy. Survivors require surgery for the oral clefts and comprehensive dental care.

*OFD II (Mohr syndrome).*   This form is named for Otto Mohr (1886–1967), dean of the medical faculty at the University of Oslo and president of the Norwegian Academy of Science, who published a description in 1941. Recognizable at birth, distinctive facial features and the presence of extra fingers or toes (polydactyly) or webbing together of fingers or toes (syndactyly) characterize this rare disorder. Affected individuals commonly exhibit a cleft tongue with ANKYLOGLOSSIA (tongue tie). In addition, the bridge of the nose is low, and the tip of the nose is broad, with an indentation. The point at which the upper and lower inner eyelids meet near the nose (canthi) may be displaced outward, and a CLEFT LIP and underdeveloped cheek and jaw bones are common.

Often an additional finger after the fifth finger is present on both hands (bilateral manual ulnar hexadactyly) and the big toe is partially reduplicated; there are two great toes fused together. In some cases three or four fingers may be webbed together with extra bones in between.

Though nervous system defects may cause mental impairment, most patients are of normal intelligence. Hearing loss (conduction DEAFNESS) is frequent due to a defect in the incus, one of the small bones of the middle ear. Respiratory infections may cause death during infancy.

Oral-facial-digital syndrome II is believed to be inherited as an AUTOSOMAL RECESSIVE trait.

The basic cause of the OFD syndromes is unknown. PRENATAL DIAGNOSIS of either may be possible by finding hand and foot abnormalities (or perhaps clefts) with ULTRASOUND (or FETOSCOPY) in at-risk pregnancies.

**ornithine transcarbamylase deficiency**
See UREA CYCLE DEFECTS.

**Osler-Weber-Rendu syndrome**   (hereditary hemorrhagic telangiectasia, HHT)   A hereditary disorder of the capillaries, characterized by vascular lesions, or telangiectasias, occurring on the skin, mucous membranes and in many internal organs. Telangiectasias are clumps of dilated blood vessels caused by deficiencies in the capillary system; the vessel walls lack elastic tissue wherever the lesions occur. When occurring near the skin's surface, well-defined areas of red skin are visible above them. Complications are caused by bleeding from these lesions and by degenerative changes the lesions may undergo.

It is named for English physicians Sir William Osler (1849–1919), author of the landmark *The Principles and Practice of Medicine*, Frederick P. Weber (1863–1962) and French physician Henri J.L. Rendu (1844–1902). They independently published descriptions in 1901, 1936 and 1896 respectively.

The characteristic telangiectasias appear as red-to-violet lesions on the cheeks, ears, lips and tongue, as well as in the mucous membranes of the nose. Internally, they may appear in the gastrointestinal tract, bladder, the lungs, brain, spinal cord and liver.

Bleeding occurs spontaneously or as a result of trauma. Bleeding from the nose (epistaxis) and the gastrointestinal tract progresses with age, often leading to chronic ANEMIA. Internally, the lesions are believed to be capable of developing into arteriovenous fistulae (anomalous connections between arteries and veins) that may appear in the lungs, pulmonary arteries, brain and liver. These give rise to an increased frequency of hemorrhages. Brain hemorrhages may give rise to seizures, transient paralysis and vision or speech difficulties. Complications may lead to death in 10% of individuals.

Treatment is directed at preventing or stopping bleeding and removing large lesions. Blood transfusions may be used if symptoms of anemia are exhibited. The disorder is generally worsened by pregnancy.

HHT is estimated to have an incidence of one in 50,000 live births in Europe, though it may be much higher due to improper diagnosis. It is inherited as an AUTOSOMAL DOMINANT trait.

For more information, contact:

HHT Foundation, Inc.
Biochemistry Dept.
University of Massachusetts
Amherst, MA 01003
(413) 545-2048
(413) 259-1515

**osteogenesis imperfecta (OI)** (brittle bone disease)   Translated from its Greek and Latin derivations as "imperfectly formed bones," in this HEREDITARY DISEASE of the connective tissue bones may be so fragile that, for example, a child can fracture a tibia (the large bone in the lower leg) merely by swinging his leg. Fractures may even occur during fetal development. In addition to fragile bones, the cardinal features are blue sclerae (that is, an abnormal blueness in the white fibrous tissue that covers the so called "white of the eye") and DEAFNESS. However, affected individuals do not always exhibit all the symptoms.

The face tends to be triangular-shaped, with yellowish-brown teeth. Stature is short and growth is stunted. Other associated features include abnormal lateral curvature of the spine (SCOLIOSIS), high pitched voice, excessive sweating, loose joints, tendency to bruise easily, respiratory problems and constipation. Those affected are also reported to exhibit euphoria and a general sense of well-being. There is great variability in symptoms and their severity. It may be limited to a few fractures in childhood, cause 50 to 100 fractures by adulthood, or cause death in the fetus or newborn.

Most deaths caused by OI are the result of associated cardiopulmonary problems. Severely affected individuals who don't succumb to these complications usually require braces, crutches or a wheelchair for mobility.

Historically, this disorder has been described under numerous names. The first case suggestive of the disorder was the mythical Danish prince, Ivar Benløs (boneless; legless), who had to be carried into battle on a shield because he was unable to walk on his soft legs. Reports of a disorder with abnormal bone brittleness and multiple fractures date to the end of the 17th century. The first description of a family exhibiting the condition was reported by a Swedish military surgeon in 1788. At one time it was speculated that French painter Toulouse-Lautrec had this affliction, but that now appears to be incorrect; he most likely had PYCNODYSOSTOSIS.

OI is now recognized to represent at least four subtypes, with incidence estimated at one in 20,000 live births. There are approximately 30,000 affected individuals in the United States. Most cases are inherited as an AUTOSOMAL DOMINANT trait (90%), though a rare AUTOSOMAL RECESSIVE form exists. Some of these cases are the result of new MUTATIONS. The cause of the disorder is unknown, but evidence points to defective development of collagen, a major protein in skin and bone. Specific abnormalities of the collagen genes have been demonstrated in some affected individuals. In other families, OI demonstrates GENETIC LINKAGE to the genes for collagen.

PRENATAL DIAGNOSIS for some forms of the disorder is possible via ULTRASOUND, and in some families by measuring fetal collagen levels or examining the collagen genes in fetal tissue collected by CHORIONIC VILLUS SAMPLING.

For more information, contact:

Osteogenesis Imperfecta Foundation
P.O. Box 14807
Clearwater, FL 34629-4807
(813) 855-7077

**osteopetrosis, infantile**   See   INFANTILE OSTEOPETROSIS.

**otitis media**   See   MIDDLE-EAR INFECTIONS.

**otosclerosis**   A slowly progressive hearing loss with its genesis in the middle and inner ear, unrelated to inflammation or disease of the middle ear. It is primarily a conductive form of DEAFNESS; that is, caused by abnormalities in the structure of the ear, rather than in the auditory nerves (sensorineural deafness). (However, abnormalities in the auditory nerves may occur and result in sensorineural deafness.) Hearing loss occurs as the ear bone composed of cartilage becomes progressively replaced by calcified abnormal bone. It occurs in young or middle-aged adults and due to slow onset is often not easily detected.

Nearly 75% of all cases affect both ears (bilateral). Those who come to medical attention may have a history of hearing best in noisy settings (paracusis Willisani) and may frequently complain about ringing in the ears (tinnitus), sometimes accompanied by an audible pulse. A small percentage experience dizziness.

The cause of this disorder is not clear, but is believed to be related to destruction of the thin membrane lining of inner surface of cochlea in the inner ear.

This disorder is inherited as an AUTOSOMAL DOMINANT trait, and appears in about 25% to 40% of those who inherit the gene. (Thus, PENETRANCE is 25% to 40%.)

Estimates for disease prevalence differ according to racial groups. For whites, it is one in 330; for blacks, it is about one in 3,300, and for Orientals, about one in 33,000.

Detectability is limited in younger individuals since this is a disease occurring during young or middle adulthood. It may be exacerbated by pregnancy. Ten percent of cases are apparent at ages 11 to 15, and 50% become apparent by the ages 21 to 25. Life span and intelligence levels are unaffected.

**oxycephaly**   See CRANIOSYNOSTOSIS.

# P

**panhypopituitarism**   See   PITUITARY DWARFISM SYNDROMES.

**papyraceous fetus**   A non-living fetus that has been retained and not immediately and spontaneously aborted following death "in utero," and that exhibits a mummified appearance when ultimately delivered. This may occur, for example, when one of a pair of twins dies during fetal development, and is not delivered until the living twin is.

**paramethadione**   See ANTICONVULSANTS.

**paraplegia**   Paralysis of both legs and the lower portion of the body, caused by damage or maldevelopment of the spinal cord. Infantile forms of paraplegia may be due to BIRTH INJURY.

**Parenti-Fraccaro type achondrogenesis**   See ACHONDROGENESIS.

**Parkinson disease**   (Parkinsonism) Disorder characterized by tremors, mostly in the upper limbs, slow voluntary movements, stooped posture, shuffling gait and other physical symptoms that grow progressively more pronounced. Onset is typically between the ages of 50 and 65 years.

While the origin of the disorder is unknown, it has been suggested that some forms may be inherited, possibly as a MULTIFACTORIAL trait, and it has reportedly appeared in multiple generations in some families. However, it has also been suggested that the disorder alluded to as familial Parkinsonism in some of these observations may actually be HUNTINGTON'S CHOREA. Most cases are SPORADIC.

**Parkinsonism**   See PARKINSON DISEASE.

**Parry's disease**   See BATTEN DISEASE.

**passive euthanasia**   Allowing an individual to succumb to a fatal condition by withholding medical treatment. This sometimes occurs in the case of infants with severe congenital defects, generally at parental request. Opposition to passive euthanasia has in some cases led to legal efforts to compel medical treatment for affected infants. (See also BABY DOE.)

**Patau syndrome**   (trisomy 13)      A CHROMOSOME ABNORMALITY resulting from an extra chromosome 13. Named for U.S. geneticist K. Patau, who published the first description in 1960, it accounts for an estimated 1% of spontaneous abortions during the first trimester of pregnancy, and occurs in about one in 12,000 to one in 24,000 live births. It is slightly more common in females than in males.

The physical characteristics are so striking that diagnosis is often possible prior to the completion of CYTOGENETIC TESTS. These characteristics include a small head (MICROCEPHALY) exhibitng scalp lesions, sloping forehead, small eyes (microphthalmia) with sparse or absent eyebrows, CLEFT LIP or palate, poorly formed ears, and deformities of the hands and feet. The hand is often clenched and may have more than five fingers (POLYDACTYLY). The heel extends back abnormally.

Internally, there are frequently cardiac and renal (kidney) defects. Both males and females often display genital abnormalities, as well. The brain shows a malformation termed HOLOPROSENCEPHALY.

Only half of affected individuals survive the first month of life, only 25% survive beyond six months and 5% more than three years. However, survival to age 35 has been reported in a single case. MENTAL RETARDATION is severe.

For more information, contact:

Support Organization for Trisomy 18, 13
   and Other Related Disorders
1522 E. Garnet
Mesa, AZ 85204-5957
(801) 882-6635

**patent ductus arteriosus   (PDA)** CONGENITAL HEART DEFECT resulting from the persistence after birth of a fetal duct that connects the pulmonary artery to the aorta. In the fetus, the duct enables blood to bypass the lungs; no air enters them during fetal life. Soon after birth the duct ordinarily closes. PDA refers to the lack of this closure. This allows already oxygenated blood to flow back into the lungs, overloading the heart's ability to keep pumping blood, which may ultimately lead to congestive heart failure. The severity of the disorder is dependent on the size of the persisting fetal duct; the larger the opening, the more serious the consequences.

PDA is most common in premature infants, with females more often affected than males by a ratio of two or three to one. It is also often associated with fetal rubella syndrome (see TORCH SYNDROME), TREACHER COLLINS SYNDROME and other single GENE disorders and CHROMOSOME ABNORMALITIES. It is usually not life-threatening and may spontaneously heal as the duct closes on its own. Infants are usually asymptomatic after one year of age. When the condition persists, affected infants are susceptible to bacterial infection of the heart (endocarditis) and may exhibit physical underdevelopment. In these cases the condition can be repaired surgically, generally resulting in complete recovery. If untreated, it may eventually cause cardiac failure and death.

PDA occurs in approximately one in 830 live births. Fifteen percent of those affected have additional cardiac abnormalities. The cause of the disorder is unknown, though MULTIFACTORIAL inheritance is suspected. It has been suggested that in some cases it may be inherited in AUTOSOMAL DOMINANT or AUTOSOMAL RECESSIVE forms.

**Peck's disease**   See AMYOTROPHIC LATERAL SCLEROSIS (ALS).

**pectus**   From the Latin, pectus refers to the chest. Consistent deformities of the chest are seen in many GENETIC DISORDERS and CONGENITAL defects.

*Pectus excavatum.* Also called "funnel breast," this is an abnormally sunken chest. Some families have exhibited the condition in a pattern consistent with AUTOSOMAL DOMINANT transmission. This deformity also occurs in hereditary disorders, including MARFAN SYNDROME.

*Pectus carinatum.* Popularly known as "pigeon breast" or "chicken breast," this is marked by an abnormal prominence of sternum. It can also occur as part of malformation syndromes such as Morquio disease (see MUCOPOLYSACCHARIDOSIS).

**pedigree**   A chart or schematic diagram detailing a family genealogy for the purpose of identifying and tracking the transmission of hereditary characteristics. The pedigree, or compendium of ancestors, is displayed through the use of symbols representing individual family members and lines representing their interrelationships.

The charts can be useful in determining if there is a genetic cause for an individual's anomalous condition, and if so, which form of MENDELIAN inheritance the trait follows: AUTOSOMAL DOMINANT, AUTOSOMAL RECESSIVE or X-LINKED. This information can then be explained to the affected individual and used as a means to assist in making family planning decisions.

Information for preparing the chart is provided from interviews with the individual(s) undergoing counseling and from medical records, family photographs and examination of other family members.

**Pelizaeus-Merzbacher disease**   An infant-onset form of progressive spasticity named for German physicians F. Pelizaeus (1850–1917), who described the disorder in 1885, and L. Merzbacher (b. 1875), who described it in 1909.

Symptoms may appear from several days to six months after birth. It begins with a characteristic rolling motion of the head and eyes (nystagmus). This uncontrolled divergence and lack of coordination of the eyes is a common feature, and affected children are known in their families as "head nodders" and "eye

# Figure III
## Symbols Commonly Used in Pedigree Construction

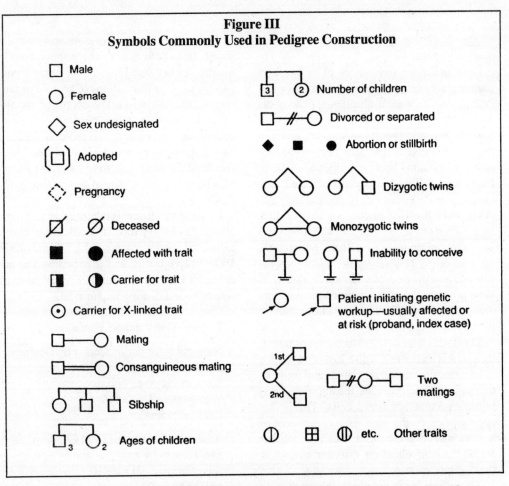

# Figure IV
## Sample Working Pedigree

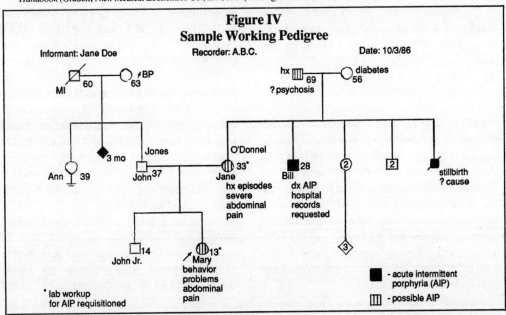

waggers." (These symptoms may later, curiously, disappear.)

Developmental milestones of sitting and standing are delayed, and speech may be delayed as well. Mental abilities appear undiminished. The progression is gradual, with lower limbs and upper limbs showing increasing deterioration of muscular control. Movements of the arms become jerky and clumsy. Fine motor skills are especially affected. Dementia and Parkinsonian symptoms may develop over the first decade or two of life. Death often occurs between the ages of 16 and 25 years, often resulting from pneumonia brought on by respiratory complications resulting from the disorder. However, due to its slow progression, some individuals may survive much longer. Pelizaeus had one patient who lived to age 52.

The basic cause of the disorder is unknown, though it is associated with a loss of myelin, a fatlike sheath composed of lipids and proteins that surrounds some axons, the impulse-transmitting portions of nerve cells. The defect appears to be in the gene for a component of myelin named proteolipid (PLP). A similar X-LINKED demyelination disorder occurs in the "jumpy" mouse.

This infant-onset disorder is inherited as an X-LINKED recessive trait and appears only in males. (Some heterozygous females, that is, CARRIERS of the recessive gene, may display symptoms of the disorder.) However, an adult-onset form has been identified as an AUTOSOMAL DOMINANT trait.

**Pendred syndrome**   Syndrome characterized by DEAFNESS in combination with an enlarged thyroid gland (goiter). While production of hormones in the thyroid is normal in most of those affected, those with deficiencies may experience a delay of skeletal maturation. A causal link between the thyroid disorder and the hearing deficit has not been established. (Hearing loss is associated with two other thyroid disorders: adult myxedema and endemic cretinism.)

The hearing impairment is sensorineural; it results from defects in the nerves involved in hearing, rather than blockage of hearing passageways or malformations of hearing organs (conductive deafness). The degree of impairment is variable, from mild to profound, though half exhibit severe to profound hearing loss. Usually both ears are affected identically (bilateral). It is present from early in life and may result in severe speech and language difficulties.

Pendred syndrome is inherited as an AUTOSOMAL RECESSIVE trait. Its incidence has been estimated at between one in 12,500 and one in 100,000 live births, and it is believed to account for between 4% and 10% of all cases of sensorineural hearing impairment.

For more information, contact:

National Information Center on Deafness
Gallaudet College
800 Florida Ave., N.E.
Washington, DC 20002
(202) 651-5000

American Society for Deaf Children
814 Thayer Avenue
Silver Spring, MD 20910
(301) 585-5400

**penetrance**   The proportion of individuals who exhibit an inherited trait for which they have inherited the necessary GENES. The term was coined by eminent German neuropathologist Otto Vogt in 1926 (who, at the same time, introduced a related term, EXPRESSIVITY). Implicit in this concept is the fact that not everyone who inherits the genes necessary to cause a hereditary disorder will exhibit the disorder. Penetrance is usually expressed as a percentage. If half of all those who possess the requisite gene(s) exhibit the disorder, penetrance is said to be 50%.

Taken as a whole, inherited conditions have a variable degree of penetrance. In disorders with a high degree of penetrance, virtually anyone who possesses the single dominant gene or the two recessive genes required for expression of the trait will exhibit it. In conditions with low penetrance, many who have the requisite genes may not exhibit any of the characteristic features of the trait. Interaction with other genes and with non-genetic factors may influence penetrance.

**periodic paralysis, familial**    A rare FA-MILIAL DISEASE characterized by attacks of weakness with flaccid paralysis, often occurring upon awakening. It is usually associated with extremely low levels of potassium in the blood (hypokalemia), though it may occur in the presence of normal or elevated potassium levels. Episodes may be precipitated in affected individuals by administration of glucose.

The disorder is inherited as an AUTOSOMAL DOMINANT trait.

**peroneal muscular atrophy**    See CHARCOT-MARIE-TOOTH DISEASE.

**pes cavus**    See CLAWFOOT.

**Peutz-Jeghers syndrome**    See Colorectal Cancer under CANCER.

**Peyronie disease**    (bent stick syndrome) A progressive deformity of the penis with onset in middle age; it results in an abnormal curvature (in any direction), especially during erection. Francois de la Peyronie (1648–1747), surgeon to King Louis XIV and a founder of the Royal Academy of Surgery in Paris, first published a description of the disorder in 1743. Inherited as an AUTOSOMAL DOMINANT trait, it is caused, as is DUPUYTREN CONTRACTURE, a condition with which it is associated, by the hardening of fibrous tissue. Although it is essentially benign and painless, it may interfere with intercourse. No effective treatment has been developed. Attempts to surgically remove fibrous masses typically result in generation of new hardened tissue.

**Pfeiffer syndrome**    (acrocephalosyndactyly)    A form of CRANIOSYNOSTOSIS, skull malformations caused by premature clo-

sure of the gaps (sutures) between one or more skull bones. Growth is thus directed in aberrant directions. This form is named for R.A. Pfeiffer, who published a description in 1964.

The characteristic head shape, observable at birth, is marked by a high forehead and squat skull (brachycephaly). Eyes are wide set (HYPERTELORISM) and the eye slits (palpebral fissures) are slanted down away from the nose (antimongoloid obliquity). The digits on hands and feet (particularly the second and third) exhibit webbing (syndactyly). The fingers are short, the thumbs and great toes are broad. However, facial features tend to attain a more normal appearance with age, and no treatment may be required. Intelligence is usually normal. This disorder is inherited as an AUTOSOMAL DOMINANT trait; many cases are new MUTATIONS.

For other forms of craniosynostoses, see APERT SYNDROME; CROUZON DISEASE; CARPENTER SYNDROME; and SAETHRE-CHOTZEN.

**phakomatosis (neurodermatosis)**    Any one of a group of CONGENITAL and hereditary disorders characterized by skin (cutaneous) and nerve (neurological) abnormalities. They include NEUROFIBROMATOSIS, VON HIPPEL-LINDAU DISEASE, STURGE-WEBER SYNDROME and TUBEROUS SCLEROSIS.

**phenobarbital**    The barbiturate phenobarbital, prescribed to prevent epileptic seizures and as a sedative, has been named as a suspected TERATOGEN, a substance capable of causing BIRTH DEFECTS. However, it is often prescribed in combination with other drugs known to cause birth defects and there is disagreement on whether phenobarbital alone can induce fetal malformations. Some studies indicate that it magnifies the risks associated with some drugs it is frequently prescribed with.

Infants born to women taking barbiturates may exhibit drug withdrawal symptoms, and their blood may not clot normally. (See also ANTICONVULSANTS.)

**phenotype** The observable or measurable characteristics associated with a gene or GENES. Most genetic conditions have characterstic physical or internal features, and the features exhibited by individuals with these conditions are said to be phenotypes. (This is in contrast to GENOTYPE, which refers only to having a particular gene or genes, not whether or how the associated traits are expressed in an individual; sometimes the gene does not manifest itself.)

The term "phenotype" was introduced in the early 1900s by Wilhelm Ludwig Johannsen (1857–1927), a pharmacist's apprentice from Copenhagen who went on to achieve considerable renown in the fields of genetics and botany. He also introduced the terms "gene" and "genotype." (See also EXPRESSIVITY and PENETRANCE.)

**phenylketonuria** An ENZYME deficiency disorder characterized by the inability to convert one AMINO ACID, phenylalanine, to another, tyrosine. (Amino acids are the building blocks of proteins.) Consequently, phenylalanine accumulates in the body, resulting in severe MENTAL RETARDATION. This disorder has been the prototype disease for newborn screening. If detected early enough through blood and urine tests, the disease can be halted. In most states it is routine to test for phenylketonuria in the first few days of life, after the infant has been exposed to a significant protein intake.

Symptoms may include severe vomiting and seizures during the first weeks of life, a "mousy" smell, dry skin or an eczema-like rash. Slightly smaller head (MICROCEPHALY), behavioral problems, abnormal hand movements and brisk reflexes may also be observed. Often, the brain-wave test (electroencephalogram or EEG) is abnormal.

Once diagnosed, the child can be treated with a diet that limits the intake of foods containing phenylalanine. With early treatment, the prognosis is excellent. Here again, this disease has been a prototype disorder for the treatment of inborn errors of metabolism

through nutritional manipulation and dietary restriction. However, once mental retardation and seizures set in, the patient's life span may be shortened. It has been previously debated as to when and if the diet can be discontinued in an affected individual. Current recommendations are to continue the diet for life. Also, the metabolic dysfunction of women with PKU can have adverse effects upon the fetus during gestation even if the fetus does not have the enzyme deficiency. These infants, with the maternal PKU syndrome, have microcephaly, mental retardation and CONGENITAL HEART DEFECTS.

Most children with the disorder have blond hair, blue eyes and fair skin. It is less likely to occur in blacks and Ashkenazi Jews (those of Eastern European ancestry). Inherited as an AUTOSOMAL RECESSIVE trait, it occurs in approximately one in 15,000 live births. The highest incidence occurs in Ireland and Scotland, lending support to the theory that the PKU gene is Celtic in origin. The PKU gene has been identified and mapped to chromosome 12.

Using molecular biologic techniques with the cloned PKU gene, PRENATAL DIAGNOSIS and CARRIER detection are possible in at-risk families.

The first case of PKU was identified by Asborn Folling in Norway in 1934. He detected and identified an abnormal substance in the urine of two mentally retarded SIBLINGS. (Coincidentally, it was later discovered that the children's mother was a distant relative of Folling's.) In a 1947 paper published in the *Journal of Biological Chemistry*, George A. Jervis identified the metabolic defect in the disease, and 20 years after Folling discovered the disease, German physician H. Bickel described the treatment of PKU. With the realization that PKU was a treatable form of mental retardation, if diagnosed early, Robert Guthrie, professor of pediatrics at the University of Buffalo, developed a simple screening test in 1963.

Today, millions of newborn children worldwide are screened for phenylketonuria, and thousands of children have been detected early, treated and are leading normal, productive lives. PKU has served as an important example of the application of genetics in public health and in the prevention of mental retardation.

**phenylthiocarbamide tasting**   Common benign trait, the result of AUTOSOMAL DOMINANT inheritance that determines an individual's ability to taste phenylthiocarbamide (PTC). About 70% of the general population possess this trait and are said to be "tasters." A taste test using a strip of paper laced with PTC can determine the presence or absence of this trait in most individuals. PTC will taste bitter to those who possess the trait, and have no taste to those without it. Due to the ubiquity of this condition and the simplicity of the test, it is frequently used in high school science courses as a genetics demonstration.

Geneticists have attempted to link the GENE for this trait with genes for various inherited disorders in order to use it as a marker for simplified screening procedures, but thus far these linkage efforts have been unsuccessful.

**phocomelia**   A CONGENITAL malformation characterized by short, flipper-like appendages. The portions of the extremities nearest (proximal) to the body are poorly developed or absent, so that hands and feet are attached almost directly to the trunk. An affected individual is said to be a "phocomelus."

This condition was associated with the use of THALIDOMIDE, a prescription sleeping pill marketed in Europe, Australia and Canada that was subsequently found to have teratogenic properties (see TERATOGENS).

**phytanic acid storage disease**   (Refsum disease)   A rare inherited disorder characterized by three symptoms: deep pigmentation of the retina of the eye (RETINITIS PIGMENTOSA), weakening of the nerves of the limbs (peripheral neuropathy) and poor coordination resulting in a staggering gait (cerebellar ataxia). It is caused by the body's inability to break down (metabolize) phytanic acid, which is present in dairy products, beef, lamb and some seafoods. The disease was first described by Norwegian physician S. Refsum in 1946. It has recently been discovered that the oxidation of phytanic acid is a function of a subcellular organelle called the peroxisome.

Inherited as an AUTOSOMAL RECESSIVE trait, the disorder is generally detected during the first 20 years of life. NIGHTBLINDNESS is usually the first symptom, due to the chemical's effect on the eye. Other symptoms include tunnel vision, muscle weakness, muscle shrinkage (atrophy) and decreased sensitivity to pain.

Because the disease affects most of the specialized nerves of the brain (cranial nerves) and spinal cord, it also results in DEAFNESS, tingling sensation in the limbs, toes and fingers (paresthesias), difficulty perceiving smells, abnormal responses of the pupil to light, and slowed reflexes. Other parts of the body affected are the heart, which may be enlarged, and the kidney. The skin may have a scaly quality, especially on the palms and soles of the feet.

In rare cases, affected individuals will die in childhood, but a substantial number survive beyond 40 years of age. Death usually results from irregular heart rhythm (arrhythmia) or respiratory difficulties. Once diagnosed, it can be treated by limiting the intake of foods that contain phytanic acid and removing it by plasmapheresis, a technique of filtering the patient's blood plasma.

The effects of phytanic acid can also be minimized by supportive therapy, such as physical therapy, orthopedic devices and cataract removal, if necessary.

Infantile Refsum disease is a more generalized disturbance of peroxisome function and resembles mild forms of ZELLWEGER SYNDROME or neonatal ADRENOLEUKODYSTROPHY.

**Pickwickian syndrome** (obesity-hypoventilation syndrome) A complication of extreme OBESITY that may result in death from interference with cardiac and respiratory functions (cardiorespiratory embarrassment). Its name is inspired by the obese character, Joe, in Charles Dickens's *The Pickwick Papers*. Individuals with PRADER-WILLI SYNDROME may develop and succumb to problems associated with this disorder.

The marked obesity causes obstruction to airflow and individuals may have restless and noisy sleep. Ultimately, as their obesity interferes with normal respiration to a severe degree, they may become so oxygen-deprived that they exhibit excessive sleepiness and may develop heart failure.

**piebald skin trait** Piebald means spotted, or of different colors. Patches of skin of affected individuals are depigmented, thus giving them a spotted, piebald appearance. Depigmented areas are most common on the front of the body, such as the forehead, chest, abdomen and extremities. The borders of these patches may be hyperpigmented. There may be a white forelock of hair, and the eyebrows may be depigmented as well. Some individuals also have eyes of different color (HETEROCHROMIA IRIDES).

A piebald Mandan was painted by George Carlin (1796–1872), an artist known for his portraits of Native Americans, and the condition was said to have been common in the tribe. Though rare in the human population, where it is inherited via AUTOSOMAL DOMINANT transmission, the piebald trait is common in the animal kingdom.

**Pierre Robin syndrome** See ROBIN ANOMALY.

**pituitary dwarfism syndrome** The pituitary gland is a small organ, located in the brain, that controls the release of hormones (chemicals necessary for growth, reproduction, nutrition and metabolism) in the body. In pituitary DWARFISM syndrome, the pituitary gland fails to function properly, resulting in subnormal growth rate, and ultimately, stunted growth (proportional dwarfism).

These conditions cause slow growth rate after the first two years of life and may also result in low blood sugar (hypoglycemia), high-pitched voice and fat pads around the chest and abdomen (truncal obesity). Because the cheekbones and jaws are small, the face is distorted.

Additionally, if sex hormones are not produced by the pituitary, the child may not undergo puberty. Females will fail to menstruate or develop adult breasts or pubic hair. Males will have a small penis and testes, and no facial hair.

Other organs affected are the thyroid gland, which plays a role in regulating growth and metabolism, and the adrenal gland, which, along with the pancreas, plays a role in the control of sugar levels in the body. As a result, the person may have low blood levels of sugar. (This condition improves as the child gets older.) Mild MENTAL RETARDATION can occur in some types of pituitary dwarfism.

There are four major types of pituitary dwarfism:

*Familial panhypopituitary dwarfism.* This is characterized by HGH (human growth hormone) deficiency and lack of one or more additional pituitary hormones, most typically gonadotropin (which regulates sexual development), ACTH (adrenocorticotropic hormone, which stimulates the adrenal gland) and TSH (thyroid-stimulating hormone). The features of this form depend on the specific hormones that are missing. Without gonadotropin, individuals will fail to mature sexually, and secondary sexual characteristics will not develop. Deficiency of ACTH may cause severe hypoglycemia. TSH deficiency may interfere with the functioning of the thyroid gland.

Most cases are not genetically influenced, though there are both AUTOSOMAL RECESSIVE and X-LINKED recessive forms of the disorder.

This form of proportional dwarfing is believed to be the condition that affected TOM THUMB, the circus dwarf.

*Congenital absence of the pituitary.* Affected individuals are born without a pituitary gland, and there is a deficiency of HGH, ACTH and TSH. Individuals exhibit mental and physical retardation. The condition is inherited as an AUTOSOMAL RECESSIVE trait.

*Isolated HGH deficiency.* Inherited in both AUTOSOMAL RECESSIVE and AUTOSOMAL DOMINANT forms, there is generally normal sexual development as well as normal functioning of the adrenal and thyroid glands. Individuals with the recessive form have hypoglycemia attacks and insulin hypersensitivity.

*Laron-type pituitary dwarfism.* Affected individuals are severely dwarfed, though normally porportioned. In females, there is normal female sexual maturation, while males exhibit delayed puberty. There may be mild MENTAL RETARDATION. This form is inherited as an AUTOSOMAL RECESSIVE trait.

Administration of hormones can alleviate some of the features associated with hormone deficiencies.

Currently, there is no method of PRENATAL DIAGNOSIS for these conditions. The exception is those families with autosomal recessive isolated but complete HGH deficiency, where a gene deletion can be found. In these families molecular diagnostic techniques may be used for prenatal diagnosis. The outlook for a normal life span is favorable.

For more information, contact:

Little People of America, Inc.
P.O. Box 633
San Bruno, CA 94066
(415) 589-0695

Human Growth Foundation
4720 Montgomery Lane, Suite 909
Bethesda, MD 20814
(301) 656-6904
(301) 656-7540

**plagiocephaly** See CRANIOSYNOSTOSIS.

**pleiotropy** The ability of one GENE or gene pair to have numerous effects, or produce various characteristics. For example, the aberrant gene that causes MARFAN SYNDROME may manifest itself in abnormalities of the skeletal, cardiovascular, or other systems, and therefore exhibits pleiotropy.

**poikiloderma atrophicans and cataracts** See ROTHMUND-THOMSON SYNDROME.

**Poland syndrome** (Poland syndactyly) Named for Alfred Poland (1822–1872), this is a sporadically-occurring developmental field defect involving muscles and tissue on one side of the chest and the hand on the same (ipsilateral) side. (A field defect is one with its origin in an isolated and localized area of the developing embryo.) Poland was a demonstrator of anatomy when he published the first account of this syndrome in 1841; he later became senior ophthalmologist at Guy's Hospital in London.

The syndrome is highly variable in expression. The constant features are abnormalities of the nipple, subcutaneous tissue and two of the major chest muscles, the pectoralis major and minor.

The breast and underlying tissue may be absent, or the nipple and breast may be displaced upward, located in the area of the armpit, for example. In both men and women, the affected breast will be smaller than the unaffected one. Portions of cartilage of the ribs may also be absent. There is usually no hair (hypotrichosis) on affected tissue. SPRENGEL DEFORMITY has been seen in some affected individuals.

The affected hand is usually smaller than the non-affected hand, and may exhibit several deformities. There may be absence of all or part of the hand. The middle bones of the fingers (phalanges) may be absent or fused with the first bone, and the skin between fingers may be webbed (SYNDACTYLY). The thumb is usually least affected.

Heredity generally does not appear to play a role in the condition, and most cases are sporadic. (However, cases have been attributed to AUTOSOMAL DOMINANT inheritance.) The syndrome has been estimated to occur in between one in 7,000 and one in 100,000 live births. Approximately 50 cases have been reported. The cause of the syndrome has been proposed to be the impairment of blood supply to the developing field structures.

Prenatally, if hand and chest deformities are severe, it may be possible to identify the condition via ULTRASOUND and FETOSCOPY.

## polycystic kidney disease (PKD)    A group of disorders characterized by fluid-filled sacs (cysts) that slowly develop in both kidneys, eventually resulting in kidney malfunctioning. A high proportion of affected individuals develop kidney failure, requiring dialysis or kidney transplant. It is the third leading cause of kidney failure in the United States.

One kidney can contain several hundred of these cysts, which form on the renal tubules, normal structures within the kidney. The cysts cause the kidneys to swell, often to several times their normal size, and can cause pain, blood in the urine, and kidney stones. They can also be associated with liver cysts and aneurysms in the brain or abdomen. Forty percent to 60% of PKD patients develop polycystic livers.

PKD is a GENETIC DISORDER and occurs in two forms: one inherited in AUTOSOMAL DOMINANT manner is slowly progressive, leading to chronic renal failure. It is a common disorder, estimated to affect as many as 300,000 to 500,000 Americans, and is found in all races and ethnic groups. Some cases may be the result of new MUTATION. The less common AUTOSOMAL RECESSIVE form causes a severe kidney disease in infancy, with death in infancy or childhood.

The dominant form, sometimes referred to as adult PKD, may remain dormant until middle age, when symptoms of abdominal pain or blood in the urine may appear. Hypertension is found in about half of all PKD patients, apparently the result of increased production of the hormone angiotensin in the kidney, which elevates blood pressure, caused by the expanding kidney cysts. It is the most common genetic kidney disease.

There is wide variability in expression of the disorder, with many affected individuals remaining unaware of the condition throughout their lives. However, there is generally consistency within families in the degree of severity and the age of onset. About half of all PKD patients ultimately develop kidney failure.

Diagnosis is made through a physical examination that may include CAT scan (computerized axial tomography) and sonogram to detect the development of cysts in the kidneys. Familial history can also play an important role in diagnosis.

The cause for the abnormal growth of kidney tubule cells that result in the disorder is unknown. However, it appears the cells that form the cysts operate in a way similar to simple benign tumors. Unlike tumors, these cells promote the accumulation of fluid as well as tissue mass.

It is believed more than one gene locus may play a role in the development of PKD. This is an example of genetic heterogeneity, whereby a single disorder may result from any one of several defects. One gene that appears responsible for PKD has been found on the short arm of CHROMOSOME 16. Other cases appear to be caused by different genes. In families where linkage to chromosome 16 can be demonstrated, GENETIC MARKERS can be used for presymptomatic or PRENATAL DIAGNOSIS.

The recessive form of PKD has been called infantile polycystic kidney disease. In addition to malfunctioning kidneys, infants may exhibit a characteristic "Potter's face" (squashed nose, small jaw and large, floppy, low-set ears), resembling a face pressed against a window pane, caused by the compression against the walls of the uterus due to lack of AMNIOTIC FLUID. (It is named for the physician who described the condition.) The amniotic fluid is mostly made up of fetal urine, which here is deficient because of the fetal kidney disease. Few affected newborns survive infancy. Often the lungs have been underdeveloped. There have been reports of successful prenatal diagnosis in this form of PKD, using ULTRASOUND. The incidence is approximately one in 40,000.

Polycystic kidneys are also associated with several genetic syndromes, including EHLERS-DANLOS SYNDROME, TUBEROUS SCLEROSIS, MECKEL SYNDROME, ZELLWEGER SYNDROME and trisomy 13.

For more information, contact:

PKR (Polycystic Kidney Research)
   Foundation
922 Walnut Street
Kansas City, MO 64106
(816) 421-1869

**polydactyly**   Having more than the normal number of fingers or toes.

This condition is seen in many GENETIC DISORDERS and also exists as an isolated malformation occurring in several forms, distinguished by the position and degree of definition of the extra digits. One inherited form, transmitted as an AUTOSOMAL DOMINANT trait, is 10 times more frequent in blacks than in whites. In this form there is an extra digit after the fifth finger. A survey in Nigeria in 1976 found incidence of approximately 18 per 1,000 for females and 27 per 1,000 for males.

Polydactyly has an important place in the history of genetics. In the 1750s French naturalist Pierre Louis Moreau de Maupertuis (1698–1759) published the pedigree of Haboc Ruhe, a surgeon of Berlin, who had extra digits on all four limbs, a trait he inherited from his mother and grandmother, and which

he transmitted to two sons out of six children. Maupertuis invoked "elementary particles" as the hereditary transmission agent, interpreting the pedigree in terms that presaged Mendel's theories of inheritance, which came over a century later.

**polygenic**   An inherited trait caused by the action of two or more GENES. Though sometimes used interchangeably with MULTI-FACTORIAL, multifactorial is more properly a term for disorders caused by the combined action of one or more genes, environmental influences and other unknown factors. In fact, most traits labeled polygenic are actually mutifactorial; that is, environment plays a role in their expression.

**polymastia**   The growth of more than two breasts or nipples. Complete extra mammary glands are rare; more commonly extra nipples appear. It is usually detectable at birth, but in some cases, development occurs only after puberty or pregnancy.

The majority of excess glands are located in the "milkline"—the area between the armpits and the groin, but, in rare instances, accessory breasts have appeared on the face, neck, arms, thighs, buttocks and back. They occur more frequently on the left side than on the right side of the body and single additional breasts or nipples are more common than multiple ones.

Accessory breasts undergo the same cyclic changes as normal breasts and are prone to the same diseases, such as breast CANCER. It is not known, however, if tumors are more common in normal breasts or in accessory breasts.

Extra breasts located above the normal breast area typically are positioned toward the outside of the body; when located below the normal breast area, the extra breasts are positioned toward the midline of the body. The outer-positioned glands are usually well-formed and can lactate, while the medial glands are imperfectly developed and cannot.

Occurrence is estimated at a remarkably high one in 100 in the general population, and reports of prevalence have ranged from one in 17 in New York females to one in 250 British children. In whites, nearly 90% of accessory breasts are located below the normal breasts and affect men more frequently than women. For the Japanese, however, about 90% of accessory breasts are located above normal breasts, and incidence for females is three times as great as males.

Polymastia is inherited as an AUTOSOMAL DOMINANT trait in some families, though the exact genetic basis in the majority of cases is unclear.

**polymorphism**    The multiple variations of a given gene or GENES; the ability of a GENETIC DISORDER to appear in more than one form.

A RESTRICTION FRAGMENT LENGTH POLY-MORPHISM is a variation in DNA sequence (see DEOXYRIBONUCLEIC ACID). These polymorphisms are often useful as GENETIC MARKERS for linkage analysis. Individual fragments can be identified on the basis of the difference in length of DNA generated after the DNA is cleaved with a RESTRICTION ENZYME.

**polyposis**    See familial polyposis syndromes under CANCER.

**polysplenia syndrome**    Malformation and duplication of internal organs characterize this rare CONGENITAL disorder. Affected individuals develop two spleens instead of the normal one, and may have one or more additional small spleens (splenules). Furthermore, in organs and organ pairs that are normally not symmetrical, the right side develops as a mirror image of the left side. For example, the right side of the lung normally has a distinctive branch of the bronchial tubes (the epiarterial bronchus), but in about 70% of individuals with this syndrome it matches the left lung. Likewise, the right and left lobes of the liver are of equal size, and the stomach

may appear on either the left or right side (situs inversus). Intestinal defects are also common.

A range of heart malformations are usually present, such as abnormal return of venous blood to the right and left atria. Defects in the membranes of the heart that separate the chambers also occur (see CONGENITAL HEART DEFECTS).

Life span depends on the severity of heart defects. In extreme cases, insufficiency of oxygen (cyanosis), difficulty breathing and feeding and congestive heart failure cause death within days or weeks of birth. When there are few or no cardiac abnormalities, individuals live to adulthood.

The basic cause and genetics of the disorder are unknown.

A similar "laterality sequence" with bilateral right-sidedness also exists and is the ASPLENIA SYNDROME, where there is no spleen but also complex heart disease.

**polysyndactyly**    The condition in which an individual has a greater than normal number of digits (fingers or toes) in association with fusion of the digits. The extra digits vary from well-formed to mere skin tags, and the fusion varies from webbing of the skin between the digits to complete joining of bones of the digits. This condition is seen in a number of genetic disorders. (POLYDACTYLY indicates having extra digits; SYNDACTYLY indicates the webbing of digits.)

**Pompe's disease**    See GLYCOGEN STORAGE DISEASE, type II.

**porencephaly**    Abnormal cavities within the brain. The condition may involve one side of the brain (unilateral) or both (bilateral).

Type I, the unilateral form, usually results from birth trauma, infection or fetal vascular occlusions and lack of blood supply. As a result of these insults there is destruction and death of brain tissue. As these necrotic regions of brain dissolve, cavities remain and become cysts within the substance of the brain.

Type II is usually bilateral and symmetrical, that is, the abnormal cavities in the cerebral hemispheres mirror each other. This form represents a primary defect in the development of embryonic nerve tissue. A familial component of this form was first reported in 1983, with inheritance suggested as AUTOSOMAL DOMINANT. Increased access to computerized axial tomography (CAT) scans may enable the identification of more affected individuals. Individuals with porencephalic cysts may exhibit neurologic deficits (including seizures or CEREBRAL PALSY) or may be completely asymptomatic with relatively normal development. The cysts may be identified by prenatal ULTRASOUND.

**porphyria** Porphyrins are a group of nitrogen-containing organic compounds that form the basis of animal and plant respiratory pigments. In humans, they form heme, the iron-containing and oxygen-carrying portion of hemoglobin, and in plants, they form chlorophyll. "Porphyria" refers to a group of inborn errors of metabolism in which porphyrin is not converted to heme in a normal fashion, resulting in the accumulation of porphyrin or "porphyrin precursors" in the body. This causes disturbances in the nervous system or the skin. The symptoms may include acute episodes of abdominal pain, psychological disturbances and photosensitivity of the skin, causing burning, blistering and scarring of areas exposed to the sun. The dermatological eruptions are thought to result from the effect of long-wave ultraviolet light on porphyrins that have accumulated in the skin.

The name of the disorder is taken from the Greek *porphyrus*, meaning purple, due to the tendency of some affected individuals to excrete purplish or reddish urine due to the presence of excess porphyrins. The urine may also darken after prolonged exposure to light.

The formation of heme is an eight-step process, each step requiring a specific enzyme.

Each form of porphyria (seven have been identified) results from a deficiency of the specific enzyme necessary for each step of this process.

Additionally, the porphyrias are subclassified in other ways. In hepatic porphyria, the excess porphyrins and porphyrin precursors originate mostly in the liver. In erythropoietic porphyria, they originate primarily in the bone marrow. Porphyrias that primarily affect the skin are referred to as cutaneous, while those involving the nervous system are referred to as acute.

There is great variability of severity among the forms of porphyria—and even of symptoms among individuals with a single form. It is believed that many who have enzyme deficiencies responsible for the disorder may never exhibit symptoms. These individuals are said to be latent, while those who exhibit symptoms are said to be active.

The great variability of symptoms often makes diagnosis difficult. While porphyrias are inherited, attacks are often triggered by non-genetic factors, an important example of genetic-environmental interaction.

Diagnosis of the porphyrias generally involves measurement of urinary and fecal porphyrias and enzyme assay in red cells, liver or fibroblasts.

*Acute intermittent porphyria (AIP).* Active cases have their onset after puberty, and are more commonly seen in women than in men. Abdominal pain, which can be severe, is the most frequent symptom. There may also be nausea, vomiting, constipation, muscle weakness, urinary retention, pain in the back, arms and legs, heart palpitations, confusion, hallucinations and seizures. Symptoms usually resolve following attacks. The skin is not affected.

Inherited as an AUTOSOMAL DOMINANT trait, it is caused by the deficiency of the ENZYME porphobilinogen deaminase (PBG-D), also known as uroporphyrinogen I-synthase. However, this deficiency alone will not cause the disorder, and it must be accompanied by hormonal drug or dietary changes in order to provoke symptoms. Most cases remain latent.

Incidence in all ethnic groups is thought to be in the order of one in 50,000 live births. However, actual incidence may be much higher, due to the number of latent cases that remain undiagnosed. As many as 90% of individuals with AIP are thought never to be detected. This form of porphyria is known to also have a high incidence in northern Sweden, perhaps as high as one in 1,000 live births.

It has been suggested that King George III of England suffered from AIP, traceable to Mary, Queen of Scots. However, many contemporary authorities doubt this contention. While he exhibited a disorder virtually indistinguishable from AIP, symptoms of skin involvement in other members of the royal family make it more plausible that "the royal malady" from which he suffered was Variegate Porphyria.

Management includes general supportive therapy, high carbohydrate intake, intravenous hematin and prevention through avoiding known precipitants.

*Congenital erythropoietic porphyria (CEP) (Gunther's disease).* Characterized by extreme photosensitivity, the disorder has its onset in infancy. Red urine may be present. Porphyrin accumulates throughout the body, and the teeth may also become red-stained. The skin may exhibit blistering, severe scarring and increased hair growth (hypertrichosis). Bacterial infection may occur at the site of skin lesions. The disease is mutilating; eventually facial features and fingers may be lost as a result of the disease process. Red blood cells have a shortened lifespan, and ANEMIA may result. Prognosis is poor; few survive beyond 40 years.

The condition is considered extremely rare. Less than 100 cases have been reported since it was first described in 1874. (H. Gunther published a more definitive description in 1911.) Inherited as an AUTOSOMAL RECESSIVE trait, the deficient enzyme is uroporphyrinogen III cosynthase. A similar disorder has been observed in several animal species, including cattle, swine and cats. It has been suggested that the "werewolves" of legend may have suffered from CEP or some severe cutaneous porphyria. It is felt that accounts of magical transformation into wolves were attempts to explain their subjects' mutilated skin, hypertrichosis, red teeth and urine, and desire to avoid light exposure.

*Porphyria cutanea tarda (PCT).* This is the most common form of porphyria, and symptoms are confined to the skin. Onset is usually between the ages of 10 and 30. Blistering after minor trauma or exposure to sunlight may occur on the hands, face and other exposed areas, often developing into chronic ulcerating lesions. There may also be increased hair growth (hypertrichosis) and darkening (hyperpigmentation) and thickening of the skin.

PCT occurs in both hereditary (AUTOSOMAL DOMINANT) and acquired forms, and results from the deficiency of uroporphyrinogen decarboxylase (URO-D). It is a hepatic (involving the liver) form of porphyria, with huge amounts of porphyrins sometimes building up in the liver when the disease becomes active. However, in most individuals with the inherited enzyme deficiency, the disorder remains latent.

The acquired form may be triggered by alcohol or estrogens such as those found in oral contraceptives and drugs for treatment of prostate cancer.

While no reliable figures for incidence are available, it may be the most common form of porphyria, and is particularly common in the Bantu of South Africa.

*Hereditary coproporphyria (HCP).* This is a hepatic form, similar to acute intermittent porphyria, though generally less severe in its manifestation. Skin photosensitivity develops in some individuals (1/3). Inherited as an AUTOSOMAL DOMINANT trait, the deficient enzyme is coproporphyrinogen oxidase.

*Variegate porphyria.*   Affected adults display variable photosensitive skin symptoms, including darkening of the skin (hyperpigmentation) and excessive hair growth (hypertrichosis). There are also protracted acute attacks similar to those of AIP, with severe abdominal pain, constipation, heart palpitations, hypertension, muscular paralysis, sensory disturbances, disorientation and psychosis. Attacks may be followed by prolonged disability.

This hepatic form is inherited as an AUTOSOMAL DOMINANT trait, and the deficient enzyme is believed to be protoporphyrinogen oxidase. While infrequent in the general population, it has a high incidence among the white population of South Africa. This disorder is a primary example of the "founder effect." It is believed that all those in South Africa suffering from the disorder inherited it either from Gerrit Jansz, a Dutch settler in the Cape, or his wife, Ariaantje Jacobs, who was one of a group of women sent from an orphanage in Rotterdam to provide wives for Dutch settlers. The prevalence among the white Afrikaans-speaking population of the Eastern Cape region may be as high as one in 250.

*Erythropoietic protoporphyria (EPP).*  As the name implies, protoporphyrin accumulates primarily in the bone marrow and red blood cells (erythrocytes; poietic is a suffix that means "making or producing"). In some cases it may accumulate in the liver as well. Onset is typically in childhood.

It is characterized by swelling, burning, itching and redness of the skin during or immediately after exposure to sunlight, even when the rays pass through a window. These symptoms typically disappear in 12 to 24 hours after exposure and leave no significant scarring or skin discoloration. However, the skin eruptions may progress to a chronic state, with lesions persisting for weeks and leaving slight scars upon healing. Attacks are usually more severe in summer and may last throughout life. Occasionally,

affected individuals may have severe liver complications.

It is inherited as an AUTOSOMAL DOMINANT trait, and the deficient enzyme is ferrochelatase.

For more information, contact:

American Porphyria Foundation
P.O. Box 11163
Montgomery, AL 36111
(205) 265-2200

**porphyria cutanea tarda**    See PORPHYRIA.

**port wine stain**    A BIRTHMARK of a well-defined patch of pink, red or purplish-colored skin, so named because the characteristic color resembles that of port wine. Most often seen on the face, it is caused by a collection of blood vessels beneath the skin that are abnormal either in their excessive number or in their degree of dilation. (Such an abnormal collection of vessels is called a HEMANGIOMA.) The increased blood flow this allows causes the discoloration in the skin over the affected area. The blood vessels are believed to be remnants of blood vessels present in the first month of embryonic life, though the cause of their retention is unknown.

Port wine stain may appear in isolation or as a feature of another condition or syndrome. It is commonly associated with STURGE-WEBER SYNDROME and KLIPPEL-TRENAUNAY-WEBER SYNDROME.

The size of the birthmark grows as the body does. After the age of 30, it may darken and become thicker than surrounding skin, and benign purplish skin growths may also appear.

Incidence of port wine stain is estimated at three per 1,000 live births. Mikhail Gorbachev, president of the Soviet Union, has a port wine stain on his forehead. The majority of cases that are not associated with other conditions appear to be SPORADIC. Recently, laser surgery has been successful in treating affected areas of skin in some individuals.

For more information, contact:

National Congenital Port Wine Stain
  Foundation
123 East 63rd Street
New York, NY 10021
(212) 755-3820

**posterior choanal atresia**     A life-threatening condition caused by the failure of the opening between the nasal passages and the airway to develop, which causes a blockage of the nasal passage. This creates a serious problem because newborns normally breathe through their nose, and must learn to breathe through their mouths. Since they have not learned mouth breathing, and the normal nasal passage is blocked, affected infants exhibit severe respiratory problems.

The genetics of this disorder are poorly understood. Like CLEFT LIP and cleft palate, it is most likely a MULTIFACTORIAL trait. It has been reported in both affected single and successive generations, with about 8% of the cases being familial. In familial cases it is inherited as an AUTOSOMAL RECESSIVE trait. It occurs twice as often in females as in males and more frequently in the right side than the left side of the nose.

Choanal atresia is a feature of the CHARGE ASSOCIATION.

**post term pregnancy**     A pregnancy that continues beyond the normal gestation period of approximately 40 weeks. Post term pregnancies are associated with an increase in complications, fetal distress and death during delivery.

It is estimated that as many as 7% of pregnant women have not delivered two weeks after their due date. If the pregnancy lasts beyond 42 weeks, the placenta ages and becomes less efficient at supplying oxygen and nutrients to the fetus. As a result, postmature babies tend to be born long and thin.

Obstetricians generally begin testing a week after the anticipated delivery date to determine if it is safe to allow the pregnancy to continue. If labor does not occur spontaneously, it may be induced with drugs, or the baby may be delivered via CESARIAN SECTION.

**Prader-Willi syndrome (PWS)**     Disorder characterized by OBESITY, MENTAL RETARDATION, poor development of the genitals and adult short stature. It is named for Swiss pediatricians Andrea Prader and H. Willi who described it in 1956, though it appears it was mentioned by Langdon-Down (for whom Down syndrome is named) in 1887. In "Mental Affections of Childhood and Youth," describing a case of what he called "polysarcia" in a retarded 25-year-old, who, with a height of little more than 4 feet 4 inches (130.2 cm), weighed over 200 pounds, Langdon-Down discussed the disparity between the small hands and feet and general obesity that is a hallmark of this condition. "Her feet and hands remained small and contrasted remarkably with the appendages they terminated . . . She had scarcely any [hair] on the pubis. She had never menstruated, nor did she exhibit the slightest sexual instinct."

At birth, individuals present a FLOPPY INFANT appearance (hypotonia), weigh a few hundred grams below average and exhibit feeding problems and poor swallowing and sucking reflexes. Their cry may be weak, and they may be unable to control their head and limbs. The face is also characteristic, with prominent forehead, poorly formed ears and a triangular-shaped upper lip. The eyes may be crossed, with uncoordinated focusing (STRABISMUS).

Developmental milestones (sitting, standing, walking, talking) are usually retarded. Physically, they lack large muscle strength and endurance and have poor balance and coordination. As infants grow, they become more lively and develop insatiable appetites. Compulsive overeating (hyperphagia) appears, on the average, at just under three years of age.

They may eat the food of house pets or food from the garbage. If eating is not controlled, obesity is usually prominent before five years of age, with a disproportionate amount of fat accumulating in the central body, lower trunk and buttocks.

The ravenous desire for food is due to a dysfunction of the central nervous system. Individuals will eat any time food is available and will not stop eating of their own accord. Additionally, they require fewer calories than average persons in order to gain weight. Exercise is difficult due to their poor muscle development.

Limiting access to food is of primary importance. In order to monitor consumption, parents are generally advised that refrigerators must be kept locked, and individuals must be monitored at all times. This becomes difficult as children age.

The degree of MENTAL RETARDATION is variable, with IQs typically in the 70s, though scores below 40 and above 100 have been found. Affected children are described as happy, friendly and cooperative, but capable of exhibiting extreme frustration, negativism and temper tantrums when denied unlimited food.

Genital abnormalities typically consist of a small penis and scrotum, often with undescended testes (CRYPTORCHISM) in males and poorly formed labia in females. Puberty is delayed and diminished. Males retain a high-pitched voice. Adult height is always below the 50th percentile.

Diabetes often appears during childhood or adolescence, and many individuals are said to exhibit excessive sleepiness (somnolence).

Independent living is rarely achieved. Life expectancy is diminished due to respiratory insufficiency. Death may also result from cardiorespiratory embarrassment (see PICKWICKIAN SYNDROME) or, more rarely, diabetic complications.

PRENATAL DIAGNOSIS is not currently available. The cause of the disorder is unknown. Almost all cases have been SPORADIC, though some have been attributed to AUTOSOMAL DOMINANT inheritance. CHROMOSOME ABNORMALITIES have been identified in about half of those screened, with an interstitial deletion of chromosome 15 the most common. Over 200 cases have been reported. Twice as many affected males as affected females have been identified, but that may be because it is easier to distinguish the genital abnormalities that help identify this condition in males than in females. (See also IMPRINTING.)

For more information, contact:

Prader-Willi Syndrome Association
6490 Excelsior Blvd., E-102
St. Louis Park, MN 55426
(612) 926-1947

**precocious puberty**    The appearance of sexual characteristics at a very early age, usually defined as before 10 years in males and 8.5 years in females. It has been reported as early as age three. Approximately one in every 10,000 children starts puberty prematurely. Boys grow facial, pubic and underarm hair, are prone to develop acne, and the penis and testicles enlarge. Viable sperm may be produced. Girls may develop breasts, grow pubic and underarm hair, menstruate and may ovulate. Adult height in both males and females is usually reduced.

Though it is usually of unknown origin (idiopathic), familial cases of precocious puberty have been observed. While in general precocious puberty is much more common in females than males, hereditary forms are more common in males.

Perhaps 5% to 10% of these males brought to medical attention have inherited precocious puberty. Two AUTOSOMAL DOMINANT forms have been identified. Less than 1% of affected females inherit the condition, and the mode of inheritance for the female form is unknown.

Precocious puberty may also be a feature of MCCUNE-ALBRIGHT SYNDROME, NEUROFIBROMATOSIS, RUSSELL-SILVER SYNDROME and disorders of the adrenal glands.

Affected individuals may encounter psychological problems due to their accelerated growth and may feel alienated from their peers. They may exhibit increased aggressiveness and hyperactivity.

For more information, contact:

National Institute of Child Health and
   Human Development
9000 Rockville Pike
Bethesda, MD 20892
(301) 496-5133

**premature birth**    See PREMATURITY;
LOW BIRTH WEIGHT.

**prematurity**    Birth before the completion of full gestational development or before the 37th week of pregnancy. (The normal human gestation period is 40 weeks.) Prematurity is associated with an increased incidence of infant health problems and death. Approximately 45,000 infant deaths are recorded annually in the United States, and two-thirds of these deaths are of infants who were born prematurely, though not all these deaths can be attributed to prematurity alone.

In 1981 the World Health Organization recommended replacing the designation "Prematurity" with LOW BIRTH WEIGHT. Low birth weight infants may be born early and thus be small, or may be born at term but be growth retarded.

For a further discussion of congenital problems associated with prematurity, see the Low Birth Weight entry.

**prenatal diagnosis**    Any of a number of procedures for identifying the presence of a CONGENITAL or HEREDITARY condition before birth.

A broad spectrum of prenatal diagnosis procedures is available, enabling physicians to confirm or rule out many fetal disorders. These diagnostic procedures can involve both invasive and noninvansive techniques. Invasive procedures include AMNIOCENTESIS, FETOSCOPY and CHORIONIC VILLUS SAMPLING, which is followed by analysis using DNA PROBES, CHROMOSOME analyses and BIO-

CHEMICAL ASSAYS. In amniocentesis, a needle is inserted through the mother's abdominal wall and a sample of the AMNIOTIC FLUID is withdrawn for analysis. In fetoscopy, a thin tube is inserted through the abdomen into the uterus to enable visual inspection of the fetus and the obtaining of fetal blood and tissue samples. Chorionic villus sampling involves the use of either a catheter inserted into the uterus or a needle inserted through the abdomen to obtain tissue samples from projections on the membrane around the fetus. Thus DNA probes, chromosome analyses and biochemical assays depend on invasive procedures to obtain the fetal samples needed.

Noninvasive procedures primarily involve testing maternal blood for the level of ALPHA-FETOPROTEIN and using ULTRASOUND to visualize an image of the fetus in the uterus. X rays may also be used for FETAL IMAGING.

Which prenatal diagnostic procedure is used depends on the type of information being sought. The physician examines not only the patient herself but also carefully checks the previous medical history and available aspects of the family medical history of both parents for clues that may indicate the need for prenatal diagnosis. GENETIC COUNSELING is therefore a critical component of prenatal diagnosis.

Not all congenital and GENETIC DISORDERS can be diagnosed prenatally, and since prenatal diagnosis procedures involve some attendant risks to the fetus, it is usually indicated as a diagnostic tool only when certain conditions exist. (At the beginning of the 1990s, approximately 250 congenital and genetic disorders could be diagnosed prenatally.) If, for example, the mother is 35 or older, prenatal diagnosis is often offered because advanced maternal age increases the risk of conceiving a child with DOWN SYNDROME. Other conditions for which prenatal diagnosis is indicated include a previous birth of a child with a chromosomal ANOMALY or one parent known to have such an anomaly; a family history of children born with NEURAL TUBE DEFECTS; a screening test that discloses elevated levels of alpha-fetoprotein; a previous birth of a SIB-LING with a genetic or metabolic disorder; and parents who are confirmed or suspected CAR-RIERS of a genetic disorder. Prenatal diagnosis is considered as one of the reproductive options available for couples at risk for genetic or congenital diseases. (See also "INTRODUC-TION.")

**primidone** See ANTICONVULSANTS.

**proband** The first person within a family who is identified as having a particular inherited disorder, or the individual who first presents a mental or physical disorder that prompts the study of the person's family in an effort to identify a potential genetic link to the abnormality. It is necessary to establish this link (if it exists) for proper diagnosis and treatment. (A synonym for the proband is the propositus, or index case.) (See also PEDIGREE.)

**progeria** (Hutchinson-Gilford progeria syndrome) A rare genetic disorder resulting in premature aging. The name is derived from Greek, meaning "prematurely old." The classic type was first described independently by English surgeons Jonathan Hutchinson (1828–1913) and Hastings Gilford (1861–1941) in 1886. Gilford coined the term progeria in 1904.

The condition is characterized by DWARF-ISM, baldness, a pinched nose, small face and small jaw (micrognathia), delayed tooth formation and aged-looking skin. Intelligence is normal or above average. The voice is thin and high-pitched. Sexual maturation does not occur. Veins of the scalp are clearly visible. Joints are stiff. There is mild flexion of the knees, producing a "horse-riding" stance. As they age, there are frequent hip dislocations, generalized hardening of the arteries (atherosclerosis) and cardiac problems. Death from coronary artery disease is common and may occur before age 10. Over 80% of deaths are due to heart attacks or congestive heart failure. The average life expectancy is 12 to 14 years of age. One affected individual was still alive at age 29.

Many Americans first became aware of this disorder in 1981, when the news media reported on the meeting of two affected children, one from South Africa and one from Texas, at Disneyland.

The cause is unknown. It is thought to be an AUTOSOMAL DOMINANT trait, with all cases being the result of new MUTATIONS occurring at the time of conception. Several facts point to dominant mutation: First-degree relatives (parents, SIBLINGS) are almost never affected, and there is a low frequency of parental CON-SANGUINITY among affected individuals. Additionally, there appears to be a correlation between incidence and increased paternal age, indicating a potential mutative effect.

Some researchers believe an understanding of the disorder could provide clues to the aging process, since it mimics some aspects of natural aging. (However, unlike normal aging, affected individuals don't exhibit degenerative joint disease, CANCER, CATARACTS, DIA-BETES MELLITUS or senile dementia.)

The syndrome has an incidence estimated at between one in four million and one in eight million live births. More than 100 cases have been described around the world since it was first described.

There is no specific diagnostic test for the condition. Diagnosis is made on the basis of the physical appearance. It is usually diagnosed in the first or second year, when skin changes and failure to gain weight become apparent. Affected individuals have been found to have elevated levels of hyaluronic acid in their urine, which can be helpful in diagnosing the condition. Currently, PRENA-TAL DIAGNOSIS for this condition is not available. (See also WERNER SYNDROME.)

For more information, contact:

Progeria International Registry
Department of Human Genetics
Institute for Basic Research in
    Developmental Disabilities

1050 Forest Hill Road
Staten Island, NY 10314
(718) 494-0600

**prolonged QT interval**   See ROMANO-
WARD SYNDROME.

**propionic acidemia**   A rare inherited
deficiency of propionyl CoA carboxylase, an
ENZYME that breaks down ketoacids. As a
result of the enzyme deficiency, ketoacids
build up to toxic levels, as identified by an
increased concentration of glycine in the
blood, elevated concentrations of propionic
acid and its precursors and metabolites in
urine, and high concentrations of ketones in
the urine.

Signs of the disorder early in infancy include recurring episodes of ketoacidosis,
characterized by nausea and vomiting, "air
hunger," or gasping for breath in an attempt to
compensate for the acidosis, a fruity odor to
the breath, abdominal tenderness and extreme
thirst and dry mucous membranes. Ketoacidosis rapidly leads to coma and death, and few
children with propionic acidosis survive infancy. Recently, a low protein diet has shown
some promise in treatment.

Those who do survive infancy exhibit MEN-
TAL RETARDATION and a variety of neurological abnormalities. Neutropenia (a decrease in
the number of blood granulocytes) leads to
frequent infections, and thrombocytopenia (a
decrease in the number of platelets) is associated with temporary episodes of purpura, a
condition characterized by multiple hemorrhages just under the skin. There may also be
thinning of the bones (osteoporosis) and subsequent fractures.

The disorder is inherited as an AUTOSOMAL
RECESSIVE trait. The definitive diagnosis is
established by demonstrating the enzyme defects in cultured skin cells. Reduced activities
have been observed in cell cultures from CAR-
RIERS, and PRENATAL DIAGNOSIS has been
carried out on cultured fetal cells collected by
AMNIOCENTESIS and CHORIONIC VILLUS SAM-
PLING.

**propositus**   See PROBAND.

**protanomaly**   See COLOR BLINDNESS.

**protanopia**   See COLOR BLINDNESS.

**protective exclusion**   The workplace
policy of excluding women who are pregnant,
fertile or of child-bearing age from jobs that
may endanger fetal health. The policy has
been adopted by some manufacturing and
chemical companies. Studies have found increased rates of msicarriage (see ABORTION)
and BIRTH DEFECTS in certain workplace en-
vironments, such as in manufacturing processes involving toxic chemicals. Protective
exclusion has also been practiced in hospitals
and research labs, the semiconductor industry
and among workers using VIDEO DISPLAY
TERMINALS.

The Equal Employment Opportunity Commission estimates at least 100,000 jobs in the
United States are closed to women due to the
risk to fetal health. (Reproductive disorders
rank in the top 10 work-related illnesses and
injuries, according to data from the National
Institute of Occupational Safety and Health,
and more than 14 million workers a year may
be exposed to known or suspected reproductive hazards on the job.) While the extent of
the reproductive risks for males in these envi-
ronments is unknown, few companies exclude
them from jobs from which they bar women
for reproductive reasons.

The legality of the policy is unclear. Title
VII of the Civil Rights Act prohibits sex discrimination in employment, but court decisions on the permissibility of protective
exclusion have varied. The issue first came to
public attention in the latter 1970s, when several women sued the American Cyanamid
Company for violating their civil rights,
claiming they had to undergo sterilization to
keep their high-paying jobs in the company's
West Virginia lead pigment plant. They settled their claims for $200,000. Subsequently,
federal courts have barred companies from
excluding women from workplace environ-

ments that present reproductive risks. More recently, however, in a case involving a Milwaukee manufacturer that prohibited all fertile women from working in its battery-making operations, appeals courts have reached contradictory verdicts.

Where companies have no policy of protective exclusion, workers have sometimes demanded the right to transfer out of jobs they perceive as presenting reproductive risks. For example, several unions, including the Communications Workers of America, have won the right for their pregnant members to temporarily transfer away from video display terminal work without a loss of pay or seniority.

**proteus syndrome**   This disorder, possibly first described in 1976, was named in 1983 by German pediatrician Hans Rudolf Wiedemann; it is characterized by grossly enlarged hands and feet, multiple nevi on the skin, distorted abnormal growth of half of the body (hemihypertrophy) and gigantism of the head. It is named for the Greek god Proteus, "the polymorphous," presumably because of the variable manifestations in the four unrelated boys first identified as having the syndrome. While it is apparently a genetic disorder, its mode of inheritance is unknown, though AUTOSOMAL DOMINANT transmission has been suggested. All cases to date have been SPORADIC.

It has been suggested that this is the condition that afflicted the Elephant Man, rather than NEUROFIBROMATOSIS, as has been generally accepted.

**prune-belly syndrome**   The most obvious manifestation of this CONGENITAL disorder in newborns is a large, thin-walled protuberant abdomen covered with many loose folds of skin (hence the name "prune belly"); caused by an abdominal muscle development deficiency (hypoplasia). The internal abdominal organs can be felt and examined with the fingers, and the wavelike and rhythmic movement (peristalsis) of the intestines can be seen through the thin abdom-

inal walls. The two other associated major congenital defects are undescended testicles (CRYPTORCHISM) and urinary tract abnormalities, which include dilation of the bladder (megalocystis), gross distension of the ureter (hydroureter) caused by blockage of the urine, swelling of the collecting systems of the kidney due to blocked urine (hydronephrosis), and abnormal development (dysplasia) of the kidneys.

Hip dysplasia is common. Approximately 40% of affected infants have CLUBFEET (talipes equinovarus), 30% have CONGENITAL HEART DEFECTS and 30% show intestinal abnormalities such as failure of the bowel to develop normally during embryonic growth, and hardening (calcification) of tissue in the colon.

This disorder occurs about once in every 50,000 births. It affects mostly males; only about 5% are females, who are mildly affected and have no severe urinary tract involvement. The exact genetic cause is not clear. It is suspected that the disorder results from a localized defect in the mesoderm, a cell layer in the embryo that develops into connective tissue.

About 20% of those affected are STILLBORN or die within a month of birth. Fifty percent die within two years, mainly due to urinary tract infection or kidney failure. Prenatal testing may disclose elevated levels of ALPHA-FETOPROTEIN produced by the fetus in the maternal blood or AMNIOTIC FLUID. ULTRASOUND examination may detect an abnormally small amount of amniotic fluid (oligohydramnios), an enlarged bladder, or pooling of fluid in the fetal abdominal cavity (ascites).

**pseudohermaphroditism**   A general term for several forms of AMBIGUOUS GENITALIA, anomalies of the external sex organs. Unlike true hermaphrodites, these individuals have the internal sexual organs of only one gender. Females exhibit various degrees of external sexual ambiguity, depending on the form, and may be raised as males. Males exhibit the same spectrum of variation and cross-gender rearing. Individuals usually come to medical attention due to abnormalities of pubertal development. (See also ADRENOGENITAL SYNDROMES; TESTICULAR FEMINIZATiON SYNDROME.)

**pseudo-Hurler polydystrophy**   See MUCOLIPIDOSIS.

**pseudohypoparathyroidism**   See ALBRIGHT HEREDITARY OSTEODYSTROPHY.

**pseudo thalidomide syndrome**   See ROBERTS SYNDROME.

**pseudoxanthoma elasticum**   A chronic degenerative skin and arterial disease, signs of which can become apparent anytime from birth to the thirties or forties. There are four different forms, two caused by AUTOSOMAL RECESSIVE inheritance (most common) and two by AUTOSOMAL DOMINANT inheritance. General characteristics of the disorder include skin alterations, failing vision brought on by retinal hemorrhages, weak pulses in the limbs, persistent high blood pressure (hypertension), severe chest pain from lack of blood flow to the heart due to coronary artery disease (angina pectoris) and dizzy spells. There are also visual and speech disturbances and other stroke symptoms (transient cerebral ischemic attacks) brought on by thickening of artery walls (arteriosclerosis). Abdominal pain is common due to constriction of the celiac artery, which supplies the abdominal region, as is severe pain in calf muscles while walking (intermittent claudication) and gastrointestinal bleeding caused by degeneration of the elastic fibers in the arteries of the walls of the gastrointestinal tract.

The skin alterations include a thickening and loss of elasticity, with raised, yellowish, pebble-like areas (nodules) appearing in mucous membranes of the mouth, cheek and inner lips, and also in the armpits, groin, around the navel and on the neck, where the skin will be loose and folded.

The combined prevalence of all four forms of this disorder is approximately one in every 40,000 live births. Intelligence is normal, though life span is significantly shortened by complications of internal bleeding and arterial blockages. The disorder involves abnormalities in connective tissue whereby the elastic fibers become fragmented and calcified, though the basic defect involved is unknown.

Currently, there is no method for PRENATAL DIAGNOSIS for this disorder or for identifying CARRIERS of the trait.

**psoriasis**   Inflammation of the skin (dermatitis) characterized by pink or dull red lesions covered by silvery scales. Demonstrated to occur in a hereditary form, it is the most common scaling skin disease, affecting 1% to 3% of the white population (and a smaller percentage of blacks) and may be severe and disabling. It is rare in Eskimos, American Indians and Japanese. Though all forms of inheritance have been reported, except for those families in which it is clearly inherited as an AUTOSOMAL DOMINANT trait, MULTIFACTORIAL inheritance seems to be the most likely cause. A survey in Denmark's Faeroe Islands found that more than 90% of those receiving medical care for the condition had affected relatives, and a large kindred exhibiting the disorder has been studied in North Carolina.

If one first-degree relative (parent, SIBLING, offspring) is affected, the recurrence risk appears to be approximately 7.5% to 17%. With both parents affected the risk may exceed 50%. The expression is variable and may be more or less severe than other affected relatives. The lesions may erupt periodically or they may be chronic. Onset is usually sometime in adulthood.

A form of arthritis may accompany familial psoriasis, resulting in painful crippling contractures of the hands or other joints, along with the eruptions of the skin. Called psoriatic arthropathy, the disorder was the model for the disease that afflicted the protagonist of a public television series of the 1980s produced in

England, "The Singing Detective." The creator of the series, Dennis Potter, a highly regarded writer, suffered from the disorder himself.

**ptosis**    The dropping or drooping of an organ or part of the body. Most commonly it is seen in the upper eyelids, which demonstrate a tendency to droop in many GENETIC DISORDERS and other disease conditions. As an isolated phenomenon, CONGENITAL ptosis of the eyelids may have a genetic basis, often demonstrating AUTOSOMAL DOMINANT transmission.

**percutaneous umbilical blood sampling (PUBS)**    See CORDOCENTESIS.

**pycnodysostosis**    Mild form of short-limb DWARFISM, first identified in 1962. Its name, taken from the Greek *pyknos*, meaning thick, refers to the increased thickness and density of the bones. A characteristic appearance results from underdevelopment of the facial bones and abnormally large cranial sutures (the gaps between the bones of the skull). This creates a relatively large head with a prominent forehead and a small face with parrot-like hooked nose, receding chin, dental and oral anomalies and bulging eyes.

French doctors Pierre Maroteaux (b. 1926) and Maurice Lamy (1895–1975) who first described it, speculated that this may have been the affliction of French artist Henri de Toulouse-Lautrec (1864–1901). His dwarfism was marked by multiple bone fractures, he had consanguinous parents (first cousins) and the top hat he habitually wore may have been an attempt to hide the marked prominence of the forehead that is a hallmark of this disorder, as well as to cover a patent fontanelle (the "soft spot" atop an infant's head that has been retained into adulthood). Similarly, his beard may have been grown to cover a receding chin.

The increased density makes the bones, particularly long bones in the limbs, prone to fracture easily and fail to grow together prop-

erly, exacerbating the natural tendency of stunted development of the limbs that is characteristic of this condition. The jawbone is also prone to breakage; for example, it can be fractured by a tooth extraction.

Though the trunk is not shortened, abnormalities of the trunk are typically present. The shoulders are narrow. The chest may be sunken (PECTUS excavatum) and the breasts may be underdeveloped in females. The spine may be curved abnormally (SCOLIOSIS) or may be humped (kyphosis) or swaybacked (lumbar lordosis). The tips of the fingers and toes may appear bulbous, and the nails may be poorly formed.

Infants display a FAILURE TO THRIVE. The persistence of the milk teeth gives an appearance of a double row of teeth in childhood. The permanent teeth are poorly formed and prone to cavities. The eyes are prone to vision problems. Adult height is usually under five feet. Lifespan is normal. MENTAL RETARDATION has been reported in about one in six cases.

The basic defect that causes the developmental failure is unknown. Pycnodysostosis is inherited as an AUTOSOMAL RECESSIVE trait. Approximately 100 cases have been reported, and about 30% involved parental CONSANGUINITY, a statistic that points to the rarity of the gene in the general population. PRENATAL DIAGNOSIS has not been achieved.

For more information, contact:

Little People of America, Inc.
P.O. Box 633
San Bruno, CA 94066
(415) 589-0695

Human Growth Foundation
4720 Montgomery Lane, Suite 909
Bethesda, MD 20814
(301) 656-6904
(301) 656-7540

**pygmy**    Studies conducted in the Central African Republic indicate the short stature observed in African pygmies may be the result of their failure to respond to somatomedin C or insulin-like growth factor I (IGF I), a human hormone growth mediator. It has been suggested that a gene for this unresponsiveness is on CHROMOSOME 12, and that the short stature of the pygmies is inherited as an AUTOSOMAL RECESSIVE trait (with almost all pygmies carrying only the recessive genes due to inbreeding). However, other research suggests that the inheritance of short stature in pygmies is MULTIFACTORIAL in nature. (See also DWARFISM.)

**pyloric stenosis**   CONGENITAL narrowing of the opening between the stomach and small intestine, the pylorus. Characteristically, an affected infant begins projectile vomiting (ejecting the stomach contents with great force) at three to four weeks of age, and as the obstruction becomes nearly complete, the infant suffers weight loss, constipation and imbalances in levels of sodium and potassium in the blood. Eagerness to nurse after vomiting is common. The enlarged and thickened pylorus can be felt through the abdominal wall as a movable mass about the size of an olive. These signs and symptoms can be confirmed by X-ray or ULTRASOUND studies.

The defect is a MULTIFACTORIAL trait involving several genes and environmental influence. It occurs in approximately one in 300 live births and is most common in whites. Males are affected four times as frequently as females. Recurrence risks are higher for SIBLINGS of females. The prognosis after surgical repair is excellent. There is some evidence that survivors have a higher incidence of peptic ulcer later in life. Though prenatal ultrasound has demonstrated distension of the stomach in congenital pyloric stenosis, the reliability of sonography for PRENATAL DIAGNOSIS of this condition has not been established.

**pyruvate carboxylase deficiency with lactic acidemia**   Rare progressive neurological disorder resulting from an absence of pyruvate carboxylase, an enzyme that is important in the cycle by which the body derives energy from food.

Newborns and infants appear normal but their development is slow, and abnormalities are evident by one year of age. They exhibit symptoms such as FAILURE TO THRIVE, vomiting, irritability, apathy, inactivity, poor muscle tone (hypotonia), absent reflexes (areflexia), spasticity, inability to coordinate muscular movements (ataxia), abnormal eye movements and seizures.

Although the signs and symptoms of the disorder are nonspecific and inconsistent, diagnosis has been made within several months of birth in some cases. It is detected by higher-than-normal lactate and pyruvate levels.

Neurological and intellectual deterioration is progressive, and death generally occurs within several years.

It is believed to be inherited as an AUTOSOMAL RECESSIVE trait. PRENATAL DIAGNOSIS is theoretically possible by measuring the amount of the ENZYME in fetal cells.

**pyruvate dehydrogenase deficiency**   Symptoms of this group of disorders vary from excessive production of lactic and pyruvic acid (acidosis) and rapidly progressive, fatal illness within the first few days of birth to uncoordinated muscle movements, growth and MENTAL RETARDATION, and muscle weakness in later infancy or childhood, often after a respiratory infection.

Inherited as an AUTOSOMAL RECESSIVE trait, it is caused by the absence of the ENZYME pyruvate dehydrogenase. (This is actually an enzyme complex of multiple individual enzymes.) The degree of enzyme deficiency corresponds to the severity of manifestations. Meals high in carbohydrates may exacerbate acidosis, a decreased alkalinity of the blood and tissues marked by sickly sweet breath, headache, nausea and vomiting, and visual disturbances. Severity of acidosis varies; lactic acidosis may cause early death.

Pyruvate dehydrogenase deficiency can be diagnosed shortly after birth by analysis of skin fibroblast cells, but the age at which it is detected is likely to depend on its severity. PRENATAL DIAGNOSIS is theoretically possible. Irreversible neurologic damage and mental retardation usually occur by the time of diagnosis.

**pyruvate kinase deficiency**    Rare hereditary ENZYME deficiency, detectable at birth and manifest as ANEMIA caused by destruction of red blood cells (hemolytic anemia). The severity of the anemia is variable, even within the same family. In addition, blood bilirubin levels are often above normal (hyperbilirubinemia).

Gallstones from chronic hyperbilirubinemia are a common complication. Infections may exacerbate anemia by preventing red blood cells from developing (erythroid hypoplasia). In severely anemic cases surgical removal of the spleen reduces or eliminates the need for blood transfusions.

The basic defect in this disorder is a low level of the enzyme pyruvate kinase in red blood cells, or production of the enzyme with an abnormal structure so that it has a low level of activity. Similar forms of this enzyme exist in different tissues of the body, an almost identical form being present in the liver. A DNA PROBE for the liver type of pyruvate kinase made it possible to clone and sequence the defective gene responsible for this hereditary disorder and to map its location to CHROMOSOME 1.

Inherited as an AUTOSOMAL RECESSIVE trait, most individuals with the disorder survive to adulthood, and those with mild anemia may have near-normal life spans, depending on complications.

# Q

**quinacrine**    Fluorescent dye used for banding (staining) CHROMOSOMES in CYTOGENETIC analysis. The Y CHROMOSOME, for example, is highly fluorescent when stained with this dye. Q banding, as this technique is called, was initially described by Torbjörn Caspersson and colleagues at the Karolinska Institute in Stockholm, Sweden in 1970; it was the first banding technique and served as the first reference for identifying individual chromosomes. (See also "INTRODUCTION.")

**quinine**    Substance used as a "folk remedy" for inducing ABORTION. It is not effective for this purpose. Large doses kill both mother and fetus. Children exposed to smaller doses as an abortifacient (any substance used to induce abortion) have had damaged nervous systems, malformed arms and legs, BLINDNESS, DEAFNESS or other vision and hearing defects. Although quinine was once the only medication for malaria, birth defects were not associated with its use for this purpose (most likely due to the lower dosage used). Less toxic drugs are now prescribed for malaria. Individuals with G6PD DEFICIENCY are susceptible to hemolytic anemia when exposed to quinine.

# R

**RA**    See RHEUMATOID ARTHRITIS.

**radial defects**    A range of defects involving arrested development and absence of bones of the thumb-side of the forearm, hand and wrist. In the mildest form, the thumb and bone in the hand leading to it (first metacarpal) are incomplete. In the next degree of severity, the first metacarpal is absent and the thumb is attached to the index finger only by soft tissue rather than by bone. In a more severe form, the radius, the bone on the outer or thumb side of the forearm is incomplete or absent with varying degrees of arrested development of the first metacarpal bone and thumb. In the most severe form, both bones of the forearm (radius and ulna) are missing, and the upper-arm bone (humerus) is defective.

Though knowledge of limb defects such as absent fingers dates back to Aristotle, radial defects are rare. The frequency at birth of radial defects has been estimated as one in 30,000. About 20% of affected persons have no other defects, and among two-thirds of these persons only one arm is affected. Most cases in which the affected person has no other defect or ANOMALY originate sporadically, that is, there is no familial or genetic tendency. Intelligence and life span are not affected.

Radial defects also occur as part of many other syndromes, including the VATER ASSOCIATION, FANCONI ANEMIA, TAR SYNDROME and HOLT-ORAM SYNDROME, as well as being associated with CRANIOSYNOSTOSIS, CONGENITAL HEART DEFECTS or CHROMOSOME ABNORMALITIES.

**radiation**    Exposure to some forms of electromagnetic radiation has potentially serious consequences for fetal development. Of major concern is ionizing radiation, which includes gamma and X rays. (Questions have also been raised regarding the consequences of long-term exposure to electromagnetic fields surrounding high tension power lines and household appliances; these questions are the subject of current research. Suggestions that radiation emitted from VIDEO DISPLAY TERMINALS may have an adverse impact on fetal development have not been demonstrated or verified.)

The discovery that X rays are capable of inducing MUTATIONS was a major advance in genetic research. It was reported by Hermann J. Muller in a 1927 paper, "Artificial Transmutation of the Gene." Prior to that time, researchers, whose primary research subject was the fly drosophila melanogaster, had to wait for natural mutations to appear, a rare occurrence. Muller reported he could increase mutation rates 15,000 times by exposure to heavy doses of X rays; he called these changes "mutations." (He was awarded the Nobel prize in 1946 for his work.) The following year, Lewis Stadler reported similar findings using maize (a corn plant) and barley.

Knowledge of the impact of radiation on human development comes primarily from studies of the infants, exposed in utero, of survivors of the atomic bombings of Hiroshima. An unexpectedly large number of these individuals had abnormally small heads (MICROCEPHALY), ocular abnormalities and mental and physical growth retardation. Additionally, high levels of radiation formerly used in CANCER treatment of some pregnant women were also associated with an increase in CONGENITAL anomalies.

Ionizing radiation appears to disrupt fetal development by interfering with the rapid cell division that characterizes early embryonic development. The extent of the damage is dependent on the size of the dose and the period of fetal development when exposure occurs. Dosage is commonly measured in rems or rads, a unit of ionizing ability. The average American is exposed to 200 millirems, or one-fifth of a rad, annually. Fetal exposure to more than 10 rads is considered to increase risks for developmental abnormalities, according to standards published by the American Academy of Radiologists in 1975. This is a level much higher than that received in diagnostic X-ray examinations. In the first two weeks of pregnancy, large doses (well above 50 rads) will either kill the fetus or have no impact at all. Exposure at two to four weeks is associated with multiple organ system malformations. Growth retardation is associated with later exposure, while the central nervous system is vulnerable throughout pregnancy.

In addition to interfering with cell division, radiation can damage GENES and CHROMOSOMES as well, creating a mutation or CHROMOSOME ABNORMALITY that may affect an individual in a later generation. However, little is known about the risks of transmitting these aberrations following adult exposure to radiation. It has been recommended that women who receive direct pelvic exposure to radiation (as in radiotherapy, therapeutic cancer treatment) defer conception for a period of several months to a year, and men are advised to wait at least a year.

The low levels of radiation associated with diagnostic X-ray procedures used during pregnancy are also considered to pose no risk to fetal development. Exposure to a dose exceeding five rads would be unusual, and thus the risks of malformations or mutations due to radiation exposure are considered to be minimal. (See TERATOGEN.)

**radioulnar synostosis** The term synostosis means the fusion of separate, adjacent bones. In this rare CONGENITAL deformity, inherited as an AUTOSOMAL DOMINANT trait, the bones of the forearm, the radius and the ulna are fused, restricting the twisting motion of the forearm to less than half of the normal range and resulting in limited function of the hand. The condition is exhibited in both forearms (bilateral) in more than 80% of those affected. It is also often seen in individuals with an XXXXXY chromosomal constitution, a rare CHROMOSOME ABNORMALITY.

**Raynaud disease** Named for French physician Maurice Raynaud (1834–1881), who published a description in 1862, this disorder is characterized by constriction of the blood vessels in the hands and feet upon exposure to cold or emotional stress. It is most frequently seen in females between the ages of 18 and 30. During episodes, the extremities, especially the fingers, may become white as the constricted blood vessels prevent blood from reaching the underlying tissue. The condition in itself is benign (except for the possibility of gangrene of the finger tips in extreme cases). However, it has been associated with the development of RHEUMATOID ARTHRITIS and SCLERODERMA.

A hereditary form was first identified in England in 1933 in an English working class family, some of whose members had periodic attacks in which their fingers turned white and became numb. This form is transmitted as an AUTOSOMAL DOMINANT trait.

**von Recklinghausen disease** See NEUROFIBROMATOSIS.

**recombinant DNA** (gene splicing) The process and result of splicing a segment of DNA (see DEOXYRIBONUCLEIC ACID) from one source into the DNA of another. When the newly combined genetic material replicates itself, the transplanted genetic material will also be copied. This technique is useful in examining the properties and action of specific genes. It is the basis for molecular diagnostic tests using DNA markers.

It is also anticipated that it may be possible to treat some GENETIC DISORDERS in the future by replacing defective segments of genetic material via this process. It is already being used for the manufacture of certain biochemical products such as insulin and growth hormone.

**Refsum disease** See PHYTANIC ACID STORAGE DISEASE.

**regional ileitis** See CROHN DISEASE.

**renal agenesis unilateral** See UNILATERAL RENAL AGENESIS.

**respiratory distress syndrome (RDS)** Respiratory insufficiency, formerly called hyaline membrane disease. It is one of the most common health problems among newborns, affecting approximately 40,000 annually in the United States. It is frequently associated with LOW BIRTH WEIGHT due to prematurity. The lungs (as well as other organs) of these infants tend to be underdeveloped and often cannot provide a sufficient supply of the lecithin-rich "pulmonary surfactant," a lubricant that helps the air sacs in the lung to inflate and prevents them from collapsing and sticking together after each breath. Without it, the alveoli collapse, leading to oxygen starvation (hypoxia) characterized by a blue or gray tint to the skin (cyanosis). Symptoms, which are usually exhibited at birth, include gulping for air (dyspnea), rapid breathing, expiratory grunt, limpness, cardiac failure and arrest. If death occurs, it is almost always within the first three days of life.

Progress has been made in diagnosis and treatment of RDS. The level of surfactant in fetal lungs can be measured by analysis of AMNIOTIC FLUID, and several hormones have been developed that may accelerate fetal lung development when taken by the mother shortly before birth. New respirator technology is helping prolong infant survival for the three to five days necessary for the lungs to produce enough surfactant for normal respiration. Trials of surfactant replacement are currently underway.

**restriction enzymes**    (restriction fragment length polymorphism, RFLP) Proteins which chemically cut DNA strands into specific fragments for use in identifying genetic defects. The first, found in 1970, was produced by the bacteria Hemophilus influenzae and capable of slicing the DNA of some viruses and bacteria at specific points.

There are now more than 200 restriction ENZYMES available for DNA analysis. Each of these enzymes will cut DNA at different locations, resulting in fragments of varying but reproducible lengths. These are termed restriction fragments. A genetic MUTATION may cause the restriction enzyme to cut an individual's DNA (or fail to cut it) at a location other than the "normal" site, producing a fragment length that differs from normal, thus indicating the presence of a genetic variation.

These variations in fragment length are called restriction fragment length polymorphisms (RFLP). By comparing the patterns of the fragments with reference patterns of genetic fragments of known length, scientists are often able to pinpoint which genetic abnormality is present. Even if the specific gene involved is not known, or what the specific defect is, diagnosis may be possible using tests involving GENETIC LINKAGE. Use of restriction enzymes has enabled more accurate PRENATAL DIAGNOSIS of a variety of genetic defects, including those that cause CYSTIC FIBROSIS and SICKLE-CELL ANEMIA. (See also DNA PROBES; "INTRODUCTION.")

**restriction fragment length polymorphism (RFLP)** See RESTRICTION ENZYME.

**retinitis pigmentosa (RP)**    A group of hereditary ocular disorders that comprise the most common forms of retinal degeneration. The retina, which forms the inner wall on the back of the eyeball, is the area where light coming into the eye registers on the photo receptor cells, called rods and cones, and is then transmitted to the brain. In RP, the retina undergoes progressive degeneration as the rods and cones stop functioning. On examination, the retina appears abnormally pigmented. The cause of this degeneration is unknown, but research has found some individuals with RP may have defective metabolism of docosahexaenoic acid, a lipid (or "fatty acid") found in high concentrations in the retinas of individuals with normal vision.

The earliest symptoms are decreased night vision (NIGHTBLINDNESS), followed by a gradual constriction of the peripheral visual field. Eventually, only a small, central portion of vision remains, as though the individual was looking through a tunnel. This progression usually occurs over many years or several decades. Onset usually occurs during childhood or young adulthood. This condition may create a sense of isolation as night driving becomes impossible, eliminating many opportunities for socializing.

Prevalence is estimated at between one in 2,000 and one in 7,000 individuals. More than 20,000 persons in the United States with this disorder are classified as legally blind, though individuals generally retain some vision.

At one time it was thought that exposure to bright light speeded the progression of the disorder, but that now appears to be incorrect. Treatment consists of visual aids to maximize the use of remaining vision. There is no cure, and ongoing ophthalmological healthcare is important.

RP is inherited in AUTOSOMAL DOMINANT, AUTOSOMAL RECESSIVE and X-LINKED recessive forms. There is a great degree of variability in the expression of the disorder, though within families the rate and severity of vision loss is generally similar. A gene responsible for the autosomal dominant form is located on CHROMOSOME 3.

RP occurs as a feature of several other syndromes, including USHER SYNDROME, BARDET-BIEDL SYNDROME, MUCOPOLYSAC-CHARIDOSIS and Refsum's disease (see PHYTANIC ACID STORAGE DISEASE). When inherited without other disorders, the most common form of RP is autosomal recessive, and it accounts for an estimated 50% to 84% of cases. The autosomal dominant form accounts for 10% to 15%, and X-linked recessive forms for 5% to 6%. Female CARRIERS of the X-linked form can often be identified. (See also BLINDNESS.)

For more information, contact:

National Retinitis Pigmentosa Foundation, Inc.
1401 Mt. Royal Avenue
Baltimore, MD 21217-4245
(301) 225-9400
(301) 225-9409 TDD for Deaf

American Foundation for the Blind, Inc.
15 West 16th Street
New York, NY 10011
(212) 620-2000

American Council of the Blind
1010 Vermont Avenue., NW
Suite 1100
Washington, DC 20005
(202) 393-3666
(800) 424-8666

**retinoblastoma**   A childhood malignant CANCER of the retina of the eye. It is estimated to develop in approximately one in 18,000 liveborn infants. Incidence is equal in blacks and whites, though other ethnic groups may have rates four times as high. Between 10% and 45% of the cases are hereditary, transmitted as an AUTOSOMAL DOMINANT trait, with PENETRANCE of over 90% (more than 90% of

those who inherit the gene for the condition will develop the associated retinal malignancy).

Hereditary cases tend to affect both eyes (bilateral). If not treated early, it may lead to death, though in some cases the cancer may go into spontaneous remission. It was not until treatment progressed to the point that affected individuals lived into adulthood and had children that the hereditary basis of many cases became clear. Treatment may consist of irradiation or removal of the affected eye(s).

Some cases have been associated with abnormalities of CHROMOSOME 13. This has led to the discovery of a GENETIC MARKER that may identify those susceptible for developing retinoblastoma and assist in PRENATAL DIAGNOSIS. A gene has been identified on chromosome 13 that appears to play a role in retinoblastoma and perhaps other cancers. It seems to be a tumor suppressor gene and MUTATIONS that inactivate it lead to the development of cancer. Affected individuals also have a risk for developing bone cancer later in life estimated to be 500 times that of the general population. (See also BLINDNESS; ONCOGENE.)

**retinopathy of prematurity (ROP)** (retrolental fibroplasia, RLF)   An excessive growth of blood vessels on the retina, the light-sensitive tissue on the back of the eyeball. The growth usually occurs between four weeks and 14 weeks of age, and can lead to retinal bleeding, scarring, retinal detachment and BLINDNESS. It is estimated that 8,000 infants born annually in the United States develop the disorder, causing vision loss in 2,600 and blindness in 650.

In the early 1950s, it was discovered the condition may occur in premature infants receiving too much oxygen in incubators. As a result, incubator oxygen use was monitored more closely, and cases of blindness caused by ROP dropped. However, increased survival rates of extremely premature infants in recent years has led to an increase in this condition. It has also become clear that multiple factors related to prematurity (and not just oxygen) are the causes of this disorder.

ROP may be treated with cryotherapy, a surgical procedure in which areas of the white (sclera) of the eye's outer surface are briefly frozen with a probe cooled to approximately minus 316° Fahrenheit. The procedure stops or slows the growth of the excessive blood vessels on the retina. It has been estimated that this treatment can reduce by half the risk of severe vision loss from ROP.

**retrolental fibroplasia**    See RETINOPA-THY OF PREMATURITY.

**Rett syndrome**    A neurological disorder observed only in females; first described in 1966 by Dr. Andreas Rett of Vienna, Austria, it was not until 1983 that the disorder came to the attention of the medical community at large.

Affected females develop normally until six to 18 months of age, at which point developmental stagnation occurs. As the condition manifests itself, the growth of the head lags behind the rest of the body, and behavioral, social and psychomotor skills begin to deteriorate. Typically, within a year and a half of onset, the condition progresses to severe to profound MENTAL RETARDATION, INFANTILE AUTISM, loss of purposeful use of the hands, and shaking of the torso and possibly the limbs, especially when the individual is upset or agitated. They may grind their teeth (bruxism) and grimace. Crying and screaming spells are sometimes exhibited and may continue intermittently over a period of days. They do not develop meaningful language skills.

One of the most striking symptoms is repetitive hand movements, such as hand "washing," wringing, clapping and hand mouthing. These may become almost constant during waking hours.

About half can walk, exhibiting an unsteady, wide-based, stiff-legged gait, sometimes walking on their toes. Seizures develop after the age of five in about 80% of cases.

Other associated medical problems include lateral curvature of the spine (SCOLIOSIS) and respiratory problems such as lung congestion and repeated respiratory infections. Abnormal respiratory control, characterized by periods of disorganized breathing and ineffective respiratory effort often resulting in poor oxygenation, is characteristic during waking hours. Deterioration typically halts by the age of 10.

While approximately 1,500 cases have been identified worldwide, incidence is thought to be as high as one in 12,000 to one in 15,000 live female births. The condition may often be misdiagnosed as autism or CEREBRAL PALSY.

There is no definitive test that can confirm the presence of this disorder. Diagnosis is made on the basis of individual clinical evaluation of symptoms.

The cause of Rett syndrome is unknown. Since only females are affected, the X CHROMOSOME is believed to be involved. It has been suggested that the syndrome is an X-LINKED dominant trait, lethal in male fetuses that possess the GENE. All cases are thought to be the result of new MUTATION. Currently, there is no method of PRENATAL DIAGNOSIS.

For more information, contact:

International Rett Syndrome Association
8511 Rose Marie Drive
Fort Washington, MD 20744
(301) 248-7031

**RFLP**    See RESTRICTION ENZYME.

**Rh blood factor**    See HEMOLYTIC DISEASE OF THE NEWBORN.

**rheumatoid arthritis (RA)**    Rheumatoid arthritis is a common autoimmune disease in which the body attacks its own tissue. It is characterized by inflammation, swelling and stiffness in the joints, causing pain and potential crippling. Occasional families show a considerable number of individuals affected with this disorder, and it has been suggested that it is transmitted as an AUTOSOMAL DOMINANT trait in these cases. However, simple MENDELIAN inheritance (dominant or recessive) has not been proven. Most often, the risks of RA to relatives are not high: They are doubled for first-degree relatives (parent, SIBLING, child) as opposed to the general population. Certain HLA-types (see HUMAN LEUKOCYTE ANTIGEN) are more frequently seen in affected individuals, and one particular type (HLA-DRW4) may be a major determinant of susceptibility to the disease in familial cases.

**rhizomelic dwarfism**    See DWARFISM.

**ribonucleic acid (RNA)**    Genetic material that controls the synthesis of protein. RNA forms on a template of DEOXYRIBONUCLEIC ACID (DNA) in the nucleus of cells. Genetic errors or MUTATIONS present in the DNA will be reflected in the RNA and possibly cause errors in protein synthesis, which may result in GENETIC DISORDERS.

**rickets**    A childhood condition primarily caused by vitamin D deficiency, which results in abnormal, stunted bone development. Other symptoms may include delayed eruption and poor development of teeth, large head and thin skull bones. It is an associated complication of many CONGENITAL and infant-onset hereditary disorders, including disorders of vitamin D metabolism such as HYPOPHOSPHATEMIA.

**Rieger syndrome**    Syndrome, first described by ophthalmologist Herwigh Rieger in 1935, consisting of an association of eye malformations and nonocular abnormalities. The eye abnormality—known as the Rieger ANOMALY, the Rieger eye malformation sequence, goniodysgenesis or mesodermal dysgenesis of the iris—is a structural defect of the anterior chamber of the eye, the fluid-filled portion of the eye between the cornea and the iris and lens. There is defective development (hypoplasia) of the iris along with other abnor-malities of the aqueous chamber (anterior chamber) of the eye, including a band that runs from the iris to the cornea. The defective development of the iris may be associated with CONGENITAL absence of all or part of the iris (aniridia) or a fissure or cleft of the iris (coloboma). Other ocular defects include unusually large or small corneas, corneal clouding or GLAUCOMA. In most cases affected individuals have slit-like pupils.

The association of this eye anomaly with hypodontia, a reduced number of teeth, has been termed the Rieger syndrome. The Rieger anomaly may also be a feature of other syndromes (see GONIODYSGENESIS).

As affected individuals grow, they tend to show common facial features. The top of the nose (nasal root) is broad and flat. They may have a prominent jaw that juts beyond the projection of the forehead (prognathism), protruding lower lip and the narrow groove between the top lip and the nose (the philtrum) is short. Teeth may be peg or cone-shaped. There is also protrusion of the skin around the umbilicus.

The basic defect that causes this syndrome is unknown. Though affected individuals may have poor vision (requiring ocular surgery in some cases), there is no impairment of intelligence, and life span is not affected.

Inherited as an AUTOSOMAL DOMINANT trait with an extreme variability of expression, Rieger syndrome is estimated to occur in approximately one in 200,000 live births. Currently, there is no method of PRENATAL DIAGNOSIS for this disorder.

In recent years Rieger has come under criticism due to his affiliation with the Nazi Party and his service in the Wehrmacht in World War II. He assumed a professorship in ophthalmology at the German University of Prague where he identified this syndrome after his predecessor had been fired for having a Jewish wife.

**Riley-Day syndrome**    See    FAMILIAL DYSAUTONOMIA.

**RNA**    See RIBONUCLEIC ACID.

**Roberts syndrome**   (pseudo thalido-mide syndrome; SC syndrome)    Named for John B. Roberts (1854–1924), a distin-guished plastic surgeon in Philadelpha who, in 1919, described the condition in three af-fected siblings of first-cousin Italian parents, this syndrome is characterized by severe mal-formations of the head and limbs.

The head is small (MICROCEPHALY), the ears are malformed and the eyes protrude abnormally (exophthalmos). Bilateral CLEFT LIP with or without cleft palate is almost always present. The skull may be shortened, and scalp hair is sparse.

The limb malformations are striking, and tend to be symmetrical. Bones of the arms and legs may be missing or severely deformed, resulting in shortening of the limbs. Hands and feet may be attached directly to the trunk (phocomelia). There are often missing digits on the hands and feet. In almost all cases, the number of digits missing is greater in the hands than in the feet. Undescended testes (CRYPTORCHIDISM) is seen in most males. There may be penile or clitorial enlargement. LOW BIRTH WEIGHT (less than five pounds) is common.

Other defects associated with this disorder include HYDROCEPHALUS, SPINA BIFIDA, short neck, atrial septal defect, polycystic kidneys and horseshoe-shaped kidney.

Most affected infants are STILLBORN or die in early infancy. Those who survive have marked growth deficiency, and many exhibit MENTAL RETARDATION.

The basic cause of this syndrome is un-known, but it may result from an abnormality of CHROMOSOME pairing and separation. Most cases have been SPORADIC, but it is thought to be inherited as an AUTOSOMAL RECESSIVE trait, based on the number of reports of af-fected SIBLINGS and parental CONSANGUIN-ITY.

**Robin anomaly**   (Pierre Robin syn-drome)    A strikingly small jaw (micro-ggnathia), protruding tongue (glossoptosis) and CLEFT PALATE are the three cardinal fea-tures of this syndrome, caused by an abnor-mality of embryonic development. Although described in medical literature as early as 1911, it bears the name of French dental sur-geon Pierre Robin (1867–1950), who pub-lished a description in 1923.

The most dangerous result of this condition is interruption of breathing at birth, due to obstruction of the newborn's airway. If artifi-cial means of breathing are not provided im-mediately, the lack of oxygen reaching the brain may cause severe MENTAL RETARDA-TION.

Other associated features in some cases are CONGENITAL HEART DEFECTS, crossed-eyes (STRABISMUS), and GLAUCOMA. The cleft pal-ate may be repaired surgically after the infant is 18 months old. By age six, the jaw reaches normal size, though it may continue to have an unusual shape.

Affecting males and females equally, it oc-curs in an estimated one in 30,000 live births.

PRENATAL DIAGNOSIS is currently not rou-tine, though it may be possible with ULTRA-SOUND. However, the ANOMALY may not be evident until late in gestation. The mode of inheritance is unknown, though it appears to be caused by the action of several genes in concert with environmental influence (MULTI-FACTORIAL). In addition, the Robin anomaly may be one feature of a number of associated syndromes, most importantly the STICKLER SYNDROME, which may account for as much as 30% of infants born with this anomaly.

**Robinow syndrome**   (fetal face syn-drome)    Rare disorder, described by American physician M. Robinow in 1969. Also known as the fetal face syndrome, the face resembles that of a fetus of about eight weeks gestation. These features include a dis-proportionately large skull, bulging forehead, curving, S-shaped lower eyelids, short, up-turned nose (anteverted nares) and flat face. The mouth may turn down at the corners, and the teeth may be misaligned or crowded. Arms may be short, and the fingers and toes short and stubby. As the affected person grows, fused vertebrae and sideways curvature of the spine (SCOLIOSIS) may become apparent. There is moderate dwarfing and the forearm bones are shortened. External genitalia may be underdeveloped, often to a severe degree.

In most cases the syndrome is transmitted as an AUTOSOMAL DOMINANT trait. The basic defect is unknown. Life expectancy and general health of affected persons are usually normal.

## Romano-Ward syndrome (prolonged Q.T. interval)

Defect characterized by sudden losses of consciousness triggered by an insufficient supply of blood to the brain (syncope). These episodes may be brief and apparently harmless, or lengthy, severe and even fatal. It was first described in Italy in 1963 by C. Romano, and in the United States in 1964 by B.C. Ward.

Usually the syncope is brought on by violent emotion or strenuous exercise. The underlying cause is an irregular or inappropriate heartbeat. Electrocardiography may show that the heart fails to increase its rate of contractions rapidly enough to meet the work demand placed on it. Frequency of these episodes ranges from several per month to only one or two in a lifetime.

This rare defect is inherited as an AUTOSOMAL DOMINANT trait. Affected individuals can be identified by characteristic electrocardiographic findings. Historically, the prognosis has been poor, with about half of those affected dying before reaching adolescence. However, modern drug therapy has improved the long-term prognosis.

The disorder is similar to JERVELL AND LANGE-NIELSEN SYNDROME but distinguished from the latter by the absence of deafness as a feature.

## Rothmund-Thomson syndrome (RTS)

(poikiloderma atrophicans and cataract) Disorder whose primary features are abnormalities of the skin and eyes. It was first described in 1868 by August von Rothmund (1830–1906), professor of ophthalmology and head of the state eye clinic in Munich, Ger-

many. Matthew S. Thomson (1894–1969), senior dermatologist at Kings College Hospital in London, described what is believed to be the same condition in 1936, and it now bears both their names.

Abnormalities of the skin may be present at birth, but usually appear between three and six months of life. Large, reddened patches caused by the dilation of capillaries near the surface of the skin (erythema) appear on the face and later involve the ears, buttocks, extremities and ultimately the entire body. Lesions form on these areas. The progression stabilizes after the first few years of life. However, skin lesions may turn cancerous in adulthood. Other skin abnormalities include brown pigmentation, depigmentation and telangiectases (prominent, dilated blood vessels). There may be sensitivity to sunlight resulting in blistering, though this is more common early in life.

About half of affected individuals have sparse hair, eyebrows and eyelashes, and some have total loss of hair (ALOPECIA). Nails of the hands and feet may be malformed. Teeth may be small, malformed or fail to erupt.

CATARACTS are the most common ocular manifestation, and usually are found in both bilateral eyes. They develop rapidly over a period of a few weeks or months. They may appear as early as four months of age, and in most cases appear by the age of five years. However, in some cases they have appeared as late as age 40.

Other features associated with the SYNDROME include short stature, SCOLIOSIS and malformation of the hands and fingers. MENTAL RETARDATION has been reported in some affected individuals. While there are no consistent skeletal deformities, maldevelopment of the arms and pelvis have been reported.

In both sexes, the development of secondary sex characteristics is poor. Females are frequently sterile.

The syndrome is inherited as an AUTOSOMAL RECESSIVE trait. It is a rare condition; over 80 cases have been reported. Seventy percent of reported cases are female, but the reason for the seeming sex predilection is unknown. Currently, PRENATAL DIAGNOSIS of this condition is not possible.

**rubella**   See TORCH SYNDROME.

**rubeola**   See MEASLES.

**Rubinstein-Taybi syndrome**   Condition first described in 1963 by U.S. physicians J.H. Rubinstein (b. 1925) and H. Taybi (b. 1919), as a syndrome with broad thumbs and toes and facial abnormalities.

The facial abnormalities consist of a small head (MICROCEPHALY), prominent forehead, eyes that slant downward away from the nose (antimongoloid obliquity), a broad nasal bridge and a beaked nose. Eyebrows may be heavy, eyelashes may be long, eyelids may droop (PTOSIS) and the eyes may be wide-set (HYPERTELORISM). The ears may be abnormally shaped, low-set or rotated. Grimacing and an unusual smile are frequently observed. A high-arched palate and dental malocclusion are also common.

In addition to the thumbs, the ends of the fingers tend to be broad, as well. An incurving (CLINODACTYLY) of the little finger and overlapping toes are other digital malformations seen in more than 50% of cases.

Skeletal abnormalities associated with this disorder include short stature, concave chest (PECTUS excavatum) and curvature of the spine (kyphoscoliosis).

**Russell-Silver syndrome**   A rare form of DWARFISM identified in about 100 cases; named for Alexander Russell, professor of pediatrics at the Hebrew University in Jerusalem, and Henry Silver, professor of pediatrics at the University of Colorado, who published descriptions in 1954 and 1953 respectively. Its most distinctive feature is asymmetry of the body. In some individuals, this asymmetry is limited to the skull or a single limb. In others, one entire side of the body is significantly larger than the other. At birth, affected individuals are unusually small for full-term infants, and throughout childhood they exhibit a pattern of growth at the lower end of the normal range.

The facial characteristics can be quite distinct: prominence of the forehead (pseudohydrocephaly, frontal bossing), prominent eyes with long eyelashes and blue tint to the white of the eye (bluish sclerae), marked underdevelopment of the jaw (micrognathia) and thin lips with the corners of the mouth turned down. Other findings include the presence of café-au-lait spots (coffee-colored flat birthmarks), bending or fusion of the fingers or toes, poor muscle development and retarded early motor performance. In about one-third of the cases, mild MENTAL RETARDATION is also seen. Some children have had low blood sugar after short periods of fasting or have had deficiency of growth hormone.

The cause of this disorder is unknown. It is believed that the basic genetic defect underlying this syndrome may be a new genetic MUTATION in the affected individual. Some recent evidence suggests the GENE may be X-LINKED, because there is more severe expression in males and mild expression in females.

PRENATAL DIAGNOSIS is not yet possible for this disorder. The prognosis for affected individuals depends on the degree of asymmetry. Most patients lead normal lives.

# S

**sacrococcygeal teratoma**   Tumors in the area of the buttocks, usually appearing during the first two months of life. "Sacrococcygeal" refers to the portion of the end of the vertebral column where these cancerous masses, or teratomas, appear. The tumors begin to develop *in utero*, and may displace or disrupt function of the bowel and bladder. Benign tumors consist of tissues similar to normal structures. The tumors may contain skin, hair, muscle, lung or pancreatic tissue and even bowel loops, teeth or limb components, such as digits. Malignant tumors are generally of "yolk sac" origin, having their genesis in early embryonic development. While most of the tumors are benign (55% to 75%), virtually all of the infants with malignancies die in infancy.

The cause of these teratoma is unknown; they occur in an estimated one in 40,000 births. Females are affected four times as frequently as males. It is the most common tumor seen in the newborn. Most occur sporadically. (See also CANCER.)

**Saethre-Chotzen syndrome**    A form of CRANIOSYNOSTOSIS, a group of disorders caused by premature closure of the gaps (sutures) between the cranial bones, resulting in an abnormal shape of the skull. It bears the names of physicians H. Saethre and F. Chotzen, who published descriptions in 1913 and 1932 respectively. In this form, the shape of the skull deformity is variable. Most typically, the head is pointed (acrocephaly), though it may be elongated (dolichocephaly) in some cases or somewhat squat (brachycephaly). Although the skull abnormality may not be evident at birth, typical facial characteristics are often present: The face tends to be lopsided, the eyes wide-set (HYPERTELORISM), the nose beaked and the ears low-set and rotated somewhat backward. Head circumference is reduced, and the hairline may be low.

This condition is also associated with vision problems and mild hearing loss. The eyes may not be coordinated, resulting in difficulty focusing (STRABISMUS). Individuals may be nearsighted (MYOPIA) and the eyelids may droop (PTOSIS).

Digital abnormalities are also common, especially a partial joining of the skin between the second and third fingers, so that the two digits appear somewhat joined (SYNDACTYLY). Shortened fingers (BRACHYDACTYLY) have also been reported. Short stature, undescended testicles (CRYPTORCHIDISM) and

renal (kidney) anomalies have also been associated with this condition.

The basic defect that results in Saethre-Chotzen syndrome is unknown. It is inherited as an AUTOSOMAL DOMINANT trait. In cases attributed to new MUTATION, an increased paternal age may play a role.

Theoretically, in an at-risk pregnancy, ULTRASOUND may be able to detect cranial abnormalities exhibited in severe cases.

**Salla disease**    (Finnish type sialuria) HEREDITARY DISEASE first reported in northeastern Finland in 1979 and named for the geographic area where the affected families lived. It is characterized by progressive deterioration of mental and physical abilities, with onset by 12 to 18 months of age. Children who have already learned to walk lose this skill. Growth is retarded in about half of those under medical care, and cardiac abnormalities have been noted. Spasticity and impaired speech are other features.

One of the hallmarks is the increased urinary excretion of free sialic acid. It is a STORAGE DISEASE and the free sialic acid (a complex sugar that is a component of mucopolysaccharides and glycoproteins) is stored in many cells of the body. Inherited as an AUTOSOMAL RECESSIVE trait, neither CARRIER detection nor PRENATAL DIAGNOSIS have been reportedly accomplished.

**Sandhoff disease**    First described by German biochemist Konrad Sandhoff in 1968, this condition is extremely similar to TAY-SACHS DISEASE and cannot be distinguished from it without laboratory testing. It is likely that some non-Jewish children diagnosed as having Tay-Sachs before the availability of definitive diagnostic procedures actually had Sandhoff disease. However, unlike Tay-Sachs, bones and abdominal organs (e.g., liver) may show signs of abnormalities.

Motor weakness begins in the first six months of life. There is an exaggerated startle response to sound, and early BLINDNESS, along with progressive motor and mental deterioration. The face is doll-like, the head is large and the CHERRY-RED SPOT in the eye, characteristic of Tay-Sachs, is also present. The loss of swallowing ability is progressive, causing difficulty in feeding (food may be inhaled) and an increased risk of lung and chest infections, which usually leads to death by three years of age.

This disorder is caused by an ENZYME deficiency of hexosaminidase A and B, which are essential for metabolizing GM2 ganglioside, a fatty material. (In Tay-Sachs disease, only hexosaminidase A is absent.) Due to the enzyme deficiency, this fatty substance (GM2 ganglioside) accumulates in the child's brain cells. This is therefore a STORAGE DISEASE, caused by an abnormal accumulation or storage of material in the cells.

The disorder is inherited as an AUTOSOMAL RECESSIVE trait. Adult CARRIERS can be identified through careful screening procedures. PRENATAL DIAGNOSIS is possible through the finding of almost total absence of hexosaminidase activity in fetal tissues collected via AMNIOCENTESIS or CHORIONIC VILLUS SAMPLING.

For more information, contact:

The National Tay-Sachs and Allied Disease
    Association
92 Washington Avenue
Cedarhurst, NY 11516
(516) 569-4300

**Sanfilippo's disease**    See MUCOPOLY-
SACCHARIDOSIS, Type III.

**SC syndrome**    See ROBERTS SYN-
DROME

**scaphocephaly**    See CRANIOSYNOSTO-
SIS.

**Scheie syndrome**    See MUCOPOLYSAC-
CHARIDOSIS.

**schizophrenia**    Term describing a variety of diseases characterized by hallucinations, delusions, disorders of thinking and irrational behavior. It is thought to affect almost 1% of the population at some time in their lives.

A familial link has long been noted; studies of affected identical (monozygotic) twins reared apart has suggested that the disorder has a genetic basis. Adoption studies also support this: The incidence in adopted chilren is close to that predicted for their natural rather than their adoptive parents. Recent research has found conclusive evidence of a genetic basis for at least one form of schizophrenia, and the location of a cluster of GENES responsible has been traced to CHROMOSOME 5. It is thought that environmental factors also play an important role in the onset of schizophrenia and that specific causes vary from individual to individual.

Effective antipsychotic drugs used to treat schizophrenia have their primary site of action in competing for dopamine receptors in the brain, leading to suspicion that an abnormality in dopamine metabolism or dopamine receptor sensitivity may be involved in the disorder. Hereditary factors may play a role in this abnormality or sensitivity.

The risks for additional family developing schizophrenia range from 2% to 3% if an aunt, uncle, nephew, niece or first cousin is affected, to 40% to 60% if an identical twin is affected. The risk if one parent is affected is 13% and 40% if both are.

The mode of inheritance is unresolved, and there is at present no method of identifying those at risk for developing schizophrenia by prenatal or presymptomatic diagnosis.

**Schmid-type metaphyseal chondrodysplasia**    See METAPHYSEAL CHONDRODYSPLASIA

**Schwartz-Jampel syndrome**    Symptoms of this rare syndrome, characterized by distortion of the facial features, short stature, muscle spasms and rigidity, and ocular problems, initially occur after the first year of life. It is thought to be caused by an interruption of the embryo's muscular and skeletal development. U.S. physicians O. Schwartz and Robert S. Jampel published the first description in 1962.

The most common skeletal effects of the disease are short neck, protruding chest (PECTUS carinatum), curvature of the spine, and small hips, which can make walking difficult. The eyes may be small in size, set far apart (HYPERTELORISM) and may have two or more rows of eyelashes. There may be drooping of the eyelids (PTOSIS), MYOPIA or CATARACTS. The chin and mouth may be small. Speech may be high-pitched or difficult to understand due to arching in the roof of the mouth. Muscles of the limbs may be thick and small, and some children may have bulges in the stomach or groin due to weak muscles (hernias). Because the muscles of the face are contracted, affected individuals appear to have no expression.

Intelligence and life span are normal. Surgery may help correct ocular or skeletal problems, and orthopedic devices may be useful as well. Some children exhibit spontaneous improvement of their muscle contractions.

The SYNDROME is inherited as an AUTOSOMAL RECESSIVE trait and occurs equally in males and females. PRENATAL DIAGNOSIS for this condition is not currently available.

**SCID**   See IMMUNE DEFICIENCY DISEASES.

**scleroderma**   A chronic disease that causes hardening (sclerosis) of the skin (dermis) and internal organs, including the gastrointestinal tract, lungs, heart and kidneys. It occurs in women four times as often as in men. The skin feels taut and leathery and is firmly bound to subcutaneous tissue. It may itch and later become hyperpigmented. Involvement of internal organs may lead to fatal complications. The cause is unknown. There have been reports of familial occurrence of scleroderma, and it has been suggested that a familial form

may be inherited as an AUTOSOMAL DOMINANT trait. There may also be an underlying genetic predisposition, as has been suggested in SYSTEMIC LUPUS ERYTHEMATOSUS and RHEUMATOID ARTHRITIS.

For more information, contact:

United Scleroderma Foundation, Inc.
  (USF)
P.O. Box 350
Watsonville, CA 95077-0350
(408) 728-2202 or 800-772-HOPE

Scleroderma Federation, Inc.
1725 York Avenue
New York, NY 10128
(212) 427-7040

**scoliosis**   A lateral, or sideways, curvature of the spine. While it is often a secondary feature of many syndromes (e.g., MARFAN SYNDROME, DYSAUTONOMIA NEUROFIBROMATOSIS, MUSCULAR DYSTROPHIES and FRIEDREICH'S ATAXIA), scoliosis occurs most frequently as an independent disorder of the musculoskeletal system.

It may be CONGENITAL, that is, present at birth, due to defective enbryonic spinal development. However, much more common is idiopathic scoliosis, which represents 80% to 90% of cases. Idiopathic (of unknown cause or origin) scoliosis is believed to be inherited as a MULTIFACTORIAL, or POLYGENIC, trait, that is, several genes may be responsible for its transmission, with expression and severity partly dependent on environmental factors. This form of scoliosis demonstrates a familial tendency, though the degree of the severity shows wide variability within affected family members. A child whose sibling has scoliosis has a 30% chance of developing the disorder.

Idiopathic scoliosis is classified by the age at which it appears: infantile (0-4 years), juvenile (4-9 years) and adolescent (10 years to skeletal maturity). Most cases fall into the adolescent category, perhaps owing to hormonal influence on development of the condition.

An estimated 4% to 10% of the adolescent population has some degree of scoliosis. Females develop the disorder more frequently than males, by a ratio of eight to one.

One of the most common signs of scoliosis is a prominent shoulder blade, most frequently the right one. One shoulder also tends to be higher, and affected children tend to list to one side. Hips may be uneven, with one higher than the other. Clothing may appear to fit improperly. This is most obvious in girls by observing an uneven hemline in skirts or dresses.

Mild cases may be unnoticeable or require no treatment. However, severe cases may result in significant skeletal deformity, and require the wearing of a brace to straighten the spine, or surgery to correct the spinal curvature.

Currently there is no method of detecting the disorder by PRENATAL DIAGNOSIS, or identifying families at high risk for having affected family members.

For more information, contact:

The Scoliosis Association, Inc.
P.O. Box 51353
Raleigh, NC 27609
(919) 846-2639

**Seckel syndrome (bird-headed dwarfism)**    "Bird-headed dwarfism" was the name used for this inherited disorder by Helmut P.G. Seckel (1900–1961), professor of pediatrics at the University of Chicago School of Medicine, who wrote the definitive description of it in 1960. Principal characteristics include LOW BIRTH WEIGHT, DWARFISM, abnormally small head (MICROCEPHALY), large eyes, a large, prominent nose with a beaklike protrusion, narrow face, receding lower jaw, small brain size, CLUBFOOT, lateral spinal deformation (SCOLIOSIS), underdeveloped thumbs, dislocation of the heads of the thigh bones out of the hip sockets, crossed eyes (STRABISMUS), malformations in the genitourinary system and MENTAL RETARDATION.

Although a normal life span is possible, mental retardation and associated body malformations make functioning difficult. Affected children tend to be friendly and pleasant but are easily distracted and hyperactive.

The incidence is estimated to be approximately one in 10,000 live births. It is inherited as an AUTOSOMAL RECESSIVE trait.

**selective IgA deficiency**    See IMMUNE DEFICIENCY DISEASES.

**selective termination**    See ABORTION.

**severe combined immunodeficiency**    See IMMUNE DEFICIENCY DISEASES

**sex chromosome**    The X and Y CHROMOSOMES. These chromosomes determine gender and carry GENES for sex-linked characteristics. In the 23 pairs of chromosomes found in the normal human KARYOTYPE, the sex chromosomes are the 23rd pair. All the non-sex chromosomes are called autosomes.

The sex chromosomes were observed as early as 1891, by German zoologist Herman Henking (1858–1942), who noted them while studying the chromosomes of the fire wasp (phyrrho coris). Their function remained unrecognized until after the rediscovery of Mendel's laws. (See also X-LINKED, AUTOSOMAL DOMINANT and AUTOSOMAL RECESSIVE, X CHROMOSOME, Y CHROMOSOME.)

**sex limited**    Expression of a genetic characteristic or trait in one sex only, in which the primary MUTATION does not involve the SEX CHROMOSOMES. These characteristics often involve a structural defect for which there is no anatomical counterpart in the opposite sex. An example is HYPOSPADIAS in the male. (See X-LINKED.)

**sex-linked**    See X-LINKED.

**sex reversal**  See XX MALE SYNDROME.

**sialidosis**  See MUCOLIPIDOSIS, NEUR-AMINIDASE DEFICIENCY.

**sialuria, Finnish type**  See SALLA DIS-EASE.

**Siamese twins.**  See CONJOINED TWINS.

**sibling (sib)**  A brother or sister; multiple children of identical parents.

Siblings have half of their GENES in common, and siblings of those affected with HE-REDITARY or CONGENITAL disorders may have increased risks of developing or being born with the same disorder, depending on the condition and its cause, whether the result of genetic or environmental influences or a combination of the two. Unaffected sibilngs of those with hereditary or congenital disorders may experience feelings of neglect and guilt as a result of familial or personal response to the affected sibling, further complicating the interpersonal dynamics in these families.

For more information, contact:

National Sibling and Adult Children
  Network
P.O. Box 19067
Minneapolis, MN 55419
(612) 872-1565

Sibling Information Network
CUAP/University of Connecticut
249 Glenbrook Road
Storrs, CT 06268
(203) 429-9435

Siblings for Significant Change
105 East 22nd Street, 7th Floor
New York, NY 10010
(212) 420-0776

**sickle-cell anemia**  This hereditary, chronic form of hemolytic ANEMIA (an anemia characterized by breakdown of the red blood cells) takes its name from the characteristic sickle or crescent shape of the red blood cells (erythrocytes) seen in those with the disorder.

Red blood cells get their color from hemoglobin, an iron-based molecule that carries oxygen in the blood, nourishing tissues throughout the body. The sickling of the red blood cells that characterizes this disorder is caused by the change in a single AMINO ACID within the hemoglobin molecule, changing it to hemoglobin-S, which makes the red blood cell collapse when deprived of oxygen. Blood cells are most likely to sickle in the capillaries, or small blood vessels, after the oxygen has been released to the body. The sickle shape causes the blood to clog these vessels, depriving organ tissue of oxygen, in turn causing more blood sickling, more oxygen deprivation, creating pain and leading to organ damage.

The identification of the basis of sickle-cell anemia, made by U.S. chemist Dr. Linus Pauling (b. 1901) in 1949, was one of the seminal events in molecular genetics. Working at the California Institute of Technology, he found the flaw in the hemoglobin molecule responsible for the condition. This change in the molecule altered its electric charge. Thus, it behaved differently in an electrical field than a normal hemoglobin, a fact Pauling used to detect the abnormal molecules. This was also the first condition linked (in 1978) to variations within a family of specific segments of DNA containing the aberrant GENE (see RE-STRICTION ENZYME). Dr. Pauling was awarded the 1954 Nobel prize in chemistry for his work. (An opponent of U.S. nuclear policy, he was also awarded the Nobel Peace Prize in 1963.)

The expression, or severity, of the disorder among individuals with sickle-cell anemia is highly variable, ranging from mild to severe. Symptoms may include growth retardation, delay in secondary sexual development, leg ulcers, fatigue, ocular abnormalities, gallstones and stroke. Affected individuals may experience recurrent attacks of pain. These episodes may require several hospitalizations a year. Life span is somewhat shortened.

The spleen is among the first internal organs affected. Sudden blood pooling in the spleen may cause death. The spleen is also important in the body's immune response to bacteria. As a result of damage to it, affected infants are prone to bacteremia, a severe infection often caused by the bacteria pneumococcus, and may develop fevers and die within 12 hours. About a third of infants with bacteremia below the age of three years succumb to it. They may also develop pneumonia or meningitis, an infection of the membrane that covers the brain.

These infections have been a major cause of mortality among infants with sickle-cell anemia, but daily doses of penicillin in at-risk infants have been found to be helpful in preventing death.

Inherited as an AUTOSOMAL RECESSIVE trait, the disorder has a high frequency among blacks, with an incidence of approximately one in 500 to one in 625 live births. Overall, 2,000 infants a year are born with sickle-cell anemia. It is estimated that one in 1,875 blacks in the United States have the disorder. One in 10 to one in 12 are thought to be CARRIERS of the gene. These carriers, who exhibit no symptoms, are said to have the sickle-cell trait. While carriers generally do not express any abnormalities of the blood, it is possible for their cells to exhibit "sickling" if subjected to prolonged oxygen deprivation, such as altitudes of 10,000 feet or more, or extreme physical exertion.

Frequency of sickle-cell anemia is also somewhat elevated in Mediterraneans and other populations originating in malaria-prone areas. It is believed that the gene for several red blood cell abnormalities (hemoglobinopathies, see HEMOGLOBIN) including sickle-cell trait, confers an increased resistance to malaria, and therefore may have been an advantage in a time and place when malaria was a greater threat than anemia.

Currently there is no cure for sickle-cell disease. Treatment generally consists of transfusions of normal red blood cells and medications to control pain and infections.

Due to its prevalence and its potentially serious consequences, it is often recommended that all newborn infants be tested for both the sickle-cell trait and sickle-cell anemia.

Carriers of the sickle-cell gene (sickle-cell trait) can be easily detected using a simple blood test. Because the specific MUTATION causing this abnormality is known (there is a single base change in the GENETIC CODE) new DEOXYRIBONUCLEIC ACID (DNA) diagnostic tests have made PRENATAL DIAGNOSIS relatively straightforward. These tests identify the change in the DNA of the ß-globin gene by analysis of that gene in fetal cells obtained by CHORIONIC VILLUS SAMPLING or AMNIOCENTESIS. A new test called the polymerase chain reaction (PCR) allows this test to be performed rapidly.

For other forms of anemia, see also ANEMIA, THALASSEMIA, GLUCOSE-6-PHOSPHATE DEHYDROGENASE DEFICIENCY.

For more information, contact:

National Association For Sickle Cell
  Disease, Inc.
4221 Wilshire Blvd., Suite 360
Los Angeles, CA 90010-3503
(213) 936-7205
(800) 421-8453

Sickle Cell Self-Help Association
P.O. Box 5610
Inglewood, CA 90310
(213) 732-4262

**SIDS**   See SUDDEN INFANT DEATH SYNDROME

**simian crease**   A single crease on the palm of the hand, resembling the transverse flexion crease found in some monkeys. Normally, at birth the palm of the hand contains several flexion creases, areas where the skin folds when the palm is manipulated. Two of these creases are separate and run generally crosswise (transverse) over the palm. When these two appear to fuse and form a single transverse crease in the middle of the palm, it is termed a simian crease.

Simian crease is often present in a variety of developmental abnormalities, including DOWN SYNDROME, FETAL ALCOHOL SYNDROME, DELANGE SYNDROME and many other syndromes. It is also found on one hand in about 4% of normal babies and in both hands in 1%. It is twice as common in males as in females.

**sirenomelia**  Taking its name from the mermaid-like lower extremities of the sirens in Homer's *Odyssey*, this rare congenital deformity is characterized by the fusion of the legs. The cause of this developmental anomaly is unknown, though it may be due to an alteration in early blood vessel development whereby blood is diverted away from the developing lower portion of the embryo. In addition to the single lower extremity, affected infants also may have other defects of the gastrointestinal and genitourinary tracts. Incidence of this rare condition is unknown.

**skin cancer**  See CANCER.

**skin tag**  A small outgrowth of skin, which is usually joined on the neck, armpit, or groin. It is often present at birth.

**Sly syndrome**  See MUCOPOLYSACCHARIDOSIS.

**Smith-Lemli-Opitz syndrome**  First described in 1964 by U.S pediatrician D.W. Smith and geneticists L. Lemli and J.M. Opitz, this syndrome is characterized by multiple CONGENITAL abnormalities, including a long narrow skull (scaphocephaly), an abnormally small head (MICROCEPHALY), drooping eyelids (PTOSIS), crossed eyes (STRABISMUS), skin folds over the inner corners of the eyes (EPICANTHUS), CATARACTS, wide-set eyes (HYPERTELORISM), a broad nasal bridge and tip, upturned nostrils (anteverted nares), increased distance between the nose and the lips, low-set ears, small jaw (micrognathia) and a short neck.

Other characterstics include hand clenching, incurving fifth fingers (CLINODACTYLY), fusion of the second and third toes (SYNDACTLYL) and a distinct single crease across the width of the palm (SIMIAN CREASE).

Male infants may have a markedly small penis, undescended testicles (CRYPTORCHIDISM) and a urinary opening on the underside of the penis (HYPOSPADIAS). Moderate to severe MENTAL RETARDATION has been observed in all infants affected with this syndrome.

Affected infants are moderately small at birth and fail to thrive. During the first 28 days after birth, the affected infants exhibit vomiting, shrill screaming and susceptibility to infection. About half of those affected die within 18 months.

Although this disorder shows evidence of AUTOSOMAL RECESSIVE inheritance, the basic defect causing the syndrome is not known. Currently, there is no method for PRENATAL DIAGNOSIS of this syndrome.

**solar sneeze reflex syndrome**  See ACHOO SYNDROME.

**sonography**  See ULTRASOUND.

**Sotos syndrome**  (cerebral gigantism) The primary features of this disorder are advanced height, weight and bone age, characteristic facial appearance and mental deficiency. It is named for J.F. Sotos, who published a description in the *New England Journal of Medicine* in 1964.

At birth, average weight is over nine pounds. Head, hands and feet are disproportionately large. Head circumference and height are typically above the 97th percentile for age, and bone age two to three years beyond chronological age.

The characteristic face consists of a large skull, prominent forehead, receding hairline, wide-set eyes (HYPERTELORISM), large jaw (prognathism) pointed chin and upturned nose (anteverted nares). Teeth are present at birth in over half of the affected infants (see NATAL TEETH).

Walking is usually delayed until after 15 months of age, and speech until after 2.5 years. Neurological dysfunction, unusual clumsiness and episodes of aggressive behavior are common. The average IQ is 60. Growth is rapid in the first years of life, though final height is often in the normal range.

The basic cause of cerebral gigantism is unknown, and the genetics of the condition are not understood, though there have been reports of families with more than one affected member. Over 100 cases have been reported, with males outnumbering females by a ratio of two to one.

PRENATAL DIAGNOSIS is not possible, though ULTRASOUND may indicate abnormal size for fetal age.

For more information, contact:

Sotos Syndrome Support Association
223 West El Moro
Mesa, AZ 85202
(602) 890-1722

**spherocytosis**　See ANEMIA.

**sphingolipidosis**　Anyone of a group of hereditary disorders characterized by defective metabolism and storage of sphingolipids. They may result in severe neurological deterioration beginning in the first few months of life, or in other significant medical problems. The disorders include SANDHOFF DISEASE, FABRY DISEASE, TAY-SACHS DISEASE, GAUCHER DISEASE, KRABBE DISEASE and NIEMANN-PICK DISEASE.

**spider fingers**　See ARACHNODACTYLY.

**Spielmeyer-Vogt-Sjögren disease**　See BATTEN DISEASE.

**spina bifida**　Meaning "split spine," spina bifida is a CONGENITAL condition that results from abnormal fetal development of the spinal cord. It is the leading disabler of newborns in America.

The condition falls into the class of disorders known as NEURAL TUBE DEFECTS. The neural tube is the embryonic structure that evolves into the brain and spinal cord. Spina bifida has its genesis in the first four weeks of pregnancy, when the neural plate, a precursor to the neural tube, is forming. Normally, the edges of the neural plate curl toward each other, joining together to form the neural tube. As the neural tube develops into the spinal cord, bone (the spine) and muscle form a protective barrier around it.

In spina bifida, part of the neural plate fails to join together, and bone and muscle are unable to grow over this open section of the developing spinal column. Nerves that relay sensation and control movement in the legs, bladder and bowel are damaged or incompletely developed. The severity of symptoms is determined by the particular nerves involved and their degree of damage or maldevelopment.

Until the 1960s, many affected infants died soon after birth due to HYDROCEPHALUS or infections of the nervous system. Today, an estimated 80% to 95% survive and grow to maturity.

The cause of spina bifida is unknown. It is believed to be a MULTIFACTORIAL trait, that is, one that both genetic and environmental factors play a role in. The incidence of spina bifida is between one and two of every 1,000 live births in North America, but there appear to be geographic, ethnographic, and socioeconomic differences reflected in the rates among various populations.

There is ample evidence supporting a genetic component. Parents with one child with spina bifida have an increased risk of giving birth to another. More females than males are born with the condition. There is variation in incidence along ethnic and racial lines. Blacks, Asians and Ashkenazi Jews have lower rates than people of Northern European origin or Egyptians.

Evidence of an environmental link comes from variations in geographic and socioeconomic incidence. In the United States, more infants with spina bifida are born in the eastern and southern states than in the West. In western Great Britain and Ireland the incidence is four in 1,000 (it was previously as high as eight in 1,000), with the highest rates found in the poorest areas. It's been suggested that maternal diet or VITAMIN deficiency may play a role, with poorly nourished expectant mothers at increased risk. Under this theory, the explanation for the higher rates of the condition found in babies conceived in winter and early spring is due to the diminished supply of fresh foods during those months.

There are two major forms of the disorder. Spina bifida occulta ("hidden") is the mildest form, with the opening of the spinal cord covered by skin. In some cases, it may manifest itself as no more than a small cavity (dermal sinus) between two adjacent vertebrae, indicating that they have not fused properly. A hairy patch or birthmark may be above the defect. In another form of spina bifida occulta, the spinal cord ends in fatty tissue, which extends through the spinal column and forms a bulge under the skin. If the abnormality is mild enough, there are usually no symptoms. But if several vertebrae are involved and a fatty area, hairy patch or dimple in the skin over the defect is noticeable, bowel, bladder or motor problems may eventually develop.

The other form is spina bifida manifesta (also called "aperta" or "cystica"), in which a sac is immediately noticeable ("manifest") on the infant's back. This form is itself divided into two categories. In the less severe, the spinal cord develops normally but bulges out through incompletely developed vertebrae, forming a sac (meningocele—*meningo* refers to membranes, *cele* means a swelling or cavity). There can be minor muscle paralysis or incontinence if nerves protrude into this sac.

The much more common and severe form of spina bifida manifesta occurs when a portion of the undeveloped spinal cord itself protrudes through the back and forms a sac (myelomeningocele—*myelo* refers to the spinal cord). This accounts for perhaps 90% of all cases and is what is generally referred to when spina bifida is discussed.

Generally, the higher up on the back this sac is located, the more severe the case, since all the nerves lower on the back are usually affected. If it occurs high on the spinal column, the lower limbs may be totally paralyzed. A sac on the bottom of the spine may result only in relatively mild paralysis and bladder and bowel problems.

The exposed sac is usually surgically closed between 24 and 48 hours after birth. Hydrocephalus is a common complication seen in between 70% and 90% of spina bifida infants, either at birth or within a few days of it. This may require additional surgery.

After the age of one, chronic bladder infections and kidney deterioration pose the greatest danger, due to the individuals' inability to control many aspects of their excretory functions. Between 8% and 15% are born with a forward bending of the lower spine (kyphosis), creating a hunchbacked appearance. Some are born with CLUB FEET and dislocated hips. A lateral bend of the spine (SCOLIOSIS) may develop in childhood. Many are confined to wheelchairs or can walk only with the assistance of braces or crutches. Approximately 30% exhibit slight to severe MENTAL RETARDATION. Muscle imbalance caused by lack of muscular control may create deformities of the hip, knee and foot joints.

Though the need for medical care is most acute during the early years, the problems created by the condition require some level of lifelong professional attention. However, with proper assistance and access to opportunities, affected individuals can lead productive and fulfilling lives.

PRENATAL DIAGNOSIS is often possible. A series of tests including AL-PHAFETOPROTEIN screening, ULTRASOUND and AMNIOCENTESIS can identify approximately eight to nine out of 10 cases of neural tube defects. (See also AN-ENCEPHALY.)

For more information, contact:

The Spina Bifida Association of America
1700 Rockville Pike, Suite 540
Rockville, MD 20852
(301) 770-7222
(800) 621-3141

**spinal muscular atrophy**    Any of a group of muscular atrophies (muscle wasting), almost always genetic in origin, characterized by degeneration of neurons (nerves) of the spinal cord. These neurons control voluntary movement. There is progressive weakness, loss of tendon reflexes, involuntary twitching of muscle fibers (fasciculation), and contractures, or permanent flexion, of joints. Intelligence and sensory organs are unaffected. Overall, they occur in about one in 10,000 live births. It is estimated that one in 60 to one in 80 individuals is a CARRIER of a GENE for one of these conditions.

The basic defect that causes them is unknown. More than 80% of these disorders are classified as proximal spinal muscular atropies, because they begin in muscles closest (proximal) to the affected nerves, later spreading to the muscles farther away (distal). While several varieties have been described, subclassification is considered somewhat arbitrary. Most are inherited as AUTOSOMAL RECESSIVE traits. Currently, there is no method of carrier detection or PRENATAL DIAGNOSIS for the disorders (except, perhaps, for lack of fetal movements by PRENATAL ULTRASOUND). However, researchers have recently mapped a gene responsible for two milder forms of the disorder to CHROMOSOME 5, a discovery that may lead to methods of GENETIC SCREENING, detection and treatment.

*Werdnig-Hoffman disease.*    This is an infantile form of spinal muscular atrophy, with general muscle weakness beginning either before birth or during the first week of life. It is named for Austrian neurologist G. Werdnig (b. 1862), who published a description in 1891, and German neurologist Johann Hoffman (1857–1919), who published in 1893.

Infants present a characteristic "frog" position with hips raised and the knees flexed. The disease's progression is rapid and inexorable, with death occurring usually by one year of age, usually due to pulmonary infection or respiratory insufficiency. However, some infants have survived as long as six years. It is estimated to occur in between one in 20,000 and one in 25,000 live births.

*Kugelberg-Welander disease.*    A childhood or adolescent-onset form first described in 1956 by Swedish neurologists E. Kugelberg and M. Welander. Early symptoms include a waddling gait and difficulty in climbing stairs. Resembling Becker's or limb-girdle MUSCULAR DYSTROPHY, the weakness spreads to the shoulders and the extremities. Some individuals may lose the ability to walk during their late teens, but others remain ambulatory for decades.

Other, non-proximal spinal muscular atrophies include juvenile progressive bulbar palsy (childhood facial palsy), distal spinal muscular atrophy, characterized by infant weakness in the distal muscles of the legs, and facioscapulohumeral spinal muscular atrophy. These differ from the proximal forms in their highly localized muscle weakness.

There is also an adult-onset form (spinal and bulbar muscular atrophy) inherited as an X-LINKED trait. Affecting only men, symptoms appear in the third decade. One of the first signs is striking enlargement of the breasts (HEREDITARY GYNECOMASTIA). It is not associated with increased mortality.

For more information, contact:

Muscular Dystrophy Association
810 Seventh Avenue
New York, NY 10019
(212) 586-0808

**spinopontine atrophy**    See AZOREAN DISEASE.

**spondylocostal dysostosis**    See SPONDYLOTHORACIC DYSPLASIA.

**spondyloepiphyseal dysplasia**    The name of this form of short-trunk DWARFISM is taken from the Greek *spondylos* for vertebra, and *epiphyseal*, referring to the bone-forming area separated from the parent bone by cartilage. As infants normally grow and mature, the cartilage is gradually replaced by bone. In this disorder, these secondary bone-forming areas of the vertebrae exhibit *dysplasia*, or abnormal tissue development. The condition has both a CONGENITAL and late childhood onset form.

*Spondyloepiphyseal dysplasia congenita.* This condition is present at birth. The ossification (formation of bones from cartilage) of the spine is retarded, causing the vertebrae to appear flattened and abnormal. Ossification of other bones may be more grossly retarded or totally absent. The hands are of normal size and shape, though ossification of the bones is retarded.

Lack of muscle tone (hypotonia) presents a FLOPPY INFANT appearance. The face tends to be flat. CLEFT PALATE or CLUBFOOT may be present. There may be moderate hearing loss, and about half of affected infants have visual defects, including MYOPIA (near-sightedness) and retinal detachment, which may lead to BLINDNESS. The chest is barrel-shaped. The bones of the limbs may be severely bent. Legs may be knock-kneed (genu valgum) or BOW-LEGGED (genu vara). Individuals walk with a waddling gait. Fully grown males are usually between 33.5 inches and 51 inches (85.1–129.5 cm) in height.

It is inherited as an AUTOSOMAL DOMINANT trait, with affected individuals exhibiting a wide variability in the severity of the characteristic defects.

*Spondyloepiphyseal dysplasia tarda.* This is a delayed onset, X-LINKED inherited form, exhibited only in males. Infants appear normal at birth. The failure of normal growth is noted between the ages of five and 10 years, when growth of the spine appears to stop. The shoulders take on a hunched-up appearance, the neck appears shortened, the chest enlarged. There is premature deterioration (os-teoarthritis) of the bones of the spine and hips, which may limit movement.

Adults are midly dwarfed, with height usually between 4 feet 4 inches and 5 feet 2 inches (130.2–155.1 cm). (Rare autosomal dominant and AUTOSOMAL RECESSIVE forms of spondyloepiphyseal dysplasia tarda have also been reported.)

For more information, contact:

The Little People of America
P.O. Box 633
San Bruno, CA 94066
(415) 589-0695

**spondylometaphyseal chondrodysplasia**    A form of moderate, juvenile-onset DWARFISM, mostly affecting the trunk. The name is taken from the Greek *spondylos* for vertebra, and *metaphyseal*, referring to primary growing area of a bone. Normally, as infants grow, cartilage (*chondro*) turns to bone. However, in this disorder, the bone-forming process of the cartilage of the vertebrae exhibits *dysplasia*, or abnormal tissue development.

The disorder was first described by Dr. K. Kozlowski, in 1967, and is sometimes referred to as spondylometaphyseal chondrodysplasia, Kozlowski type.

Dwarfing usually becomes apparent between ages one and four years and is progressive. There are deformities of the spine, including pronounced hump (kyphosis), lateral bend (SCOLIOSIS) or both (kyphoscoliosis). Joints may exhibit severe deterioration. Individuals have a waddling gait. Adult height is about 4 feet 7 inches (147.8 cm). Life expectancy and intelligence are normal.

Inherited as an AUTOSOMAL DOMINANT trait, more than 40 cases have been documented.

For more information, contact:

The Little People of America
P.O. Box 633

San Bruno, CA 94066
(415) 589-0695

**spondylothoracic dysplasia**  (Jarcho-Levin syndrome, spondylocostal dysostosis)   A rare and generally lethal form of CONGENITAL DWARFISM characterized by a markedly shortened trunk, protuberant abdomen and limbs that may appear relatively long, though they are of normal length. The face is round and appears puffy. The neck is short, and the chin appears to rest on the chest.

The name of the disorder is taken from *spondylo*, Greek for vertebra, and *thoracic*, referring to the chest. Both the vertebral column (spine) and the rib cage exhibit dysplasia, or abnormal development. The typical appearance of the chest on X ray is described as "crab-like." Death is usually from respiratory insufficiency or pneumonia as a result of a small chest.

It is believed to be inherited as an AUTOSOMAL RECESSIVE trait. Most affected individuals have been Puerto Rican, with more female than male cases in the literature. PRENATAL DIAGNOSIS may be possible by ULTRASOUND, though the characteristic changes may not be obvious until late in gestation.

There are probably two other forms of spondylothoracic dysplasia: another autosomal recessive form with a better prognosis and an AUTOSOMAL DOMINANT form with milder manifestations.

**spongy degeneration of the brain**  See CANAVAN DISEASE.

**sporadic**   The random appearance of a BIRTH DEFECT or CONGENITAL condition that results from an unknown cause or from a new MUTATION.

**Sprengel deformity**   (high scapula) The scapula is the large, flat, triangular bone that forms the back of the shoulder, the "shoulder blade." In this rare developmental abnormality, named for German surgeon Otto Sprengel (1852–1915), the scapula is poorly formed and displaced higher and more toward the midline of the back than when normally positioned. This, in turn, may restrict the ability to raise the arm. The condition may be in one (unilateral) or both (bilateral) of the scapulae. Surgery may help alleviate both restrictions of movement and cosmetic aspects of the disorder.

About two-thirds of the cases exhibit associated abnormalities, including lateral curvature of the spine (SCOLIOSIS), fused vertebrae, missing ribs and poor development of the shoulder muscles.

Most cases are SPORADIC, but some are believed to be transmitted as an AUTOSOMAL DOMINANT trait.

**Steinert disease**   See MYOTONIC DYSTROPHY.

**Stein-Leventhal syndrome**   Named for U.S. gynecologists Irving F. Stein, Sr. (b. 1887) and Michael L. Leventhal (1901–1971), who published a description in 1935, this disorder is characterized by the development of multiple cysts in the ovaries (polycystic ovaries). Affected females are usually infertile (see INFERTILITY), and some may have excessive body hair (hirsutism). Fathers of affected individuals also tend to have excessive body hair, and sisters and mothers may exhibit menstrual irregularities. It is believed to be inherited as an AUTOSOMAL DOMINANT trait.

**sterility**   See INFERTILIITY.

**Stickler syndrome**  (hereditary progressive arthroophthalmopathy)   Progressive near-sightedness (MYOPIA) and abnormalities of the joints. The myopia, beginning in the first decade of life, often eventually results in retinal detachment and BLINDNESS. This rare hereditary syndrome was first recognized in 1965 by Gunnar B. Stickler, chairman of pediatrics at the Mayo Medical School in Minnesota.

Enlarged ankles, knees and wrists as well as a developmental defect involving a small jaw, relatively large tongue and cleft palate (ROBIN ANOMALY) are among the first signs of this disorder in newborns. Typically, affected individuals have rounded, asymmetrical faces, depressed bridge of the nose, folds of skin at the inner corners of the eye (EPICANTHUS) and a marked undergrowth of one side of the jaw compared to the other. They may also have a flat midface and cleft palate.

During childhood, stiffness and soreness in the joints may occur after overuse, accompanied by swelling and redness, leading to temporary locking of the joints. Crepitation, a soft, fine crackling sound, may be heard over the joints through a stethoscope.

If the thigh bone is involved, the individual may experience difficulty walking. Frequently there may also be problems of premature and progressive arthritis. About 25% of all patients experience problems with outward curvature of the spine (thoracic kyphosis) or sideward curvature (SCOLIOSIS) and 40% will have excessive joint mobility.

Prognosis for a normal life span is favorable, though affected individuals must be particularly careful of ocular problems such as GLAUCOMA, CATARACTS and retinal degeneration.

The basic defect causing this SYNDROME is unknown, though it may involve one of the GENES for collagen, the major structural protein of connective tissue. It is inherited as an AUTOSOMAL DOMINANT trait, with highly variable EXPRESSIVITY.

There is currently no available method of PRENATAL DIAGNOSIS; however, in at least one large PEDIGREE there was linkage of Stickler syndrome to one of the collagen genes. This may prove helpful in presymptomatic and prenatal diagnosis.

**stillbirth**    The birth of a dead infant. This may be caused by CHROMOSOME ABNORMAL-ITIES, lethal GENETIC DISORDERS, physical conditions within the uterus or injuries associated with childbirth. In many cases the cause may be unclear.

Approximately 20% of stillbirths or neonatal deaths have CONGENITAL ANOMALIES, compared with incidence in the general newborn population of between 2% and 3%. An estimated 5% to 10% have chromosome abnormalities, while only 0.5% of all newborns do (TRISOMY 18 is the most common). However, these are not necessarily the cause of death. Postmortem examinations can sometimes reveal the cause and be of assistance in GENETIC COUNSELING and management of future pregnancies.

**storage disease**    Genetic disorders caused by enzyme deficiencies. Due to these deficiencies, the body is unable to metabolize, or break down, substances that then accumulate, or are stored, within cells. Examples include TAY SACHS DISEASE, GAUCHER DISEASE, FABRY DISEASE, MUCOPOLYSACCHARIDOSIS and GLYCOGEN STORAGE DISEASE.

**strabismus**    The inability to direct the axis of the eyes in tandem; each appears to be looking in a different direction. In common terminology, it is referred to as being "cross-eyed."

Strabismus is seen in many GENETIC DISORDERS. As an isolated anomaly, a familial link has been recognized in medical literature since Hippocrates. No simple MENDELIAN inheritance pattern (dominant or recessive) is established, and it is thought to be a POLYGENIC (caused by the action of several genes) trait. SIBLINGS of affected infants have a 15% chance of exhibiting the disorder. If a parent is affected as well, risk rises to 40%.

**strawberry mark**    See NEVUS.

**Sturge-Weber syndrome**    A non-familial, CONGENITAL condition characterized by large areas of facial discoloration and neurological abnormalities. Abnormalities of the eye and internal organs may also be present.

The disorder bears the names of English physicians W.A. Sturge (1850–1919) and F.P. Weber (1863–1962). Sturge, who sometimes attended Queen Victoria, described the disorder in 1879, and Weber, the son of noted physician H.D. Weber, published a description in 1922.

The facial discoloration (PORT WINE STAIN; NEVUS) typically involves at least one upper eyelid and the forehead, though there is great variability among affected individuals. It is usually on one side (unilateral) of the face but may be on both (bilateral). The nevus can extend down the neck and onto the chest or back. The color, which rarely fades with age, ranges from light pink to deep purple and is caused by an overabundance of aberrant capillaries just beneath the surface of the skin. (Laser treatments have shown promise in reducing skin discoloration.)

Excessive blood vessels also develop on the surface of the brain (angiomas), usually on the back of the brain on the same side as the facial discoloration, and can cause abnormal brain activity. Seizures often begin by one year of age, with convulsions occurring on the side of the body opposite from the affected side of the face. MENTAL RETARDATION occurs in 30% of cases, most typically in individuals with frequent seizures.

Common visual problems include GLAUCOMA (in 30% of those under medical care), a buildup in pressure within the eyeball that damages the optic nerve. It is usually confined to the side of the face with the characteristic birthmark. The eye may also become enlarged (buphthalmos), and there may be opacity or clouding of the lens (CATARACT). The neurologic and ocular complications occur only in those patients where the lesion is on that part of the face that gets its stimulation from the first branch of the fifth cranial nerve (trigeminal nerve).

The condition has its origins in the sixth week of fetal development. A mass of blood vessel tissue forms in the area that will develop into the head, beneath the layer of embryonic tissue that will become facial skin. Normally, this mass of blood vessels diminishes during the ninth week of gestation but, in this condition, it remains.

All cases of this rare SYNDROME have been SPORADIC, with no gender or ethnic predilection. There is no method of PRENATAL DIAGNOSIS. Theoretically, an extensive nevus could be observed via FETOSCOPY. (See also KLIPPEL-TRENAUNAY-WEBBER SYNDROME.)

For more information, contact:

The Sturge-Weber Foundation
P.O. Box 460931
Aurora, CO 80015
(303) 693-2986

National Association for the Craniofacially Handicapped
P.O. Box 11082
Chattenooga, TN 37401
(615) 266-1632

Let's Face It
P.O. Box 711
Concord, MA 01742
(508) 371-3186

**stuttering** (stammering)   A hesitant or faltering speech disorder, apparently genetically influenced. Mentioned in Mesopotamian clay tablets, Chinese poems and Egyptian hieroglyphics, it is said to be unusually frequent in Japanese, infrequent in Polynesians and virtually absent in American Indians. A family from India was described in 1979 in which there were 12 stutterers in five generations. In the United States, it is estimated that at least 4% of children and 1.1% of adults stutter. Among identical twins, CONCORDANCE for stuttering is between 76% and 90% (that is, in from 76% to 90% of identical twins, if one stutters, the other will also). Among fraternal twins, concordance is 20%. These figures suggest hereditary transmission. It has also been suggested that, in some cases, this is an AUTOSOMAL DOMINANT trait.

Synonyms: anarthria literalis; spasmophemia.

For more information, contact:

American Speech-Language-Hearing
  Association
10801 Rockville Pike
Rockville, MD 20852
(301) 897-5700
(800) 638-8255

## sudden infant death syndrome (SIDS)

(crib death)   The sudden and unexplained death of an infant with no apparent disease. This is the leading cause of death in infants between one month and 12 months of age, claiming an estimated 7,000 to 8,000 lives annually in the United States. It affects blacks three times as frequently as whites. Ninety percent to 95% die before six months of age, with the peak incidence between two and four months. Most deaths occur during the winter months and between the hours of midnight and 8 A.M. (In most cases, the infants die during normal sleep periods. This is the origin of its secondary name, "crib death.") Premature and LOW BIRTH WEIGHT infants, those born to teenagers, smokers and drug addicted mothers, and those with a SIBLING who succumbed to SIDS, are all at increased risk. SIDS is slightly more common in males.

The cause of SIDS is unknown. Recognized since biblical times, it was once thought to be caused by inadvertent suffocation of the infant by the mother while sleeping, a belief now known to be incorrect. (The Old Testament story of King Solomon ordering a baby cut in half to learn the identity of its true mother is thought to represent an account of both SIDS and this erroneous suffocation assumption. Each of the women had a baby, but one of the infants died during the night. As related in the bible: "and this woman's died in the night because she overlaid it ... And she arose at midnight and beheld it was dead" [I Kings 3:19].) Many other suspected causes have also been ruled out, including choking, allergic reactions, infection, parental neglect and immunizations. Periodic cessation of breathing (apnea) during sleep has been suggested as a cause, though the true nature of SIDS appears to be more complex. Current hypotheses are focusing in defects in the interplay of several regulatory systems required to maintain life. Abnormalities in the brainstem tissue, which have recently been found in SIDS infants, may also play a role.

Efforts have been made to identify the "typical" SIDS infant, family and environment. One research project involved the tape recording of heart and breathing functions of 9,000 newborns, 22 of whom eventually died of SIDS. Researchers hope analysis of the tapes may hold clues that will help in the prevention of SIDS.

Many infants have been outfitted with monitors that sound an alarm if their breathing becomes irregular during sleep. However, these devices have been ineffective in assuring survival; parents may be unable to revive infants despite training in resuscitation techniques. Monitors are currently recommended only for a very small proportion of at-risk infants.

A number of previously unrecognized defects in fatty acid and organic acid metabolism have only recently been discovered to be the cause of some instances of SIDS. Recognition of a possible biochemical basis of some cases of SIDS is important since there is effective therapy by dietary manipulation, and since these disorders are inherited in an AUTOSOMAL RECESSIVE manner. Thus, in those families recurrence in another sibling is possible (25%) but PRENATAL DIAGNOSIS is also available. The frequency of these disorders among infants with SIDS is as yet unknown.

For more information, contact:

National Sudden Infant Death Syndrome
  (SIDS) Foundation
8200 Professional Plaza, Suite 104
Landover, MD 20785
(301) 459-3388
(800)-221-SIDS

**supernumerary teeth** Having more than the normal number of teeth. Approximately 2% of the population have extra teeth, almost always upper incisors. This condition is also associated with dental developmental abnormalities, such as CLEFT PALATE.

**sweaty feet syndrome (isovaleric acidemia)** A characteristic odor resembling that of sweaty feet, apparent within the first few weeks of life, gives this rare syndrome its name. It is caused by the inability of the body to metabolize adequately the AMINO ACID leucine. As a result, infection or ingestion of protein produces abnormally high levels of isovaleric acid in the blood.

Signs of this disorder usually become apparent within the first few weeks of life. In addition to the characteristic odor, they include intermittent acute attacks of vomiting, loss of muscular coordination (ataxia), seizures, lethargy and coma. Half of affected infants die within a few weeks of birth.

The defect, the inability to degrade leucine, is probably due to a flaw in the ENZYME isovaleryl-CoA dehydrogenase and is believed to be inherited as an AUTOSOMAL RECESSIVE trait. Laboratory tests can reveal the defective enzyme in a newborn, and PRENATAL DIAGNOSIS by enzyme assay of fetal cells is possible.

**syndactyly** Fusion of the digits of the fingers or toes. The extent of the fusion varies from webbing of skin tissue between the digits to complete joining of the bones of adjacent digits.

Syndactyly is a common feature of many CONGENITAL conditions, and it is also believed to occur in five hereditary forms as an isolated or featured characteristic. Most are believed to be AUTOSOMAL DOMINANT traits, though recessive forms also exist.

A survey of approximately 600,000 consecutive births in Latin America conducted in 1980 found incidence of syndactyly at approximately three per 10,000 live births.

**syndrome** A recognizable pattern or group of multiple signs, symptoms or malformations that characterize a particular disorder. Syndromes are thought to arise from a common origin and result from more than one developmental error during fetal growth.

**synophrys** The joining together of the eyebrows over the bridge of the nose, giving the suggestion of one long, continuous eyebrow. This condition is seen in many GENETIC DISORDERS, including CORNELIA DE LANGE SYNDROME, Sanfilippo syndrome (see MUCOPOLYSACCHARIDOSIS) and WAARDENBURG SYNDROME.

**syphilis** A veneral disease caused by the spirochetal bacteria, treponema pallidum. Though usually transmitted sexually, syphilis can be passed from an infected mother to the fetus through the placenta from the fourth month of pregnancy until birth.

Syphilis progresses in three stages: The first symptoms are painless skin sores, often on the genitals. Three months or longer after the sores heal, a rash appears, accompanied by swollen glands, headache and fever. The final stage begins three to 10 years after the first infection and damages most organs and tissues in the body.

Risk to the fetus depends on which stage of the disease the mother is in. Those in the first stage who are more than four months pregnant are assumed to have transmitted the infection to the fetus. Treatment with penicillin and erythromycin can cure the fetus before birth. As many as half of the infants born to syphilitic women in the second and third stages of the disease may be healthy, but the chances of STILLBIRTH or premature birth (see PREMATURITY) are high, and 10% to 40% are born with syphilis. Ninety-eight percent of those who receive treatment after birth survive.

Syphilitic infants may have skin sores, particularly around the mouth, genitals or anus, though physical signs of infection often are not manifest for months or years. Other early symptoms include mucous discharge from the nose and throat ("snuffles"), bone problems, skin rash, enlarged liver and spleen, and ANEMIA. Ocular problems, including GLAUCOMA, as well as DEAFNESS, abnormal teeth and bones, a deformed nose, MENTAL RETARDATION, and central nervous system disorders, develop if the disease remains untreated.

Although largely brought under control after World War II—with the ready availability of penicillin—rates of congenital syphilis began to rise in the late 1980s. This trend has been attributed to promiscuity and lack of prenatal health care among female abusers of crack and cocaine. In 1988, the U.S. Centers for Disease Control reported 691 cases of congenital syphilis, more than 50% above the previous year, and the highest to that time since the advent of penicillin. In 1989, New York became the first state to institute mandatory testing for syphilis among all newborns. The test, which costs about 30 cents in materials, uses a blood sample taken from the umbilical cord.

**systemic lupus erythematosus** See LUPUS.

# T

**talipes** See CLUBFOOT.

**talipes cavus** See CLUBFOOT.

**Tangier disease** Rare disorder named for Tangier Island in the Chesapeake Bay, whose inhabitants exhibit a higher than normal incidence of this hereditary condition. The primary defect is an abnormally low level of high-density lipoprotein (HDL), due to the complete absence of a protein component of HDL, termed apolipoprotein A-I. This protein, found in blood plasma, carries cholesterol and other fats from the blood to the tissues. The defect is presumably present at birth, though the disease may first be detected

at any time during infancy to late adulthood. Affected individuals can absorb and store dietary fat in the form of triglycerides, a fatty substance, but there is a delay in clearing the triglycerides from the blood once they are made, and high triglyceride blood levels result. Though elevated triglyceride and diminished HDL blood levels suggest increased risk for premature heart disease, life span expectations for affected individuals are not reduced.

The hallmark of the disorder is enlarged orange tonsils. Other symptoms include enlarged spleen (splenomegaly) and, in many cases, neurologic symptoms such as muscle wasting and loss of sensation in the skin.

Tangier disease is inherited as an AUTOSOMAL RECESSIVE trait. CARRIERS have half the normal lipoprotein levels, allowing for carrier detection. (See also CORONARY ARTERY DISEASE.)

**TAR syndrome** (thrombocytopenia-aplasia of radius syndrome) At birth, this syndrome is easily recognizable due to deformities of the upper and lower limbs. They include absence or shortening of the outer forearm bone (radius), often accompanied by malformation or absence of the inner forearm bone (ulna) and upper arm bone (humerus), as well as deformity of the wrist, hands, legs or feet. The thumbs are always present. The defects are usually bilateral, that is, affect the limbs on both sides of the body.

Small, purplish spots (petechiae) appear on the body from bleeding due to the abnormal decrease in the number of platelets (thrombocytopenia). The platelets are the blood cells involved in initiation of blood clotting. Internal examination often discloses an enlarged liver and spleen (hepatosplenomegaly), and a host of other abnormalities may be found; about one-third of affected infants have a CONGENITAL HEART DEFECT. Testing of the blood and bone marrow reveals defects, including a deficiency in the large bone marrow cells that produce the platelets (megakaryocytes), a decrease in red blood cells (ANEMIA) and an abnormal increase in certain white blood cells (granulocytosis and eosinophilia).

Approximately 40% of those affected with this disorder die in infancy because of hemorrhaging. The basic defect causing the syndrome is unknown, although AUTOSOMAL RECESSIVE inheritance is suspected. Use of ULTRASOUND prenatally may disclose the upper limb defects.

For more information, contact:

TARSA: TAR Syndrome Association
312 Sherwood Drive, R.D. 1
Linwood, NJ 08221
(609) 927-0418

**Tay-Sachs disease (TSD)**    A fatal degenerative disease of the nervous system that is found primarily but not exclusively among Ashkenazi Jews, those of Eastern European ancestry. (There is a noticeable incidence of TSD among non-Jewish French Canadians living near the St. Lawrence River.) It is named for Warren Tay (1843–1927), a British ophthalmologist who in 1881 first described the CHERRY-RED SPOT on the retina of the eye that is one of the characteristic symptoms of the disorder, and Bernard Sachs (1858–1944), a New York neurologist who described the cellular changes of Tay-Sachs and noted its increased prevalence in the Eastern European Jewish population in 1887.

Inherited as an AUTOSOMAL RECESSIVE trait, TSD is one of a group of STORAGE DISEASES: Due to a deficiency of the enzyme hexosaminidase A (Hex-A), there is an accumulation of $GM_2$ ganglioside, a fatty substance, in the nerve cells of the brain. The storage of this substance causes nerve degeneration. Though the process begins during pregnancy, the child appears healthy at birth and develops normally until about six months of age.

Among the first symptoms are a slowing of development, loss of vision, abnormal startle response and convulsions. Examination of the retina reveals the characteristic cherry-red spot. As the disease progresses, there is a deterioration of all functions, leading to BLINDNESS, MENTAL RETARDATION, paralysis and death, usually by the age of three to four years.

Researchers have concluded that the proliferation of the TSD GENE occurred after the second Diaspora (70 A.D.) and before the major migrations to regions of Poland and Russia (1100 A.D. and later).

Some researchers believe that CARRIERS of the TSD gene may be at some selective advantage for resistance to tuberculosis, though this is a controversial hypothesis.

TSD affects about one in every 2,500 newborn Ashkenazic Jews, and it is estimated that approximately one in every 25 Jews in the United States is a carrier of the TSD gene. TSD screening has been the prototype for carrier screening programs designed to permit the prevention of GENETIC DISORDERS. Carriers can be identified through GENETIC SCREENING. By 1985 over half a million persons had been screened, resulting in the identification of more than 20,000 carriers.

PRENATAL DIAGNOSIS is possible by assay for Hex A activity in cultured fetal cells obtained via AMNIOCENTESIS or CHORIONIC VILLUS SAMPLING.

For more information, contact:

National Tay-Sachs and Allied Diseases
    Association, Inc.
385 Elliot Street
Newton, MA 02164
(617) 964-5508

Center for Jewish Genetic Disease
Division of Medical Genetics of
    Mount Sinai Medical Center
100 Street at Fifth Avenue
New York, NY 10029
(212) 241-6947

**teratogen**    With its etymological origin in the Greek work *teras*, meaning monster, a teratogen is any substance (drug, chemical, viral or environmental agent) that can trigger malformation of the fetus. Maternal medical conditions associated with birth defects, such as DIABETES MELLITUS or PHENYLKETONURIA, are also considered teratogens. (The term "teratology," which refers to the study of human malformations, was coined by zoologist Isidore Geoffroy Saint-Hilaire [1805–1861], who was among the first to scientifically investigate these conditions.)

A teratogen may damage the embryo directly or by disrupting normal functioning of the placenta by which the fetus receives nutrients, thereby creating an abnormal uterine environment.

The impact on fetal development is in general dependent on the amount of exposure to a given teratogen and the stage of fetal development at which the exposure occurs. The greater the exposure, the greater the risk to the fetus. However, the susceptibility to the effect of a given teratogen varies greatly from individual to individual.

The first two weeks after conception is called the "all-or-none" period; exposure to a teratogen at this critical period will generally either kill the embryo or have no impact at all. During the third through eighth weeks of pregnancy, the embryo's cells begin to develop characteristics of specific organ systems, and exposure to teratogens during this period can result in damage to specific organs. The central nervous system is susceptible to teratogens throughout pregnancy.

Most substances recognized as teratogens produce a particular pattern of defects. The now-banned drug THALIDOMIDE, for example, led to missing limb bones; in some cases the entire limb failed to develop so that the hand or foot was attached directly to the body. Epileptics who take ANTICONVULSANTS during pregnancy sometimes give birth to babies with distinctive facial features and heart defects caused by the drugs. Some infections during pregnancy can also lead to birth defects. Rubella (German measles [see TORCH SYNDROME]) can cause CATARACTS, DEAFNESS, CONGENITAL HEART DEFECTS and MENTAL RETARDATION in the infant.

Teratogens may also cause birth defects in concert with genetic influences in families predisposed toward certain malformations. CLEFT LIP, cleft palate, NEURAL TUBE DEFECTS, such as SPINA BIFIDA and ANENCEPHALY, pyloric stenosis (an abnormally small passage between the stomach and the intestine), CONGENITAL HIP DISLOCATION and some congenital heart defects are examples. About 20% of birth defects are estimated to be caused in this MULTIFACTORIAL (combination of genes and environmental agents) manner.

For information on specific agents, see: ACCUTANE, AGENT ORANGE, CAFFEINE, CIGARETTES, COCAINE, FETAL ALCOHOL SYNDROME, LEAD, MARIJUANA, MEASLES, PHENOBARBITAL, QUININE, RADIATION, SYPHILIS, VARICELLA (Chicken Pox), VIDEO DISPLAY TERMINALS, WARFARIN EMBRYOPATHY.

**teratoma of head and neck**    See DERMATOID CYST (OR TERATOMA) OF HEAD AND NECK.

**testes, absent**    See ABSENT TESTES.

**testicular feminization syndrome** (complete androgen insensitivity)    A form of PSEUDOHERMAPHRODITISM. Affected individuals are born with female external genitalia and and are thought to be females at birth. At puberty, their breasts develop, and though they usually have little body hair, they otherwise have normal female appearance. They typically come to medical attention when they fail to begin menstruating at the time of puberty.

Upon examination, the vagina is shallow, and there are no Fallopian tubes or uterus. The testicles may be in the abdominal area and are incapable of producing viable sperm.

Despite the overwhelmingly feminine appearance, the chromosomes are those of a male—an XY chromosome pair, rather than the XX found in normal females.

The testes are generally removed, and plastic surgery can enlarge the size of the vagina, enabling continued female gender identification. (Some genetic counselors suggest that affected males never be told their true genetic sex for psychological reasons though counseling in each case should be individual.)

Following treatment and continued estrogen therapy, affected individuals live as normal women, although they are sterile. Life span and intelligence are normal.

It has been proposed by one genetic researcher that Joan of Arc was actually a male with this syndrome. The suggestion is based on examination of extensive documentation of her physical characteristics presented at her trial for heresy in 1431 and at her posthumous Trial of Rehabilitation in 1456. This documentation includes accounts by those who lived in close quarters with her that while she had well-developed breasts, she had no pubic hair and did not menstruate. This hypothesis has led to speculation concerning elevated testosterone levels and her behavior.

Testicular feminization syndrome is thought to occur in approximately one in 70,000 live male births. It is inherited as an X-LINKED trait that results from a new MUTATION. PRENATAL DIAGNOSIS is theoretically possible. A male KARYOTYPE identified via AMNIOCENTESIS, with no penis or scrotum found via ULTRASOUND, would suggest a possible case.

**tetralogy of Fallot**    A complex of four associated CONGENITAL HEART DEFECTS (CHD): ventricular septal defect; an enlarged (hypertrophied) right ventricle; a malpositioned aorta, the major artery leading from the heart; and a narrowing (stenosis) of the pulmonary artery.

Named for French physician Etienne L.A. Fallot (1850–1911), it accounts for approximately 10% of all CHDs, with males more often affected than females by a ratio of 3 to 2.

Affected infants exhibit bluish skin (cyanosis), feeding difficulties and FAILURE TO THRIVE. Older children display a characteristic squatting position and clubbed fingers and toes. Without surgery to correct the cardiac defects, prognosis is poor.

Besides occurring in isolation, this condition may be associated with GOLDENHAR SYNDROME and KLIPPEL-FEIL ANOMALY, as well as with some TERATOGENS, such as THALIDOMIDE, maternal PHENYLKETONURIA and TRIMETHADIONE.

**thalassemia**  (Cooley's anemia; Mediterranean anemia)    The thalassemias are a group of inherited disorders involving defective production of HEMOGLOBIN, the oxygen-carrying component of red blood, resulting in ANEMIA, a generally debilitating condition marked by weakness and fatigue. Thalassemia is taken from the Greek *thalassa*, meaning "sea." The names "thalassemia" and "Mediterranean anemia" are indicative of its high incidence in populations bordering on the Mediterranean Sea, particularly in Italy and Greece. As in other red blood cell disorders with origins in populations from malaria-prone areas, it appears that asymptomatic CARRIERS of the trait have an increased resistance to malaria. The disorder is also prevalent in Southeast Asia, India, the Middle East and parts of Africa.

Hemoglobin occurs in several forms. It is composed of heme, the oxygen-carrying respiratory pigment that gives blood its red color, and globin chains, designated alpha, beta, gamma and delta. Specific combinations of globin chains determine the form of hemoglobin.

The thalassemias have their origin in abnormal production of hemoglobin A, the main form of adult hemoglobin, which normally contains two alpha and two beta globin chains. Beta-thalassemias, the most common type, involve abnormalities in the beta chain synthesis. These were among the first human GENETIC DISORDERS to be examined by RECOMBINANT DNA analysis techniques.

The thalassemias are inherited as AUTOSOMAL RECESSIVE traits.

*Cooley's anemia (beta-thalassemia major).*    This is the most severe form of beta-thalassemia, first described in 1925 by Dr. Thomas Benton Cooley (1871–1945), an American pediatrician. In this disorder, beta chains are absent from hemoglobin A, or their synthesis is greatly reduced.

Infants appear normal at birth. Onset is usually in the first few months of life. Early signs are paleness, fatigue, irritability and FAILURE TO THRIVE. There may also be fever, feeding problems, diarrhea and gastrointestinal complications. Symptoms become progressively more severe, leading to an enlarged spleen (splenomegaly), severe anemia, enlargement of the heart, slight jaundice and leg ulcers.

Under examination, the red blood cells appear pale, thin and misshapen, and most are unusually small. While normal red blood cells survive for four months, these break down within a few weeks. The need for more red blood cells causes the bone marrow, where they are produced, to expand dramatically, thinning the surrounding bone, especially the bones of the skull and face. This gives affected infants a characteristic facial appearance, with prominent cheek bones, eyes slanted toward the nose, overgrowth of the upper jaw and dental malformations of the upper teeth. Bones fracture easily.

Additionally, the iron and waste products from the breakdown of the red blood cells accumulate in organs, damaging the spleen, liver and heart. The iron overload that results causes many of the life-threatening problems of the disease. Without treatment, Cooley's anemia is invariably fatal. Current management consists of blood transfusion of packed red blood cells in concert with iron chelators, an agent that binds with excess iron in the body, so that it can be excreted. Removal of the spleen (splenectomy) may be necessary in some cases. The prognosis for life expectancy using these modern treatment methods is currently unknown, though some affected individuals are surviving into their twenties and thirties. Experimental research on the effectiveness of bone marrow transplantation as a means of stimulating healthy red blood cell production is in progress. In general, the younger the child is when the disease appears, the more unfavorable the prognosis.

In the United States, it is estimated that one in 800 to one in 2,500 individuals of Greek or Italian descent have this disorder. Carrier screening is available. Prenatal diagnosis is now possible using recombinant DNA techniques through analysis of the globin chain genes in fetal cells obtained by CHORIONIC VILLUS SAMPLING or AMNIOCENTESIS. Since a variety of different MUTATIONS cause thalassemia, the specific mutation in a given family must be known before prenatal diagnosis is possible.

*Beta-thalassemia minor (thalassemia trait).*   This is a mild, often completely asymptomatic trait that results from having only one recesssive GENE for the condition, rather than the two recessive genes necessary for full expression of the disorder. It is estimated that over 2,000,000 Americans, and 4% of all individuals of Greek or Italian descent, are CARRIERS of this trait. The incidence of the gene is also higher among blacks than in the general population, and may play a role in the expression of the SICKLE-CELL ANEMIA trait. While blacks may have an increased incidence of beta-thalassemia minor (the beta-thalassemia trait), they rarely have thalassemia major.

*Alpha-thalassemia.*   This disorder is seen mainly in Asian populations and involves defective synthesis of alpha chains in hemoglobin. As with beta thalassemias, it appears in major and minor forms. Alpha-thalassemia major frequently results in fetal death.

Alpha-thalassemia commonly results from the deletion of one or more of the four genes that code for alpha chains. If all four are deleted this is lethal in utero, or affected infants are stillborn with hydrops fetalis. If there are three deletions, hemoglobin H disease results, with hemolytic anemia of variable severity. Only one or two deletions results in alpha-thalassemia minor, the carrier state, with no clinial abnormalities.

For more information, contact:

Cooley's Anemia Foundation, Inc.
105 East 22nd St., Suite 911
New York, NY 10010
(212) 598-9011
(800) 221-3571

**thalidomide**  A sedative widely prescribed in the late 1950s in Europe, Australia
and Canada to prevent nausea in pregnant
women; subsequently found to cause severe
limb deformities. Affected infants typically
had incompletely developed arms or legs,
with hands or feet attached almost directly to
the trunk (PHOCOMELIA). Although several
thousand thalidomide babies were born, initial
suggestions of a link between the drug and the
defects were discounted; prior to that time, it
was believed the placenta protected the fetus
from harmful influences, and therefore that
drugs could not cause birth defects. Though
animal studies had been conducted with thalidomide, the drug did not have the same effect
on laboratory animals as on humans.

Never approved for use in the United States
by the Food and Drug Administration,
thalidomide's use as a sedative was halted in
1962. However, it is still used outside the
United States as an immunosuppressive agent,
treating autoimmune disorders (see IMMUNE
DEFICIENCY DISEASES) by suppressing the immune system. In Canada it is available as an
"emergency status" agent, requiring special
permission from the Health Protection Branch
for use. It is also a major medication used to
treat one form of leprosy, and is available in
England for use in treating some skin diseases,
discoid lupus (see LUPUS ERYTHEMATOSUS)
and RHEUMATOID ARTHRITIS. It has also been
renamed in England due to the negative associations of the name thalidomide; it is now
known as "sauramide." (See also TERATO-
GEN.)

**thanatophoric dwarfism**  A rare and
severe form of short-limbed DWARFISM that
results in death soon after birth, primarily due
to respiratory insufficiency caused by the abnormally small rib cage. It is believed to be
inherited as an AUTOSOMAL DOMINANT disorder, with all affected infants resulting from
new MUTATIONS. Named in 1967, and incor-
porating the Greek *thanatos*, "death," in its
designation, the first report of a condition that
fits this description was published in 1898.

Incidence has been estimated at between one
in 6,400 and one in 8,900 births.

**thrombasthenia of Glanzmann and
Naegeli** (Glanzmann thrombasthenia,
GTA)  Taken from the Greek *thrombos*,
for "clot," and *asthenia*, "weakness,"
"thrombasthenia" denotes a hemorrhagic
(bleeding) disorder characterized by prolonged bleeding and abnormal platelet function studies. When viewed microscopically,
blood smears show little evidence of platelet
aggregation. It was first described by Swiss
pediatrician E. Glanzmann (1887–1959) in
1918. It also bears the name of Swiss hematologist Otto Naegeli (1871–1938).

Multiple blood factors (in the platelets,
plasma and tissues) have been identified as
being necessary for proper platelet function.
In this disorder, the factor that makes platelets
adhere to the walls of injured vessels is missing. This factor is a complex of platelet membrane proteins called GP II b and GP III a.
(VON WILLEBRAND's disease is caused by the
absence of another of these, a plasma factor.)

While almost all cases are considered the
result of AUTOSOMAL RECESSIVE inheritance,
there is likely more than one form of the
disorder. It has been reported as being the
second most common bleeding disorder in
Jordan, and frequent among Iraqi Jews.

Affected individuals have a lifelong tendency of mild to severe bleeding from mucous
membranes (e.g., nosebleeds, gums etc.) and
prolonged bleeding after injury.

In some cases, PRENATAL DIAGNOSIS has
been possible by studying fetal blood samples
obtained by FETOSCOPY or CORDOCENTESIS.
Heterozygotes (CARRIERS), those who have
only one of the two GENES required for the
expression of this disorder, may exhibit mild
clotting abnormalities, though upon examination their blood appears normal.

**thrombocytopenia-aplasia of radius
syndrome**  See TAR SYNDROME.

**thumb sign**   The protrusion of the thumb, when bent, across the palm and beyond the clenched fist. It is seen in children with MARFAN SYNDROME.

**thymic alymphoplasia**   See DI GEORGE SYNDROME.

**tobacco**   See CIGARETTES.

**Tom Thumb**   "General" Tom Thumb, born Charles Stratton, was the most famous dwarf of the 19th century, an era in which there were a great many "prodigies" whose physical abnormalities formed the basis of performing careers that often brought them considerable renown and fortune. The name "Tom Thumb" is taken from a legend, probably Scandinavian in origin but common to several European countries, of an extremely small person. This mythical person is limned in the 1630 poem, "Tom Thumbe: His Life and Death."

> In Arthur's court Tom Thumbe did live
> A man of mickle might,
> The best of all the table round,
> And eke a doughty knight;
> His stature but an inch in height
> Or quarter of a span;
> Then thinke you not this little knight
> Was prov'd a valiant man?

Born January 11, 1832, Stratton reached 25 inches in length at five months, and then stopped growing for several years. His condition is believed to have been panhypopituitary dwarfism (see PITUITARY DWARFISM SYNDROMES). His parents were first cousins (see CONSANGUINITY) and thus he probably had an AUTOSOMAL RECESSIVE disorder interfering with the synthesis of growth hormone. He was first exhibited by P.T. Barnum at his American Museum in New York, and created an immediate sensation, drawing 30,000 attendees. A crowd estimated at 10,000 saw him off when he set sail for his first European tour in January of 1844, and his reception in Europe was even more tumultuous than in New York. He was received by Queen Victoria and other European heads of state.

His act consisted of posing himself in the attitude of various famous Greek statues, or impersonations of Cupid with wings and bow, the gladiator Hercules and Napoleon Bonaparte. In this last role he would appear in deep meditation or strut about the stage in a miniature uniform. He was presented to the Duke of Wellington, who asked what he was thinking about while seeming so lost in thought during the impersonation. "I was thinking of the loss of the battle of Waterloo," Tom replied.

After his last visit to Europe in 1878, Tom Thumb retired and lived on the large fortune earned from his European tours.

**tongue folding or rolling**   The ability to fold the tongue backward or roll it into a tubular shape, two independent traits, are inherited by AUTOSOMAL DOMINANT transmission. The conditions are benign. In samples of various population groups, the majority of those surveyed were able to roll their tongues.

**tongue-tie**   See ANKYLOGLOSSIA.

**tooth-and-nail syndrome**   (dysplasia of the nails with hypodontia)   As the name implies, this disorder involves underdevelopment of the teeth and nails. Though rare, it has been reported as being frequent among Dutch Mennonites in Canada. Some teeth are absent (most often absent are the mandibular incisors, second molars and maxillary canines). Nails on fingers and especially toes form poorly. (Nails grow normally following childhood.) The condition has usually been detected when teeth failed to erupt. It is inherited as an AUTOSOMAL DOMINANT trait.

The group of disorders that are characterized by ANOMALIES of dental development and skin appendages (nails, hair, sweat glands) are termed ECTODERMAL DYSPLASIAS (ED). Tooth-and-nail syndrome differs from other forms of ED in not exhibiting abnormal sweat gland function and in a lesser severity of dental abnormalities.

**TORCH Syndrome**    An acronym for four infectious diseases that are known to cause similar birth defects: Toxoplasmosis, Rubella and infections with Cytomegalovirus (CMV) and Herpes simplex virus. PRENATAL DIAGNOSIS of fetal infection with these organisms is now possible using new invasive diagnostic techniques of fetal blood sampling, such as CORDOCENTESIS.

## Toxoplasmosis

This common infection is caused by the parasitic microscopic organism Toxoplasma gondii. Humans contract the disease by eating or handling raw meat or coming in contact with cat feces containing the organism. Outdoor cats that hunt are more likely to be infected.

Women who have had the infection before pregnancy (about 35%) are immune to it, and they confer this immunity to their unborn child. However, if a woman becomes infected during pregnancy, particularly between the 10th and 24th weeks, the fetus may be affected. Infection in early pregnancy carries a lower risk of the infection spreading to the fetus than infection later in pregancy; however, early infection carries a higher risk of severe abnormalities. In the United States, approximately one in 1,000 newborns is infected with toxoplasmosis. Premature birth (see PREMATURITY) is common among such infants, although only 10% to 20% of infected infants show signs of illness. Among those with severe infection, over 80% suffer MENTAL RETARDATION and have seizures. Other abnormalities include ocular defects, such as inflammation of the retina (seen in about 25% of cases), accumulation of fluid in the brain (HYDROCEPHALUS), convulsions, calcium deposits in the brain, an abnormally small head (MICROCEPHALY) and yellowish skin color (jaundice). However, about 60% of infants born with toxoplasmosis exhibit no, or only minor, health problems.

## Rubella

Maternal infection with rubella (German measles) during pregnancy may cause CATA-RACTS and GLAUCOMA, CONGENITAL HEART DEFECTS, DEAFNESS, delayed motor development or CEREBRAL PALSY, and MENTAL RETARDATION. It may also result in miscarriage or STILLBIRTH. Infants with rubella often develop other infections, such as pneumonia, meningitis and encephalitis. Endocrine abnormalities such as DIABETES may result. The abnormalities seen vary with the time in gestation during which infection occurred.

About 10% to 20% of infants with CONGENITAL rubella die within their first year. It is preventable by immunization against rubella prior to pregnancy.

Rubella epidemics used to occur approximately every six to nine years, with major epidemics occurring at intervals of up to 30 years. The most recent of these major outbreaks occurred between 1962 and 1965. Beginning in Europe, it reached the United States in 1964. This 1964–65 epidemic in the United States resulted in an estimated 12.5 million cases of rubella, and more than 11,000 cases of fetal death by miscarriage or therapeutic ABORTION. Approximately 20,000 infants were born with congenital rubella syndrome. Of these, an estimated 2,100 died in early infancy and almost 12,000 were deaf. The economic cost of this epidemic was placed at approximately $1.5 billion.

The development of a live attenuated rubella vaccine in 1969 greatly reduced the incidence of this viral infection. No large epidemics have subsequently occurred in areas where the vaccine is in wide use, though limited outbreaks continue to occur in settings such as schools, where large groups of susceptible individuals are in close contact with one another. All 50 of the states require rubella vaccinations prior to school entry.

## Cytomegalovirus Syndrome (CMV)

A very common and usually asymptomatic infection, this is a variety of the herpes virus. Nearly everyone has been infected by the age of 40, but unlike rubella and measles, CMV can recur. Contracting CMV for the first time during pregnancy presents a greater risk to the fetus than a recurring infection. The mother can transmit the virus to her newborn before birth through the placenta as well as during the birth process or through breast milk.

Approximately 1% of infants in the United States are born with CMV. About 90% are asymptomatic at birth. In those who show signs of infection, enlarged liver and spleen (HEPATOSPLENOMEGALY), a purplish rash from multiple area of bleeding (purpura), a yellowish skin color (jaundice) and a form of ANEMIA are common. MENTAL RETARDATION, seizures and hearing loss may also occur.

No treatment is available but most infants with mild cases recover completely. As with the previous two infections, the effects vary depending on the time of infection.

### Herpes simplex virus (HSV)

There are two types of this common infection; one primarily causes sores around the mouth, the other, transmitted sexually, primarily causes genital sores. Herpes can be transmitted from mother to infant during birth. If a woman contracts herpes during pregnancy, the risk of miscarriage or stillbirth is greatly increased.

Symptoms of herpes at birth include blisters on the skin or eyes (cutaneous or conjunctival vesicles), fever, jaundice and seizures. About half of infants with herpes die within a week of birth. Of those who survive, 25% to 30% have eye defects, abnormal motor development or MENTAL RETARDATION.

Birth by cesarian section can prevent infection of the newborn in women known to harbor the virus in their genital tracts.

**torsion dystonia**    See DYSTONIA.

**Tourette syndrome** (Gilles de la Tourette syndrome)    Named for Georges Gilles de la Tourette, who first described the syndrome in 1885, Tourette syndrome (TS) is a neurological disorder characterized by rap-

idly repetitive multiple movements called tics and by involuntary vocalizations.

The tics may include eye blinking, shoulder shrugging, head jerking, facial twitches or repetitive movements of the torso or limbs. The vocalizations may include repeated sniffing, throat clearing, coughing, grunting, barking or shrieking. Some affected individuals repeat other people's words (echolalia), stutter, repeat their own words (palilalia) or utter inappropriate or obscene words (coprolalia). (Though coprolalia occurs in only 5% to 40% of patients, it is the most well-known symptom of the disorder.) These body movements and vocalizations are the result of a chemical imbalance in the brain.

The disorder usually appears between the ages of two and 16 years and lasts throughout life. About three-quarters of patients are male, and 10% of affected individuals have a family history of the disorder. Those most at risk are sons of mothers with TS, where the percentage who develop it may be as high as 30%. The specific mode of genetic transmission has not been established. Some familial cases suggest that TS is an AUTOSOMAL DOMINANT trait with sex thresholds that affect the expression of the disorder. However, many SPORADIC cases have been reported. The incidence of full-blown cases of TS is estimated to be one in 2,000 live births. Mild cases may appear as frequently as one in 200 or one in 300 live births. It is said to be unusually frequent in a Mennonite religious isolate population in Canada.

Compulsive behaviors, seen in 40% of cases, include repeated touching, rubbing, incessant thoughts, imitating other people's movements, distractibility, ritualistic actions, and self-mutilation. Some compulsive behavior may be dangerous, e.g., the compulsion to run across the street before oncoming cars. Learning disabilities are present in 60% of cases.

Affected individuals rarely exhibit all the symptoms. There may be tremendous variability over time in the symptoms, their frequency and severity. In mild cases, a few tics or twitches may be confined to the face or eyes. In more severe cases, individuals may exhibit arm flapping, foot stamping or stomach jerks. The symptoms wax and wane, usually over three to four month periods. New symptoms may join old symptoms or take their place. Stress usually aggravates the condition. Events like birthdays, holidays, the beginning of a new school year may exacerbate the disorder. Symptoms also tend to get worse during puberty and sometimes stabilize during adulthood. However, it's estimated that 5% to 16% of cases go into remission at puberty.

While the vocalizations or body movements are involuntary, some affected individuals can suppress them, or substitute less socially inappropriate tics for brief periods of time, such as in a classroom, at work or when being examined by a physician. However, their symptoms usually emerge more explosively when they return to less threatening surroundings. A variety of medications may be useful in suppressing the symptoms.

Currently, there is no method of PRENATAL DIAGNOSIS or CARRIER screening.

It should be noted that perhaps 15% of all children exhibit transient tic disorders during their early school years, such as eye blinking, nose puckering, grimacing or squinting, and it may be especially noticeable with excitement or fatigue. Therefore, tics by themselves should not be taken as an indication of the presence of TS.

For more information, contact:

Tourette Syndrome Association
41-02 Bell Boulevard
Bayside, NY 11361
(718) 224-2999

**Townes syndrome**    Described in 1972 by U.S. physician Philip L. Townes (b. 1927) and his colleague E.R. Brocks, this syndrome was first observed in one family, affecting a father and five of his seven children. All six had IMPERFORATE ANUS (failure of develop-ment of the opening of the end of the intestinal tract to allow passage of the bowel contents), malformed ears and MENTAL RETARDATION. Most also had malformations of the thumb and other digits and mild to moderate deafness. By 1978, at least 36 affected individuals had been reported.

Inherited as an AUTOSOMAL DOMINANT trait, the ANOMALIES of the anus and rectum and malformed thumb and ears can be surgically treated. The outlook for a normal life span appears to be favorable.

**toxoplasmosis**    See TORCH SYNDROME.

**tracheoesophageal fistula**    An abnormal opening, present at birth, between the branches of the esophagus leading to the lungs and the digestive system. As a result, ingested liquids and foods may enter the lungs, causing respiratory infections and feeding difficulties. Once diagnosis is made, it can be repaired surgically.

This disorder has its genesis in the fourth week of embryonic development, though the cause of this maldevelopment is unknown. It occurs in an estimated one in 100,000 births, and may be seen alone or in association with other defects, for example, in infants with the VATER syndrome or in some CHROMOSOME ABNORMALITIES such as trisomy 18.

**Treacher Collins syndrome**    (mandibulo-facial dysostosis)    Inherited condition evident at birth due to its characteristic facial appearance. It is named for Edward Treacher Collins (1862–1932), an ophthalmologist at the Royal Eye Hospital in London, who described the condition in 1900, although a case may have been described in 1846. Its secondary name refers to malformations of the individual bones (DYSOSTOSIS) of the jaw and face (mandibulofacial).

The slits of the eyes (palpebral fissures) slant downward away from the nose (antimongoloid obliquity). The outer portion of the lower eyelid may be fissured (COLOBOMA), with a deficiency of eyelashes on the lower lid.

The cheek bones are underdeveloped, giving the nose a large appearance. The nasal bridge may be raised, the nostrils narrowed and the jaw very small (micrognathia). The ears may show several developmental abnormalities; the outer ear may appear grossly malformed or misplaced. The auditory canal may be missing, or the bones of the inner ear may be anomalous. CLEFT PALATE, dental malocclusion and high-arched palate are common.

Non-facial features occasionally associated with this primarily craniofacial disorder include CONGENITAL HEART DEFECTS, deformities of the spinal cord, congenital anomalies of the extremities, undescended testicles (CRYPTORCHIDISM) and renal (kidney) abnormalities.

Plastic surgery can correct some of the cosmetic manifestations of the syndrome.

The syndrome is inherited as an AUTOSOMAL DOMINANT trait and displays a high degree of variability in severity of expression. Over half of the cases are thought to arise from new MUTATION. Life span is normal, except in rare occasions where severe cardiac or renal abnormalities are present, leading to potentially fatal complications. Intelligence appears normal. (Reports of mental retardation in some cases may be due to the hearing disorder that usually accompanies this syndrome.)

In at-risk pregnancies, FETOSCOPY and ULTRASOUND may be able to detect some of the facial features that characterize Treacher Collins syndrome.

For more information, contact:

National Association for the Craniofacially Handicapped
P.O. Box 11082
Chattanooga, TN 37401
(615) 266-1632

National Foundation for Facial Reconstruction
550 First Avenue
New York, NY 10016
(212) 340-5400

Let's Face It
P.O. Box 711
Concord, MA 01742
(617) 371-3186

**tremor, hereditary essential**  See HEREDITARY ESSENTIAL TREMOR.

## trichorrhinophalangeal syndrome

This syndrome involves abnormalities of the face, hair and joints of the fingers. At birth affected infants have sparse scalp hair, eyelashes and eyebrows, a bulbous nose with tented (dilated) nostrils, large protruding ears and a thin upper lip. The infant may also have a high forehead, a long indentation between the nose and the mouth (philtrum) and a horizontal groove on the chin.

From mid-childhood until puberty the fingers and possibly the toes become progressively deformed due to abnormal growth of the bones. The fingers appear tapered. Flat feet are also common. Bone age is often several years behind chronological age and many adults with this disorder tend to be short, with approximately 40% below the third percentile in height.

Other features may include small teeth, problems with the bite (dental malocclusions), abnormal curvature of the spine (SCOLIOSIS), winging of the shoulder blades and CONGENITAL HEART DEFECTS.

The basic defect causing this syndrome is not known. Both AUTOSOMAL DOMINANT and RECESSIVE forms of the disorder exist, though most cases are dominantly inherited.

Life expectancy is normal. However, during infancy and early childhood affected individuals have an increased susceptibility to upper respiratory tract infections. A degenerative hip disease often develops in young adulthood.

The LANGER-GIEDION SYNDROME is a similar trichorrhinophalangeal syndrome but is distinguished by the presence of multiple exostoses, or bony outgrowths.

**trigonocephaly**  See CRANIOSYNOSTO-SIS.

**trimethadione**  See ANTICONVUL-SANTS.

**triploidy**  The condition of having a complete extra set of CHROMOSOMES, that is, having three rather than the normal complement of two of each of the 23 chromosomes. Therefore, instead of having 46 chromosomes (2 X 23), individuals with triploidy have 69 (3 X 23) (see CHROMOSOME ABNORMALITIES). Pure triploidy can result from the fertilization of one egg by two sperm (dispermy) or a failure of disjunction during meiosis, the process whereby pairs of chromosomes split during the formation of sperm and egg. However, some individuals may exhibit triploidy in only some cells of the body (see MOSAICISM), resulting from an error in cell division shortly after conception.

Approximately two-thirds to three-quarters of triploidy cases result from dispermy. About one-quarter of cases arise from fertilization of a normal ovum by a diploid sperm, and about 10% are the result of a diploid ovum. Mosaic cases of triploidy are very rare; only 14 have been reported.

Pure triploidy is lethal, resulting in spontaneous ABORTION, stillbirth or death within days of birth. However, individuals who have mosaic triploidy may have prolonged survival, though they usually exhibit MENTAL RETARDATION.

Newborns with pure triploidy as well as mosaics are typically premature and exhibit LOW BIRTH WEIGHT. Abnormalities of skull development are common, as are wide-set eyes (HYPERTELORISM) that are unusually small (microphthalmia). The ears are often low-set and malformed. The tongue may be enlarged (MACROGLOSSIA) and protrude from the mouth, and the chin is small (MICROGNATHIA). Fine, downy hair (lanugo) may be visible on the cheeks and forehead.

Some of the fingers and toes may be webbed (SYNDACTYLY), the feet may be clubbed (talipes equinovarus) and in males the external genitalia may be small. Part of the intestine may protrude through a defective wall of the abdomen (OMPHALOCELE). A host of other internal malformations may be found of nervous system, heart, kidney, digestive tract or genitalia.

This condition may occur as frequently as one in 2,500 live births and in approximately 2% of conceptions. Most are lost as miscarriages and account for approximately 20% of all chromosomally abnormal spontaneous abortions.

While there is no specific prenatal diagnostic procedure for this condition, fetuses with omphalocele or NEURAL TUBE DEFECTS will cause elevated maternal ALPHA-FETOPROTEIN levels. Triploidy can then be detected prenatally by chromosome analysis of fetal cells obtained via CHORIONIC VILLUS SAMPLING or AMNIOCENTESIS.

**trisomy 13**  See PATAU SYNDROME.

**trisomy 18**  See EDWARD SYNDROME.

**trisomy 21**  See DOWN SYNDROME.

**tritanopia**  See COLOR BLINDNESS.

**tuberous sclerosis**  An AUTOSOMAL DOMINANT hereditary disease characterized by epileptic seizures, MENTAL RETARDATION, tumors that may appear on internal organs, and a variety of skin manifestations. Affected individuals may exhibit one or more of these symptoms.

Seizures occur in more than 85% of cases. Lesions and tumors are often found in the brain, kidneys and retina. They may also occur in the heart, bone, lungs and liver. A common skin manifestation in growing children consists of reddish, seed-like bumps that appear in a butterfly pattern across the cheeks and nose (angiofibroma). Depigmented areas on the skin (hypomelanotic macules), commonly called "white spots" or "ash leaf spots," are present at birth in 90% of affected infants.

Café-au-lait spots (coffee-colored patches of skin) may also be evident. Collagenous patches of slightly elevated, yellowish-brown skin with the texture of an orange peel (shagreen patches) may also be present. Nail beds of the fingers and toes may have wart-like growths.

Affected individuals may display unusual behavior or may exhibit delayed speech, slow motor development and learning disabilities. Mental retardation of a moderate to severe degree is seen in about two out of three patients.

There is a great variability in expression of this disorder, even within a family with a history of the condition. While some affected individuals lead normal and productive lives and may remain undiagnosed, severe cases may result in premature death due to seizures, tumors or infections. The disorder is slowly progressive, and most individuals who come to the attention of physicians die by the age of 25.

There seems to be a correlation between the age of onset and the severity of seizures and the degree of mental retardation. For that reason, early diagnosis, and treatment with anticonvulsant drugs is important in reducing the potential severity of the condition.

The disorder is inherited as an autosomal dominant trait, with a high percentage being the result of new MUTATION. When first identified in 1862 by F.D. von Recklinghausen, it was considered to be rare, but now incidence is estimated at approximately one in 10,000 to one in 100,000 live births. The wide range reflects the possibility of many new cases remaining unrecognized.

Diagnosis is made on the basis of seizures, behavioral symptoms and computerized axial tomography (CAT) scanning, which can reveal hallmark internal manifestations of the disorder. The basic cause of tuberous sclerosis is unknown. Recently, GENETIC MARKERS have been found on both CHROMOSOME 9 and CHROMOSOME 11 that appear to be linked to the disease. Additional experimental work is underway to further define the location of the tuberous sclerosis GENE and determine whether marker studies are useful in pre-symptomatic or PRENATAL DIAGNOSIS. However, at present there is no accepted prenatal diagnostic procedure.

For more information, contact:

National Tuberous Sclerosis Association, Inc.
4351 Garden City Drive
Landover, MD 20785
(301) 459-9888
(800) 225-NTSA

**Turner syndrome**    The total absence of one of the two X CHROMOSOMES normally found in all of a female's cells, or the structural alteration of one of the two X chromosomes in some or all of a female's cells. This condition, exclusively seen in females, is characterized by short stature, failure to develop secondary sex characteristics and INFERTILITY.

It carries the name of U.S. physician Henry H. Turner (b. 1892), who first identified the characteristics of the disorder in 1928. The chromosomal aberration that causes it was discovered by Dr. C.E. Ford in 1959.

Turner syndrome is estimated to occur in one of every 2,500 live female births, though only about 2% of Turner's fetuses survive to full term. In addition to the features described above, there may be malformations and/or health problems in the eyes, ears, heart, kidneys and thyroid. Other typical physical characteristics include low-set ears, low hairline, webbed neck, broad chest with wide-spaced nipples, puffy hands and feet and pronounced bending out of the elbows. The average height at full growth is 4 feet 8 inches (150.3 cm).

Turner syndrome does not affect intelligence, but affected individuals tend to have poor spatial perceptual abilities and an increased incidence of specific learning disabilities. The need for psychological care and support for those affected can be as important as medical attention for the physical complications arising out of this disorder.

Most affected individuals do not have ovaries. Hormone therapy can replace the estrogen normally produced in these reproductive organs. However, while infertility is the rule, there have been exceptions, with isolated cases of women with Turner syndrome giving birth. Though the risk in such cases has been said to be high, with an increased risk of miscarriage, STILLBIRTH, CHROMOSOME ABNORMALITIES and malformations, some of this increased risk may be due to ascertainment bias. That is, the mother was found to have Turner syndrome only after investigation because of the adverse outcomes of childbirth.

Approximately one-third of those identified are diagnosed in the neonatal period (the first six weeks of life), one-third during childhood and one-third during the late teens when they fail to sexually mature. Diagnosis is made by chromosomal analysis, which reveals the chromosomal aberration that causes the disorder.

PRENATAL DIAGNOSIS is accomplished by chromosome analysis, which may be prompted by an elevated maternal serum ALPHA-FETOPROTEIN or abnormal ULTRASOUND. Individuals with Turner syndrome have normal life expectancies and can lead full and productive lives.

For more information, contact:

Turner's Syndrome Society
York UniversityAdministrative Studies
    Building
Toronto, Ontario M3J 1P3
Canada
(416) 736-5023

Little People of America, Inc.
P.O. Box 633
San Bruno, CA 94066
(415) 589-0695

Parents of Dwarfed Children
11524 Colt Terrace
Silver Spring, MD 20902
(301) 649-3275

**turricephaly**     See CRANIO SYNOSTOSIS.

**twins**     The result of the simultaneous gestation of two embryos in one mother. Twins occur in approximately one in 70 to one in 100 deliveries and may be either identical or fraternal. About 30% are identical and 70% fraternal. Twinning is also associated with increased risks for fetal development or structural defects due to uterine crowding.

Identical twins are monozygotic (MZ), the product of a single egg that divides into separate embryos soon after conception. Therefore, the twins share identical genetic endowments: All their genes are the same. (Genetically, the children of identical co-twins are half-siblings, rather than cousins.) Identical twins occur in 3.5 to four of every 1,000 deliveries in all populations and ethnic groups.

Fraternal twins are dizygotic (DZ). They originate from two separate eggs: Genetically, they are no more alike than siblings and may be either of the same or opposite sexes. The frequency of fraternal twins ranges from 16 per 1,000 in blacks to eight per 1,000 in white and four per 1,000 in Asians. There is also a familial tendency: women who have had fraternal twins have a 3% chance of having fraternal twins again, about four times the rate found in the general population. The incidence of fraternal twins also increases with maternal age. Conceptions that occur soon after puberty have essentially a 0% chance of producing fraternal twins, rising to 15 per 1,000 births by the age of 37 and falling to 0% again shortly before menopause.

Twins have commanded attention in cultures around the world throughout history. Mythical twins have often been depicted as healing gods or magicians, and in many fables they have the power to foretell the future, control fire and flood, promote fertility and cure disease. Mystical powers were imputed to the twins Castor and Polydeuces (Pollux among Romans) of Greek legend, who are represented in the constellation Gemini. The mythical founders of Rome, Romulus and Remus, were twins as well.

In other primitive societies, however, twins were considered dangerous aberrations, and mothers of twins, and in some cultures one or both twins as well, were immediately killed.

Genetically, twins are important in determining genetic components of traits, particularly those that do not demonstrate clear MENDELIAN inheritance patterns, such as CLEFT PALATE and blood pressure. (The degree to which twins both exhibit any given trait exhibited in one is called "concordance" and is expressed as a percentage. If the trait is always present in both members of a twin pair when it is present in one, CONCORDANCE is 100%.) Yet the potential importance of twin studies was not recognized until 1875, when Galton raised the question of the comparative influence of "nature and nurture" in twins' physical and mental character. Since that time, studies of twins have indicated that hereditary factors often exert more influence than environmental factors in shaping behavior.

**tyrosinemia**    A group of rare disorders of the metabolism of tyrosine, an AMINO ACID.

Tyrosinemia type I, hepatorenal tyrosinemia, manifests itself in early infancy with FAILURE TO THRIVE, vomiting and diarrhea, and enlargement of the liver (hepatomegaly). Death results from liver failure. Some patients have a more chronic form, with chronic liver disease (cirrhosis), kidney abnormalities and RICKETS. This form is thought to be due to the deficiency of the ENZYME fumaryl acetoacetase. Measure of the enzyme allows PRENATAL DIAGNOSIS. Though it is rare in the general population, tyrosinemia I has been reported to have an incidence as high as one in 1,500 births in an isolated French Canadian population.

Tyrosinemia type II is caused by a deficiency of the enyzme tyrosine aminotransferase. Termed oculocutaneous tyrosinemia, it is characterized by skin and ocular lesions and MENTAL RETARDATION in some individuals. The ocular findings include increased tearing, intolerance to bright light (photopobia) and inflammation and ulceration of the cornea. There is no liver or kidney disease. Many cases are of Mediterranean origin, particularly Italian. Both forms are inherited as AUTOSOMAL RECESSIVE traits.

# U

**Ultrasonography**    See ULTRASOUND.

**ultrasound** (ultrasonography)    An imaging procedure for viewing a developing fetus in the womb using high-frequency sound waves. It is one of the most common prenatal diagnostic procedures in use today. The sound waves, above the range of human hearing, are directed into the uterus. The echoes, reflected by the various densities of the fetal tissues encountered, are displayed on a TV-like monitor, forming an image. This image, interpreted by a skilled operator, can be useful for PRENATAL DIAGNOSIS, by itself or as a component of other prenatal diagnostic procedures.

Diagnoses using ultrasound are based on the images displayed and concern mostly structural details, although fine distinctions can be made in this respect. Ultrasound has proved useful, for example, in prenatal diagnosis of the enlarged skull caused by excessive fluid in the cranium (HYDROCEPHALY) and of an absence of brain tissue accompanied by a failure of the skull to close (ANENCEPHALY). Also, stunted limbs and some heart, kidney and intestinal defects can be disclosed by ultrasound. However, the inherent nature of ultrasound does not allow for genetic determinations through ultrasound itself.

Ultrasound is of vital importance in guiding the movement of the instruments employed in prenatal diagnostic procedures that are invasive in nature: AMNIOCENTESIS, CHORIONIC VILLUS SAMPLING, FETOSCOPY and fetal blood and tissue sampling.

Other uses of ultrasound fetal images include evaluating the age of the fetus, locating the placenta, determining fetal size, monitoring fetal growth, evaluating the amount of amniotic fluid in the sac, determining if the pregnancy will produce twins or triplets and indicating the sex of the fetus.

The small exposure to ultrasound as used has not proved dangerous to either the mother or the fetus, and this procedure is considered relatively safe. However, physicians have cautioned that it should not be routinely performed unless suspected defects or other medical conditions warrant its use. Using ultrasound to determine the sex of the fetus or to show the mother an image or provide educational demonstrations is not generally recommended.

**unilateral renal agenesis**    Affected individuals are born with only one kidney (usually on the right side). While the condition is rare, it may remain undiagnosed in the absence of other CONGENITAL ANOMALIES or future dysfunciton of the remaining kidney. First-degree relatives (parents, children, SIBLINGS) of affected individuals should be examined for this condition, as it demonstrates a familial aggregation, though the cause and mode of transmission are unknown. It should be distinguished from Potter syndrome, a fatal condition in which infants are born without either kidney (bilateral renal agenesis). First-degree relatives of a child with bilateral renal agenesis have a 13% chance of having silent unilateral renal agenesis. This increases to 30% in families in which two infants with Potter syndrome are born. In families in which unilateral renal agenesis has occurred, there is an increase in bilateral agenesis, as well. In other words, though the two defects are distinct, in families in which one of these anomalous conditions occurs, there is also an increased incidence of the other condition, in addition to other developmental abnormalities of the kidney.

**urea cycle defects**    A group of rare hereditary ENZYME disorders characterized by the accumulation of very high levels of ammonia in the blood and tissues (hyperammonemia). Symptoms include vomiting, lethargy, seizures, respiratory distress and coma, possibly leading to death in the first weeks of life, though some may be less severely affected. MENTAL RETARDATION and

neurologic defects are common resultant disorders in the survivors.

Ammonia is a byproduct of the metabolism of protein and its constituents, the AMINO ACIDS. The only way the body can eliminate ammonia is by converting it to urea (through the urea cycle) so that it can be excreted in urine. Most of this activity occurs in the liver. Several enzymes are necessary for this conversion, and an inherited deficiency of any one of the enzymes will result in a specific urea cycle disorder. These disorders, in total, have an estimated incidence of approximately one in 30,000 births.

*Argininemia.*  This deficiency of the enzyme arginase may result in mental retardation, seizures and progressive spastic diplegia. It is diagnosed by the finding of elevated levels of arginine in the urine and blood, which may be reduced by low protein diets. Inherited as an AUTOSOMAL RECESSIVE trait, parents of affected infants have been reported to have subnormal arginase activity in red blood cells, which may allow CARRIER detection and PRENATAL DIAGNOSIS in some cases.

*Argininosuccinic aciduria.*  Characterized by severe symptoms of hyperammonemia in the majority of affected infants, a significant proportion may be less severely affected and may come to medical attention due to mild mental retardation and a natural aversion to protein. Affected individuals often have hair and skin abnormalities as well.

Inherited as an autosomal recessive trait, both prenatal diagnosis and carrier detection are possible.

*Carbamyl phosphate synthetase deficiency (CPS-I).*  Diagnosis is made based on examination of enzyme activity of CPS-I in liver tissue. A low-protein diet and a complex regimen of drug therapy may be beneficial for some affected. Inherited as an autosomal recessive trait, prenatal diagnosis may be possible using GENETIC LINKAGE studies.

*Citrullinemia.*  This may manifest itself with severe symptoms soon after birth, or may have onset in later childhood and exhibit a much more benign course. The variations are thought to be due to varying levels of reduced enzyme activity among affected individuals. Protein-restricted diets are recommended. Diagnosis is easily made from the massive amounts of citrulline excreted in the urine and its higher levels in the blood.

It is inherited as an autosomal recessive disorder and may be diagnosed prenatally.

*Ornithine transcarbamylase (OTC) deficiency.* This X-LINKED disorder is often lethal in males during early infancy. They may have a complete absence, or less than 1% of normal levels, of the enzyme OTC. Surviving males are treated similarly to those with CPS deficiency. Females are much more mildly and variably affected. Enzyme activity is 10% to 40% of normal level. They may be entirely asymptomatic, have lethargy and nausea after eating a high protein meal or be as symptomatic as affected males.

Affected females are typically placed on low-protein diets. CARRIER identification for females is possible in some cases, and prenatal diagnosis is now available using restriction fragment length POLYMORPHISM studies with the cloned OTC GENE.

## Usher syndrome (retinitis pigmentosa and congenital deafness)    An inherited disorder characterized by hearing loss and deteriorating vision. The hearing loss is usually profound and present at birth, but may be more mild and occur soon after birth. If the DEAFNESS is not profound, it usually does not deteriorate beyond the deficit first exhibited. The loss of vision is a result of RETINITIS PIGMENTOSA, a group of disorders resulting in retinal degeneration and possibly leading to BLINDNESS.

The relationship of hearing loss to RP is not well understood. The combination was first reported in 1858 by von Graefe, but is named for the Scottish ophthalmologist Charles H. Usher (1865–1942), who first emphasized the hereditary nature of the disorder in 1914.

Usher syndrome is typically classified as either type I or type II, with type I being the more severe, with profound deafness present at birth and an earlier onset of vision problems.

Approximately 30% of all RP patients report some degree of hearing impairment. RP may result in total blindness in some cases of Usher, but though they may be classified as legally blind, most individuals retain some vision. There are an estimated 10,000 individuals with Usher syndrome in the United States. The condition, inherited as an AUTOSOMAL RECESSIVE trait, is estimated to occur in between one in 15,000 and one in 30,000 live births, and accounts for 1% to 3% of individuals with profound deafness. A high frequency has been reported in the Louisiana Cajun population (where the GENE appears to be linked to GENETIC MARKERS on CHROMOSOME 4).

There is no cure for the loss of hearing, which results from an inner ear problem, or for the loss of vision. The hearing of some patients has reportedly benefited from cochlear implants.

The combination of deafness and blindness creates problems both in diagnosing the condition and coping with psychological implications. Deteriorating vision, which typically begins in the late teen years, may go unrecognized for a long period of time. Individuals have no way of knowng that what they see is different from what others see. Individuals may exhibit clumsiness and bump into people and objects. They may have many small auto accidents, be labeled as inattentive and stupid and be unable to follow group conversations in sign language because of the inability to see more than one person at a time. There is a strong tendency toward denial of visual problems among those first diagnosed with Usher, and care must be taken to help individuals cope with the eventual condition of deaf-blindness. Patients require extensive counseling and information about the condition.

For more information, contact:

Retinitis Pigmentosa Foundation, Inc.
1401 Mt. Royal Ave., 4th Floor
Baltimore, MD 21217
(301) 225-9409
(800) 638-2300

Helen Keller National Center for Deaf-
  Blind Children

Bureau of Education of Handicapped
Dept. of Education
400 Maryland Ave., S.W.
Washington, DC 20202

---

# V

---

**varicella (chicken pox)**   Fetal exposure during the first 20 weeks of pregnancy to varicella, the virus that causes chicken pox, may cause severe skin scarring, malformed arms and legs, eye abnormalities, MENTAL RETARDATION and retarded growth. About 5% to 10% of infants of women who had varicella during their first trimester of pregnancy exhibit these anomalies. Infection after the 21st week of pregnancy rarely causes birth defects. Infants may be born with a severe case of varicella if maternal infection occurs shortly before delivery. (See also TERATOGEN.)

**variegate porphyria**   See PORPHYRIA.

**VATER association**   The acronym VATER describes a group of abnormalities that are found together more frequently than would be expected at random: Vertebral anomalies; Anal malformations (IMPERFORATE ANUS); an abnormal passage from the trachea to the esophagus (TracheoEsophageal fistula); and thumb and forearm (Radial limb) abnormalities. At least three of these abnormalities must be present to be considered an example of the VATER association.

About 60% of affected individuals also have CONGENITAL HEART DEFECTS, and kidney abnormalities (most often absence of one kidney) are also common. In addition, half-formed vertebrae and spinal deformities near the pelvis frequently occur, as well as an absent or malformed radius bone in the forearm. Because of the kidney and cardiac involvement, the acronym VACTERL, with *c* for *c*ardiac, *r* for *r*enal and *l* for *l*imb anomalies, is sometimes used.

About 75% of affected individuals survive infancy. Heart failure is the most common cause of death. Although surviving infants tend to be small and usually require surgery, they grow to the normal range of height and weight by four or five years of age.

Almost all cases have been SPORADIC. The basic cause of the abnormalities is not known, although they are believed to result from an event during the second month of gestation, when differentiation of organ systems (morphogenesis) takes place in the fetus. No drug or virus has been implicated, and no CHROMOSOME ABNORMALITY has been found in the majority of cases, but the components of the association can be found in some infants with chromosome ANOMALIES. PRENATAL DIAGNOSIS of this disorder is currently unavailable, but ULTRASOUND may detect skeletal, kidney or heart defects.

**VDT**   See VIDEO DISPLAY TERMINALS.

**ventricular septal defects**   See CONGENITAL HEART DEFECTS.

**video display terminals (VDTs)**   The potential link between maternal exposure to video display terminals during pregnancy and an increased risk of miscarriage has received a great deal of attention, though there is no clear consensus on the actual danger. While some studies have found an increased miscarriage rate among women who report that their jobs include heavy use of VDTs, the VDTs have yet to be isolated as the cause, and general working conditions and other factors have been suggested as the potential culprit. An early major study of more than 1,500 women who reported working more than 20 hours a week on VDTs found they had twice the rate of miscarriage (see ABORTION) as working women who did not use VDTs. They also reported a slightly increased rate of BIRTH DEFECTS, though the increase was considered statistically insignificant.

Both the American College of Obstetricians and Gynecologists and the American

Medical Association have concluded that the levels of radiation emitted by VDTs are insufficient to cause birth defects or miscarriage. However, animal studies have found that very low frequency, pulsed, non-ionizing electromagnetic radiation emitted by VDTs can interfere with embryonic cellular growth. Little is actually known about the effects of this type of radiation; furthermore, most of the radiation is emitted from the back and sides of the terminal, so that the individual sitting in front of the terminal may be less exposed than an individual in back of it.

Legislation has been introduced in a number of states in the United States that would regulate exposure to VDTs for all workers, and include provisions for pregnant women. Additionally, some unions representing clerical workers have negotiated contracts allowing women to transfer to jobs that don't involve VDT exposure should they become pregnant.

If a link is ultimately found between VDT use and miscarriage, it may be due not to radiation emitted but to the stress and strain associated with the monotony or pressure of VDT work.

**vitamins**   Multivitamin use in early pregnancy has been linked to a decreased incidence of NEURAL TUBE DEFECTS (NTDs), which include SPINA BIFIDA and ANENCEPHALY. One pioneering study found women who take multivitamins at the time of conception had 60% less risk of giving birth to an infant with a neural tube defect than women who did not use vitamins. A later study by Boston University's Center for Human Genetics, published in 1989 and involving 23,000 pregnant women, found those who reported taking multivitamins in the first six weeks of pregnancy had rates of NTDs in their offspring only one-quarter the rates of women who did not use vitamins. (NTD incidence was 0.9 per 1,000 births among vitamin users vs. 3.5 per 1,000 births among non-vitamin users.)

NTDs are more common in the offspring of women in lower socioeconomic groups and women who have poor diets. Additionally, there was an "epidemic" of neural tube defects during the Depression, a time when many people, including women of child-bearing age, received substandard nutrition. However, the potential link between vitamin deficiencies and neural tube defects did not receive scientific attention until after World War II, when it was noted that women in England, Holland and Germany who had been malnourished gave birth to an unexpectedly large number of infants with these developmental defects.

Despite the evidence, there is no conclusive proof that vitamins do reduce incidence of NTDs; data from other studies has not always suported this conclusion. No detrimental side effects have been noted from maternal use of normal doses of vitamins during pregnancy; thus many medical experts advise women contemplating pregnancy to take multivitamins. However, some vitamins can cause birth defects when taken in large quantities. For example, concern has been raised regarding vitamin A, especially since a vitamin A derivative, ACCUTANE, is known to be teratogenic. Recommendations for or against the use of vitamins to prevent CONGENITAL defects must await the results of ongoing collaborative studies.

**vitiligo**   A benign condition characterized by well-defined patches of depigmented skin. Similar to PIEBALD SKIN TRAIT its only impact is cosmetic. However, vitiligo is distinguished from the piebald trait by its onset after birth, and tendency to progress or regress. It has been suggested that this is an AUTOSOMAL DOMINANT trait, though few familial cases have been reported. Supporting evidence for genetic transmission is the fact that vitiligo patterns observed on opposite sides of the body and in identical twins are generally similar.

**von Gierke disease**   See GLYCOGEN STORAGE DISEASE.

**von Hippel-Lindau syndrome** The hallmark of this hereditary disorder is the abnormal growth and proliferation of blood vessels (HEMANGIOMA) on the retina of the eye and the cerebellum of the brain. Onset is in early adulthood, with initial symptoms of headaches, dizziness and visual disturbances, progressing to uncontrolled clumsy movements on one side of the body (unilateral ataxia), BLINDNESS and permanent brain damage. The disorder is frequently associated with cysts and CANCERS in the kidneys and pancreas. Hemangiomas of lung and liver and adrenal tumors (pheochromocytomas) may also be seen. Cryotherapy (a surgical procedure involving ultra-cold temperatures) of the retina may alleviate some ocular symptoms. Cysts may be treated with conventional surgical techniques.

Inherited as an AUTOSOMAL DOMINANT trait, it is named for E. von Hippel (1867–1939), a German ophthalmologist, and Swedish pathologist A. Lindau (b. 1892), who published descriptions in 1895 and 1926, respectively. Recent evidence points to the short arm of CHROMOSOME 3 as the site of the GENE for this disorder.

**von Recklinghausen disease** See NEUROFIBROMATOSIS.

**von Willebrand disease** The first hereditary bleeding disorder distinguished from HEMOPHILIA. Inherited (usually) as an AUTOSOMAL DOMINANT trait, this relatively common disorder is characterized by prolonged bleeding and easy bruising, which manifests at an early age, excessive bleeding after dental extractions or surgery, and excess blood loss during menstruation. The severity of symptoms decreases with age. It is named for Finnish physician E.A. von Willebrand (1879–1949), who found the condition among the inhabitants of the Aland Islands in the Sea of Bothnia between Sweden and Finland. He published a description of the condition in 1926, calling it "pseudohemophilia."

It has been demonstrated that the platelets responsible for clotting are normal, but they have reduced adhesiveness due to a factor VIII deficiency.

A variety of blood factor replacement measures may treat bleeding episodes successfully.

# W

**Waardenburg syndrome** The most striking features of this inherited condition are the abnormal pigmentation seen in the hair, skin and eyes, though its most serious feature is CONGENITAL sensorineural DEAFNESS. Named for Dutch physician P.J. Waardenburg, who first described it in 1951, it is estimated to account for 2% of congenital deafness.

In its classic form there is a white forelock of depigmented hair, premature graying, milky white patches of skin (VITILIGO) and eyes of differing colors (HETEROCHROMIA IRIDES). The white forelock may be present at birth and later disappear. The inner portion of the eye slits (palpebral fissures) may not extend toward the nose as far as would normally be expected (lateral displacement of inner canthi). The eyebrows may grow together (SYNOPHRYS) over a broad nasal bridge. CLEFT PALATE may also be present.

Two forms of this disorder, labeled as type I and type II, have been documented. In type I there is lateral displacement of the inner canthi; in type II, there is not. Mild to profound hearing loss is reported in an estimated 25% of those affected with type I and 50% of those with type II. Diagnosis may be made at birth or soon after based on pigmentary and facial manifestations. Hearing aids and educational assistance are usually recommended when hearing impairment is present. Life expectancy and intelligence are unaffected, though apparent MENTAL RETARDATION may be associated with signifcant hearing impairment.

Inherited as an AUTOSOMAL DOMINANT trait, Waardenburg syndrome is estimated to occur in about one in 40,000 live births, though there is a wide variability of expression; affected, yet apparently asymptomatic individuals can transmit the disorder to offspring. Advanced paternal age has been associated with sporadic new MUTATIONS.

It has been reported in American blacks, Maoris (aboriginal New Zealanders) and whites. In South Australia, this is a leading cause of deafness and holds a position similar to that of PORPHYRIA in South Africa, having been introduced by early settlers (with many descendants).

**Walt Disney dwarfism** (geroderma osteodysplastica)    First described in a Swiss family in 1950, in addition to short stature, characteristic features of this disorder include changes in the skin that suggest premature aging, and osseous (bone) changes, including osteoporosis, susceptibility to fractures and multiple lines on bones that appear like growth rings of trees.

A physical appearance similar to the characters in *Snow White and the Seven Dwarfs*, Walt Disney's animated film, was noted in affected family members, hence the name of the disorder. Inherited as an AUTOSOMAL RECESSIVE trait, it is very rare.

**warfarin embryopathy**    Warfarin is an anticoagulant that is prescribed to treat and prevent blood clots, certain cardiac conditions and strokes. Taken during the first trimester of pregnancy, warfarin increases the risk of miscarriage (see ABORTION) and STILLBIRTH, and causes a syndrome of CONGENITAL defects in 5% to 25% of infants exposed *in utero*. Infants with warfarin embryopathy have an abnormally small nose with deformed cartilage. Nasal passages are small and in some cases blocked, creating breathing difficulties. LOW BIRTH WEIGHT, slow development, BLINDNESS and other ocular problems, and bone deformities such as shortened fingers are also seen.

Though exposure during the sixth to ninth weeks after conception carries the greatest risk of ANOMALIES, when taken during the second and third trimester of pregnancy, warfarin still may cause MENTAL RETARDATION, an abnormally small head (MICROCEPHALY) and vision problems.

**Watson-Alagille syndrome**    See ALAGILLE SYNDROME.

**Werdnig-Hoffmann disease**    See SPINAL MUSCULAR ATROPHY.

**Werner syndrome (WS)**    Also called "PROGERIA of the adult," WS has several features resembling premature aging. Affected individuals appear normal during childhood but stop growing during their early teenage years. There is a premature graying or whitening of hair, early CATARACT formation, development of aged-looking skin with hard, scaly patches (SCLERODERMA), a high-pitched voice, weakening of muscles, poor wound healing, chronic leg and ankle ulcers, hardening and loss of elasticity of the walls of the arteries (atherosclerosis), loss of calcium from bones (osteoporosis) and DIABETES MELLITUS. About 10% of affected individuals develop CANCERS.

The syndrome is named for Otto Werner (1879–1936), a general practitioner in Eddelak, West Germany, who first described it in 1904.

Several studies have suggested immune system abnormalities may also be present in this disorder. The condition is usually diagnosed during the third decade, and death usually occurs in the fourth decade due to complications of atherosclerosis. While there is no specific diagnostic test, affected individuals exhibit elevated levels of hyaluronic acid in their urine, as do individuals with PROGERIA. Currently, there is no method to identify CARRIERS or for PRENATAL DIAGNOSIS of this disorder.

The basic defect that causes WS is unknown. It is inherited as an AUTOSOMAL RECESSIVE trait and is very rare. More than 125 cases have been reported.

For more information, contact:

Progeria International Registry
Department of Human Genetics
N.Y. State Institute for Basic Research in
  Developmental Disabilities
1050 Forest Hill Road
Staten Island, NY 10314
(718) 494-5230

**whistling face syndrome** (Freeman-Sheldon syndrome; craniocarpotarsal dysplasia)    Taking its name from its characteristic facial appearance, features consist of a masklike, immobile expression, with a flat midface, deeply-set, widely spaced eyes (HYPERTELORISM), a long philtrum (the groove extending from the upper lip to the nose), small nose, receding chin, and small mouth (microstomia) fixed in a puckered position, as if whistling. Additional abnormalities are flexion contractures of the hands and CLUBFOOT deformities: The ankles are twisted inward, and the sole turned upward, so that the heel is the lowest part of the foot (talipes equinovarus).

The syndrome was first described in 1938 by Ernest A. Freeman (1900–1975) and Joseph H. Sheldon (1893–1972), senior orthopedic surgeon and senior physician at the Royal Wolverhampton Hospital in England. They called the condition "craniocarpotarsal DYSPLASIA" in their original report of two unrelated children that they presented at the Royal Society of Medicine in London. It is sometimes referred to by that name, or as Freeman-Sheldon syndrome.

The basic defect that causes this disorder is unknown. Most of the approximately 50 cases reported have been SPORADIC, but there is evidence that it can be inherited as an AUTOSOMAL DOMINANT trait with variable EXPRES-SIVITY. An AUTOSOMAL RECESSIVE form has also been reported.

The diagnosis of the condition is made by the distinctive facial appearance combined with the characteristic musculoskeletal abnormalities, although some cases have been mistaken as ARTHROGRYPOSIS multiplex congenita.

Intelligence and lifespan are normal in this disorder. However, vomiting and swallowing difficulties may lead to FAILURE TO THRIVE in infancy, and retarded growth and short stature are common features. Surgical treatment may improve facial appearance and functioning of the hands and feet.

There is no accepted method of PRENATAL DIAGNOSIS, though ULTRASOUND and FETOSCOPY have been used in some pregnancies to detect severe skeletal abnormalities.

For more information, contact:

Freeman-Sheldon Parent Support Group
1459 East Maple Hills Drive
Bountiful, UT 84010
(801) 298-3149

**Williams syndrome** (elfin facies with hypercalcemia)    The two major features of this syndrome are a characteristic, elfin facial appearance and CONGENITAL HEART DEFECTS. Affected individuals often have LOW BIRTHWEIGHT and exhibit FAILURE TO THRIVE and developmental delays in sitting, walking, talking, as well as in development of motor skills.

The classic characteristics were first described in 1961 by Dr. J.C.P. Williams of New Zealand.

The facial features include flat midface with full cheeks, thick, wide lips with open mouth, upturned nostrils (anteverted nares), broad forehead, widely spaced teeth, small chin, puffiness around the eyes, and depressed nasal bridge. The head tends to be small. The ears may be prominent. These features become more striking with age.

Ocular findings may be present, including a star-like pattern in the iris (stellate iris pattern) of blue and green-eyed children, and sometimes corneal opacities or crossed eyes (STRABISMUS).

Any of several cardiovascular abnormalities may be present, and include narrowing (stenosis) of the aorta just above the aortic valve, narrowing of the pulmonic valve or pulmonary arteries, and atrial or ventricular septal defects.

Children with Williams syndrome may also have hypersensitivity to sound and exhibit friendly, talkative, impulsive personalities. MENTAL RETARDATION and attention-deficit disorders are common features. They have specific psychological problems, with perceptual and motor function being more impaired than memory or verbal performance.

The basic cause of Williams syndrome is unknown, though affected individuals often show an inability to handle calcium, and this may play a role in the disorder. The incidence is estimated to be approximately one in 20,000 live births. Though almost all cases have been SPORADIC, it has also been suggested that classic Williams syndrome might be an AUTOSOMAL DOMINANT characteristic.

Currently, there is no method for PRENATAL DIAGNOSIS of this disorder. Treatment for the various conditions that comprise the syndrome often require a team approach that includes physician, speech and language therapist, occupational and physical therapy and vocational training. Surgery may be required for correction of cardiac abnormalities.

For more information, contact:
Williams Syndrome Association
16211 N. Greenfield Drive
Klein, TX 77379
(713) 376-7072

Williams Syndrome Clinic
Baylor University
Texas Children's Hospital
1730 Mayweather Lane
Richmond, TX 77469
(713) 342-8488

**Wilms tumor**    Infant-onset CANCER of the kidney(s), one of the most common forms of childhood cancer. Wilms tumor accounts for 15% of all tumors diagnosed before the age of 15 years. Fifty percent of cases occur before age three and 90% are diagnosed before the age of 10. Approximately one-third of those affected have inherited the tendency to develop the tumor. Incidence is estimated at between one in 10,000 and one in 25,000 live births in the human population, with no ethnic or other predilection. Despite its ubiquity, it was only after effective therapy became available that affected families were noted with regularity. A little over 60% of those who inherit the tendency develop the disorder. (One inherits a predisposition to develop cancer rather than the cancer itself.) Its eponymic designation refers to German surgeon M. Wilms (1867–1918), who published the seminal description in 1899.

Familial cases (see FAMILIAL DISEASE) have a greater likelihood than SPORADIC cases of affecting both kidneys (bilateral) and tend to have an earlier onset than sporadic cases. Initial symptoms include abdominal distension, an abdominal or flank mass, weight loss and hypertension.

Wilms tumor is also associated with other abnormalities. It is seen in one-third of individuals affected with absence of the iris of the eye (ANIRIDIA). It has also been associated with a SYNDROME involving both aniridia and male PSEUDOHERMAPHRODITISM, with BECKWITH-WIEDEMANN SYNDROME and with HEMIHYPERTROPHY.

Some affected individuals exhibit a deletion of chromosomal material on the short arm on one of their two CHROMOSOME 11s. This may serve as a basis for chromosomal analysis for PRENATAL DIAGNOSIS.

It also appears that the gender of the parent this damaged chromosome was inherited from may influence development of the disorder through the process of IMPRINTING. When found in those affected, the chromosome 11 exhibiting this deletion (see CHROMOSOME ABNORMALITIES) is almost always inherited from the mother. This suggests that maternal GENES normally play some role in suppressing tumor development, and that the loss of this suppressor function is apparently not compensated for by the gene(s) carried on the paternally derived chromosome 11.

The long-term outlook for affected individuals was previously uniformly poor. Currently, with early diagnosis and treatment, there is a high probability of cure.

## Wilson disease (hepatolenticular degeneration)

A genetic disorder characterized by the accumulation of copper in body tissues, particularly in the liver, kidneys, brain, and cornea of the eyes. Essentially, it results in chronic copper poisoning. Eventually, the buildup of copper causes degenerative changes in the brain, liver and nerves, resulting in incoordination, drooling, slurred speech, tremors, muscular rigidity, spastic movements, lack of balance, double vision, difficulty in swallowing (dysphagia) and masklike facial appearance. The symptoms progress over months, and in the most advanced stages, weakness and emaciation leave affected individuals totally helpless, unable to walk or talk.

Psychiatric manifestation may be prominent and differ from case to case. They include depression, bizarre behavior, mania, psychosis, hysteria or even SCHIZOPHRENIA. Drugs typically prescribed to control these psychic disturbances may only exacerbate neurologic and psychiatric problems in individuals with Wilson disease.

Left untreated, or if diagnosed too late, the condition is ultimately fatal. However, with early diagnosis and therapy, affected individuals can recover fully. Therapy typically consists of drugs known as chelators, which have the ability to combine with metals. Copper binds with the drugs and is eliminated in the urine. Treatment must continue throughout the individual's life. Liver transplants have been successful in some patients with severe liver damage who haven't responded to drug therapy.

The first case was possibly described as early as 1861, with later reports calling the disorder "pseudosclerosis." It is named for British neurologist Samuel A. Kinnier Wilson, who made the first detailed study of the disease and provided the classic description of the condition in 1912.

The scientific name "hepatolenticular degeneration" refers to the degenerative effects on the liver (hepato), which mimic cirrhosis, and lenticular nuclei, a region of the brain.

Wilson disease has been observed in all races and ethnic groups. Symptoms typically begin between the ages of six and 20, though they may appear as early as four or as late as 40. Unfortunately, it is difficult to diagnose, as the symptoms present themselves in many different ways and are similar to several different neurological and psychiatric disorders, liver diseases and blood, kidney and bone disorders. The corneal accumulation of copper is one of the most indicative signs of the disorder, creating a rusty brown ring in each eye, known as a Kayser-Fleischer ring. However, this may not be present in early stages of the disease process, and it is difficult to observe in brown-eyed individuals.

Inherited as an AUTOSOMAL RECESSIVE trait, Wilson disease is estimated to have an incidence of approximately one in 200,000 live births. However, due to the difficulty of diagnosing the condition, some studies suggest that the incidence may be much higher, perhaps as much as one in 35,000 live births, with one in 100 people being CARRIERS of the disorder. There are approximately 1,000 known cases in the United States.

The GENE for Wilson disease has recently been mapped to the long arm of CHROMOSOME 13, and CARRIER detection and presymptomatic and PRENATAL DIAGNOSIS have been accomplished using linked DNA 'GENETIC MARKERS. However, it is not known whether these markers are applicable to all cases of the disease.

For more information, contact:

Wilson's Disease Association
P.O. Box 75324

Washington, DC 20013
(703) 636-3003
(703) 636-3014

Foundation for the Study of
 Wilson's Disease, Inc.
5447 Palisade Avenue
Bronx, NY 10471
(212) 430-2091

**Wiskott-Aldrich syndrome**    A severe
hereditary IMMUNE DEFICIENCY DISEASE with
onset in infancy or childhood. Affected children also have platelet abnormalities and eczema. Death usually results from repeated
infections or massive bleeding. Those who
survive infancy often succumb to various
CANCERS of the lymph system, though some
have lived into their teens. An X-LINKED recessive disorder, it is exhibited only in males.
Bone marrow transplantation can correct the
condition.

It is named for German pediatrician A.
Wiskott, who first reported the disorder in
1937, and U.S. pediatrician R.A. Aldrich, who
published a second report in 1954.

**Wolf-Hirschhorn syndrome (4p-)**    A
CHROMOSOME ABNORMALITY caused by the
deletion of the most distal, or end, portion of
the short arm of chromosome 4. It is characterized by severe motor, growth and MENTAL
RETARDATION. Birthweight is low (see LOW
BIRTHWEIGHT), generally well under five
pounds. Infants have seizures and exhibit poor
muscle tone (hypotonia) from birth.

It is named for German geneticist Dr. Ul-
rich Wolf and U.S. geneticist Dr. Kurt
Hirschhorn (b. 1926) of Mt. Sinai Medical
Center in New York City, who simultaneously
published separate descriptions in
*Humangenetik* (now *Human Genetics*) in
1965. (Dr. Hirschhorn also published an earlier description in 1961.)

The head is markedly small
(MICROENCEPHALY), the trunk is long and
the limbs thin. Facially, the forehead is high,
the eyes wide-set (HYPERTELORISM) and

often down-slanting and the eyelids may
droop (PTOSIS). The eyebrows are sparse, the
nasal bridge wide, the corners of the mouth
downturned. The groove extending from beneath the nose to the top lip (philtrum) is
short and deep. CLEFT LIP and cleft palate are
noted in over half of the cases, as are CON-
GENITAL HEART DEFECTS. The ears are low-
set, and the ear lobes adhere to the side of
the head.

Over 100 cases have been reported, and this
abnormality is estimated to occur in about one
in 50,000 live births, affecting females twice
as often as males. In approximately 10% to
15% of cases the deletion is due to a translocation. At least one-third of affected infants
die within two years of birth, though some
may survive into adulthood.

**Wolman disease**    An inborn error of
lipid metabolism (lysosomal acid lipase deficiency) causing lipids (fatty substances) to
accumulate in the spleen, liver and other organs, with fatal consequences. It is inherited
as an AUTOSOMAL RECESSIVE trait. Onset occurs in the first few weeks of life, beginning
with vomiting and diarrhea. The liver and
spleen enlarge (hepatosplenomegaly) due to
the accumulation of lipids. Death usually occurs by two to four months of age, due to
nutritional failure.

Israeli pathologist M. Wolman (b. 1914)
coauthored a report describing the disorder,which now bears his name, in 1956.

CHOLESTERYL ESTER STORAGE DISEASE is
a more benign form of this STORAGE DISEASE.

# X

**X chromosome**    The "female" SEX
CHROMOSOME. Females have only X sex chromosomes and no Y CHROMOSOMEs, and the
presence of two X chromosomes is responsible for their gender. A pair of X chromosomes
can be found in every somatic cell of the

normal female, and characteristics transmitted on the X chromosome are said to be X-LINKED, or sex-linked. However, only one of the two X GENES is active; the other is inactive, and it can be identified by a small dark mass within the nucleus of the cell called a "Barr body" for its discoverer, Canadian anatomist Murray L. Barr.

X chromosomes were observed as early as 1891, by German zoologist Hermann Henking (1858–1942), who noted them while studying chromosomes of the fire wasp (pyrrhocoris). Henking was unable to identify the nature of these chromosomes, hence he labeled them "X" chromosomes. Their function remained unrecognized until after the rediscovery of Mendel's laws. The X (and Y) chromosomes were first identified as sex chromosomes in 1910, from a study of sex-linked traits in the fly Drosophila melanogaster by Thomas Hunt Morgan at Columbia University.

**xeroderma pigmentosum**   A rare, progressive disorder characterized by sensitivity to sunlight, abnormal pigmentation and freckling of the skin, and the development of numerous growths, lesions and tumors on areas of the skin exposed to the sun. Degenerative changes also occur in the eyes.

The condition was first described in Vienna by Hungarian dermatologist Moriz Kaposi in 1863. He called it "xeroderma," or parchment skin, and added the term "pigmentosum" in 1882 to emphasize the striking pigmentary abnormalities.

Xeroderma pigmentosum is inherited as an AUTOSOMAL RECESSIVE trait. Incidence is estimated to be about one in from 60,000 to 100,000 individuals. (One in 250,000 in Europe and the United States and one in 40,000 in Japan.) Malignant melanoma has been associated with affected individuals from Europe and the United States, but not from Japan.

Onset is typically in the first few years of life. Acute sun sensitivity occurs in early infancy, with minimal exposure to sunlight causing severe blistering. Copious freckles begin to appear on the skin, especially on sun-exposed areas, prior to the age of two

years. Hyperpigmented areas may also appear on the lips, tongue, palms and soles. The skin becomes dry, wrinkled, scaly and parchment-like. It may tighten, especially at the center of the face, making severely affected individuals unable to fully open their mouths. Benign growths, warts and lesions appear on exposed areas, especially the face. Lesions may become malignant over a period of years. Similar growths may occur on the surface of the eye.

In acute forms, the first exposure to sunlight triggers the development of malignant growths on the skin, which lead to death in childhood. The basic defect involves the inability of DNA (see DEOXYRIBONUCLEIC ACID) to repair damage done by ultraviolet radiation from the sun or other sources.

There is a delayed onset form of the disorder, with slow progression, in which individuals may live to an old age, as well as a severe form, which includes progressive neurological degeneration, MENTAL RETARDATION and dwarfing.

Affected individuals must be constantly protected from exposure to sources of ultraviolet radiation, including sunlight, germicidal lamps, sunlamps and to a small extent from common, unfiltered, cool white fluorescent lamps. Light from incandescent lamps or sunlight passing through windows is not known to be harmful.

PRENATAL DIAGNOSIS is possible by cultivating fetal skin fibroblasts obtained at AMNIOCENTESIS to test their reaction to exposure to ultraviolet radiation. CARRRIER detection by similar assays is not always reliable.

For more information, contact:

Xeroderma Pigmentosum Registry
Medical Science Building
UMDNJ-NJ Medical School
185 South Orange Avenue
Newark, NJ 07103
(201) 456-4405

**X-linked**   (sex-linked)   A method of genetic transmission of hereditary traits. It is the confirmed mode of transmission of approximately 140 genetic disorders, and the sus-

**Figure V**

## how X-linked inheritance works

In the most common form, the female sex chromosomes of an unaffected mother carry one faulty gene (**X**) and one normal one (x). The father has normal male x and y chromosome complement.

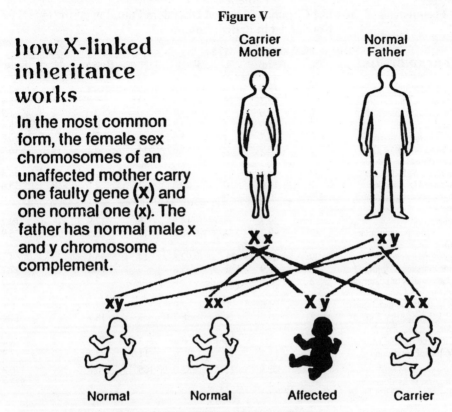

Carrier Mother   Normal Father

X x      x y

xy       xx       X y       X x

Normal   Normal   Affected   Carrier

The odds for each *male* child are 50/50:
1. 50% risk of inheriting the faulty **X** and the disorder
2. 50% chance of inheriting normal x and y chromosomes
For each *female* child, the odds are:
1. 50% risk of inheriting one faulty **X**, to be a carrier like mother
2. 50% chance of inheriting no faulty gene

Source: March of Dimes Birth Defects Foundation, *Genetics Counseling* (January 1987).

pected mode of over 170 more. Like non-X-linked traits (that is, autosomal traits), X-linked disorders may be either dominant or recessive, though the majority are recessive. (Some X-linked disorders have not yet been clearly fit into either dominant or recessive categories.)

These disorders are called X-linked because they have their origins in MUTATIONS or defects in individual GENES found on the X CHROMOSOME, which is found in the 23rd chromosome pair in humans. Due to the nature of this chromosome pair, many X-linked dis-

orders are exhibited only in males, while only females are silent carriers. Classic X-linked disorders include COLOR BLINDNESS and HEMOPHILIA.

Though inheritance of X-linked traits such as color blindness and hemophilia has been recognized for some time, the link between sex chromosomes and X-linked traits was established in 1910 by Thomas Hunt Morgan in experiments with the fly Drosophilia melanogaster (see introductory section, "The History of Genetics").

## Table XX
## Frequencies of the Most Common X-linked Disorders Found in a Survey
## Conducted in British Columbia*

| X-LINKED CONDITION | 1952–63 | | 1964–73 | | 1974–83 | | TOTAL | |
|---|---|---|---|---|---|---|---|---|
| | N | Rate[a] | N | Rate[a] | N | Rate[a] | N | Rate[a] |
| Other testicular dysfunction | 8 | 18.3 | 0 | 0.0 | 7 | 18.1 | 15 | 12.8 |
| Disorders of urea-cycle metabolism | 1 | 2.3 | 0 | 0.0 | 3 | 7.7 | 4 | 3.4 |
| Disorders of calcium metabolism | 0 | 0.0 | 2 | 5.8 | 0 | 0.0 | 2 | 1.7 |
| Mucopolysaccharidosis | 3 | 6.9 | 3 | 8.7 | 0 | 0.0 | 6 | 5.1 |
| Deficiency of humoral immunity | 6 | 13.7 | 2 | 5.8 | 0 | 0.0 | 8 | 6.8 |
| Anemia due to disorder of gluta-thione metabolism | 3 | 6.9 | 2 | 5.8 | 14 | 36.1 | 19 | 16.2 |
| Congenital factor VIII disorder | 28 | 64.0 | 24 | 69.6 | 14 | 36.1 | 66 | 56.4 |
| Congenital factor IX disorder | 7 | 16.0 | 10 | 29.0 | 1 | 2.6 | 18 | 15.4 |
| Functional disorder of neutrophil polymorphs | 0 | 0.0 | 0 | 0.0 | 3 | 7.7 | 3 | 2.6 |
| Mental retardation | 13 | 29.7 | 5 | 14.5 | 5 | 12.9 | 23 | 19.7 |
| Hereditary progressive muscular dystrophy | 43 | 98.3 | 34 | 98.6 | 13 | 33.5 | 90 | 76.9 |
| Color-vision deficiencies | 29 | 66.3 | 32 | 92.8 | 14 | 36.1 | 75 | 64.1 |
| Nephrogenic diabetes insipidus | 3 | 6.9 | 2 | 5.8 | 4 | 10.3 | 9 | 7.7 |
| Congenital anomalies of posterior segment | 2 | 4.6 | 2 | 5.8 | 3 | 7.7 | 7 | 6.0 |
| Anomalies of skull and face bones | 2 | 4.6 | 1 | 2.9 | 3 | 7.7 | 6 | 5.1 |
| Other specified congenital anoma-lies of skin | 3 | 6.9 | 3 | 8.7 | 7 | 18.1 | 13 | 11.1 |
| Other specified congenital anomalies | 1 | 2.3 | 0 | 0.0 | 3 | 7.7 | 4 | 3.4 |
| All other X-linked conditions[b] | 5 | 11.4 | 10 | 29.0 | 11 | 28.4 | 26 | 22.2 |
| Total | 157 | 358.9 | 13.2 | 383.0 | 105 | 270.8 | 394 | 336.8 |
| Sum of highest individual rates | | | | | | | | 532.4 |

N—Number of patients.
[a] Per 1 million live births.
[b] Each individual rate was used to get the sum of highest individual rates for these conditions.
*Statistics reflect local population bias.

Source: Patricia A. Baird, "A Population Study of Genetic Disorders in Children and Young Adults," *American Journal of Human Genetics*, 42 (1988), pp. 677-693.

Females have two X CHROMOSOMES while males have one X and one Y CHROMOSOME. The Y chromosome has fewer genes than the X chromosome, and in X-linked disorders, a recessive, aberrant gene on the X chromosome has no normal counterpart on the Y chromosome to override its influence. Any male that inherits an X chromosome with such a mutation will therefore exhibit the trait, while a female, with two X chromosomes, will almost always have a normal gene to mask the influence of the aberrant recessive one. These women are said to be CARRIERS. (Inheritance of two recessive genes or two dominant genes for an X-linked disorder may be lethal in utero for females.)

Classic X-linked disorders can never be passed from father to son, since the aberrant gene is on the X chromosome, and the affected father must pass on the Y chromosome to have male offspring. However, all daughters will be carriers. Screening can identify carriers in some of these disorders. (See Figure V.)

X-linked dominant disorders are very rare. In some, they follow inheritance patterns of AUTOSOMAL DOMINANT transmission, with no transmission from father to son. Some may be seen only in females, as inheritance of the single dominant mutant gene is lethal in utero for males.

Female carriers may exhibit mild symptoms in some X-linked disorders. In females, in any individual cell, only one X chromosome is active (see MOSAICISM).

## X-linked agammaglobulinemia    See
IMMUNE DEFICIENCY DISEASES.

## XX male syndrome (sex reversal)
Individuals exhibiting the PHENOTYPE, or typical appearance, of a normal male, though chromosomally (GENOTYPE) they are females, having two X CHROMOSOMES instead of one X and one Y CHROMOSOME found in males. The penis, scrotum and testes are usually small but well-differentiated, but the individuals fail to exhibit normal pubertal development. Breasts develop (GYNECOMASTIA) in about one-third of those affected. Pubic hair may grow in a characteristic female pattern, and body and facial hair is decreased. Affected individuals are infertile, as well.

It has recently been theorized that the translocation of a particular region of the Y chromosome, termed testis determining factor, is involved in causing this disorder. This is the "master switch" for determining male characteristics. In affected individuals the genes are present on one of the X chromosomes due to chromosomal translocation. Some familial cases of this syndrome have been reported. In some cases there is evidence of a translocation of chromosomal material from the Y chromosome onto a chromosome other than the X chromosome. (See also CHROMOSOME ABNORMALITIES.)

## XXXXX
CHROMOSOME ABNORMALITY exhibited only in females, characterized by MENTAL RETARDATION (of varying severity), failure to mature sexually at puberty, and sterility. (For the male equivalent of this disorder, see XXXXY.) Individuals have 49 chromosomes, with five X chromosomes. Approximately 20 cases have been reported.

At birth, the external genitalia appear normal. Non-genital physical characterstics are similar to those exhibited by males with XXXXY. Infants display poor muscle tone (hypotonia) and are short, with height often below the third percentile. The head tends to be mildly undersized. The face is usually rounded. They may resemble babies with trisomy 21 (DOWN SYNDROME). The eyes are often wide-set (HYPERTELORISM) and frequently exhibit ocular abnormalities, including inability to focus the eyes in concert (STRABISMUS or crossed-eyes), nearsightedness (MYOPIA) and mild upward slant (obliquity) of the eye slits (palpebral fissures).

As infants age, the roundness of the face disappears, but midface growth is retarded, creating a rather pronounced, jutting jaw (mandibular prognathism), particularly after puberty.

The breasts and uterus remain infantile, and there is scant pubic hair growth at the time of puberty. In some individuals, microscopic examination of the ovaries reveals no abnormalities. Lifespan is normal.

## XXXXY
CHROMOSOME ABNORMALITY, exhibited only in males; characterized by MENTAL RETARDATION, poor development of external genitalia and STERILITY. (For the female equivalent of this disorder, see XXXXX.) The penis, scrotum and testes are very small, and the testes are undescended (CRYPTORCHIDISM). These individuals have 49 chromosomes, with four X chromosomes and one Y.

At birth, infants exhibit poor muscle tone (hypotonia) and are short, with height often below the third percentile. The head tends to be mildly undersized. The face is usually oval-shaped. Most infants exhibit wide-set eyes (HYPERTELORISM), frequently accompanied by ocular abnormalities, including inability to focus the eyes in concert (STRABISMUS or crossed-eyes) and mild upward slant (antimongoloid obliquity) of the eye slits (palpebral fissures). The neck is short and webbed.

As infants age, midface growth is retarded, creating a rather pronounced, jutting jaw (mandibular prognathism), particularly after puberty. Abnormalities of the upper limbs are characterstic, especially inability to bend the elbow. Life span is normal. Retardation is present and severe in all cases.

Over 100 cases have been reported and it is believed to be at the least 10 times more frequent than XXXXX.

**XY syndrome**    The normal male genotype. It has semi-facetiously been suggested by one genetic researcher that this is a SYNDROME in which affected individuals have an increased susceptibility to stroke, hypertension and cardiovascular disease, as well as a tendency to exhibit aggressive behaviors associated with increased mortality rates.

**XYY syndrome**    CHROMOSOME ABNORMALITY characterized by the presence of an additional Y CHROMOSOME, the sex chromosome that determines male gender. Affected individuals are sometimes referred to as "hypermasculine" or "supermales."

It occurs as frequently as one in 840 live male births but may remain undiagnosed throughout life, as the features are subtle. They include accelerated growth in mid-childhood, potentially explosive, antisocial behavior, relative weakness, poor coordination of fine motor skills and low intelligence; IQ is usually 10 to 15 points below unaffected SIBLINGS. Physically, affected individuals tend to be tall and thin, with mildly sunken chests (PECTUS excavatum). Severe acne may develop in adolescence.

It has been suggested that individuals with this KARYOTYPE are more prone to criminal behavior, but studies have not corroborated this speculation, though among institutionalized male juvenile delinquents, incidence has been reported as much as 24 times above that in the general population.

Affected individuals have passed the condition on to their sons only in very rare instances, though the majority of XYY individuals are fertile.

# Y

**Y chromosome**    The male sex chromosome. Males have one X CHROMOSOME and one Y SEX CHROMOSOME, and the presence of the Y chromosome is responsible for their gender. (Females have two X chromosomes.) While only an X chromosome can be inherited from the mother, the father may pass on either an X or Y chromosome. If he passes on a Y chromosome, the offspring will be a male. The XY chromosome pair can be found in every somatic cell of the normal male.

The only sex-linked characteristic, in addition to the male determining factor (termed TDF or testis determining factor), that is known to be on the Y chromosome is the trait for HAIRY EARS.

The Y (and X) chromosomes were first identified as sex chromosomes in 1910, arising from a study of sex-linked traits in the fly Drosophila melanogaster by Thomas Hunt Morgan at Columbia University.

# Z

**Zellweger syndrome**    (cerebro-hepato-renal syndrome, CHRS)    First described in 1964 by Hans V. Zellweger (b. 1908) and colleagues at Johns Hopkins University, this disorder is marked at birth by LOW BIRTHWEIGHT, a FLOPPY INFANT appearance due to lack of muscle tone (hypotonia), and characterstic facial features. Most infants are relatively motionless. The forehead is high and bulging, the face is round, the eyes are wide-set (HYPERTELORISM) and slanted toward the nose (mongoloid obliquity with epicanthal folds (see EPICANTHUS). The eyelids are puffy, and other ocular abnormalities may include GLAUCOMA, corneal clouding and CATARACTS. The nose is upturned (anteverted nares) and ears are poorly formed, low-set and rotated slightly backward. The jaw is small (micrognathia).

The liver is almost always enlarged (hepatomegaly). Males frequently exhibit undescended testes (CRYPTORCHIDISM), while the clitoris is often enlarged in females. There are microscopic cysts in the kidneys that can be confirmed only by biopsy. There are also stippled calcifications, dot-like flecks of calcium deposits, seen on X rays of the knees.

Fingers and knees may exhibit permanent bending (flexion contractures). Mental and physical development is extremely limited, and seizures are common. Death, most often from pneumonia, usually occurs before the age of six months. There is no effective therapy.

CHRS is inherited as an AUTOSOMAL RECESSIVE trait. The basic defect that causes it lies in an organelle (a componenet of the cell) known as the peroxisome. Only about 65 cases have been reported, though it has been estimated to occur in one in 100,000 live births. However, recent discovery of new cases indicates the incidence may be as high as one in 25,000 to one in 50,000 newborns. Twice as many affected females as males have been identified. PRENATAL DIAGNOSIS is currently not possible.

Neonatal ALD (see ADRENO-LEUKODYSTROPHY) is a related disorder that is also a defect in peroxisomal assembly. This disorder has facial dysmorphic features and hypotonia (floppiness) in common with CHRS. But it is a separate disorder, with absence of renal cysts, cataracts or bony involvement. Adrenal gland dysfunction, a major feature of neonatal ALD, does not occur in CHRS.

**zygodactyly**    The fusion of the second and third toes or the third and fourth fingers by a web of skin. It is the mildest form of SYNDACTYLY (the fusion of the digits). It may be SPORADIC or AUTOSOMAL DOMINANTly inherited and may be seen in normal children as well as those with other associated problems.

# Appendixes

# 1.
# CONGENITAL
# MALFORMATION STATISTICS

**Figure 1**
**Percentage of United States Live Births in the BDMP/CPHA (Birth Defects Monitoring Program/Commission of Professional Hospital Activities)**

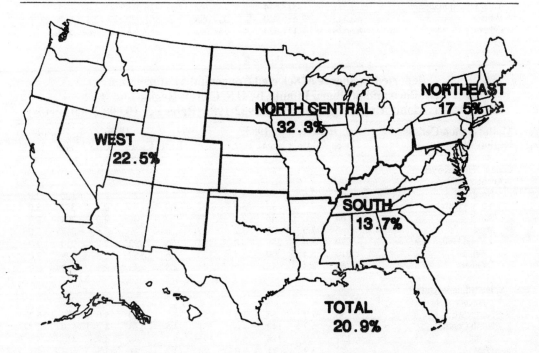

NORTHEAST
17.5%

NORTH CENTRAL
32.3%

WEST
22.5%

SOUTH
13.7%

TOTAL
20.9%

Sources: Centers for Disease Control, *Congenital Malformations Surveillance Report, January 1982-December 1985* (Atlanta: CDC, March 1988); *Morbidity and Mortality Weekly Report* (Atlanta: CDC, 1988).

## Table 1

### Number of Monitored Births (Live-Born and Stillborn)
### By U.S. Census Region and Races
### Birth Defects Monitoring Program/CPHA, 1982-1985

| Census Region/Race | 1982 | 1983 | 1984 | 1985 | Total |
|---|---|---|---|---|---|
| Northeast | 118,076 | 126,933 | 119,079 | 119,553 | 483,641 |
| North Central | 307,208 | 312,043 | 282,090 | 277,630 | 1,178,971 |
| South | 210,245 | 195,206 | 157,009 | 140,273 | 702,733 |
| West | 187,742 | 179,662 | 184,104 | 179,522 | 731,030 |
| Total United States | 823,271 | 813,844 | 742,282 | 716,978 | 3,096,375 |
| White | 640,643 | 636,220 | 583,088 | 561,737 | 2,421,688 |
| Other | 182,628 | 177,624 | 159,194 | 155,241 | 674,687 |

## Table 2

### Reported Incidence of Selected Congenital Malformations
### Live-Born and Stillborn Infants, by U.S. Census Region and Race
### Birth Defects Monitoring Program/CPHA, 1982-1985 (Rates Per 10,000 Total Births)

| Malformation/Census Region/Race | 1982 Cases | Rate | 1983 Cases | Rate | 1984 Cases | Rate | 1985 Cases | Rate | Total Cases | Rate |
|---|---|---|---|---|---|---|---|---|---|---|
| **Central Nervous System** | | | | | | | | | | |
| Anencephalus | | | | | | | | | | |
| Northeast | 42 | 3.6 | 39 | 3.1 | 27 | 2.3 | 28 | 2.3 | 136 | 2.8 |
| North Central | 107 | 3.5 | 93 | 3.0 | 77 | 2.7 | 76 | 2.7 | 353 | 3.0 |
| South | 64 | 3.0 | 56 | 2.9 | 43 | 2.7 | 41 | 2.9 | 204 | 2.9 |
| West | 66 | 3.5 | 57 | 3.2 | 47 | 2.6 | 47 | 2.6 | 217 | 3.0 |
| Total United States | 279 | 3.4 | 245 | 3.0 | 194 | 2.6 | 192 | 2.7 | 910 | 2.9 |
| White | 219 | 3.4 | 200 | 3.1 | 150 | 2.6 | 159 | 2.8 | 728 | 3.0 |
| Other | 60 | 3.3 | 45 | 2.5 | 44 | 2.8 | 33 | 2.1 | 182 | 2.7 |
| **Spina Bifida W/Out Anencephalus** | | | | | | | | | | |
| Northeast | 58 | 4.9 | 54 | 4.3 | 54 | 4.5 | 60 | 5.0 | 226 | 4.7 |
| North Central | 161 | 5.2 | 142 | 4.6 | 131 | 4.6 | 116 | 4.2 | 550 | 4.7 |
| South | 127 | 6.0 | 116 | 5.9 | 105 | 6.7 | 66 | 4.7 | 414 | 5.9 |
| West | 73 | 3.9 | 71 | 4.0 | 78 | 4.2 | 81 | 4.5 | 303 | 4.1 |
| Total United States | 419 | 5.1 | 383 | 4.7 | 368 | 5.0 | 323 | 4.5 | 1493 | 4.8 |
| White | 356 | 5.6 | 303 | 4.8 | 304 | 5.2 | 270 | 4.8 | 1233 | 5.1 |
| Other | 63 | 3.4 | 80 | 4.5 | 64 | 4.0 | 53 | 3.4 | 260 | 3.9 |
| **Hydrocephalus W/Out Spina Bifida** | | | | | | | | | | |
| Northeast | 71 | 6.0 | 84 | 6.6 | 72 | 6.0 | 72 | 6.0 | 299 | 6.2 |
| North Central | 162 | 5.3 | 208 | 6.7 | 164 | 5.8 | 162 | 5.8 | 696 | 5.9 |
| South | 137 | 6.5 | 125 | 6.4 | 100 | 6.4 | 102 | 7.3 | 464 | 6.6 |
| West | 99 | 5.3 | 75 | 4.2 | 82 | 4.5 | 66 | 3.7 | 322 | 4.4 |
| Total United States | 469 | 5.7 | 492 | 6.0 | 418 | 5.6 | 402 | 5.6 | 1781 | 5.8 |
| White | 343 | 5.4 | 363 | 5.7 | 322 | 5.5 | 300 | 5.3 | 1328 | 5.5 |
| Other | 126 | 6.9 | 129 | 7.3 | 96 | 6.0 | 102 | 6.6 | 453 | 6.7 |
| **Encephalocele** | | | | | | | | | | |
| Northeast | 10 | 0.8 | 17 | 1.3 | 11 | 0.9 | 8 | 0.7 | 46 | 1.0 |
| North Central | 35 | 1.1 | 31 | 1.0 | 37 | 1.3 | 24 | 0.9 | 127 | 1.1 |
| South | 21 | 1.0 | 24 | 1.2 | 20 | 1.3 | 21 | 1.5 | 86 | 1.2 |
| West | 21 | 1.1 | 25 | 1.4 | 17 | 0.9 | 19 | 1.1 | 82 | 1.1 |
| Total United States | 87 | 1.1 | 97 | 1.2 | 85 | 1.1 | 72 | 1.0 | 341 | 1.1 |
| White | 65 | 1.0 | 77 | 1.2 | 67 | 1.1 | 58 | 1.0 | 267 | 1.1 |
| Other | 22 | 1.2 | 20 | 1.1 | 18 | 1.1 | 14 | 0.9 | 74 | 1.1 |

## Table 2 (continued)

| Malformation/Census Region/Race | 1982 Cases | Rate | 1983 Cases | Rate | 1984 Cases | Rate | 1985 Cases | Rate | Total Cases | Rate |
|---|---|---|---|---|---|---|---|---|---|---|
| **Microcephalus** | | | | | | | | | | |
| Northeast | 31 | 2.6 | 36 | 2.8 | 34 | 2.9 | 36 | 3.0 | 137 | 2.8 |
| North Central | 85 | 2.8 | 84 | 2.7 | 72 | 2.6 | 71 | 2.6 | 312 | 2.6 |
| South | 30 | 1.4 | 56 | 2.9 | 48 | 3.1 | 41 | 2.9 | 175 | 2.5 |
| West | 43 | 2.3 | 47 | 2.6 | 32 | 1.7 | 39 | 2.2 | 161 | 2.2 |
| Total United States | 189 | 2.3 | 223 | 2.7 | 186 | 2.5 | 187 | 2.6 | 785 | 2.5 |
| White | 122 | 1.9 | 154 | 2.4 | 119 | 2.0 | 134 | 2.4 | 529 | 2.2 |
| Other | 67 | 3.7 | 69 | 3.9 | 67 | 4.2 | 53 | 3.4 | 256 | 3.8 |
| **Eye** | | | | | | | | | | |
| **Anophthalmos/Microphthalmos** | | | | | | | | | | |
| Northeast | 14 | 1.2 | 15 | 1.2 | 6 | 0.5 | 9 | 0.8 | 44 | 0.9 |
| North Central | 20 | 0.7 | 36 | 1.2 | 24 | 0.9 | 14 | 0.5 | 94 | 0.8 |
| South | 16 | 0.8 | 18 | 0.9 | 12 | 0.8 | 8 | 0.6 | 54 | 0.8 |
| West | 8 | 0.4 | 13 | 0.7 | 18 | 1.0 | 14 | 0.8 | 53 | 0.7 |
| Total United States | 58 | 0.7 | 82 | 1.0 | 60 | 0.8 | 45 | 0.6 | 245 | 0.8 |
| White | 42 | 0.7 | 60 | 0.9 | 42 | 0.7 | 40 | 0.7 | 184 | 0.8 |
| Other | 16 | 0.9 | 22 | 1.2 | 18 | 1.1 | 5 | 0.3 | 61 | 0.9 |
| **Congenital Cataract** | | | | | | | | | | |
| Northeast | 10 | 0.8 | 17 | 1.3 | 22 | 1.8 | 16 | 1.3 | 65 | 1.3 |
| North Central | 32 | 1.0 | 34 | 1.1 | 31 | 1.1 | 33 | 1.2 | 130 | 1.1 |
| South | 19 | 0.9 | 23 | 1.2 | 14 | 0.9 | 15 | 1.1 | 71 | 1.0 |
| West | 18 | 1.0 | 12 | 0.7 | 24 | 1.3 | 12 | 0.7 | 66 | 0.9 |
| Total United States | 79 | 1.0 | 86 | 1.1 | 91 | 1.2 | 76 | 1.1 | 332 | 1.1 |
| White | 55 | 0.9 | 64 | 1.0 | 72 | 1.2 | 53 | 0.9 | 244 | 1.0 |
| Other | 24 | 1.3 | 22 | 1.2 | 19 | 1.2 | 23 | 1.5 | 88 | 1.3 |
| **Coloboma of Eye** | | | | | | | | | | |
| Northeast | 3 | 0.3 | 7 | 0.6 | 3 | 0.3 | 2 | 0.2 | 15 | 0.3 |
| North Central | 10 | 0.3 | 9 | 0.3 | 11 | 0.4 | 8 | 0.3 | 38 | 0.3 |
| South | 3 | 0.1 | 4 | 0.2 | 2 | 0.1 | 1 | 0.1 | 10 | 0.1 |
| West | 4 | 0.2 | 5 | 0.3 | 7 | 0.4 | 6 | 0.3 | 22 | 0.3 |
| Total United States | 20 | 0.2 | 25 | 0.3 | 23 | 0.3 | 17 | 0.2 | 85 | 0.3 |
| White | 18 | 0.3 | 18 | 0.3 | 20 | 0.3 | 14 | 0.2 | 70 | 0.3 |
| Other | 2 | 0.1 | 7 | 0.4 | 3 | 0.2 | 3 | 0.2 | 15 | 0.2 |
| **Aniridia** | | | | | | | | | | |
| Northeast | 0 | 0.0 | 0 | 0.0 | 0 | 0.0 | 0 | 0.0 | 0 | 0.0 |
| North Central | 2 | 0.1 | 2 | 0.1 | 1 | 0.0 | 5 | 0.2 | 10 | 0.1 |
| South | 2 | 0.1 | 0 | 0.0 | 0 | 0.0 | 1 | 0.1 | 3 | 0.0 |
| West | 2 | 0.1 | 2 | 0.1 | 0 | 0.0 | 2 | 0.1 | 6 | 0.1 |
| Total United States | 6 | 0.1 | 4 | 0.0 | 1 | 0.0 | 8 | 0.1 | 19 | 0.1 |
| White | 6 | 0.1 | 4 | 0.1 | 1 | 0.0 | 8 | 0.1 | 19 | 0.1 |
| Other | 0 | 0.0 | 0 | 0.0 | 0 | 0.0 | 0 | 0.0 | 0 | 0.0 |
| **Cardiovascular** | | | | | | | | | | |
| **Common Truncus** | | | | | | | | | | |
| Northeast | 6 | 0.5 | 2 | 0.2 | 4 | 0.3 | 0 | 0.0 | 12 | 0.2 |
| North Central | 8 | 0.3 | 6 | 0.2 | 7 | 0.2 | 7 | 0.3 | 28 | 0.2 |
| South | 1 | 0.0 | 1 | 0.1 | 5 | 0.3 | 8 | 0.6 | 15 | 0.2 |
| West | 8 | 0.4 | 4 | 0.2 | 11 | 0.6 | 2 | 0.1 | 25 | 0.3 |
| Total United States | 23 | 0.3 | 13 | 0.2 | 27 | 0.4 | 17 | 0.2 | 80 | 0.3 |
| White | 17 | 0.3 | 13 | 0.2 | 23 | 0.4 | 14 | 0.2 | 67 | 0.3 |
| Other | 6 | 0.3 | 0 | 0.0 | 4 | 0.3 | 3 | 0.2 | 13 | 0.2 |
| **Transposition of Great Arteries** | | | | | | | | | | |
| Northeast | 10 | 0.8 | 12 | 0.9 | 20 | 1.7 | 17 | 1.4 | 59 | 1.2 |

## Table 2 (continued)

| Malformation/Census Region/Race | 1982 Cases | Rate | 1983 Cases | Rate | 1984 Cases | Rate | 1985 Cases | Rate | Total Cases | Rate |
|---|---|---|---|---|---|---|---|---|---|---|
| North Central | 36 | 1.2 | 34 | 1.1 | 36 | 1.3 | 40 | 1.4 | 146 | 1.2 |
| South | 14 | 0.7 | 20 | 1.0 | 9 | 0.6 | 19 | 1.4 | 62 | 0.9 |
| West | 16 | 0.9 | 16 | 0.9 | 28 | 1.5 | 21 | 1.2 | 81 | 1.1 |
| Total United States | 76 | 0.9 | 82 | 1.0 | 93 | 1.3 | 97 | 1.4 | 348 | 1.1 |
| White | 60 | 0.9 | 64 | 1.0 | 77 | 1.3 | 87 | 1.5 | 288 | 1.2 |
| Other | 16 | 0.9 | 18 | 1.0 | 16 | 1.0 | 10 | 0.6 | 60 | 0.9 |
| **Tetralogy of Fallot** | | | | | | | | | | |
| Northeast | 15 | 1.3 | 10 | 0.8 | 17 | 1.4 | 18 | 1.5 | 60 | 1.2 |
| North Central | 38 | 1.2 | 31 | 1.0 | 34 | 1.2 | 42 | 1.5 | 145 | 1.2 |
| South | 12 | 0.6 | 20 | 1.0 | 13 | 0.8 | 29 | 2.1 | 74 | 1.1 |
| West | 13 | 0.7 | 17 | 0.9 | 13 | 0.7 | 24 | 1.3 | 67 | 0.9 |
| Total United States | 78 | 0.9 | 78 | 1.0 | 77 | 1.0 | 113 | 1.6 | 346 | 1.1 |
| White | 62 | 1.0 | 62 | 1.0 | 64 | 1.1 | 88 | 1.6 | 276 | 1.1 |
| Other | 16 | 0.9 | 16 | 0.9 | 13 | 0.8 | 25 | 1.6 | 70 | 1.0 |
| **Ventricular Septal Defect** | | | | | | | | | | |
| Northeast | 265 | 22.4 | 276 | 21.7 | 240 | 20.2 | 306 | 25.6 | 1087 | 22.5 |
| North Central | 517 | 16.8 | 520 | 16.7 | 548 | 19.4 | 542 | 19.5 | 2127 | 18.0 |
| South | 244 | 11.6 | 227 | 11.6 | 200 | 12.7 | 230 | 16.4 | 901 | 12.8 |
| West | 282 | 15.0 | 273 | 15.2 | 296 | 16.1 | 321 | 17.9 | 1172 | 16.0 |
| Total United States | 1308 | 15.9 | 1296 | 15.9 | 1284 | 17.3 | 1399 | 19.5 | 5287 | 17.1 |
| White | 1045 | 16.3 | 1023 | 16.1 | 1056 | 18.1 | 1126 | 20.0 | 4250 | 17.5 |
| Other | 263 | 14.4 | 273 | 15.4 | 228 | 14.3 | 273 | 17.6 | 1037 | 15.4 |
| **Atrial Septal Defect** | | | | | | | | | | |
| Northeast | 19 | 1.6 | 15 | 1.2 | 24 | 2.0 | 39 | 3.3 | 97 | 2.0 |
| North Central | 58 | 1.9 | 73 | 2.3 | 56 | 2.0 | 91 | 3.3 | 278 | 2.4 |
| South | 35 | 1.7 | 39 | 2.0 | 32 | 2.0 | 49 | 3.5 | 155 | 2.2 |
| West | 26 | 1.4 | 15 | 0.8 | 46 | 2.5 | 38 | 2.1 | 125 | 1.7 |
| Total United States | 138 | 1.7 | 142 | 1.7 | 158 | 2.1 | 217 | 3.0 | 655 | 2.1 |
| White | 111 | 1.7 | 115 | 1.8 | 124 | 2.1 | 170 | 3.0 | 520 | 2.1 |
| Other | 27 | 1.5 | 27 | 1.5 | 34 | 2.1 | 47 | 3.0 | 135 | 2.0 |
| **Endocardial Cushion Defect** | | | | | | | | | | |
| Northeast | 9 | 0.8 | 14 | 1.1 | 4 | 0.3 | 15 | 1.3 | 42 | 0.9 |
| North Central | 17 | 0.6 | 23 | 0.7 | 24 | 0.9 | 27 | 1.0 | 91 | 0.8 |
| South | 8 | 0.4 | 9 | 0.5 | 14 | 0.9 | 19 | 1.4 | 50 | 0.7 |
| West | 12 | 0.6 | 12 | 0.7 | 14 | 0.8 | 14 | 0.8 | 52 | 0.7 |
| Total United States | 46 | 0.6 | 58 | 0.7 | 56 | 0.8 | 75 | 1.0 | 235 | 0.8 |
| White | 37 | 0.6 | 46 | 0.7 | 40 | 0.7 | 58 | 1.0 | 181 | 0.7 |
| Other | 9 | 0.5 | 12 | 0.7 | 16 | 1.0 | 17 | 1.1 | 54 | 0.8 |
| **Pulmonary Valve Stenosis and Atresia** | | | | | | | | | | |
| Northeast | 43 | 3.6 | 21 | 1.7 | 22 | 1.8 | 43 | 3.6 | 129 | 2.7 |
| North Central | 32 | 1.0 | 59 | 1.9 | 63 | 2.2 | 73 | 2.6 | 227 | 1.9 |
| South | 20 | 1.0 | 23 | 1.2 | 39 | 2.5 | 62 | 4.4 | 144 | 2.0 |
| West | 19 | 1.0 | 16 | 0.9 | 24 | 1.3 | 26 | 1.4 | 85 | 1.2 |
| Total United States | 114 | 1.4 | 119 | 1.5 | 148 | 2.0 | 204 | 2.8 | 585 | 1.9 |
| White | 72 | 1.1 | 81 | 1.3 | 81 | 1.4 | 119 | 2.1 | 353 | 1.5 |
| Other | 42 | 2.3 | 38 | 2.1 | 67 | 4.2 | 85 | 5.5 | 232 | 3.4 |
| **Tricuspid Valve Stenosis and Atresia** | | | | | | | | | | |
| Northeast | 2 | 0.2 | 2 | 0.2 | 5 | 0.4 | 2 | 0.2 | 11 | 0.2 |
| North Central | 5 | 0.2 | 5 | 0.2 | 8 | 0.3 | 8 | 0.3 | 26 | 0.2 |
| South | 3 | 0.1 | 5 | 0.3 | 8 | 0.5 | 15 | 1.1 | 31 | 0.4 |
| West | 5 | 0.3 | 5 | 0.3 | 7 | 0.4 | 4 | 0.2 | 21 | 0.3 |

Table 2 (continued)

| Malformation/Census Region/Race | 1982 Cases | Rate | 1983 Cases | Rate | 1984 Cases | Rate | 1985 Cases | Rate | Total Cases | Rate |
|---|---|---|---|---|---|---|---|---|---|---|
| Total United States | 15 | 0.2 | 17 | 0.2 | 28 | 0.4 | 29 | 0.4 | 89 | 0.3 |
| White | 12 | 0.2 | 14 | 0.2 | 25 | 0.4 | 19 | 0.3 | 70 | 0.3 |
| Other | 3 | 0.2 | 3 | 0.2 | 3 | 0.2 | 10 | 0.6 | 19 | 0.3 |
| **Aortic Valve Stenosis and Atresia** | | | | | | | | | | |
| Northeast | 8 | 0.7 | 7 | 0.6 | 7 | 0.6 | 9 | 0.8 | 31 | 0.6 |
| North Central | 17 | 0.6 | 25 | 0.8 | 12 | 0.4 | 27 | 1.0 | 81 | 0.7 |
| South | 6 | 0.3 | 5 | 0.3 | 4 | 0.3 | 10 | 0.7 | 25 | 0.4 |
| West | 8 | 0.4 | 11 | 0.6 | 9 | 0.5 | 8 | 0.4 | 36 | 0.5 |
| Total United States | 39 | 0.5 | 48 | 0.6 | 32 | 0.4 | 54 | 0.8 | 173 | 0.6 |
| White | 31 | 0.5 | 38 | 0.6 | 28 | 0.5 | 43 | 0.8 | 140 | 0.6 |
| Other | 8 | 0.4 | 10 | 0.6 | 4 | 0.3 | 11 | 0.7 | 33 | 0.5 |
| **Hypoplastic Left Heart Syndrome** | | | | | | | | | | |
| Northeast | 8 | 0.7 | 11 | 0.9 | 5 | 0.4 | 18 | 1.5 | 42 | 0.9 |
| North Central | 23 | 0.7 | 27 | 0.9 | 23 | 0.8 | 33 | 1.2 | 106 | 0.9 |
| South | 18 | 0.9 | 18 | 0.9 | 10 | 0.6 | 15 | 1.1 | 61 | 0.9 |
| West | 11 | 0.6 | 13 | 0.7 | 7 | 0.4 | 11 | 0.6 | 42 | 0.6 |
| Total United States | 60 | 0.7 | 69 | 0.8 | 45 | 0.6 | 77 | 1.1 | 251 | 0.8 |
| White | 47 | 0.7 | 48 | 0.8 | 30 | 0.5 | 61 | 1.1 | 186 | 0.8 |
| Other | 13 | 0.7 | 21 | 1.2 | 15 | 0.9 | 16 | 1.0 | 65 | 1.0 |
| **Patent Ductus Arteriosus** | | | | | | | | | | |
| Northeast | 347 | 29.4 | 400 | 31.5 | 355 | 29.8 | 370 | 30.9 | 1472 | 30.4 |
| North Central | 917 | 29.8 | 930 | 29.8 | 770 | 27.3 | 941 | 33.9 | 3558 | 30.2 |
| South | 460 | 21.9 | 531 | 27.2 | 544 | 34.6 | 541 | 38.6 | 2076 | 29.5 |
| West | 605 | 32.2 | 429 | 23.9 | 543 | 29.5 | 493 | 27.5 | 2070 | 28.3 |
| Total United States | 2329 | 28.3 | 2290 | 28.1 | 2212 | 29.8 | 2345 | 32.7 | 9176 | 29.6 |
| White | 1592 | 24.9 | 1640 | 25.8 | 1578 | 27.1 | 1696 | 30.2 | 6506 | 26.9 |
| Other | 737 | 40.4 | 650 | 36.6 | 634 | 39.8 | 649 | 41.8 | 2670 | 39.6 |
| **Coarctation of Aorta** | | | | | | | | | | |
| Northeast | 13 | 1.1 | 8 | 0.6 | 11 | 0.9 | 10 | 0.8 | 42 | 0.9 |
| North Central | 22 | 0.7 | 15 | 0.5 | 25 | 0.9 | 31 | 1.1 | 93 | 0.8 |
| South | 9 | 0.4 | 9 | 0.5 | 8 | 0.5 | 10 | 0.7 | 36 | 0.5 |
| West | 16 | 0.9 | 11 | 0.6 | 16 | 0.9 | 15 | 0.8 | 58 | 0.8 |
| Total United States | 60 | 0.7 | 43 | 0.5 | 60 | 0.8 | 66 | 0.9 | 229 | 0.7 |
| White | 50 | 0.8 | 37 | 0.6 | 50 | 0.9 | 56 | 1.0 | 193 | 0.8 |
| Other | 10 | 0.5 | 6 | 0.3 | 10 | 0.6 | 10 | 0.6 | 36 | 0.5 |
| **Pulmonary Artery Anomaly** | | | | | | | | | | |
| Northeast | 19 | 1.6 | 24 | 1.9 | 16 | 1.3 | 18 | 1.5 | 77 | 1.6 |
| North Central | 88 | 2.9 | 67 | 2.1 | 80 | 2.8 | 99 | 3.6 | 334 | 2.8 |
| South | 28 | 1.3 | 23 | 1.2 | 15 | 1.0 | 31 | 2.2 | 97 | 1.4 |
| West | 15 | 0.8 | 27 | 1.5 | 34 | 1.8 | 22 | 1.2 | 98 | 1.3 |
| Total United States | 150 | 1.8 | 141 | 1.7 | 145 | 2.0 | 170 | 2.4 | 606 | 2.0 |
| White | 89 | 1.4 | 92 | 1.4 | 82 | 1.4 | 83 | 1.5 | 346 | 1.4 |
| Other | 61 | 3.3 | 49 | 2.8 | 63 | 4.0 | 87 | 5.6 | 260 | 3.9 |
| **Lung Agenesis and Hypoplasia** | | | | | | | | | | |
| Northeast | 55 | 4.7 | 75 | 5.9 | 53 | 4.5 | 66 | 5.5 | 249 | 5.1 |
| North Central | 68 | 2.2 | 86 | 2.8 | 81 | 2.9 | 111 | 4.0 | 346 | 2.9 |
| South | 44 | 2.1 | 56 | 2.9 | 33 | 2.1 | 57 | 4.1 | 190 | 2.7 |
| West | 53 | 2.8 | 43 | 2.4 | 47 | 2.6 | 54 | 3.0 | 197 | 2.7 |
| Total United States | 220 | 2.7 | 260 | 3.2 | 214 | 2.9 | 288 | 4.0 | 982 | 3.2 |
| White | 174 | 2.7 | 198 | 3.1 | 173 | 3.0 | 233 | 4.1 | 778 | 3.2 |
| Other | 46 | 2.5 | 62 | 3.5 | 41 | 2.6 | 55 | 3.5 | 204 | 3.0 |

## Table 2 (continued)

| Malformation/Census Region/Race | 1982 Cases | Rate | 1983 Cases | Rate | 1984 Cases | Rate | 1985 Cases | Rate | Total Cases | Rate |
|---|---|---|---|---|---|---|---|---|---|---|
| **Orofacial** | | | | | | | | | | |
| Cleft Palate W/Out Cleft Lip | | | | | | | | | | |
| Northeast | 58 | 4.9 | 69 | 5.4 | 62 | 5.2 | 77 | 64 | 266 | 5.5 |
| North Central | 170 | 5.5 | 187 | 6.0 | 170 | 6.0 | 189 | 6.8 | 716 | 6.1 |
| South | 93 | 4.4 | 104 | 5.3 | 83 | 5.3 | 61 | 4.3 | 341 | 4.9 |
| West | 97 | 5.2 | 108 | 6.0 | 104 | 5.6 | 102 | 5.7 | 411 | 5.6 |
| Total United States | 418 | 5.1 | 468 | 5.8 | 419 | 5.6 | 429 | 6.0 | 1734 | 5.6 |
| White | 349 | 5.4 | 392 | 6.2 | 341 | 5.8 | 345 | 6.1 | 1427 | 5.9 |
| Other | 69 | 3.8 | 76 | 4.3 | 78 | 4.9 | 84 | 5.4 | 307 | 4.6 |
| Cleft Lip with and W/Out Cleft Palate | | | | | | | | | | |
| Northeast | 94 | 8.0 | 115 | 9.1 | 107 | 9.0 | 97 | 8.1 | 413 | 8.5 |
| North Central | 328 | 10.7 | 274 | 8.8 | 252 | 8.9 | 270 | 9.7 | 1124 | 9.5 |
| South | 168 | 8.0 | 165 | 8.5 | 125 | 8.0 | 118 | 8.4 | 576 | 8.2 |
| West | 178 | 9.5 | 196 | 10.9 | 180 | 9.8 | 152 | 8.5 | 706 | 9.7 |
| Total United States | 768 | 9.3 | 750 | 9.2 | 664 | 8.9 | 637 | 8.9 | 2819 | 9.1 |
| White | 631 | 9.8 | 626 | 9.8 | 564 | 9.7 | 534 | 9.5 | 2355 | 9.7 |
| Other | 137 | 7.5 | 124 | 7.0 | 100 | 6.3 | 103 | 6.6 | 464 | 6.9 |
| **Gastrointestinal** | | | | | | | | | | |
| Tracheo-Esophageal Anomalies | | | | | | | | | | |
| Northeast | 33 | 2.8 | 15 | 1.2 | 37 | 3.1 | 33 | 2.8 | 118 | 2.4 |
| North Central | 70 | 2.3 | 58 | 1.9 | 52 | 1.8 | 83 | 3.0 | 263 | 2.2 |
| South | 24 | 1.1 | 27 | 1.4 | 25 | 1.6 | 39 | 2.8 | 115 | 1.6 |
| West | 30 | 1.6 | 47 | 2.6 | 30 | 1.6 | 51 | 2.8 | 158 | 2.2 |
| Total United States | 157 | 1.9 | 147 | 1.8 | 144 | 1.9 | 206 | 2.9 | 654 | 2.1 |
| White | 134 | 2.1 | 121 | 1.9 | 119 | 2.0 | 188 | 3.3 | 562 | 2.3 |
| Other | 23 | 1.3 | 26 | 1.5 | 25 | 1.6 | 18 | 1.2 | 92 | 1.4 |
| Rectal and Intestinal Atresia | | | | | | | | | | |
| Northeast | 40 | 3.4 | 52 | 4.1 | 40 | 3.4 | 48 | 4.0 | 180 | 3.7 |
| North Central | 102 | 3.3 | 86 | 2.8 | 92 | 3.3 | 129 | 4.6 | 409 | 3.5 |
| South | 66 | 3.1 | 59 | 3.0 | 61 | 3.9 | 56 | 4.0 | 242 | 3.4 |
| West | 59 | 3.1 | 64 | 3.6 | 73 | 4.0 | 60 | 3.3 | 256 | 3.5 |
| Total United States | 267 | 3.2 | 261 | 3.2 | 266 | 3.6 | 293 | 4.1 | 1087 | 3.5 |
| White | 210 | 3.3 | 219 | 3.4 | 216 | 3.7 | 236 | 4.2 | 881 | 3.6 |
| Other | 57 | 3.1 | 42 | 2.4 | 50 | 3.1 | 57 | 3.7 | 206 | 3.1 |
| **Genitourinary** | | | | | | | | | | |
| Renal Agenesis | | | | | | | | | | |
| Northeast | 25 | 2.1 | 30 | 2.4 | 25 | 2.1 | 32 | 2.7 | 112 | 2.3 |
| North Central | 42 | 1.4 | 59 | 1.9 | 44 | 1.6 | 55 | 2.0 | 200 | 1.7 |
| South | 46 | 2.2 | 32 | 1.6 | 19 | 1.2 | 24 | 1.7 | 121 | 1.7 |
| West | 34 | 1.8 | 25 | 1.4 | 32 | 1.7 | 30 | 1.7 | 121 | 1.7 |
| Total United States | 147 | 1.8 | 146 | 1.8 | 120 | 1.6 | 141 | 2.0 | 554 | 1.8 |
| White | 111 | 1.7 | 119 | 1.9 | 109 | 1.9 | 124 | 2.2 | 463 | 1.9 |
| Other | 36 | 2.0 | 27 | 1.5 | 11 | 0.7 | 17 | 1.1 | 91 | 1.3 |
| Bladder Exstrophy | | | | | | | | | | |
| Northeast | 4 | 0.3 | 5 | 0.4 | 7 | 0.6 | 0 | 0.0 | 16 | 0.3 |
| North Central | 10 | 0.3 | 10 | 0.3 | 8 | 0.3 | 7 | 0.3 | 35 | 0.3 |
| South | 5 | 0.2 | 4 | 0.2 | 5 | 0.3 | 7 | 0.5 | 21 | 0.3 |
| West | 3 | 0.2 | 7 | 0.4 | 6 | 0.3 | 2 | 0.1 | 18 | 0.2 |
| Total United States | 22 | 0.3 | 26 | 0.3 | 26 | 0.4 | 16 | 0.2 | 90 | 0.3 |

## Table 2 (continued)

| Malformation/Census Region/Race | 1982 Cases | Rate | 1983 Cases | Rate | 1984 Cases | Rate | 1985 Cases | Rate | Total Cases | Rate |
|---|---|---|---|---|---|---|---|---|---|---|
| White | 17 | 0.3 | 23 | 0.4 | 24 | 0.4 | 12 | 0.2 | 76 | 0.3 |
| Other | 5 | 0.3 | 3 | 0.2 | 2 | 0.1 | 4 | 0.3 | 14 | 0.2 |

**Musculoskeletal**

*Clubfoot W/Out CNS Defects*

| | | | | | | | | | | |
|---|---|---|---|---|---|---|---|---|---|---|
| Northeast | 353 | 29.9 | 353 | 27.8 | 310 | 26.0 | 320 | 26.8 | 1336 | 27.6 |
| North Central | 1049 | 34.1 | 991 | 31.8 | 780 | 27.7 | 838 | 30.2 | 3658 | 31.0 |
| South | 419 | 19.9 | 429 | 22.0 | 306 | 19.5 | 281 | 20.0 | 1435 | 20.4 |
| West | 369 | 19.7 | 404 | 22.5 | 444 | 24.1 | 425 | 23.7 | 1642 | 22.5 |
| Total United States | 2190 | 26.6 | 2177 | 26.7 | 1840 | 24.8 | 1864 | 26.0 | 8071 | 26.1 |
| White | 1809 | 28.2 | 1766 | 27.8 | 1519 | 26.1 | 1553 | 27.6 | 6647 | 27.4 |
| Other | 381 | 20.9 | 411 | 23.1 | 321 | 20.2 | 311 | 20.0 | 1424 | 21.1 |

*Reduction Deformity Upper Limbs*

| | | | | | | | | | | |
|---|---|---|---|---|---|---|---|---|---|---|
| Northeast | 11 | 0.9 | 21 | 1.7 | 19 | 1.6 | 24 | 2.0 | 75 | 1.6 |
| North Central | 48 | 1.6 | 57 | 1.8 | 43 | 1.5 | 39 | 1.4 | 187 | 1.6 |
| South | 32 | 1.5 | 19 | 1.0 | 22 | 1.4 | 26 | 1.9 | 99 | 1.4 |
| West | 38 | 2.0 | 39 | 2.2 | 24 | 1.3 | 35 | 1.9 | 136 | 1.9 |
| Total United States | 129 | 1.6 | 136 | 1.7 | 108 | 1.5 | 124 | 1.7 | 497 | 1.6 |
| White | 107 | 1.7 | 115 | 1.8 | 92 | 1.6 | 96 | 1.7 | 410 | 1.7 |
| Other | 22 | 1.2 | 21 | 1.2 | 16 | 1.0 | 28 | 1.8 | 87 | 1.3 |

*Reduction Deformity Lower Limbs*

| | | | | | | | | | | |
|---|---|---|---|---|---|---|---|---|---|---|
| Northeast | 7 | 0.6 | 12 | 0.9 | 12 | 1.0 | 10 | 0.8 | 41 | 0.8 |
| North Central | 19 | 0.6 | 20 | 0.6 | 23 | 0.8 | 33 | 1.2 | 95 | 0.8 |
| South | 18 | 0.9 | 20 | 1.0 | 8 | 0.5 | 6 | 0.4 | 52 | 0.7 |
| West | 19 | 1.0 | 27 | 1.5 | 13 | 0.7 | 22 | 1.2 | 81 | 1.1 |
| Total United States | 63 | 0.8 | 79 | 1.0 | 56 | 0.8 | 71 | 1.0 | 269 | 0.9 |
| White | 50 | 0.8 | 61 | 1.0 | 47 | 0.8 | 60 | 1.1 | 218 | 0.9 |
| Other | 13 | 0.7 | 18 | 1.0 | 9 | 0.6 | 11 | 0.7 | 51 | 0.8 |

*Congenital Arthrogryposis*

| | | | | | | | | | | |
|---|---|---|---|---|---|---|---|---|---|---|
| Northeast | 34 | 2.9 | 44 | 3.5 | 25 | 2.1 | 23 | 1.9 | 126 | 2.6 |
| North Central | 55 | 1.8 | 81 | 2.6 | 88 | 3.1 | 63 | 2.3 | 287 | 2.4 |
| South | 25 | 1.2 | 24 | 1.2 | 22 | 1.4 | 28 | 2.0 | 99 | 1.4 |
| West | 29 | 1.5 | 40 | 2.2 | 41 | 2.2 | 51 | 2.8 | 161 | 2.2 |
| Total United States | 143 | 1.7 | 189 | 2.3 | 176 | 2.4 | 165 | 2.3 | 673 | 2.2 |
| White | 122 | 1.9 | 155 | 2.4 | 151 | 2.6 | 143 | 2.5 | 571 | 2.4 |
| Other | 21 | 1.1 | 34 | 1.9 | 25 | 1.6 | 22 | 1.4 | 102 | 1.5 |

**Chromosomal**

*Trisomy 13*

| | | | | | | | | | | |
|---|---|---|---|---|---|---|---|---|---|---|
| Northeast | 5 | 0.4 | 8 | 0.6 | 8 | 0.7 | 9 | 0.8 | 30 | 0.6 |
| North Central | 35 | 1.1 | 21 | 0.7 | 26 | 0.9 | 15 | 0.5 | 97 | 0.8 |
| South | 10 | 0.5 | 8 | 0.4 | 14 | 0.9 | 10 | 0.7 | 42 | 0.6 |
| West | 20 | 1.1 | 16 | 0.9 | 14 | 0.8 | 14 | 0.8 | 64 | 0.9 |
| Total United States | 70 | 0.9 | 53 | 0.7 | 62 | 0.8 | 48 | 0.7 | 233 | 0.8 |
| White | 58 | 0.9 | 43 | 0.7 | 51 | 0.9 | 40 | 0.7 | 192 | 0.8 |
| Other | 12 | 0.7 | 10 | 0.6 | 11 | 0.7 | 8 | 0.5 | 41 | 0.6 |

*Down Syndrome*

| | | | | | | | | | | |
|---|---|---|---|---|---|---|---|---|---|---|
| Northeast | 91 | 7.7 | 108 | 8.5 | 88 | 7.4 | 133 | 11.1 | 420 | 8.7 |
| North Central | 304 | 9.9 | 286 | 9.2 | 216 | 7.7 | 244 | 8.8 | 1050 | 8.9 |
| South | 132 | 6.3 | 128 | 6.6 | 107 | 6.8 | 110 | 7.8 | 477 | 6.8 |
| West | 176 | 9.4 | 145 | 8.1 | 164 | 8.9 | 210 | 11.7 | 695 | 9.5 |

## Table 2 (continued)

| Malformation/Census Region/Race | 1982 Cases | 1982 Rate | 1983 Cases | 1983 Rate | 1984 Cases | 1984 Rate | 1985 Cases | 1985 Rate | Total Cases | Total Rate |
|---|---|---|---|---|---|---|---|---|---|---|
| Total United States | 703 | 8.5 | 667 | 8.2 | 575 | 7.7 | 697 | 9.7 | 2642 | 8.5 |
| White | 557 | 8.7 | 529 | 8.3 | 462 | 7.9 | 554 | 9.9 | 2102 | 8.7 |
| Other | 146 | 8.0 | 138 | 7.8 | 113 | 7.1 | 143 | 9.2 | 540 | 8.0 |
| Trisomy 18 | | | | | | | | | | |
| Northeast | 14 | 1.2 | 14 | 1.1 | 13 | 1.1 | 18 | 1.5 | 59 | 1.2 |

## Table 3

### Number of Monitored Births (Live-Born) by U.S. Census Region and Race Birth Defects Monitoring Program/MDHIS, 1982-1985

| Census Region/Race | 1982 | 1983 | 1984 | 1985 | Total |
|---|---|---|---|---|---|
| Northeast | 54,858 | 43,102 | 38,044 | 29,221 | 165,225 |
| North Central | 161,613 | 158,412 | 135,883 | 121,829 | 577,737 |
| South | 158,327 | 181,480 | 162,936 | 143,910 | 646,653 |
| West | 217,660 | 218,442 | 177,781 | 147,472 | 761,355 |
| Total United States | 592,458 | 601,436 | 514,644 | 442,432 | 2,150,970 |
| White | 479,042 | 483,035 | 418,058 | 352,384 | 1,732,519 |
| Other | 113,416 | 118,401 | 96,586 | 90,048 | 418,451 |

**Figure 2**
**Percentage of United States Live Births in the BDMP/MDHIS**
**by United States Census Region, 1982-1985**

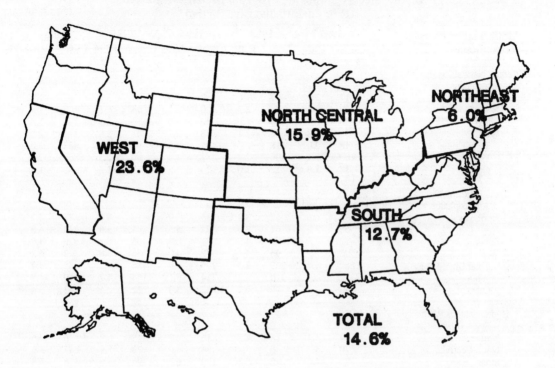

Table 4
Reported Incidence of Selected Congenital Malformations
Live-Born and Stillborn Infants, by U.S. Census Region and Race
Birth Defects Monitoring Program/MDHIS, 1982-1985
(Rates per 10,000 Live Births)

| Malformation/Census Region/Race | 1982 Cases | Rate | 1983 Cases | Rate | 1984 Cases | Rate | 1985 Cases | Rate | Total Cases | Rate |
|---|---|---|---|---|---|---|---|---|---|---|
| **Central Nervous System** | | | | | | | | | | |
| Anencephalus | | | | | | | | | | |
| Northeast | 11 | 2.0 | 7 | 1.6 | 7 | 1.8 | 7 | 2.4 | 32 | 1.9 |
| North Central | 39 | 2.4 | 36 | 2.3 | 20 | 1.5 | 14 | 1.1 | 109 | 1.9 |
| South | 29 | 1.8 | 29 | 1.6 | 30 | 1.8 | 30 | 2.1 | 118 | 1.8 |
| West | 39 | 1.8 | 46 | 2.1 | 48 | 2.7 | 41 | 2.8 | 174 | 2.3 |
| Total United States | 118 | 2.0 | 118 | 2.0 | 105 | 2.0 | 92 | 2.1 | 433 | 2.0 |
| White | 100 | 2.1 | 106 | 2.2 | 81 | 1.9 | 80 | 2.3 | 367 | 2.1 |
| Other | 18 | 1.6 | 12 | 1.0 | 24 | 2.5 | 12 | 1.3 | 66 | 1.6 |
| Spina Bifida W/Out Anencephalus | | | | | | | | | | |
| Northeast | 36 | 6.6 | 17 | 3.9 | 15 | 3.9 | 10 | 3.4 | 78 | 4.7 |
| North Central | 56 | 3.5 | 61 | 3.9 | 72 | 5.3 | 44 | 3.6 | 233 | 4.0 |
| South | 72 | 4.5 | 85 | 4.7 | 87 | 5.3 | 76 | 5.3 | 320 | 4.9 |
| West | 98 | 4.5 | 96 | 4.4 | 72 | 4.0 | 56 | 3.8 | 322 | 4.2 |
| Total United States | 262 | 4.4 | 259 | 4.3 | 246 | 4.8 | 186 | 4.2 | 953 | 4.4 |
| White | 222 | 4.6 | 210 | 4.3 | 214 | 5.1 | 164 | 4.7 | 810 | 4.7 |
| Other | 40 | 3.5 | 49 | 4.1 | 32 | 3.3 | 22 | 2.4 | 143 | 3.4 |
| Hydrocephalus W/Out Spina Bifida | | | | | | | | | | |
| Northeast | 24 | 4.4 | 18 | 4.2 | 16 | 4.2 | 18 | 6.2 | 76 | 4.6 |
| North Central | 70 | 4.3 | 86 | 5.4 | 54 | 4.0 | 72 | 5.9 | 282 | 4.9 |
| South | 73 | 4.6 | 96 | 5.3 | 109 | 6.7 | 98 | 6.8 | 376 | 5.8 |
| West | 110 | 5.1 | 115 | 5.3 | 81 | 4.6 | 80 | 5.4 | 386 | 5.1 |
| Total United States | 277 | 4.7 | 315 | 5.2 | 260 | 5.1 | 268 | 6.1 | 1120 | 5.2 |
| White | 225 | 4.7 | 250 | 5.2 | 202 | 4.8 | 199 | 5.6 | 876 | 5.1 |
| Other | 52 | 4.6 | 65 | 5.5 | 58 | 6.0 | 69 | 7.7 | 244 | 5.8 |
| Encephalocele | | | | | | | | | | |
| Northeast | 5 | 0.9 | 1 | 0.2 | 1 | 0.3 | 3 | 1.0 | 10 | 0.6 |
| North Central | 10 | 0.6 | 11 | 0.7 | 10 | 0.7 | 11 | 0.9 | 42 | 0.7 |
| South | 12 | 0.8 | 18 | 1.0 | 15 | 0.9 | 13 | 0.9 | 58 | 0.9 |
| West | 25 | 1.1 | 14 | 0.6 | 21 | 1.2 | 17 | 1.2 | 77 | 1.0 |
| Total United States | 52 | 0.9 | 44 | 0.7 | 47 | 0.9 | 44 | 1.0 | 187 | 0.9 |
| White | 42 | 0.9 | 40 | 0.8 | 39 | 0.9 | 39 | 1.1 | 160 | 0.9 |
| Other | 10 | 0.9 | 4 | 0.3 | 8 | 0.8 | 5 | 0.6 | 27 | 0.6 |
| Microcephalus | | | | | | | | | | |
| Northeast | 16 | 2.9 | 9 | 2.1 | 10 | 2.6 | 12 | 4.1 | 47 | 2.8 |
| North Central | 29 | 1.8 | 44 | 2.8 | 27 | 2.0 | 21 | 1.7 | 121 | 2.1 |
| South | 51 | 3.2 | 37 | 2.0 | 44 | 2.7 | 61 | 4.2 | 193 | 3.0 |
| West | 42 | 1.9 | 56 | 2.6 | 63 | 3.5 | 72 | 4.9 | 233 | 3.1 |
| Total United States | 138 | 2.3 | 146 | 2.4 | 144 | 2.8 | 166 | 3.8 | 594 | 2.8 |
| White | 99 | 2.1 | 98 | 2.0 | 89 | 2.1 | 79 | 2.2 | 365 | 2.1 |
| Other | 39 | 3.4 | 48 | 4.1 | 55 | 5.7 | 87 | 9.7 | 229 | 5.5 |
| **Eye** | | | | | | | | | | |
| Anophthalmos/Microphthalmos | | | | | | | | | | |
| Northeast | 2 | 0.4 | 5 | 1.2 | 5 | 1.3 | 0 | 0.0 | 12 | 0.7 |
| North Central | 9 | 0.6 | 11 | 0.7 | 7 | 0.5 | 7 | 0.6 | 34 | 0.6 |
| South | 10 | 0.6 | 15 | 0.8 | 12 | 0.7 | 6 | 0.4 | 43 | 0.7 |
| West | 14 | 0.6 | 18 | 0.8 | 16 | 0.9 | 12 | 0.8 | 60 | 0.8 |

## Table 4 (continued)

| Malformation/Census Region/Race | 1982 Cases | Rate | 1983 Cases | Rate | 1984 Cases | Rate | 1985 Cases | Rate | Total Cases | Rate |
|---|---|---|---|---|---|---|---|---|---|---|
| Total United States | 35 | 0.6 | 49 | 0.8 | 40 | 0.8 | 25 | 0.6 | 149 | 0.7 |
| White | 29 | 0.6 | 38 | 0.8 | 30 | 0.7 | 19 | 0.5 | 116 | 0.7 |
| Other | 6 | 0.5 | 11 | 0.9 | 10 | 1.0 | 6 | 0.7 | 33 | 0.8 |
| **Congenital Cataract** | | | | | | | | | | |
| Northeast | 5 | 0.9 | 3 | 0.7 | 8 | 2.1 | 4 | 1.4 | 20 | 1.2 |
| North Central | 14 | 0.9 | 12 | 0.8 | 8 | 0.6 | 10 | 0.8 | 44 | 0.8 |
| South | 14 | 0.9 | 11 | 0.6 | 12 | 0.7 | 17 | 1.2 | 54 | 0.8 |
| West | 17 | 0.8 | 21 | 1.0 | 19 | 1.1 | 23 | 1.6 | 80 | 1.1 |
| Total United States | 50 | 0.8 | 47 | 0.8 | 47 | 0.9 | 54 | 1.2 | 198 | 0.9 |
| White | 37 | 0.8 | 39 | 0.8 | 34 | 0.8 | 41 | 1.2 | 151 | 0.9 |
| Other | 13 | 1.1 | 8 | 0.7 | 13 | 1.3 | 13 | 1.4 | 47 | 1.1 |
| **Coloboma of Eye** | | | | | | | | | | |
| Northeast | 1 | 0.2 | 1 | 0.2 | 1 | 0.3 | 0 | 0.0 | 3 | 0.2 |
| North Central | 4 | 0.2 | 5 | 0.3 | 5 | 0.4 | 4 | 0.3 | 18 | 0.3 |
| South | 6 | 0.4 | 3 | 0.2 | 6 | 0.4 | 3 | 0.2 | 18 | 0.3 |
| West | 2 | 0.1 | 2 | 0.1 | 2 | 0.1 | 9 | 0.6 | 15 | 0.2 |
| Total United States | 13 | 0.2 | 11 | 0.2 | 14 | 0.3 | 16 | 0.4 | 54 | 0.3 |
| White | 10 | 0.2 | 9 | 0.2 | 13 | 0.3 | 13 | 0.4 | 45 | 0.3 |
| Other | 3 | 0.3 | 2 | 0.2 | 1 | 0.1 | 3 | 0.3 | 9 | 0.2 |
| **Aniridia** | | | | | | | | | | |
| Northeast | 1 | 0.2 | 1 | 0.2 | 0 | 0.0 | 0 | 0.0 | 2 | 0.1 |
| North Central | 2 | 0.1 | 1 | 0.1 | 1 | 0.1 | 0 | 0.0 | 4 | 0.1 |
| South | 2 | 0.1 | 1 | 0.1 | 1 | 0.1 | 0 | 0.0 | 4 | 0.1 |
| West | 2 | 0.1 | 0 | 0.0 | 1 | 0.1 | 0 | 0.0 | 3 | 0.0 |
| Total United States | 7 | 0.1 | 3 | 0.0 | 3 | 0.1 | 0 | 0.0 | 13 | 0.1 |
| White | 5 | 0.1 | 1 | 0.0 | 2 | 0.0 | 0 | 0.0 | 8 | 0.0 |
| Other | 2 | 0.2 | 2 | 0.2 | 1 | 0.1 | 0 | 0.0 | 5 | 0.1 |
| **Cardiovascular** | | | | | | | | | | |
| **Common Truncus** | | | | | | | | | | |
| Northeast | 1 | 0.2 | 0 | 0.0 | 2 | 0.5 | 0 | 0.0 | 3 | 0.2 |
| North Central | 5 | 0.3 | 2 | 0.1 | 3 | 0.2 | 1 | 0.1 | 11 | 0.2 |
| South | 0 | 0.0 | 0 | 0.0 | 2 | 0.1 | 4 | 0.3 | 6 | 0.1 |
| West | 3 | 0.1 | 5 | 0.2 | 6 | 0.3 | 5 | 0.3 | 19 | 0.2 |
| Total United States | 9 | 0.2 | 7 | 0.1 | 13 | 0.3 | 10 | 0.2 | 39 | 0.2 |
| White | 9 | 0.2 | 5 | 0.1 | 12 | 0.3 | 9 | 0.3 | 35 | 0.2 |
| Other | 0 | 0.0 | 2 | 0.2 | 1 | 0.1 | 1 | 0.1 | 4 | 0.1 |
| **Transposition of Great Arteries** | | | | | | | | | | |
| Northeast | 9 | 1.6 | 4 | 0.9 | 3 | 0.8 | 3 | 1.0 | 19 | 1.1 |
| North Central | 13 | 0.8 | 11 | 0.7 | 8 | 0.6 | 15 | 1.2 | 47 | 0.8 |
| South | 9 | 0.6 | 18 | 1.0 | 17 | 1.0 | 14 | 1.0 | 58 | 0.9 |
| West | 11 | 0.5 | 13 | 0.6 | 10 | 0.6 | 18 | 1.2 | 52 | 0.7 |
| Total United States | 42 | 0.7 | 46 | 0.8 | 38 | 0.7 | 50 | 1.1 | 176 | 0.8 |
| White | 34 | 0.7 | 42 | 0.9 | 33 | 0.8 | 46 | 1.3 | 155 | 0.9 |
| Other | 8 | 0.7 | 4 | 0.3 | 5 | 0.5 | 4 | 0.4 | 21 | 0.5 |
| **Tetralogy of Fallot** | | | | | | | | | | |
| Northeast | 7 | 1.3 | 8 | 1.9 | 9 | 2.4 | 1 | 0.3 | 25 | 1.5 |
| North Central | 11 | 0.7 | 13 | 0.8 | 10 | 0.7 | 17 | 1.4 | 51 | 0.9 |
| South | 7 | 0.4 | 13 | 0.7 | 19 | 1.2 | 22 | 1.5 | 61 | 0.9 |
| West | 17 | 0.8 | 25 | 1.1 | 12 | 0.7 | 17 | 1.2 | 71 | 0.9 |
| Total United States | 42 | 0.7 | 59 | 1.0 | 50 | 1.0 | 57 | 1.3 | 208 | 1.0 |
| White | 36 | 0.8 | 45 | 0.9 | 35 | 0.8 | 34 | 1.0 | 150 | 0.9 |

## Table 4 (continued)

| Malformation/Census Region/Race | 1982 Cases | Rate | 1983 Cases | Rate | 1984 Cases | Rate | 1985 Cases | Rate | Total Cases | Rate |
|---|---|---|---|---|---|---|---|---|---|---|
| Other | 6 | 0.5 | 14 | 1.2 | 15 | 1.6 | 23 | 2.6 | 58 | 1.4 |
| **Ventricular Septal Defect** | | | | | | | | | | |
| Northeast | 113 | 20.6 | 73 | 16.9 | 54 | 14.2 | 54 | 18.5 | 294 | 17.8 |
| North Central | 227 | 14.0 | 240 | 15.2 | 248 | 18.3 | 227 | 18.6 | 942 | 16.3 |
| South | 127 | 8.0 | 200 | 11.0 | 177 | 10.9 | 209 | 14.5 | 713 | 11.0 |
| West | 274 | 12.6 | 318 | 14.6 | 274 | 15.4 | 235 | 15.9 | 1101 | 14.5 |
| Total United States | 741 | 12.5 | 831 | 13.8 | 753 | 14.6 | 725 | 16.4 | 3050 | 14.2 |
| White | 608 | 12.7 | 681 | 14.1 | 639 | 15.3 | 570 | 16.2 | 2498 | 14.4 |
| Other | 133 | 11.7 | 150 | 12.7 | 114 | 11.8 | 155 | 17.2 | 552 | 13.2 |
| **Atrial Septal Defect** | | | | | | | | | | |
| Northeast | 6 | 1.1 | 4 | 0.9 | 3 | 0.8 | 3 | 1.0 | 16 | 1.0 |
| North Central | 31 | 1.9 | 28 | 1.8 | 17 | 1.3 | 19 | 1.6 | 95 | 1.6 |
| South | 8 | 0.5 | 15 | 0.8 | 20 | 1.2 | 37 | 2.6 | 80 | 1.2 |
| West | 34 | 1.6 | 38 | 1.7 | 41 | 2.3 | 39 | 2.6 | 152 | 2.0 |
| Total United States | 79 | 1.3 | 85 | 1.4 | 81 | 1.6 | 98 | 2.2 | 343 | 1.6 |
| White | 59 | 1.2 | 66 | 1.4 | 66 | 1.6 | 78 | 2.2 | 269 | 1.6 |
| Other | 20 | 1.8 | 19 | 1.6 | 15 | 1.6 | 20 | 2.2 | 74 | 1.8 |
| **Endocardial Cushion Defect** | | | | | | | | | | |
| Northeast | 2 | 0.4 | 3 | 0.7 | 5 | 1.3 | 4 | 1.4 | 14 | 0.8 |
| North Central | 9 | 0.6 | 4 | 0.3 | 9 | 0.7 | 9 | 0.7 | 31 | 0.5 |
| South | 4 | 0.3 | 9 | 0.5 | 9 | 0.6 | 13 | 0.9 | 35 | 0.5 |
| West | 12 | 0.6 | 22 | 1.0 | 19 | 1.1 | 16 | 1.1 | 69 | 0.9 |
| Total United States | 27 | 0.5 | 38 | 0.6 | 42 | 0.8 | 42 | 0.9 | 149 | 0.7 |
| White | 20 | 0.4 | 29 | 0.4 | 28 | 0.7 | 28 | 0.7 | 105 | 0.6 |
| Other | 7 | 0.6 | 9 | 0.8 | 14 | 1.4 | 14 | 1.6 | 44 | 1.1 |
| **Pulmonary Valve Stenosis and Atresia** | | | | | | | | | | |
| Northeast | 2 | 0.4 | 2 | 0.5 | 3 | 0.8 | 6 | 2.1 | 13 | 0.8 |
| North Central | 19 | 1.2 | 34 | 2.1 | 22 | 1.6 | 19 | 1.6 | 94 | 1.6 |
| South | 14 | 0.9 | 15 | 0.8 | 21 | 1.3 | 26 | 1.8 | 76 | 1.2 |
| West | 28 | 1.3 | 44 | 2.0 | 24 | 1.3 | 18 | 1.2 | 114 | 1.5 |
| Total United States | 63 | 1.1 | 95 | 1.6 | 70 | 1.4 | 69 | 1.6 | 297 | 1.4 |
| White | 38 | 0.8 | 75 | 1.6 | 52 | 1.2 | 39 | 1.1 | 204 | 1.2 |
| Other | 25 | 2.2 | 20 | 1.7 | 18 | 1.9 | 30 | 3.3 | 93 | 2.2 |
| **Tricuspid Valve Stenosis and Atresia** | | | | | | | | | | |
| Northeast | 0 | 0.0 | 1 | 0.2 | 1 | 0.3 | 1 | 0.3 | 3 | 0.2 |
| North Central | 3 | 0.2 | 3 | 0.2 | 2 | 0.1 | 3 | 0.2 | 11 | 0.2 |
| South | 3 | 0.2 | 1 | 0.1 | 3 | 0.2 | 6 | 0.4 | 13 | 0.2 |
| West | 2 | 0.1 | 5 | 0.2 | 4 | 0.2 | 6 | 0.4 | 17 | 0.2 |
| Total United States | 8 | 0.1 | 10 | 0.2 | 10 | 0.2 | 16 | 0.4 | 44 | 0.2 |
| White | 6 | 0.1 | 8 | 0.2 | 5 | 0.1 | 10 | 0.3 | 29 | 0.2 |
| Other | 2 | 0.2 | 2 | 0.2 | 5 | 0.5 | 6 | 0.7 | 15 | 0.4 |
| **Aortic Valve Stenosis and Atresia** | | | | | | | | | | |
| Northeast | 1 | 0.2 | 4 | 0.9 | 2 | 0.5 | 1 | 0.3 | 8 | 0.5 |
| North Central | 9 | 0.6 | 6 | 0.4 | 9 | 0.7 | 4 | 0.3 | 28 | 0.5 |
| South | 3 | 0.2 | 6 | 0.3 | 6 | 0.4 | 11 | 0.8 | 26 | 0.4 |
| West | 6 | 0.3 | 11 | 0.5 | 7 | 0.4 | 4 | 0.3 | 28 | 0.4 |
| Total United States | 19 | 0.3 | 27 | 0.4 | 24 | 0.5 | 20 | 0.5 | 90 | 0.4 |
| White | 16 | 0.3 | 22 | 0.5 | 20 | 0.5 | 17 | 0.5 | 75 | 0.4 |
| Other | 3 | 0.3 | 5 | 0.4 | 4 | 0.4 | 3 | 0.3 | 15 | 0.4 |

## Table 4 (continued)

| Malformation/Census Region/Race | 1982 Cases | Rate | 1983 Cases | Rate | 1984 Cases | Rate | 1985 Cases | Rate | Total Cases | Rate |
|---|---|---|---|---|---|---|---|---|---|---|
| **Hypoplastic Left Heart Syndrome** | | | | | | | | | | |
| Northeast | 3 | 0.5 | 1 | 0.2 | 2 | 0.5 | 5 | 1.7 | 11 | 0.7 |
| North Central | 7 | 0.4 | 16 | 1.0 | 14 | 1.0 | 8 | 0.7 | 45 | 0.8 |
| South | 7 | 0.4 | 4 | 0.2 | 8 | 0.5 | 10 | 0.7 | 29 | 0.4 |
| West | 18 | 0.8 | 20 | 0.9 | 17 | 1.0 | 10 | 0.7 | 65 | 0.9 |
| Total United States | 35 | 0.6 | 41 | 0.7 | 41 | 0.8 | 33 | 0.7 | 150 | 0.7 |
| White | 28 | 0.6 | 32 | 0.7 | 30 | 0.7 | 25 | 0.7 | 115 | 0.7 |
| Other | 7 | 0.6 | 9 | 0.8 | 11 | 1.1 | 8 | 0.9 | 35 | 0.8 |
| **Patent Ductus Arteriosus** | | | | | | | | | | |
| Northeast | 98 | 17.9 | 97 | 22.5 | 98 | 25.8 | 55 | 18.8 | 348 | 21.1 |
| North Central | 331 | 20.5 | 324 | 20.5 | 291 | 21.4 | 252 | 20.7 | 1198 | 20.7 |
| South | 280 | 17.7 | 377 | 20.8 | 453 | 27.8 | 438 | 30.4 | 1548 | 23.9 |
| West | 521 | 23.9 | 612 | 28.0 | 473 | 26.6 | 437 | 29.6 | 2043 | 26.8 |
| Total United States | 1230 | 20.8 | 1410 | 23.4 | 1315 | 25.6 | 1182 | 26.7 | 5137 | 23.9 |
| White | 917 | 19.1 | 1068 | 22.1 | 993 | 23.8 | 866 | 24.6 | 3844 | 22.2 |
| Other | 313 | 27.6 | 342 | 28.9 | 322 | 33.3 | 316 | 35.1 | 1293 | 30.9 |
| **Coarctation of Aorta** | | | | | | | | | | |
| Northeast | 4 | 0.7 | 6 | 1.4 | 4 | 1.1 | 1 | 0.3 | 15 | 0.9 |
| North Central | 20 | 1.2 | 11 | 0.7 | 13 | 1.0 | 10 | 0.8 | 54 | 0.9 |
| South | 7 | 0.4 | 14 | 0.8 | 8 | 0.5 | 10 | 0.7 | 39 | 0.6 |
| West | 16 | 0.7 | 14 | 0.6 | 20 | 1.1 | 19 | 1.3 | 69 | 0.9 |
| Total United States | 47 | 0.8 | 45 | 0.7 | 45 | 0.9 | 40 | 0.9 | 177 | 0.8 |
| White | 34 | 0.7 | 40 | 0.8 | 36 | 0.9 | 31 | 0.9 | 141 | 0.8 |
| | 13 | 1.1 | 5 | 0.4 | 9 | 0.9 | 9 | 1.0 | 36 | 0.9 |
| **Pulmonary Artery Anomaly** | | | | | | | | | | |
| Northeast | 7 | 1.3 | 8 | 1.9 | 6 | 1.6 | 4 | 1.4 | 25 | 1.5 |
| North Central | 25 | 1.5 | 27 | 1.7 | 20 | 1.5 | 22 | 1.8 | 94 | 1.6 |
| South | 15 | 0.9 | 19 | 1.0 | 27 | 1.7 | 25 | 1.7 | 86 | 1.3 |
| West | 30 | 1.4 | 39 | 1.8 | 28 | 1.6 | 24 | 1.6 | 121 | 1.6 |
| Total United States | 77 | 1.3 | 93 | 1.5 | 81 | 1.6 | 75 | 1.7 | 326 | 1.5 |
| White | 57 | 1.2 | 59 | 1.2 | 57 | 1.4 | 52 | 1.5 | 225 | 1.3 |
| Other | 20 | 1.8 | 34 | 2.9 | 24 | 2.5 | 23 | 2.6 | 101 | 2.4 |
| **Lung Agenesis and Hypoplasia** | | | | | | | | | | |
| Northeast | 15 | 2.7 | 10 | 2.3 | 17 | 4.5 | 10 | 3.4 | 52 | 3.1 |
| North Central | 41 | 2.5 | 43 | 2.7 | 30 | 2.2 | 21 | 1.7 | 135 | 2.3 |
| South | 17 | 1.1 | 50 | 2.8 | 51 | 3.1 | 55 | 3.8 | 173 | 2.7 |
| West | 35 | 1.6 | 61 | 2.8 | 48 | 2.7 | 41 | 2.8 | 185 | 2.4 |
| Total United States | 108 | 1.8 | 164 | 2.7 | 146 | 2.8 | 127 | 2.9 | 545 | 2.5 |
| White | 84 | 1.8 | 136 | 2.8 | 111 | 2.7 | 102 | 2.9 | 433 | 2.5 |
| Other | 24 | 2.1 | 28 | 2.4 | 35 | 3.6 | 25 | 2.8 | 112 | 2.7 |
| **Orofacial** | | | | | | | | | | |
| **Cleft Palate W/Out Cleft Lip** | | | | | | | | | | |
| Northeast | 34 | 6.2 | 22 | 5.1 | 21 | 5.5 | 13 | 4.4 | 90 | 5.4 |
| North Central | 85 | 5.3 | 89 | 5.6 | 63 | 4.6 | 61 | 5.0 | 298 | 5.2 |
| South | 85 | 5.4 | 77 | 4.2 | 96 | 5.9 | 79 | 5.5 | 337 | 5.2 |
| West | 112 | 5.1 | 120 | 5.5 | 107 | 6.0 | 77 | 5.2 | 416 | 5.5 |
| Total United States | 316 | 5.3 | 308 | 5.1 | 287 | 5.6 | 230 | 5.2 | 1141 | 5.3 |
| White | 254 | 5.3 | 268 | 5.5 | 244 | 5.8 | 191 | 5.4 | 957 | 5.5 |
| Other | 62 | 5.5 | 40 | 3.4 | 43 | 4.5 | 39 | 4.3 | 184 | 4.4 |
| **Cleft Lip With and W/Out Cleft Palate** | | | | | | | | | | |

## Table 4 (continued)

| Malformation/Census Region/Race | 1982 Cases | Rate | 1983 Cases | Rate | 1984 Cases | Rate | 1985 Cases | Rate | Total Cases | Rate |
|---|---|---|---|---|---|---|---|---|---|---|
| Northeast | 50 | 9.1 | 35 | 8.1 | 32 | 8.4 | 28 | 9.6 | 145 | 8.8 |
| North Central | 131 | 8.1 | 131 | 8.3 | 114 | 8.4 | 109 | 8.9 | 485 | 8.4 |
| South | 109 | 6.9 | 149 | 8.2 | 142 | 8.7 | 123 | 8.5 | 523 | 8.1 |
| West | 189 | 8.7 | 217 | 9.9 | 157 | 8.8 | 144 | 9.8 | 707 | 9.3 |
| Total United States | 479 | 8.1 | 532 | 8.8 | 445 | 8.6 | 404 | 9.1 | 1860 | 8.6 |
| White | 408 | 8.5 | 469 | 9.7 | 385 | 9.2 | 343 | 9.7 | 1605 | 9.3 |
| Other | 71 | 6.3 | 63 | 5.3 | 60 | 6.2 | 61 | 6.8 | 255 | 6.1 |

**Gastrointestinal**

**Tracheo-Esophageal Anomalies**

| | 1982 Cases | Rate | 1983 Cases | Rate | 1984 Cases | Rate | 1985 Cases | Rate | Total Cases | Rate |
|---|---|---|---|---|---|---|---|---|---|---|
| Northeast | 8 | 1.5 | 19 | 4.4 | 10 | 2.6 | 7 | 2.4 | 44 | 2.7 |
| North Central | 27 | 1.7 | 35 | 2.2 | 31 | 2.3 | 22 | 1.8 | 115 | 2.0 |
| South | 21 | 1.3 | 24 | 1.3 | 29 | 1.8 | 38 | 2.6 | 112 | 1.7 |
| West | 54 | 2.5 | 45 | 2.1 | 39 | 2.2 | 28 | 1.9 | 166 | 2.2 |
| Total United States | 110 | 1.9 | 123 | 2.0 | 109 | 2.1 | 95 | 2.1 | 437 | 2.0 |
| White | 90 | 1.9 | 105 | 2.2 | 103 | 2.5 | 79 | 2.2 | 377 | 2.2 |
| Other | 20 | 1.8 | 18 | 1.5 | 6 | 0.6 | 16 | 1.8 | 60 | 1.4 |

**Rectal and Intestinal Atresia**

| | 1982 Cases | Rate | 1983 Cases | Rate | 1984 Cases | Rate | 1985 Cases | Rate | Total Cases | Rate |
|---|---|---|---|---|---|---|---|---|---|---|
| Northeast | 18 | 3.3 | 15 | 3.5 | 16 | 4.2 | 8 | 2.7 | 57 | 3.4 |
| North Central | 63 | 3.9 | 57 | 3.6 | 91 | 6.7 | 65 | 5.3 | 276 | 4.8 |
| South | 47 | 3.0 | 58 | 3.2 | 48 | 2.9 | 48 | 3.3 | 201 | 3.1 |
| West | 63 | 2.9 | 79 | 3.6 | 59 | 3.3 | 48 | 3.3 | 249 | 3.3 |
| Total United States | 191 | 3.2 | 209 | 3.5 | 214 | 4.2 | 169 | 3.8 | 783 | 3.6 |
| White | 162 | 3.4 | 173 | 3.6 | 166 | 4.0 | 127 | 3.6 | 628 | 3.6 |
| Other | 29 | 2.6 | 36 | 3.0 | 48 | 5.0 | 42 | 4.7 | 155 | 3.7 |

**Genitourinary**

**Renal Agenesis**

| | 1982 Cases | Rate | 1983 Cases | Rate | 1984 Cases | Rate | 1985 Cases | Rate | Total Cases | Rate |
|---|---|---|---|---|---|---|---|---|---|---|
| Northeast | 9 | 1.6 | 7 | 1.6 | 4 | 1.1 | 3 | 1.0 | 23 | 1.4 |
| North Central | 26 | 1.6 | 22 | 1.4 | 17 | 1.3 | 21 | 1.7 | 86 | 1.5 |
| South | 21 | 1.3 | 24 | 1.3 | 24 | 1.5 | 36 | 2.5 | 105 | 1.6 |
| West | 28 | 1.3 | 35 | 1.6 | 31 | 1.7 | 23 | 1.6 | 117 | 1.5 |
| Total United States | 84 | 1.4 | 88 | 1.5 | 76 | 1.5 | 83 | 1.9 | 331 | 1.5 |
| White | 67 | 1.4 | 71 | 1.5 | 63 | 1.5 | 70 | 2.0 | 271 | 1.6 |
| Other | 17 | 1.5 | 17 | 1.4 | 13 | 1.3 | 13 | 1.4 | 60 | 1.4 |

**Bladder Exstrophy**

| | 1982 Cases | Rate | 1983 Cases | Rate | 1984 Cases | Rate | 1985 Cases | Rate | Total Cases | Rate |
|---|---|---|---|---|---|---|---|---|---|---|
| Northeast | 0 | 0.0 | 2 | 0.5 | 1 | 0.3 | 0 | 0.0 | 3 | 0.2 |
| North Central | 6 | 0.4 | 5 | 0.3 | 2 | 0.1 | 7 | 0.6 | 20 | 0.3 |
| South | 3 | 0.2 | 7 | 0.4 | 4 | 0.2 | 4 | 0.3 | 18 | 0.3 |
| West | 5 | 0.2 | 8 | 0.4 | 3 | 0.2 | 7 | 0.5 | 23 | 0.3 |
| Total United States | 14 | 0.2 | 22 | 0.4 | 10 | 0.2 | 18 | 0.4 | 64 | 0.3 |
| White | 13 | 0.3 | 20 | 0.4 | 8 | 0.2 | 15 | 0.4 | 56 | 0.3 |
| Other | 1 | 0.1 | 2 | 0.2 | 2 | 0.2 | 3 | 0.3 | 8 | 0.2 |

**Musculoskeletal**

**Clubfoot W/Out CNS Defects**

| | 1982 Cases | Rate | 1983 Cases | Rate | 1984 Cases | Rate | 1985 Cases | Rate | Total Cases | Rate |
|---|---|---|---|---|---|---|---|---|---|---|
| Northeast | 134 | 24.4 | 83 | 19.3 | 96 | 25.2 | 46 | 15.7 | 359 | 21.7 |
| North Central | 454 | 28.1 | 487 | 30.7 | 440 | 32.4 | 312 | 25.6 | 1693 | 29.3 |
| South | 299 | 18.9 | 371 | 20.4 | 338 | 20.7 | 319 | 22.2 | 1327 | 20.5 |
| West | 503 | 23.1 | 553 | 25.3 | 383 | 21.5 | 324 | 22.0 | 1763 | 23.2 |
| Total United States | 1390 | 23.5 | 1494 | 24.8 | 1257 | 24.4 | 1001 | 22.6 | 5142 | 23.9 |

**Table 4 (continued)**

| Malformation/Census Region/Race | 1982 Cases | Rate | 1983 Cases | Rate | 1984 Cases | Rate | 1985 Cases | Rate | Total Cases | Rate |
|---|---|---|---|---|---|---|---|---|---|---|
| White | 1193 | 24.9 | 1239 | 25.7 | 1049 | 25.1 | 826 | 23.4 | 4307 | 24.9 |
| Other | 197 | 17.4 | 255 | 21.5 | 208 | 21.5 | 175 | 19.4 | 835 | 20.0 |
| **Reduction Deformity Upper Limbs** | | | | | | | | | | |
| Northeast | 13 | 2.4 | 8 | 1.9 | 4 | 1.1 | 3 | 1.0 | 28 | 1.7 |
| North Central | 31 | 1.9 | 27 | 1.7 | 18 | 1.3 | 17 | 1.4 | 93 | 1.6 |
| South | 29 | 1.8 | 16 | 0.9 | 17 | 1.0 | 21 | 1.5 | 83 | 1.3 |
| West | 31 | 1.4 | 32 | 1.5 | 19 | 1.1 | 29 | 2.0 | 111 | 1.5 |
| Total United States | 104 | 1.8 | 83 | 1.4 | 58 | 1.1 | 70 | 1.6 | 315 | 1.5 |
| White | 85 | 1.8 | 67 | 1.4 | 52 | 1.2 | 58 | 1.6 | 262 | 1.5 |
| Other | 19 | 1.7 | 16 | 1.4 | 6 | 0.6 | 12 | 1.3 | 53 | 1.3 |
| **Reduction Deformity Lower Limbs** | | | | | | | | | | |
| Northeast | 5 | 0.9 | 5 | 1.2 | 6 | 1.6 | 1 | 0.3 | 17 | 1.0 |
| North Central | 12 | 0.7 | 17 | 1.1 | 13 | 1.0 | 7 | 0.6 | 49 | 0.8 |
| South | 9 | 0.6 | 5 | 0.3 | 11 | 0.7 | 11 | 0.8 | 36 | 0.6 |
| West | 27 | 1.2 | 27 | 1.2 | 19 | 1.1 | 12 | 0.8 | 85 | 1.1 |
| Total United States | 53 | 0.9 | 54 | 0.9 | 49 | 1.0 | 31 | 0.7 | 187 | 0.9 |
| White | 44 | 0.9 | 43 | 0.9 | 38 | 0.9 | 25 | 0.7 | 150 | 0.9 |
| Other | 9 | 0.8 | 11 | 0.9 | 11 | 1.1 | 6 | 0.7 | 37 | 0.9 |
| **Congenital Arthrogryposis** | | | | | | | | | | |
| Northeast | 9 | 1.6 | 9 | 2.1 | 10 | 2.6 | 4 | 1.4 | 32 | 1.9 |
| North Central | 22 | 1.4 | 45 | 2.8 | 45 | 3.3 | 23 | 1.9 | 135 | 2.3 |
| South | 13 | 0.8 | 14 | 0.8 | 26 | 1.6 | 26 | 1.8 | 79 | 1.2 |
| West | 28 | 1.3 | 36 | 1.6 | 16 | 0.9 | 24 | 1.6 | 104 | 1.4 |
| Total United States | 72 | 1.2 | 104 | 1.7 | 97 | 1.9 | 77 | 1.7 | 350 | 1.6 |
| White | 60 | 1.3 | 94 | 1.9 | 86 | 2.1 | 59 | 1.7 | 299 | 1.7 |
| Other | 12 | 1.1 | 10 | 0.8 | 11 | 1.1 | 18 | 2.0 | 51 | 1.2 |
| **Chromosomal** | | | | | | | | | | |
| **Trisomy 13** | | | | | | | | | | |
| Northeast | 2 | 0.4 | 1 | 0.2 | 2 | 0.5 | 2 | 0.7 | 7 | 0.4 |
| North Central | 13 | 0.8 | 7 | 0.4 | 8 | 0.6 | 2 | 0.2 | 30 | 0.5 |
| South | 3 | 0.2 | 14 | 0.8 | 13 | 0.8 | 15 | 1.0 | 45 | 0.7 |
| West | 14 | 0.6 | 18 | 0.8 | 11 | 0.6 | 10 | 0.7 | 53 | 0.7 |
| Total United States | 32 | 0.5 | 40 | 0.7 | 34 | 0.7 | 29 | 0.7 | 135 | 0.6 |
| White | 25 | 0.5 | 32 | 0.7 | 29 | 0.7 | 19 | 0.5 | 105 | 0.6 |
| Other | 7 | 0.6 | 8 | 0.7 | 5 | 0.5 | 10 | 1.1 | 30 | 0.7 |
| **Down Syndrome** | | | | | | | | | | |
| Northeast | 61 | 11.1 | 48 | 11.1 | 37 | 9.7 | 38 | 13.0 | 184 | 11.1 |
| North Central | 127 | 7.9 | 130 | 8.2 | 108 | 7.9 | 93 | 7.6 | 458 | 7.9 |
| South | 114 | 7.2 | 136 | 7.5 | 120 | 7.4 | 128 | 8.9 | 498 | 7.7 |
| West | 205 | 9.4 | 206 | 9.4 | 177 | 10.0 | 141 | 9.6 | 729 | 9.6 |
| Total United States | 507 | 8.6 | 520 | 8.6 | 442 | 8.6 | 400 | 9.0 | 1869 | 8.7 |
| White | 412 | 8.6 | 449 | 9.3 | 371 | 8.9 | 329 | 9.3 | 1561 | 9.0 |
| Other | 95 | 8.4 | 71 | 6.0 | 71 | 7.4 | 71 | 7.9 | 308 | 7.4 |
| **Trisomy 18** | | | | | | | | | | |
| Northeast | 4 | 0.7 | 2 | 0.5 | 10 | 2.6 | 4 | 1.4 | 20 | 1.2 |
| North Central | 13 | 0.8 | 12 | 0.8 | 4 | 0.3 | 14 | 1.1 | 43 | 0.7 |
| South | 13 | 0.8 | 12 | 0.7 | 9 | 0.6 | 13 | 0.9 | 47 | 0.7 |
| West | 26 | 1.2 | 20 | 0.9 | 15 | 0.8 | 22 | 1.5 | 83 | 1.1 |
| Total United States | 56 | 0.9 | 46 | 0.8 | 38 | 0.7 | 53 | 1.2 | 193 | 0.9 |
| White | 44 | 0.9 | 35 | 0.7 | 30 | 0.7 | 46 | 1.3 | 155 | 0.9 |

## Table 5

### Selected Congenital Malformations Live-Born and Stillborn Infants, By Race
### Metropolitan Atlanta Congenital Defects Program
### (Rates Per 10,000 Live Births) 1982-1985

| Malformation/Race | 1982 | | 1983 | | 1984 | | 1985 | | Total 1982–1985 | | Total 1968–1985 | |
|---|---|---|---|---|---|---|---|---|---|---|---|---|
| | Cases | Rate | Cases | Rate | Cases | Rate | Cases | Rate | Cases | Rate | Cases | Rate |
| **Central Nervous System** | | | | | | | | | | | | |
| Anencephalus | | | | | | | | | | | | |
| White | 6 | 3.5 | 8 | 4.6 | 6 | 3.3 | 9 | 4.7 | 29 | 4.0 | 237 | 7.6 |
| Other | 1 | 0.9 | 2 | 1.9 | 6 | 5.5 | 0 | 0.0 | 9 | 2.1 | 48 | 2.9 |
| Total, All Races | 7 | 2.5 | 10 | 3.6 | 12 | 4.1 | 9 | 2.9 | 38 | 3.3 | 285 | 6.0 |
| Spina Bifida W/Out Anencephalus | | | | | | | | | | | | |
| White | 12 | 7.0 | 14 | 8.1 | 11 | 6.0 | 14 | 7.3 | 51 | 7.1 | 317 | 10.2 |
| Other | 3 | 2.8 | 7 | 6.6 | 10 | 9.2 | 5 | 4.3 | 25 | 5.7 | 83 | 5.0 |
| Total, All Races | 15 | 5.4 | 21 | 7.5 | 21 | 7.2 | 19 | 6.1 | 76 | 6.5 | 400 | 8.4 |
| Hydrocephalus W/Out Spina Bifida | | | | | | | | | | | | |
| White | 7 | 4.1 | 7 | 4.0 | 14 | 7.6 | 20 | 10.4 | 48 | 6.6 | 264 | 8.5 |
| Other | 10 | 9.4 | 7 | 6.6 | 12 | 11.0 | 12 | 10.3 | 41 | 9.4 | 177 | 10.8 |
| Total, All Races | 17 | 6.1 | 14 | 5.0 | 26 | 8.9 | 32 | 10.3 | 89 | 7.7 | 441 | 9.3 |
| Encephalocele | | | | | | | | | | | | |
| White | 2 | 1.2 | 2 | 1.2 | 1 | 0.5 | 5 | 2.6 | 10 | 1.4 | 58 | 1.9 |
| Other | 5 | 4.7 | 3 | 2.8 | 4 | 3.7 | 3 | 2.6 | 15 | 3.4 | 36 | 2.2 |
| Total, All Races | 7 | 2.5 | 5 | 1.8 | 5 | 1.7 | 8 | 2.6 | 25 | 2.2 | 94 | 2.0 |
| Microcephalus | | | | | | | | | | | | |
| White | 0 | 0.0 | 9 | 5.2 | 4 | 2.2 | 7 | 3.6 | 20 | 2.8 | 101 | 3.2 |
| Other | 6 | 5.7 | 9 | 8.5 | 11 | 10.1 | 16 | 13.7 | 42 | 9.6 | 131 | 8.0 |
| Total, All Races | 6 | 2.2 | 18 | 6.4 | 15 | 5.1 | 23 | 7.4 | 62 | 5.3 | 232 | 4.9 |
| **Eye** | | | | | | | | | | | | |
| Anophthalmos/Microphthalmos | | | | | | | | | | | | |
| White | 5 | 2.9 | 5 | 2.9 | 4 | 2.2 | 6 | 3.1 | 20 | 2.8 | 92 | 2.9 |
| Other | 0 | 0.0 | 11 | 10.4 | 6 | 5.5 | 6 | 5.1 | 23 | 5.2 | 74 | 4.5 |
| Total, All Races | 5 | 1.8 | 16 | 5.7 | 10 | 3.4 | 12 | 3.9 | 43 | 3.7 | 166 | 3.5 |
| Congenital Cataract | | | | | | | | | | | | |
| White | 2 | 1.2 | 2 | 1.2 | 4 | 2.2 | 3 | 1.6 | 11 | 1.5 | 56 | 1.8 |
| Other | 4 | 3.8 | 0 | 0.0 | 1 | 0.9 | 4 | 3.4 | 9 | 2.1 | 46 | 2.8 |
| Total, All Races | 6 | 2.2 | 2 | 0.7 | 5 | 1.7 | 7 | 2.3 | 20 | 1.7 | 102 | 2.1 |

## Table 5 (continued)

| Malformation/Race | 1982 Cases | 1982 Rate | 1983 Cases | 1983 Rate | 1984 Cases | 1984 Rate | 1985 Cases | 1985 Rate | Total 1982–1985 Cases | Total 1982–1985 Rate | Total 1968–1985 Cases | Total 1968–1985 Rate |
|---|---|---|---|---|---|---|---|---|---|---|---|---|
| **Coloboma of Eye** | | | | | | | | | | | | |
| White | 1 | 0.6 | 2 | 1.2 | 1 | 0.5 | 0 | 0.0 | 4 | 0.6 | 28 | 0.9 |
| Other | 2 | 1.9 | 2 | 1.9 | 0 | 0.0 | 0 | 0.0 | 4 | 0.9 | 8 | 0.5 |
| Total, All Races | 3 | 1.1 | 4 | 1.4 | 1 | 0.3 | 0 | 0.0 | 8 | 0.7 | 36 | 0.8 |
| **Aniridia/Other Anomalies of Iris** | | | | | | | | | | | | |
| White | 2 | 1.2 | 2 | 1.2 | 0 | 0.0 | 3 | 1.6 | 7 | 1.0 | 15 | 0.5 |
| Other | 1 | 0.9 | 1 | 0.9 | 0 | 0.0 | 1 | 0.9 | 3 | 0.7 | 9 | 0.5 |
| Total, All Races | 3 | 1.1 | 3 | 1.1 | 0 | 0.0 | 4 | 1.3 | 10 | 0.9 | 24 | 0.5 |
| **Cardiovascular** | | | | | | | | | | | | |
| **Common Truncus** | | | | | | | | | | | | |
| White | 3 | 1.7 | 1 | 0.6 | 1 | 0.5 | 1 | 0.5 | 6 | 0.8 | 31 | 1.0 |
| Other | 1 | 0.9 | 0 | 0.0 | 1 | 0.9 | 0 | 0.0 | 2 | 0.5 | 10 | 0.6 |
| Total, All Races | 4 | 1.4 | 1 | 0.4 | 2 | 0.7 | 1 | 0.3 | 8 | 0.7 | 41 | 0.9 |
| **Transposition of Great Arteries** | | | | | | | | | | | | |
| White | 10 | 5.8 | 11 | 6.3 | 11 | 6.0 | 8 | 4.1 | 40 | 5.5 | 143 | 4.6 |
| Other | 4 | 3.8 | 3 | 2.8 | 5 | 4.6 | 3 | 2.6 | 15 | 3.4 | 52 | 3.2 |
| Total, All Races | 14 | 5.0 | 14 | 5.0 | 16 | 5.5 | 11 | 3.5 | 55 | 4.7 | 195 | 4.1 |
| **Tetralogy of Fallot** | | | | | | | | | | | | |
| White | 7 | 4.1 | 6 | 3.5 | 6 | 3.3 | 6 | 3.1 | 25 | 3.5 | 96 | 3.1 |
| Other | 2 | 1.9 | 2 | 1.9 | 3 | 2.7 | 5 | 4.3 | 12 | 2.7 | 40 | 2.4 |
| Total, All Races | 9 | 3.2 | 8 | 2.9 | 9 | 3.1 | 11 | 3.5 | 37 | 3.2 | 136 | 2.9 |
| **Ventricular Septal Defect** | | | | | | | | | | | | |
| White | 29 | 16.8 | 36 | 20.8 | 34 | 18.6 | 38 | 19.7 | 137 | 19.0 | 527 | 16.9 |
| Other | 14 | 13.2 | 11 | 10.4 | 23 | 21.1 | 29 | 24.8 | 77 | 17.6 | 323 | 19.6 |
| Total, All Races | 43 | 15.4 | 47 | 16.8 | 57 | 19.5 | 67 | 21.6 | 214 | 18.4 | 850 | 17.8 |
| **Atrial Septal Defect** | | | | | | | | | | | | |
| White | 19 | 11.0 | 26 | 15.0 | 40 | 21.8 | 30 | 15.5 | 115 | 15.9 | 314 | 10.1 |
| Other | 9 | 8.5 | 11 | 10.4 | 23 | 21.1 | 20 | 17.1 | 63 | 14.4 | 185 | 11.3 |
| Total, All Races | 28 | 10.0 | 37 | 13.2 | 63 | 21.5 | 50 | 16.1 | 178 | 15.3 | 499 | 10.5 |

Table 5 (continued)

| Malformation/Race | 1982 Cases | 1982 Rate | 1983 Cases | 1983 Rate | 1984 Cases | 1984 Rate | 1985 Cases | 1985 Rate | Total 1982–1985 Cases | Total 1982–1985 Rate | Total 1968–1985 Cases | Total 1968–1985 Rate |
|---|---|---|---|---|---|---|---|---|---|---|---|---|
| Pulmonary Artery Anomaly | | | | | | | | | | | | |
| White | 9 | 5.2 | 8 | 4.6 | 10 | 5.5 | 3 | 1.6 | 30 | 4.2 | 74 | 2.4 |
| Other | 6 | 5.7 | 4 | 3.8 | 15 | 13.7 | 10 | 8.6 | 35 | 8.0 | 73 | 4.4 |
| Total, All Races | 15 | 5.4 | 12 | 4.3 | 25 | 8.5 | 13 | 4.2 | 65 | 5.6 | 147 | 3.1 |
| Conus Arteriosus | | | | | | | | | | | | |
| White | 20 | 11.6 | 18 | 10.4 | 17 | 9.3 | 15 | 7.8 | 70 | 9.7 | 267 | 8.6 |
| Other | 7 | 6.6 | 5 | 4.7 | 8 | 7.3 | 8 | 6.8 | 28 | 6.4 | 100 | 6.1 |
| Total, All Races | 27 | 9.7 | 23 | 8.2 | 25 | 8.5 | 23 | 7.4 | 98 | 8.4 | 367 | 7.7 |
| Lung Agenesis and Hypoplaia | | | | | | | | | | | | |
| White | 8 | 4.6 | 7 | 4.0 | 9 | 4.9 | 11 | 5.7 | 35 | 4.8 | 119 | 3.8 |
| Other | 6 | 5.7 | 7 | 6.6 | 5 | 4.6 | 11 | 9.4 | 29 | 6.6 | 101 | 6.1 |
| Total, All Races | 14 | 5.0 | 14 | 5.0 | 14 | 4.8 | 22 | 7.1 | 64 | 5.5 | 220 | 4.6 |
| Orofacial | | | | | | | | | | | | |
| Cleft Palate W/Out Cleft Lip | | | | | | | | | | | | |
| White | 8 | 4.6 | 7 | 4.0 | 9 | 4.9 | 5 | 2.6 | 29 | 4.0 | 179 | 5.7 |
| Other | 3 | 2.8 | 4 | 3.8 | 7 | 6.4 | 6 | 5.1 | 20 | 4.6 | 85 | 5.2 |
| Total, All Races | 11 | 3.9 | 11 | 3.9 | 16 | 5.5 | 11 | 3.5 | 49 | 4.2 | 264 | 5.5 |
| Cleft Lip With and W/Out Cleft Palate | | | | | | | | | | | | |
| White | 23 | 13.3 | 21 | 12.1 | 16 | 8.7 | 23 | 11.9 | 83 | 11.5 | 395 | 12.7 |
| Other | 5 | 4.7 | 14 | 13.2 | 12 | 11.0 | 11 | 9.4 | 42 | 9.6 | 131 | 8.0 |
| Total, All Races | 28 | 10.0 | 35 | 12.5 | 28 | 9.6 | 34 | 11.0 | 125 | 10.8 | 526 | 11.0 |
| Gastrointestinal | | | | | | | | | | | | |
| Tracheo-Esophageal Anomalies | | | | | | | | | | | | |
| White | 2 | 1.2 | 4 | 2.3 | 5 | 2.7 | 8 | 4.1 | 19 | 2.6 | 91 | 2.9 |
| Other | 3 | 2.8 | 0 | 0.0 | 1 | 0.9 | 4 | 3.4 | 8 | 1.8 | 20 | 1.2 |
| Total, All Races | 5 | 1.8 | 4 | 1.4 | 6 | 2.1 | 12 | 3.9 | 27 | 2.3 | 111 | 2.3 |
| Rectal and Intestinal Atresia | | | | | | | | | | | | |
| White | 6 | 3.5 | 5 | 2.9 | 8 | 4.4 | 11 | 5.7 | 30 | 4.2 | 141 | 4.5 |
| Other | 2 | 1.9 | 5 | 4.7 | 2 | 1.8 | 4 | 3.4 | 13 | 3.0 | 54 | 3.3 |
| Total, All Races | 8 | 2.9 | 10 | 3.6 | 10 | 3.4 | 15 | 4.8 | 43 | 3.7 | 195 | 4.1 |

| Malformation/Race | 1982 Cases | 1982 Rate | 1983 Cases | 1983 Rate | 1984 Cases | 1984 Rate | 1985 Cases | 1985 Rate | Total 1982–1985 Cases | Total 1982–1985 Rate | Total 1968–1985 Cases | Total 1968–1985 Rate |
|---|---|---|---|---|---|---|---|---|---|---|---|---|
| **Genitourinary** | | | | | | | | | | | | |
| Renal Agenesis | | | | | | | | | | | | |
| White | 7 | 4.1 | 8 | 4.6 | 8 | 4.4 | 5 | 2.6 | 28 | 3.9 | 112 | 3.6 |
| Other | 1 | 0.9 | 3 | 2.8 | 2 | 1.8 | 4 | 3.4 | 10 | 2.3 | 47 | 2.9 |
| Total, All Races | 8 | 2.9 | 11 | 3.9 | 10 | 3.4 | 9 | 2.9 | 38 | 3.3 | 159 | 3.3 |
| Bladder Exstrophy | | | | | | | | | | | | |
| White | 0 | 0.0 | 0 | 0.0 | 0 | 0.0 | 1 | 0.5 | 1 | 0.1 | 12 | 0.4 |
| Other | 0 | 0.0 | 0 | 0.0 | 0 | 0.0 | 0 | 0.0 | 0 | 0.0 | 5 | 0.3 |
| Total, All Races | 0 | 0.0 | 0 | 0.0 | 0 | 0.0 | 1 | 0.3 | 1 | 0.1 | 17 | 0.4 |
| **Musculoskeletal** | | | | | | | | | | | | |
| Clubfoot W/Out CNS Defects | | | | | | | | | | | | |
| White | 49 | 28.4 | 47 | 27.1 | 39 | 21.3 | 45 | 23.3 | 180 | 24.9 | 1301 | 41.7 |
| Other | 25 | 23.6 | 29 | 27.3 | 24 | 22.0 | 33 | 28.2 | 111 | 25.3 | 441 | 26.8 |
| Total, All Races | 74 | 26.6 | 76 | 27.2 | 63 | 21.5 | 78 | 25.2 | 291 | 25.1 | 1742 | 36.6 |
| Reduction Deformity Upper Limbs | | | | | | | | | | | | |
| White | 10 | 5.8 | 6 | 3.5 | 13 | 7.1 | 5 | 2.6 | 34 | 4.7 | 161 | 5.2 |
| Other | 5 | 4.7 | 5 | 4.7 | 3 | 2.7 | 3 | 2.6 | 16 | 3.7 | 73 | 4.4 |
| Total, All Races | 15 | 5.4 | 11 | 3.9 | 16 | 5.5 | 8 | 2.6 | 50 | 4.3 | 234 | 4.9 |
| Reduction Deformity Lower Limbs | | | | | | | | | | | | |
| White | 1 | 0.6 | 5 | 2.9 | 2 | 1.1 | 2 | 1.0 | 10 | 1.4 | 62 | 2.0 |
| Other | 1 | 0.9 | 3 | 2.8 | 0 | 0.0 | 4 | 3.4 | 8 | 1.8 | 41 | 2.5 |
| Total, All Races | 2 | 0.7 | 8 | 2.9 | 2 | 0.7 | 6 | 1.9 | 18 | 1.6 | 103 | 2.2 |
| Congenital Arthrogryposis | | | | | | | | | | | | |
| White | 3 | 1.7 | 3 | 1.7 | 0 | 0.0 | 0 | 0.0 | 6 | 0.8. | 58 | 1.9 |
| Other | 2 | 1.9 | 6 | 5.7 | 2 | 1.8 | 5 | 4.3 | 15 | 3.4 | 50 | 3.0 |
| Total, All Races | 5 | 1.8 | 9 | 3.2 | 2 | 0.7 | 5 | 1.6 | 21 | 1.8 | 108 | 2.3 |
| Omphalocele | | | | | | | | | | | | |
| White | 11 | 6.4 | 6 | 3.5 | 2 | 1.1 | 9 | 4.7 | 28 | 3.9 | 122 | 3.9 |
| Other | 0 | 0.0 | 2 | 1.9 | 2 | 1.8 | 3 | 2.6 | 7 | 1.6 | 46 | 2.8 |
| Total, All Races | 11 | 3.9 | 8 | 2.9 | 4 | 1.4 | 12 | 3.9 | 35 | 3.0 | 168 | 3.5 |

Table 5 (continued)

| Malformation/Race | 1982 | | 1983 | | 1984 | | 1985 | | Total 1982–1985 | | Total 1968–1985 | |
|---|---|---|---|---|---|---|---|---|---|---|---|---|
| | Cases | Rate | Cases | Rate | Cases | Rate | Cases | Rate | Cases | Rate | Cases | Rate |
| Gastroschisis | | | | | | | | | | | | |
| White | 3 | 1.7 | 6 | 3.5 | 2 | 1.1 | 4 | 2.1 | 15 | 2.1 | 52 | 1.7 |
| Other | 4 | 3.8 | 2 | 1.9 | 1 | 0.9 | 1 | 0.9 | 8 | 1.8 | 17 | 1.0 |
| Total, All Races | 7 | 2.5 | 8 | 2.9 | 3 | 1.0 | 5 | 1.6 | 23 | 2.0 | 69 | 1.4 |
| Chromosomal | | | | | | | | | | | | |
| Trisomy 13 | | | | | | | | | | | | |
| White | 2 | 1.2 | 3 | 1.7 | 1 | 0.5 | 1 | 0.5 | 7 | 1.0 | 18 | 0.6 |
| Other | 0 | 0.0 | 0 | 0.0 | 2 | 1.8 | 3 | 2.6 | 5 | 1.1 | 19 | 1.2 |
| Total, All Races | 2 | 0.7 | 3 | 1.1 | 3 | 1.0 | 4 | 1.3 | 12 | 1.0 | 37 | 0.8 |
| Down Syndrome | | | | | | | | | | | | |
| White | 16 | 9.3 | 17 | 9.8 | 21 | 11.5 | 20 | 10.4 | 74 | 10.2 | 307 | 9.8 |
| Other | 11 | 10.4 | 14 | 13.2 | 5 | 4.6 | 9 | 7.7 | 39 | 8.9 | 163 | 9.9 |
| Total, All Races | 27 | 9.7 | 31 | 11.1 | 26 | 8.9 | 29 | 9.4 | 113 | 9.7 | 470 | 9.9 |
| Trisomy 18 | | | | | | | | | | | | |
| White | 3 | 1.7 | 4 | 2.3 | 2 | 1.1 | 3 | 1.6 | 12 | 1.7 | 31 | 1.0 |
| Other | 0 | 0.0 | 1 | 0.9 | 6 | 5.5 | 4 | 3.4 | 11 | 2.5 | 21 | 1.3 |
| Total, All Races | 3 | 1.1 | 5 | 1.8 | 8 | 2.7 | 7 | 2.3 | 23 | 2.0 | 52 | 1.1 |

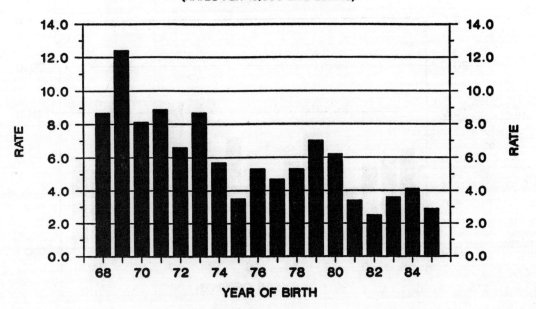

### Figure 3
### Anencephalus

**TRENDS IN REPORTED INCIDENCE AMONG LIVE AND STILLBIRTHS,
METROPOLITAN ATLANTA CONGENITAL DEFECTS PROGRAM
JAN 1968 – DEC 1985**

**(RATES PER 10,000 LIVE BIRTHS)**

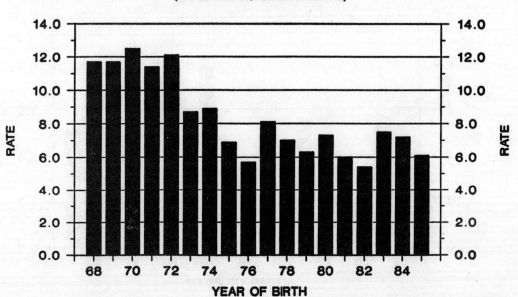

### Figure 4
### Spina Bifida W/Out Anencephalus

**TRENDS IN REPORTED INCIDENCE AMONG LIVE AND STILLBIRTHS,
METROPOLITAN ATLANTA CONGENITAL DEFECTS PROGRAM
JAN 1968 – DEC 1985**

**(RATES PER 10,000 LIVE BIRTHS)**

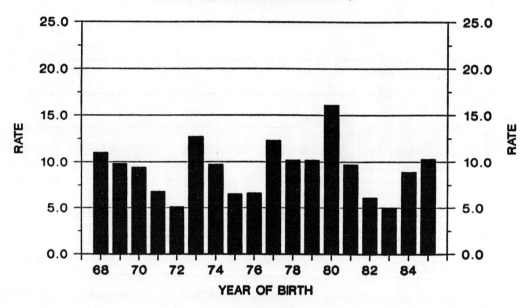

**Figure 5**
**Hydrocephalus W/Out Spina Bifida**

TRENDS IN REPORTED INCIDENCE AMONG LIVE AND STILLBIRTHS,
METROPOLITAN ATLANTA CONGENITAL DEFECTS PROGRAM
JAN 1968 – DEC 1985

(RATES PER 10,000 LIVE BIRTHS)

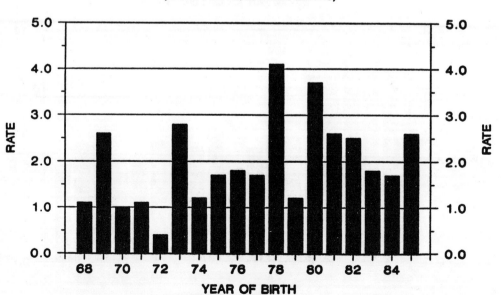

**Figure 6**
**Encephalocele**

TRENDS IN REPORTED INCIDENCE AMONG LIVE AND STILLBIRTHS,
METROPOLITAN ATLANTA CONGENITAL DEFECTS PROGRAM
JAN 1968 – DEC 1985

(RATES PER 10,000 LIVE BIRTHS)

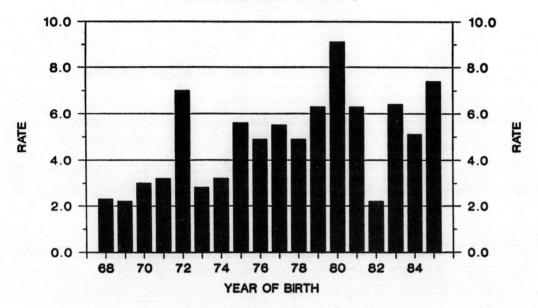

**Figure 7**
**Microcephalus**

TRENDS IN REPORTED INCIDENCE AMONG LIVE AND STILLBIRTHS,
METROPOLITAN ATLANTA CONGENITAL DEFECTS PROGRAM
JAN 1968 – DEC 1985

(RATES PER 10,000 LIVE BIRTHS)

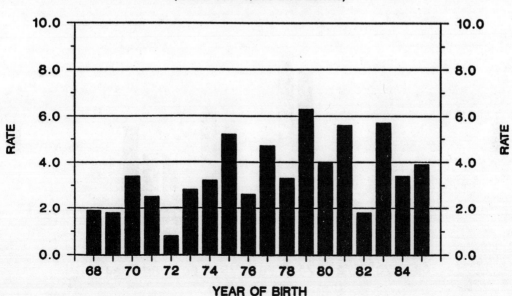

**Figure 8**
**Anophthalmos/Microphthalmos**

TRENDS IN REPORTED INCIDENCE AMONG LIVE AND STILLBIRTHS,
METROPOLITAN ATLANTA CONGENITAL DEFECTS PROGRAM
JAN 1968 – DEC 1985

(RATES PER 10,000 LIVE BIRTHS)

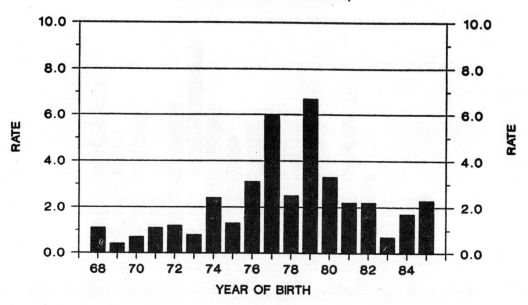

**Figure 9**
**Congenital Cataract**

TRENDS IN REPORTED INCIDENCE AMONG LIVE AND STILLBIRTHS,
METROPOLITAN ATLANTA CONGENITAL DEFECTS PROGRAM
JAN 1968 – DEC 1985

(RATES PER 10,000 LIVE BIRTHS)

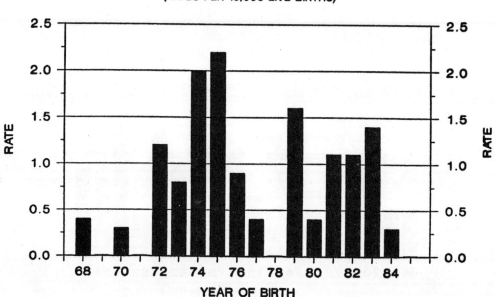

**Figure 10**
**Coloboma of Eye**

TRENDS IN REPORTED INCIDENCE AMONG LIVE AND STILLBIRTHS,
METROPOLITAN ATLANTA CONGENITAL DEFECTS PROGRAM
JAN 1968 – DEC 1985

(RATES PER 10,000 LIVE BIRTHS)

## Figure 11
## Ventricular Septal Defect

TRENDS IN REPORTED INCIDENCE AMONG LIVE AND STILLBIRTHS,
METROPOLITAN ATLANTA CONGENITAL DEFECTS PROGRAM
JAN 1968 – DEC 1985

(RATES PER 10,000 LIVE BIRTHS)

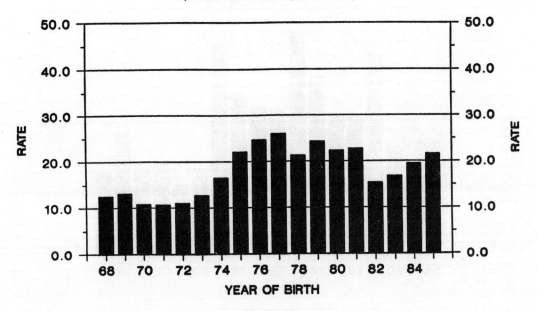

## Figure 12
## Atrial Septal Defect

TRENDS IN REPORTED INCIDENCE AMONG LIVE AND STILLBIRTHS,
METROPOLITAN ATLANTA CONGENITAL DEFECTS PROGRAM
JAN 1968 – DEC 1985

(RATES PER 10,000 LIVE BIRTHS)

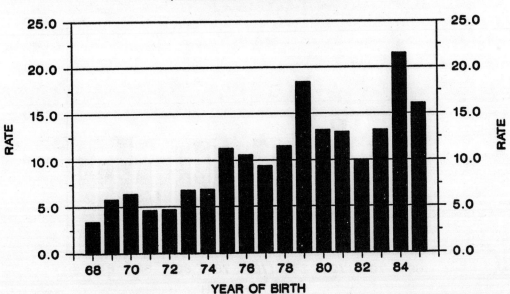

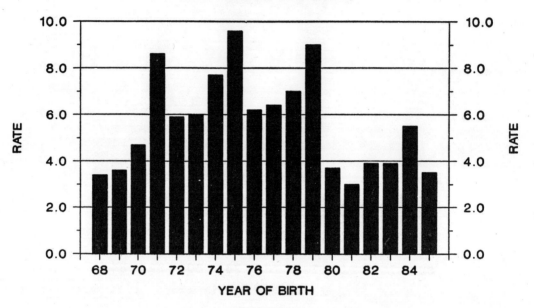

**Figure 13**
**Cleft Palate W/Out Cleft Lip**

TRENDS IN REPORTED INCIDENCE AMONG LIVE AND STILLBIRTHS,
METROPOLITAN ATLANTA CONGENITAL DEFECTS PROGRAM
JAN 1968 – DEC 1985

(RATES PER 10,000 LIVE BIRTHS)

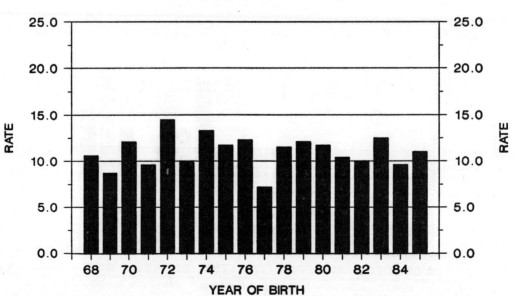

**Figure 14**
**Clept Lip With and W/Out Cleft Palate**

TRENDS IN REPORTED INCIDENCE AMONG LIVE AND STILLBIRTHS,
METROPOLITAN ATLANTA CONGENITAL DEFECTS PROGRAM
JAN 1968 – DEC 1985

(RATES PER 10,000 LIVE BIRTHS)

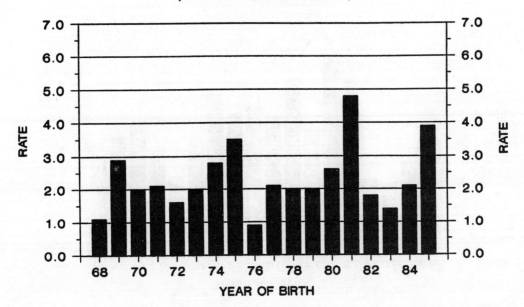

**Figure 15**
**Tracheo-Esophageal Anomalies**

TRENDS IN REPORTED INCIDENCE AMONG LIVE AND STILLBIRTHS,
METROPOLITAN ATLANTA CONGENITAL DEFECTS PROGRAM
JAN 1968 – DEC 1985

(RATES PER 10,000 LIVE BIRTHS)

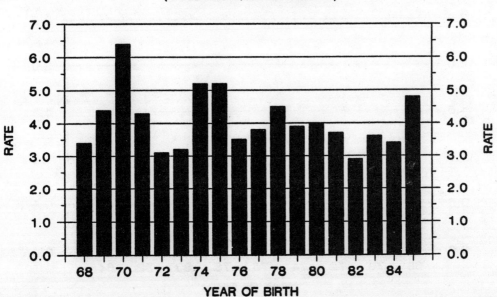

**Figure 16**
**Rectal and Intestinal Atresia**

TRENDS IN REPORTED INCIDENCE AMONG LIVE AND STILLBIRTHS,
METROPOLITAN ATLANTA CONGENITAL DEFECTS PROGRAM
JAN 1968 – DEC 1985

(RATES PER 10,000 LIVE BIRTHS)

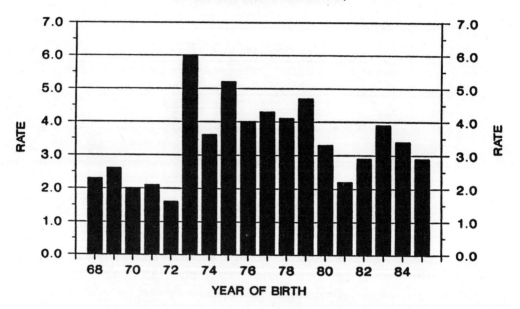

**Figure 17**
**Renal Agenesis**

TRENDS IN REPORTED INCIDENCE AMONG LIVE AND STILLBIRTHS,
METROPOLITAN ATLANTA CONGENITAL DEFECTS PROGRAM
JAN 1968 – DEC 1985

(RATES PER 10,000 LIVE BIRTHS)

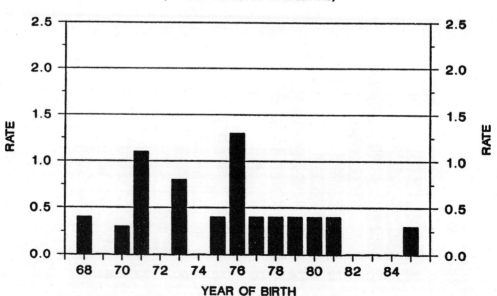

**Figure 18**
**Bladder Exstrophy**

TRENDS IN REPORTED INCIDENCE AMONG LIVE AND STILLBIRTHS,
METROPOLITAN ATLANTA CONGENITAL DEFECTS PROGRAM
JAN 1968 – DEC 1985

(RATES PER 10,000 LIVE BIRTHS)

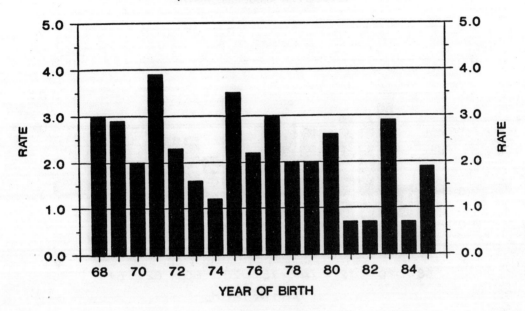

**Figure 19**
**Reduction Deformity Lower Limbs**

TRENDS IN REPORTED INCIDENCE AMONG LIVE AND STILLBIRTHS,
METROPOLITAN ATLANTA CONGENITAL DEFECTS PROGRAM
JAN 1968 – DEC 1985

(RATES PER 10,000 LIVE BIRTHS)

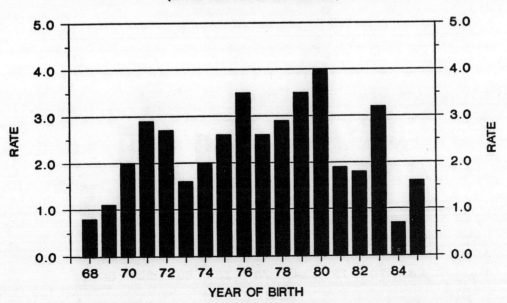

**Figure 20**
**Congenital Arthrogryposis**

TRENDS IN REPORTED INCIDENCE AMONG LIVE AND STILLBIRTHS,
METROPOLITAN ATLANTA CONGENITAL DEFECTS PROGRAM
JAN 1968 – DEC 1985

(RATES PER 10,000 LIVE BIRTHS)

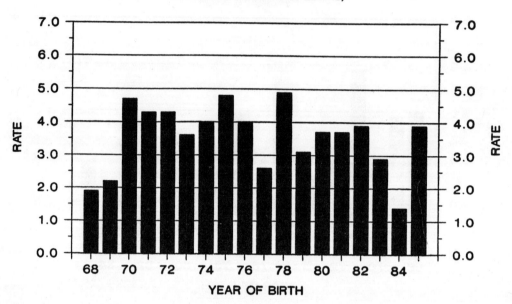

### Figure 21
### Omphalocele

TRENDS IN REPORTED INCIDENCE AMONG LIVE AND STILLBIRTHS,
METROPOLITAN ATLANTA CONGENITAL DEFECTS PROGRAM
JAN 1968 – DEC 1985

(RATES PER 10,000 LIVE BIRTHS)

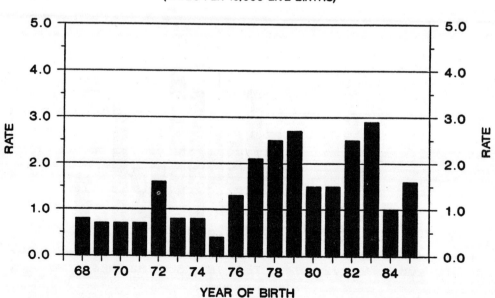

### Figure 22
### Gastroschisis

TRENDS IN REPORTED INCIDENCE AMONG LIVE AND STILLBIRTHS,
METROPOLITAN ATLANTA CONGENITAL DEFECTS PROGRAM
JAN 1968 – DEC 1985

(RATES PER 10,000 LIVE BIRTHS)

## Figure 23
### Trisomy 13

TRENDS IN REPORTED INCIDENCE AMONG LIVE AND STILLBIRTHS,
METROPOLITAN ATLANTA CONGENITAL DEFECTS PROGRAM
JAN 1968 – DEC 1985

(RATES PER 10,000 LIVE BIRTHS)

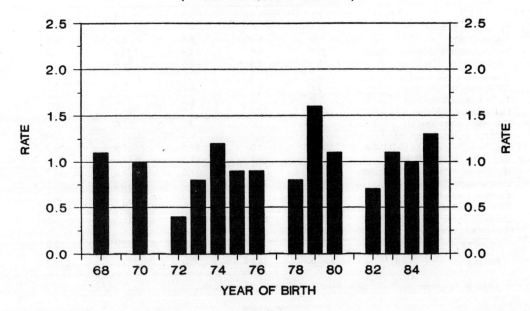

## Figure 24
### Down Syndrome

TRENDS IN REPORTED INCIDENCE AMONG LIVE AND STILLBIRTHS,
METROPOLITAN ATLANTA CONGENITAL DEFECTS PROGRAM
JAN 1968 – DEC 1985

(RATES PER 10,000 LIVE BIRTHS)

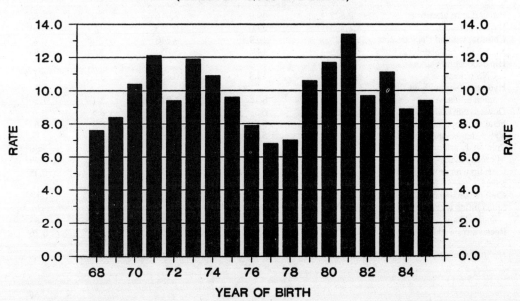

### Table 6

### Rates of major congenital malformations, by race/ethnicity, United States, 1981–1986

| | Rates[†] | | | | |
|---|---|---|---|---|---|
| | | | American | | |
| Malformation[*] | Blacks | Hispanics | Indians | Asians | Whites |
| Anencephaly | 2.1 | 4.4 | 3.6 | 4.4 | 3.0 |
| Spina bifida without anencephaly | 3.3 | 5.9 | 4.1 | 1.8 | 5.1 |
| Hydrocephalus without spina bifida | 8.1 | 4.6 | 10.8 | 4.8 | 5.4 |
| Microcephalus | 4.8 | 2.8 | 2.6 | 1.9 | 2.1 |
| Ventricular septal defect | 14.4 | 13.8 | 19.1 | 21.0 | 17.4 |
| Atrial septal defect | 2.1 | 1.2 | 4.1 | 2.5 | 2.1 |
| Valve stenosis and atresia | 5.9 | 1.9 | 8.2 | 2.8 | 3.2 |
| Patent ductus arteriosus | 49.9 | 20.7 | 33.5 | 25.1 | 26.5 |
| Pulmonary artery stenosis | 5.4 | 1.4 | 0 | 1.8 | 1.5 |
| Cleft palate without cleft lip | 3.7 | 3.7 | 9.8 | 4.6 | 5.9 |
| Cleft lip with or without cleft palate | 4.4 | 8.6 | 17.5 | 12.9 | 9.7 |
| Clubfoot without CNS[§] defects | 19.9 | 19.1 | 15.5 | 14.4 | 27.5 |
| Hip dislocation without CNS defects | 13.8 | 24.0 | 31.4 | 25.0 | 32.3 |
| Hypospadias | 24.6 | 14.9 | 17.5 | 16.5 | 32.7 |
| Rectal atresias and stenosis | 2.8 | 3.0 | 4.6 | 3.8 | 3.7 |
| Fetal alcohol syndrome | 6.0 | 0.8 | 29.9 | 0.3 | 0.9 |
| Down syndrome | 6.5 | 11.6 | 6.7 | 11.3 | 8.5 |
| Autosomal abnormalities, excluding Down syndrome | 2.1 | 2.1 | 3.1 | 2.9 | 2.2 |
| Total | 179.9 | 144.4 | 222.0 | 157.8 | 189.8 |

*By organ and/or system.      [†]Per 10,000 total births.      §Central nervous system.

### Table 7

### Cases and rates of 15 leading major congenital malformations among blacks, by comparison with those among whites, United States, 1981–1986

| | Blacks (N = 565,455) | | Whites (N = 3,361,963) | | Rate |
|---|---|---|---|---|---|
| Malformation | Cases | Rate* | Cases | Rate | Ratio[†] |
| Patent ductus arteriosus | 2,822 | 49.9 | 8,916 | 26.5 | 1.88[§] |
| Hypospadias | 1,393 | 24.6 | 10,995 | 32.7 | 0.75[§] |
| Clubfoot without CNS[¶] defects | 1,125 | 19.9 | 9,240 | 27.5 | 0.72[§] |
| Ventricular septal defect | 815 | 14.4 | 5,854 | 17.4 | 0.83[§] |
| Hip dislocation without CNS defects | 783 | 13.8 | 10,850 | 32.3 | 0.43[§] |
| Hydrocephalus without spina bifida | 458 | 8.1 | 1,816 | 5.4 | 1.50[§] |
| Down syndrome | 368 | 6.5 | 2,872 | 8.5 | 0.76[§] |
| Fetal alcohol syndrome | 340 | 6.0 | 302 | 0.9 | 6.67[§] |
| Valve stenosis and atresia | 336 | 5.9 | 1,060 | 3.2 | 1.84[§] |
| Pulmonary artery stenosis | 308 | 5.4 | 489 | 1.5 | 3.60[§] |
| Microcephalus | 273 | 4.8 | 706 | 2.1 | 2.29[§] |
| Cleft lip with or without cleft palate | 248 | 4.4 | 3,270 | 9.7 | 0.45[§] |
| Cleft palate without cleft palate | 211 | 3.7 | 1,991 | 5.9 | 0.63[§] |
| Spina bifida without anencephaly | 184 | 3.3 | 1,716 | 5.1 | 0.65[§] |
| Rectal atresia and stenosis | 156 | 2.8 | 1,252 | 3.7 | 0.76[§] |

*Per 10,000 total births.      [†]Rate for blacks divided by the rate for whites.      §p<0.05.      [¶]Central nervous system.

## Table 8

**Cases and rates of 15 leading major congenital malformations among Hispanics, by comparison with those among whites, United States, 1981–1986**

| Malformation | Hispanics (N = 261,810) | | Whites (N = 3,361,963) | | Rate Ratio[†] |
|---|---|---|---|---|---|
| | Cases | Rate* | Cases | Rate | |
| Hip dislocation without CNS[§] defects | 628 | 24.0 | 10,850 | 32.3 | 0.74[¶] |
| Patent ductus arteriosus | 542 | 20.7 | 8,916 | 26.5 | 0.78[¶] |
| Clubfoot without CNS defects | 499 | 19.1 | 9,240 | 28/5 | 0.69[¶] |
| Hypospadias | 390 | 14.9 | 10,995 | 32.7 | 0.46[¶] |
| Ventricular septal defect | 360 | 13.8 | 5,854 | 17.4 | 0.79[¶] |
| Down syndrome | 305 | 11.6 | 2,872 | 8.5 | 1.36[¶] |
| Cleft lip with or without cleft palate | 226 | 8.6 | 3,270 | 9.7 | 0.89 |
| Spina bifida without anencephaly | 154 | 5.9 | 1,716 | 5.1 | 1.16 |
| Hydrocephalus without spina bifida | 120 | 4.6 | 1,816 | 5.4 | 0.85 |
| Anencephaly | 115 | 4.4 | 1,003 | 3.0 | 1.47[¶] |
| Cleft palate without cleft lip | 98 | 3.7 | 1,991 | 5.9 | 0.63[¶] |
| Rectal atresia and stenosis | 79 | 3.0 | 1,252 | 3.7 | 0.81 |
| Microcephalus | 73 | 2.8 | 706 | 2.2 | 1.33[¶] |
| Autosomal abnormalities excluding Down syndrome | 54 | 2.1 | 748 | 2.2 | 0.95 |
| Valve stenosis and atresia | 49 | 1.9 | 1,060 | 3.2 | 0.59[¶] |

*Per 10,000 total births.  [†]Rate for Hispanics divided by the rate for whites.  [§]Central nervous system.  [¶]p<0.05.

## Table 9

**Cases and rates of 15 leading major congenital malformations among Hispanics, by comparison with those among whites, United States, 1981-1986**

| Malformation | American Indians (N = 19,412) | | Whites (N = 3,361,963) | | Rate Ratio[†] |
|---|---|---|---|---|---|
| | Cases | Rate* | Cases | Rate | |
| Patent ductus arteriosus | 65 | 33.5 | 8,916 | 26.5 | 1.26 |
| Hip dislocation without CNS[§] defects | 61 | 31.4 | 10,850 | 32.3 | 0.97 |
| Fetal alcohol syndrome | 58 | 29.9 | 302 | 0.9 | 33.22[¶] |
| Ventricular septal defect | 37 | 19.1 | 5,854 | 17.4 | 1.10 |
| Cleft lip with or without cleft palate | 34 | 17.5 | 3,270 | 9.7 | 1.80[¶] |
| Hypospadias | 34 | 17.5 | 10,995 | 32.7 | 0.54[¶] |
| Clubfoot without CNS defects | 30 | 15.5 | 9,240 | 27.5 | 0.56[¶] |
| Hydrocephalus without spina bifida | 21 | 10.8 | 1,816 | 5.4 | 2.00[¶] |
| Cleft palate without cleft lip | 19 | 9.8 | 1,991 | 5.9 | 1.66[¶] |
| Valve stenosis and atresia | 16 | 8.2 | 1,060 | 3.2 | 2.56[¶] |
| Down syndrome | 13 | 6.7 | 2,872 | 8.5 | 0.79 |
| Rectal atresia and stenosis | 9 | 4.6 | 1,252 | 3.7 | 1.24 |
| Atrial septal defect | 8 | 4.1 | 718 | 2.1 | 1.95 |
| Spina bifida without anencephaly | 8 | 4.1 | 1,716 | 5.1 | 0.80 |
| Anencephaly | 7 | 3.6 | 1,003 | 3.0 | 1.20 |

*Per 10,000 total births.  [†]Rate for American Indians divided by the rate for whites.  [§]Central nervous system.  [¶]p<0.05.

## Table 10

### Cases and rates of 15 leading major congenital malformations among Asians, by comparison with those among whites, United States, 1982–1986

| Malformation | Asians (N = 68,063) | | Whites (N = 3,361,963) | | Rate Ratio[†] |
|---|---|---|---|---|---|
| | Cases | Rate* | Cases | Rate | |
| Patent ductus arteriosus | 171 | 25.1 | 8,916 | 26.5 | 0.95 |
| Hip dislocation without CNS[§] defects | 170 | 25.0 | 10,850 | 32.3 | 0.77[¶] |
| Ventricular septal defect | 143 | 21.0 | 5,854 | 17.4 | 1.21[¶] |
| Hypospadias | 112 | 16.5 | 10,995 | 32.7 | 0.50[¶] |
| Clubfoot without CNS defects | 98 | 14.4 | 9,240 | 27.5 | 0.52[¶] |
| Cleft lip with or without cleft palate | 88 | 12.9 | 3,270 | 9.7 | 1.33[¶] |
| Down syndrome | 77 | 11.3 | 2,872 | 8.5 | 1.33[¶] |
| Hydrocephalus without spina bifida | 33 | 4.8 | 1,816 | 5.4 | 0.89 |
| Cleft palate without cleft lip | 31 | 4.6 | 1,991 | 5.9 | 0.78 |
| Anencephaly | 30 | 4.4 | 1,003 | 3.0 | 1.47[¶] |
| Rectal atresia and stenosis | 26 | 3.8 | 1,252 | 3.7 | 1.03 |
| Autosomal abnormalities, excluding Down syndrome | 20 | 2.9 | 748 | 2.2 | 1.32 |
| Valve stenosis and atresia | 19 | 2.8 | 1,060 | 3.2 | 0.88 |
| Atrial septal defect | 17 | 2.5 | 718 | 2.1 | 1.19 |
| Microcephalus | 13 | 1.9 | 706 | 2.1 | 0.90 |

*Per 10,000 total births.   †Rate for Asians divided by the rate for whites.   §Central nervous system.   ¶p<0.05.

## Table 11

### Years of potential life lost before age 65 due to congenital anomalies, by type of defect and race—United States, 1985

| Cases of mortality | White | | Other | | Total | |
|---|---|---|---|---|---|---|
| | No. | (%) | No. | (%) | No. | (%) |
| Agenesis, hypoplasia and dysplasia of lung | 48,765 | (8.9) | 12,903 | (9.8) | 61,667 | (9.1) |
| Anencephalus | 39,008 | (7.2) | 5,733 | (4.3) | 44,741 | (6.6) |
| Hypoplastic left heart syndrome | 35,505 | (6.5) | 7,725 | (5.8) | 43,230 | (6.4) |
| Edwards' syndrome (Trisomy 18) | 23,054 | (4.2) | 5,661 | (4.3) | 28,715 | (4.2) |
| Anomalies of diaphragm | 23,545 | (4.3) | 3,831 | (2.9) | 27,376 | (4.0) |
| Renal agenesis and dysgenesis | 22,695 | (4.2) | 4,421 | (3.3) | 27,116 | (4.0) |
| Ventricular septal defect | 14,903 | (2.7) | 4,098 | (3.1) | 19,001 | (2.8) |
| Congenital hydrocephalus | 13,369 | (2.5) | 4,753 | (3.6) | 18,122 | (2.7) |
| Patau's syndrome (Trisomy 13) | 13,014 | (2.4) | 3,138 | (2.4) | 16,152 | (2.4) |
| Transposition of great vessels | 12,003 | (2.2) | 1,442 | (1.1) | 13,444 | (2.0) |
| Tetralogy of Fallot | 10,386 | (1.9) | 2,519 | (1.9) | 12,905 | (1.9) |
| Down syndrome | 8,442 | (1.6) | 1,722 | (1.3) | 10,214 | (1.5) |
| Endocardial cushion defects | 7,808 | (1.4) | 2,246 | (1.7) | 10,053 | (1.5) |
| Spina bifida | 8,730 | (1.6) | 1,294 | (1.0) | 10,024 | (1.5) |
| Common truncus | 6,364 | (1.2) | 1,067 | (0.8) | 7,430 | (1.1) |
| Other anomalies | 258,200 | (47.3) | 69,664 | (52.7) | 327,868 | (48.4) |
| **Total anomalies** | 545,791 | (100.0) | 132,267 | (100.0) | 678,058 | (100.0) |

# 2.
# INFANT MORTALITY STATISTICS

## Table 12
### Mortality Rates in the First Year of Life and Low-Birthweight Births, All Races, 1986

| State | Infant Mortality | | Neonatal Mortality | | Postneonatal Mortality | | Low Birthweight | |
|---|---|---|---|---|---|---|---|---|
| | Rate | Rank | Rate | Rank | Rate | Rank | Rate | Rank |
| Alabama | 13.3 | 49 | 9.1 | 50 | 4.2 | 36 | 8.0 | 46 |
| Alaska | 10.8 | 33 | 6.2 | 22 | 4.5 | 42 | 4.6 | 1 |
| Arizona | 9.4 | 16 | 5.5 | 9 | 3.9 | 29 | 6.2 | 18 |
| Arkansas | 10.3 | 28 | 5.7 | 16 | 4.6 | 44 | 7.6 | 41 |
| California | 8.9 | 8 | 5.6 | 13 | 3.3 | 10 | 6.0 | 17 |
| Colorado | 8.6 | 5 | 5.3 | 6 | 3.3 | 9 | 7.7 | 43 |
| Connecticut | 9.1 | 9 | 6.8 | 30 | 2.3 | 1 | 6.6 | 23 |
| Delaware | 11.5 | 41 | 8.8 | 49 | — | — | 7.4 | 37 |
| District of Columbia | 21.1 | 51 | 16.1 | 51 | 5.0 | 47 | 12.2 | 51 |
| Florida | 11.0 | 35 | 7.3 | 36 | 3.7 | 23 | 7.6 | 40 |
| Georgia | 12.5 | 47 | 8.5 | 47 | 4.0 | 30 | 8.1 | 47 |
| Hawaii | 9.3 | 14 | 6.3 | 23 | 3.1 | 5 | 6.9 | 29 |
| Idaho | 11.3 | 39 | 6.7 | 29 | 4.6 | 43 | 5.2 | 7 |
| Illinois | 12.1 | 45 | 8.1 | 45 | 4.0 | 31 | 7.4 | 39 |
| Indiana | 11.3 | 38 | 7.5 | 40 | 3.8 | 24 | 6.4 | 20 |
| Iowa | 8.5 | 3 | 5.6 | 11 | 2.9 | 4 | 5.2 | 10 |
| Kansas | 8.9 | 7 | 5.1 | 5 | 3.8 | 26 | 6.2 | 19 |
| Kentucky | 9.8 | 23 | 6.4 | 24 | 3.5 | 14 | 7.1 | 35 |
| Louisiana | 11.9 | 44 | 7.8 | 43 | 4.1 | 35 | 8.6 | 49 |
| Maine | 8.8 | 6 | 5.6 | 14 | 3.2 | 6 | 5.1 | 5 |
| Maryland | 11.7 | 43 | 8.3 | 46 | 3.5 | 13 | 7.7 | 42 |
| Massachusetts | 8.5 | 2 | 5.8 | 18 | 2.6 | 2 | 5.8 | 15 |
| Michigan | 11.4 | 40 | 7.8 | 44 | 3.5 | 17 | 6.9 | 31 |
| Minnesota | 9.2 | 12 | 5.5 | 10 | 3.7 | 22 | 5.1 | 3 |
| Mississippi | 12.4 | 46 | 7.7 | 42 | 4.6 | 45 | 8.7 | 50 |
| Missouri | 10.7 | 32 | 6.8 | 32 | 3.9 | 28 | 6.8 | 25 |
| Montana | 9.6 | 20 | 5.6 | 12 | 4.0 | 32 | 5.9 | 16 |
| Nebraska | 10.1 | 25 | 6.6 | 28 | 3.5 | 15 | 5.5 | 14 |
| Nevada | 9.1 | 11 | 4.9 | 3 | 4.2 | 38 | 7.4 | 38 |
| New Hampshire | 9.1 | 10 | 5.9 | 19 | 3.2 | 8 | 5.2 | 9 |
| New Jersey | 9.8 | 21 | 6.6 | 26 | 3.2 | 7 | 6.8 | 26 |
| New Mexico | 9.5 | 19 | 5.4 | 8 | 4.1 | 34 | 7.1 | 34 |
| New York | 10.7 | 31 | 7.3 | 37 | 3.4 | 11 | 7.3 | 36 |
| North Carolina | 11.5 | 42 | 7.7 | 41 | 3.9 | 27 | 7.9 | 44 |
| North Dakota | 8.4 | 1 | 4.1 | 1 | 4.3 | 39 | 4.9 | 2 |
| Ohio | 10.6 | 30 | 6.9 | 33 | 3.8 | 25 | 6.7 | 24 |
| Oklahoma | 10.4 | 29 | 6.2 | 21 | 4.2 | 37 | 6.5 | 22 |
| Oregon | 9.4 | 17 | 4.7 | 2 | 4.7 | 46 | 5.1 | 4 |
| Pennsylvania | 10.2 | 26 | 6.8 | 31 | 3.4 | 12 | 6.9 | 30 |
| Rhode Island | 9.4 | 15 | 6.5 | 25 | 2.9 | 3 | 6.4 | 21 |
| South Carolina | 13.2 | 48 | 8.8 | 48 | 4.4 | 41 | 8.6 | 48 |
| South Dakota | 13.3 | 50 | 7.1 | 35 | 6.2 | 49 | 5.3 | 11 |
| Tennessee | 11.0 | 36 | 6.9 | 34 | 4.1 | 33 | 7.9 | 45 |
| Texas | 9.5 | 18 | 6.0 | 20 | 3.5 | 18 | 6.8 | 28 |
| Utah | 8.6 | 4 | 5.1 | 4 | 3.5 | 16 | 5.4 | 13 |
| Vermont | 10.0 | 24 | 7.5 | 39 | — | — | 5.2 | 6 |
| Virginia | 11.1 | 37 | 7.5 | 38 | 3.6 | 20 | 7.0 | 33 |
| Washington | 9.8 | 22 | 5.4 | 7 | 4.4 | 40 | 5.2 | 8 |
| West Virginia | 10.2 | 27 | 6.6 | 27 | 3.6 | 21 | 7.0 | 32 |
| Wisconsin | 9.2 | 13 | 5.7 | 15 | 3.6 | 19 | 5.4 | 12 |
| Wyoming | 10.9 | 34 | 5.8 | 17 | 5.1 | 48 | 6.8 | 27 |
| | | | | | | | | |
| United States | 10.4 | — | 6.7 | — | 3.6 | — | 6.8 | — |

Source: National Center for Health Statistics, Hyattsville, Maryland; calculations by Children's Defense Fund, Washington, D.C.

### Table 13
### Mortality Rates in the First Year of Life and Low-Birthweight Births, White, 1986

| State | Infant Mortality Rate | Infant Mortality Rank | Neonatal Mortality Rate | Neonatal Mortality Rank | Postneonatal Mortality Rate | Postneonatal Mortality Rank | Low Birthweight Rate | Low Birthweight Rank |
|---|---|---|---|---|---|---|---|---|
| Alabama | 9.8 | 43 | 6.9 | 46 | 2.9 | 11 | 6.0 | 39 |
| Alaska | 10.1 | 46 | 6.0 | 26 | 4.2 | 41 | 3.9 | 1 |
| Arizona | 9.0 | 27 | 5.4 | 12 | 3.6 | 38 | 6.0 | 41 |
| Arkansas | 8.9 | 21 | 5.3 | 8 | 3.6 | 37 | 6.3 | 44 |
| California | 8.6 | 10 | 5.4 | 14 | 3.1 | 20 | 5.2 | 15 |
| Colorado | 8.3 | 5 | 5.1 | 6 | 3.2 | 22 | 7.3 | 51 |
| Connecticut | 7.8 | 3 | 5.9 | 23 | 2.0 | 1 | 5.6 | 25 |
| Delaware | 9.6 | 40 | 7.4 | 49 | — | — | 6.0 | 38 |
| District of Columbia | — | — | — | — | — | — | 5.0 | 7 |
| Florida | 8.8 | 18 | 5.9 | 25 | 2.8 | 7 | 6.0 | 35 |
| Georgia | 9.4 | 35 | 6.5 | 41 | 2.9 | 12 | 6.0 | 36 |
| Hawaii | 8.6 | 14 | — | — | — | — | 5.4 | 20 |
| Idaho | 11.3 | 50 | 6.6 | 44 | 4.7 | 46 | 5.1 | 12 |
| Illinois | 9.3 | 34 | 6.4 | 40 | 2.9 | 13 | 5.5 | 22 |
| Indiana | 10.1 | 45 | 6.7 | 45 | 3.4 | 32 | 5.7 | 28 |
| Iowa | 8.3 | 6 | 5.5 | 16 | 2.9 | 8 | 5.0 | 8 |
| Kansas | 8.4 | 7 | 4.8 | 3 | 3.6 | 39 | 5.6 | 23 |
| Kentucky | 9.6 | 38 | 6.3 | 39 | 3.3 | 27 | 6.5 | 46 |
| Louisiana | 8.7 | 15 | 5.9 | 24 | 2.7 | 5 | 5.8 | 31 |
| Maine | 9.0 | 24 | 5.8 | 21 | 3.2 | 24 | 5.1 | 10 |
| Maryland | 9.5 | 37 | 6.5 | 42 | 3.0 | 15 | 5.5 | 21 |
| Massachusetts | 7.7 | 1 | 5.3 | 10 | 2.4 | 3 | 5.3 | 16 |
| Michigan | 9.0 | 26 | 6.0 | 30 | 3.0 | 14 | 5.4 | 19 |
| Minnesota | 8.9 | 20 | 5.5 | 18 | 3.3 | 29 | 4.7 | 3 |
| Mississippi | 9.0 | 22 | 6.1 | 31 | 2.9 | 9 | 6.0 | 40 |
| Missouri | 9.3 | 32 | 6.0 | 27 | 3.3 | 28 | 5.7 | 27 |
| Montana | 8.7 | 17 | 5.3 | 11 | 3.4 | 31 | 5.9 | 34 |
| Nebraska | 9.2 | 31 | 6.2 | 37 | 3.1 | 18 | 5.2 | 14 |
| Nevada | 8.6 | 9 | 4.9 | 4 | 3.6 | 36 | 6.6 | 47 |
| New Hampshire | 9.1 | 28 | 5.8 | 22 | 3.3 | 26 | 5.2 | 13 |
| New Jersey | 7.8 | 2 | 5.4 | 15 | 2.4 | 2 | 5.4 | 18 |
| New Mexico | 9.0 | 25 | 5.5 | 17 | 3.5 | 35 | 7.2 | 50 |
| New York | 9.2 | 29 | 6.5 | 43 | 2.7 | 4 | 5.8 | 30 |
| North Carolina | 9.2 | 30 | 6.2 | 38 | 3.0 | 16 | 6.1 | 43 |
| North Dakota | 8.3 | 4 | 4.1 | 1 | 4.2 | 42 | 4.7 | 4 |
| Ohio | 9.5 | 36 | 6.1 | 34 | 3.3 | 30 | 5.7 | 29 |
| Oklahoma | 10.1 | 44 | 6.0 | 29 | 4.1 | 40 | 5.9 | 33 |
| Oregon | 9.3 | 33 | 4.6 | 2 | 4.8 | 47 | 5.0 | 9 |
| Pennsylvania | 8.6 | 12 | 5.7 | 20 | 2.9 | 10 | 5.6 | 26 |
| Rhode Island | 8.8 | 19 | 6.1 | 32 | 2.8 | 6 | 6.0 | 37 |
| South Carolina | 10.1 | 47 | 6.9 | 47 | 3.2 | 23 | 6.1 | 42 |
| South Dakota | 10.4 | 48 | 6.1 | 35 | 4.3 | 43 | 4.9 | 6 |
| Tennessee | 8.7 | 16 | 5.6 | 19 | 3.1 | 19 | 6.5 | 45 |
| Texas | 8.6 | 11 | 5.4 | 13 | 3.2 | 21 | 5.9 | 32 |
| Utah | 8.6 | 13 | 5.1 | 5 | 3.5 | 34 | 5.3 | 17 |
| Vermont | 9.7 | 41 | 7.3 | 48 | — | — | 5.1 | 11 |
| Virginia | 9.0 | 23 | 6.0 | 28 | 3.0 | 17 | 5.6 | 24 |
| Washington | 9.8 | 42 | 5.3 | 9 | 4.5 | 44 | 4.8 | 5 |
| West Virginia | 9.6 | 39 | 6.2 | 36 | 3.5 | 33 | 6.8 | 49 |
| Wisconsin | 8.5 | 8 | 5.2 | 7 | 3.3 | 25 | 4.7 | 2 |
| Wyoming | 10.8 | 49 | 6.1 | 33 | 4.6 | 45 | 6.8 | 48 |
| United States | 8.9 | — | 5.8 | — | 3.1 | — | 5.6 | — |

Source: National Center for Health Statistics, Hyattsville, Maryland; calculations by Children's Defense Fund, Washington, D.C.

## Table 14
## Mortality Rates in the First Year of Life and Low-Birthweight Births, Black, 1986

| State | Infant Mortality | | Neonatal Mortality | | Postneonatal Mortality | | Low Birthweight | |
|---|---|---|---|---|---|---|---|---|
| | Rate | Rank | Rate | Rank | Rate | Rank | Rate | Rank |
| Alabama | 20.0 | 29 | 13.4 | 24 | 6.7 | 19 | 11.9 | 15 |
| Alaska | — | — | — | — | — | — | 8.0 | 2 |
| Arizona | 14.7 | 3 | — | — | — | — | 11.2 | 9 |
| Arkansas | 15.3 | 5 | 7.3 | 1 | 8.0 | 25 | 12.0 | 18 |
| California | 16.2 | 7 | 9.9 | 6 | 6.3 | 12 | 11.9 | 16 |
| Colorado | 17.2 | 12 | 10.4 | 8 | — | — | 14.4 | 43 |
| Connecticut | 18.4 | 23 | 13.9 | 26 | — | — | 12.9 | 36 |
| Delaware | 17.6 | 18 | 13.3 | 22 | — | — | 12.1 | 21 |
| District of Columbia | 24.0 | 33 | 18.4 | 30 | 5.6 | 4 | 14.2 | 42 |
| Florida | 18.2 | 21 | 11.6 | 16 | 6.5 | 16 | 12.7 | 34 |
| Georgia | 18.4 | 22 | 12.4 | 19 | 5.9 | 5 | 12.1 | 23 |
| Hawaii | — | — | — | — | — | — | 8.0 | 1 |
| Idaho | — | — | — | — | — | — | — | — |
| Illinois | 22.3 | 31 | 14.4 | 27 | 7.8 | 24 | 14.2 | 41 |
| Indiana | 21.5 | 30 | 14.9 | 28 | 6.6 | 18 | 11.9 | 14 |
| Iowa | — | — | — | — | — | — | 12.1 | 22 |
| Kansas | 15.0 | 4 | 9.2 | 3 | — | — | 12.0 | 17 |
| Kentucky | 12.7 | 1 | 7.7 | 2 | — | — | 12.5 | 28 |
| Louisiana | 17.0 | 11 | 10.7 | 9 | 6.3 | 13 | 12.9 | 35 |
| Maine | — | — | — | — | — | — | — | — |
| Maryland | 17.3 | 14 | 12.6 | 21 | 4.7 | 1 | 12.6 | 32 |
| Massachusetts | 18.5 | 24 | 13.6 | 25 | 4.9 | 2 | 10.8 | 7 |
| Michigan | 22.8 | 32 | 16.6 | 29 | 6.2 | 11 | 13.9 | 39 |
| Minnesota | 16.4 | 9 | — | — | — | — | 13.1 | 7 |
| Mississippi | 16.2 | 8 | 9.7 | 4 | 6.6 | 17 | 11.7 | 12 |
| Missouri | 18.5 | 26 | 11.5 | 15 | 7.0 | 21 | 12.6 | 29 |
| Montana | — | — | — | — | — | — | — | — |
| Nebraska | — | — | — | — | — | — | 11.2 | 8 |
| Nevada | — | — | — | — | — | — | 14.0 | 40 |
| New Hampshire | — | — | — | — | — | — | — | — |
| New Jersey | 18.5 | 25 | 11.7 | 17 | 6.8 | 20 | 12.7 | 33 |
| New Mexico | — | — | — | — | — | — | 8.9 | 3 |
| New York | 16.7 | 10 | 10.8 | 10 | 6.0 | 7 | 12.6 | 30 |
| North Carolina | 17.4 | 17 | 11.5 | 14 | 6.0 | 8 | 12.2 | 25 |
| North Dakota | — | — | — | — | — | — | — | — |
| Ohio | 17.4 | 16 | 11.2 | 11 | 6.2 | 10 | 12.1 | 24 |
| Oklahoma | 17.3 | 13 | 10.2 | 7 | 7.1 | 22 | 11.4 | 11 |
| Oregon | — | — | — | — | — | — | 10.0 | 5 |
| Pennsylvania | 19.8 | 28 | 13.3 | 23 | 6.5 | 15 | 13.9 | 38 |
| Rhode Island | — | — | — | — | — | — | 12.1 | 19 |
| South Carolina | 18.1 | 20 | 11.8 | 18 | 6.3 | 14 | 12.4 | 27 |
| South Dakota | — | — | — | — | — | — | — | — |
| Tennessee | 18.6 | 27 | 11.3 | 13 | 7.2 | 23 | 12.6 | 31 |
| Texas | 15.9 | 6 | 9.9 | 5 | 5.9 | 6 | 12.3 | 26 |
| Utah | — | — | — | — | — | — | 9.3 | 4 |
| Vermont | — | — | — | — | — | — | — | — |
| Virginia | 18.0 | 19 | 12.5 | 20 | 5.5 | 3 | 11.3 | 10 |
| Washington | 13.5 | 2 | — | — | — | — | 10.7 | 6 |
| West Virginia | — | — | — | — | — | — | 11.8 | 13 |
| Wisconsin | 17.3 | 15 | 11.3 | 12 | 6.0 | 9 | 12.1 | 20 |
| Wyoming | — | — | — | — | — | — | — | — |
| United States | 18.0 | — | 11.7 | — | 6.3 | — | 12.5 | — |

Source: National Center for Health Statistics, Hyattsville, Maryland; calculations by Children's Defense Fund, Washington, D.C.

## Table 15
## Mortality Rates in the First Year of Life and Low-Birthweight Births

| State | Infant Mortality Rate | Infant Mortality Rank | Neonatal Mortality Rate | Neonatal Mortality Rank | Postneonatal Mortality Rate | Postneonatal Mortality Rank | Low Birthweight Rate | Low Birthweight Rank |
|---|---|---|---|---|---|---|---|---|
| Alabama | 19.8 | 34 | 13.2 | 30 | 6.5 | 22 | 11.8 | 32 |
| Alaska | 12.2 | 11 | — | — | — | — | 6.2 | 2 |
| Arizona | 11.2 | 5 | 5.8 | 1 | 5.5 | 10 | 7.0 | 7 |
| Arkansas | 14.7 | 16 | 7.1 | 7 | 7.7 | 29 | 11.7 | 30 |
| California | 10.4 | 3 | 6.3 | 3 | 4.1 | 2 | 8.8 | 14 |
| Colorado | 11.9 | 8 | 7.4 | 10 | — | — | 12.0 | 36 |
| Connecticut | 16.3 | 21 | 12.1 | 26 | — | — | 12.2 | 40 |
| Delaware | 17.0 | 27 | 13.0 | 29 | — | — | 11.7 | 29 |
| District of Columbia | 22.6 | 39 | 17.3 | 34 | 5.4 | 9 | 13.6 | 48 |
| Florida | 17.4 | 28 | 11.1 | 22 | 6.3 | 21 | 12.4 | 42 |
| Georgia | 17.9 | 31 | 12.1 | 27 | 5.8 | 11 | 11.9 | 35 |
| Hawaii | 9.6 | 1 | 6.6 | 5 | 3.0 | 1 | 7.3 | 10 |
| Idaho | — | — | — | — | — | — | 7.3 | 9 |
| Illinois | 21.1 | 37 | 13.7 | 31 | 7.4 | 28 | 13.6 | 47 |
| Indiana | 20.3 | 36 | 14.2 | 32 | 6.1 | 19 | 11.5 | 25 |
| Iowa | — | — | — | — | — | — | 10.2 | 19 |
| Kansas | 12.4 | 12 | 7.3 | 8 | — | — | 10.7 | 21 |
| Kentucky | 12.2 | 10 | 7.3 | 9 | — | — | 12.1 | 38 |
| Louisiana | 16.5 | 23 | 10.3 | 15 | 6.1 | 18 | 12.6 | 44 |
| Maine | — | — | — | — | — | — | — | — |
| Maryland | 16.1 | 19 | 11.8 | 25 | 4.3 | 4 | 12.0 | 37 |
| Massachusetts | 14.6 | 15 | 10.4 | 16 | 4.2 | 3 | 9.5 | 16 |
| Michigan | 21.2 | 38 | 15.4 | 33 | 5.8 | 12 | 13.1 | 45 |
| Minnesota | 13.1 | 13 | 5.8 | 2 | 7.3 | 27 | 9.2 | 15 |
| Mississippi | 16.2 | 20 | 9.6 | 13 | 6.6 | 23 | 11.6 | 27 |
| Missouri | 17.6 | 29 | 10.9 | 20 | 6.6 | 24 | 12.2 | 39 |
| Montana | — | — | — | — | — | — | 5.4 | 1 |
| Nebraska | 20.2 | 35 | — | — | — | — | 9.5 | 17 |
| Nevada | 11.7 | 7 | — | — | — | — | 11.3 | 23 |
| New Hampshire | — | — | — | — | — | — | — | — |
| New Jersey | 16.4 | 22 | 10.5 | 17 | 5.9 | 15 | 11.8 | 33 |
| New Mexico | 12.0 | 9 | — | — | 6.9 | 25 | 6.4 | 3 |
| New York | 15.0 | 17 | 9.7 | 14 | 5.3 | 7 | 11.7 | 28 |
| North Carolina | 16.6 | 24 | 10.8 | 19 | 5.8 | 13 | 11.8 | 34 |
| North Dakota | — | — | — | — | — | — | 6.5 | 5 |
| Ohio | 16.7 | 26 | 10.8 | 18 | 6.0 | 16 | 11.8 | 31 |
| Oklahoma | 11.4 | 6 | 6.7 | 6 | 4.7 | 5 | 8.5 | 13 |
| Oregon | 10.4 | 4 | — | — | — | — | 6.5 | 4 |
| Pennsylvania | 18.4 | 33 | 12.5 | 28 | 6.0 | 17 | 13.3 | 46 |
| Rhode Island | — | — | — | — | — | — | 10.2 | 18 |
| South Carolina | 17.9 | 30 | 11.7 | 24 | 6.2 | 20 | 12.3 | 41 |
| South Dakota | 27.5 | 40 | — | — | 15.5 | 30 | 7.1 | 8 |
| Tennessee | 18.3 | 32 | 11.1 | 21 | 7.2 | 26 | 12.4 | 43 |
| Texas | 14.3 | 14 | 9.0 | 11 | 5.4 | 8 | 11.6 | 26 |
| Utah | — | — | — | — | — | — | 6.8 | 6 |
| Vermont | — | — | — | — | — | — | — | — |
| Virginia | 16.7 | 25 | 11.5 | 23 | 5.2 | 6 | 10.9 | 22 |
| Washington | 9.7 | 2 | 6.4 | 4 | — | — | 7.9 | 12 |
| West Virginia | — | — | — | — | — | — | 11.3 | 24 |
| Wisconsin | 15.3 | 18 | 9.4 | 12 | 5.8 | 14 | 10.4 | 20 |
| Wyoming | — | — | — | — | — | — | 7.8 | 11 |
| United States | 15.7 | — | 10.1 | — | 5.6 | — | 11.2 | — |

Source: National Center for Health Statistics, Hyattsville, Maryland; calculations by Children's Defense Fund, Washington, D.C.

## Table 16.
### Infant Mortality Rates for Cities of 500,000+ Population, 1986

| City | Total | White | Black | Nonwhite |
|------|-------|-------|-------|----------|
| Baltimore | 16.2 | 12.6 | 18.2 | 17.8 |
| Boston | 13.9 | 8.4 | 23.0 | 20.7 |
| Chicago | 16.6 | 10.7 | 22.9 | 22.2 |
| Cleveland | 16.3 | 11.9 | 20.3 | 20.3 |
| Columbus | 12.3 | 11.9 | 13.8 | 13.0 |
| Dallas | 11.8 | 9.8 | 16.0 | 15.3 |
| Detroit | 20.3 | 9.7 | 24.0 | 23.6 |
| District of Columbia | 21.1 | — | 24.0 | 22.6 |
| Houston | 11.3 | 9.2 | 17.2 | 15.7 |
| Indianapolis | 14.2 | 10.7 | 24.6 | 24.0 |
| Jacksonville | 13.1 | 10.0 | 19.7 | 19.0 |
| Los Angeles | 10.1 | 8.0 | 21.2 | 15.9 |
| Memphis | 15.8 | 10.7 | 18.4 | 18.6 |
| Milwaukee | 12.2 | 9.0 | 17.2 | 16.2 |
| New Orleans | 15.5 | 12.5 | 16.8 | 16.4 |
| New York City | 12.4 | 11.2 | 15.5 | 14.0 |
| Philadelphia | 15.5 | 9.6 | 21.8 | 20.7 |
| Phoenix | 11.0 | 10.3 | — | 16.0 |
| San Antonio | 10.2 | 9.6 | — | — |
| San Diego | 9.4 | 8.7 | 14.3 | 11.1 |
| San Francisco | 8.8 | 10.1 | — | 7.6 |
| San Jose | 7.3 | 7.3 | — | — |
| United States | 10.4 | 8.9 | 18.0 | 15.7 |

Source: National Center for Health Statistics, Hyattsville, Maryland; calculations by Children's Defense Fund, Washington, D.C.

## Table 17.
### Infant Mortality Rates, Selected Countries, 1986

| Rank | Country | Rate[1] | Rank | Country | Rate[1] |
|------|---------|---------|------|---------|---------|
| 1 | Japan | 6 | 18 | Austria | 10 |
| 1 | Finland | 6 | 18 | Australia | 10 |
| 1 | Sweden | 6 | 18 | United States | 10 |
| 4 | Denmark | 7 | 21 | Italy | 11 |
| 4 | Switzerland | 7 | 21 | New Zealand | 11 |
| 4 | Norway | 7 | 23 | Greece | 12 |
| 7 | Netherlands | 8 | 24 | Israel | 14 |
| 7 | France | 8 | 24 | Czechoslovakia | 14 |
| 7 | Canada | 8 | 26 | Cuba | 15 |
| 10 | Hong Kong | 9 | 26 | Bulgaria | 15 |
| 10 | Singapore | 9 | 28 | Poland | 18 |
| 10 | German Dem. Rep. | 9 | 28 | Hungary | 18 |
| 10 | Belgium | 9 | 28 | Portugal | 18 |
| 10 | German Fed. Rep. | 9 | 28 | Costa Rica | 18 |
| 10 | United Kingdom | 9 | | U.S. (Black) | 18 |
| 10 | Spain | 9 | | | |
| 10 | Ireland | 9 | | | |
| | U.S. (White) | 9 | | | |

[1]Deaths per 1,000 live births.
Source: UNICEF, New York, N.Y.

## Table 18
### Infant Mortality Rates[1] for 15 of the Leading Causes of Infant Death, by Race, U.S., 1986

| | | | Nonwhite | | Ratio of Black to White |
| --- | --- | --- | --- | --- | --- |
| | **All Races** | **White** | **Black** | **Total** | |
| All Causes | 1,035.3 | 894.3 | 1,803.5 | 1,568.1 | 2.0 |
| 1. Congenital anomalies | 219.5 | 219.5 | 232.1 | 219.4 | 1.1 |
| 2. Sudden infant death syndrome | 140.5 | 123.0 | 233.6 | 206.6 | 1.9 |
| 3. Respiratory distress syndrome | 90.6 | 81.5 | 144.2 | 124.8 | 1.8 |
| 4. Disorders relating to short gestation and low birthweight | 86.4 | 60.3 | 225.4 | 185.1 | 3.7 |
| 5. Maternal complications of pregnancy | 36.1 | 31.9 | 61.0 | ·51.8 | 1.9 |
| 6. Intrauterine hypoxia and birth asphyxia | 26.2 | 22.2 | 47.6 | 41.3 | 2.1 |
| 7. Infections specific to the perinatal period | 24.4 | 20.7 | 44.1 | 38.7 | 2.1 |
| 8. Complications of placenta, cord or membranes | 22.3 | 19.6 | 37.8 | 32.4 | 1.9 |
| 9. Accidents and adverse effects | 24.2 | 20.3 | 43.1 | 39.1 | 2.1 |
| 10. Pneumonia and influenza | 17.6 | 14.2 | 35.9 | 30.8 | 2.5 |
| 11. Neonatal hemorrhage | 9.2 | 7.4 | 18.8 | 16.2 | 2.5 |
| 12. Septicemia | 8.0 | 6.4 | 16.7 | 14.4 | 2.6 |
| 13. Homicide | 7.4 | 5.4 | 18.2 | 15.0 | 3.4 |
| 14. Birth trauma | 7.1 | 6.3 | 12.1 | 9.9 | 1.9 |
| 15. Meningitis | 5.9 | 4.5 | 11.9 | 10.8 | 2.6 |

[1]Deaths per 100,000 live births.
Source: National Center for Health Statistics, Hyattsville, Maryland.

## Table 19
### Neonatal Mortality for the 15 Leading Causes of Death

| | **Number** | **Rate[1]** | **Percent of Total Deaths** |
| --- | --- | --- | --- |
| All Causes | 25,212 | 671.1 | 100.0 |
| 1. Congenital anomalies | 6,155 | 163.8 | 24.4 |
| 2. Disorders relating to short gestation and low birthweight | 3,202 | 85.2 | 12.7 |
| 3. Respiratory distress syndrome | 3,179 | 84.6 | 12.6 |
| 4. Maternal complications of pregnancy | 1,344 | 35.8 | 5.3 |
| 5. Intrauterine hypoxia and birth asphyxia | 909 | 24.2 | 3.6 |
| 6. Infections specific to the perinatal period | 869 | 23.1 | 3.4 |
| 7. Complications of placenta, cord, or membranes | 825 | 22.0 | 3.3 |
| 8. Sudden infant death syndrome | 362 | 9.6 | 1.4 |
| 9. Neonatal hemorrhage | 341 | 9.1 | 1.4 |
| 10. Birth trauma | 256 | 6.8 | 1.0 |
| 11. Pneumonia and influenza | 152 | 4.0 | 0.6 |
| 12. Maternal conditions that may be unrelated to present pregnancy | 111 | 3.0 | 0.4 |
| 13. Accidents and adverse effects | 89 | 2.4 | 0.4 |
| 14. Other complications of labor and delivery | 71 | 1.9 | 0.3 |
| 15. Viral diseases | 48 | 1.3 | 0.2 |

[1]Deaths per 100,000 live births.
Source: National Center for Health Statistics, Hyattsville, Maryland.

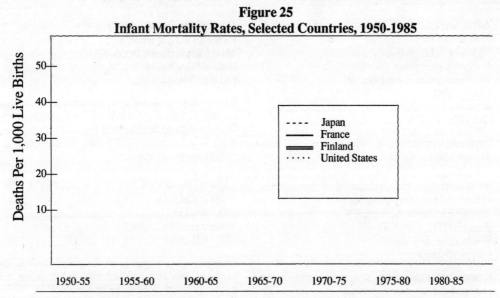

**Figure 25**
**Infant Mortality Rates, Selected Countries, 1950-1985**

Source: Children's Defense Fund, *The Health of America's Children: Maternal and Child Health Data Book* (Washington, D.C.: Children's Defense Fund, 1987).

# 3.
# FEDERAL ORGANIZATIONS

**Administration for Children, Youth,
   and Families**
Office of Public Affairs
Hubert H. Humphrey Building
200 Independence Avenue, SW
Room 329D
Washington, DC 20201
(202) 472-7257

Responds to inquiries on topics such as child abuse,
day care, domestic violence and Head Start.

**Administration on Developmental Disabilities**
Hubert H. Humphrey Building
200 Independence Avenue, SW
Room 351D
Washington, DC 20201
(202) 245-2888

Responds to inquiries and provides information and
publications on developmental disabilities. Produces and distributes a directory of services for
training handicapped persons.

**Centers for Disease Control**
Center for Health Promotion and Education
1600 Clifton Road, NE
Atlanta, GA 30333
(404) 639-3492

Responds to inquiries from professionals and consumers and provides leadership and program direction for the prevention of disease, disability,
premature death and other health problems. A catalog of publications is available.

**Centers for Disease Control**
Division of Birth Defects and
   Developmental Disabilities
CEH-KOGER
1600 Clifton Road, NE
Atlanta, GA 30333
(404) 488-4717

Responds to inquiries from consumers and professionals with information and reports on birth defects
and developmental disabilities.

**Centers for Disease Control**
Immunization Division
1600 Tullie Circle
Freeway Park
Atlanta, GA 30333
(404) 329-1880

Responds to inquiries and provides information and
publications regarding immunization against vac-
cine-preventable diseases of young children.

**Centers for Disease Control**
Public Inquiries, Building 1
1600 Clifton Road, Room B63
Atlanta, GA 30333
(404) 639-3534

Responds to inquiries and requests for information
on areas of preventive medicine, immunization, disease control and health education. Collects and com-
piles a wide variety of health-related data and
distributes publications.

**Clearinghouse on Child Abuse and Neglect In-
   formation**
P.O. Box 1182
Washington, DC 20013
(703) 821-2086

Responds to inquiries from the general public and
professionals and disseminates information and
publications on child abuse and neglect.

**Clearinghouse on Health Indexes**
3700 East-West Highway, Room 2-27
Hyattsville, MD 20782
(301) 436-7035

Responds to inquiries and provides bibliographic
and other informational assistance in the development of health measures for health researchers, ad-
ministrators and planners.

**Clearinghouse on the Handicapped**
330 C Street, SW, Room 3132
Washington, DC 20202
(202) 732-1245

Responds to inquiries and provides information on
government services for the disabled. Offers access
to a number of publications.

**Consumer Information Center**
Pueblo, CO 81009
(202) 566-1794

Distributes consumer publications on topics such as
prenatal care, parenting, nutrition, exercise, weight
control and child safety. The Consumer Information
Catalog and a list of Federal Information Centers are
available free from the center.

**Eric Clearinghouse on Handicapped and
   Gifted Children**
CEC Information Center
The Council for Exceptional Children
1920 Association Drive
Reston, VA 22091
(703) 620- 3660

Provides publications, bibliographies and customized computer searches on topics related to the education of handicapped and gifted children and youth. Produces abstracts for the ERIC database.

**Family Life Information Exchange**
P.O Box 10716
Rockville, MD 20850
(301) 770-3662

Responds to inquiries from consumers and professionals on family planning topics such as contraception and infant adoption; produces and distributes informational materials and publications, and makes referrals to other information centers.

**Food and Drug Administration**
Office of Consumer Affairs
5600 Fishers Lane (HFN- 88)
Rockville, MD 20857
(301) 443-3170

Responds to consumers' inquiries and provides information and publications concerning foods, drugs and medications.

**Food and Nutrition Information Center**
National Agricultural Library
Room 304
Beltsville, MD 20705
(301) 344-3719

Responds to inquiries and provides information, publications and audiovisual materials on topics such as nutrition, food service management, food technology, and nutrition for adolescents with particular emphasis on adolescent pregnancy. Publications are geared for professionals, educators and consumers.

**Food and Nutrition Service**
Office of Public Information
3101 Park Center Drive
Alexandria, VA 22302
(703) 756-3281

Responds to inquiries and provides information and publications on federal maternal and child nutrition programs such as the Special Supplemental Food Programs for Women, Infants and Children (WIC).

**Health Care Financing Administration**
Office of Public Affairs
Hubert H. Humphrey Building
330 Independence Avenue, SW
Room 4235
Washington, DC 20201
(202) 245-6161

Responds to questions concerning financing of health care for chronically ill children.

**National Cancer Institute**
Cancer Information Center
9000 Rockville Pike
Bethesda, MD 20892
(800) 4-CANCER
(301) 496-5583

Responds to inquiries from the general public and professionals and disseminates publications on cancer.

**National Center for Clinical Infant Programs**
733 15th Street, NW
Suite 912
Washington, DC 20005
(202) 347-0308

Supports professional initiatives in infant health, mental health and development. Project Zero to Three, funded by the Bureau of Maternal and Child Health and Resources Development, focuses on infants who are disabled or at risk. Publications are available on clinical issues targeted at disciplines concerned with infants, toddlers and their families.

**National Center for Education in Maternal and Child Health**
38th and R Streets, NW
Washington, DC 20057
(202) 625-8400

Responds to inquiries with publications, information packets and referrals for questions concerning pregnancy and childbirth, adolescent health and pregnancy, child health and development, disorders and disabling conditions, genetic disorders, genetic counseling, prenatal diagnosis and women's health topics. Provides a number of services, including maintaining a resource center of educational materials and publishing a variety of guides, directories, bibliographies and newsletters. Serves as a major link between sources of information and services and the professional in areas of maternal and child health.

**National Center for Health Services Research and Health Care Technology Assessment**
5600 Fishers Lane
Room 1812
Rockville, MD 20857
(301) 443-4100

Evaluates health services, assesses technologies and sponsors and conducts research on health care delivery. Findings are disseminated through publications and bibliographies.

**National Center for Health Statistics**
Scientific and Technical Information Branch
Division of Data Services
3700 East-West Highway
Room 1- 57
Hyattsville, MD 20782
(301) 436-8500

Responds to inquiries from consumers and professionals; maintains data files containing information on vital statistics, birth and mortality surveys and utilization of health resources; collects statistical data on low birthweight infants and infant mortality; produces statistical reports and publications on high risk infants. Data from surveys and studies are presented in a variety of publications.

**National Center for Youth with Disabilities**
Adolescent Health Program
University of Minnesota
Box 721 - UMHC
Harvard Street at East River Road
Minneapolis, MN 55455
(612) 626-2825

Provides a library that includes major health publications since 1980 relating to youth with chronic illness and/or disability, model programs and projects, and training and educational materials pertaining to these issues; provides a network of professionals with expert knowledge in these areas.

**National Clearinghouse for Alcohol and Drug Information**
P.O. Box 2345
Rockville, MD 20852
(301) 468-2600

Collects and disseminates information for professionals and consumers on prevention of alcohol and drug abuse and on alcohol and drug use during pregnancy.

**National Diabetes Information Clearinghouse**
Box NDIC
Bethesda, MD 20892
(301) 468-2162

Responds to inquiries and disseminates patient education materials. Coordinates the development of materials and programs for diabetes education.

**National Digestive Diseases Information Clearinghouse**
1255 23rd Street, NW
Suite 275
Washington, DC 20037
(202) 296-1138

Develops and distributes educational materials, responds to requests for information and provides central information and educational resources on digestive diseases.

**National Eye Institute**
9000 Rockville Pike
Building 31
Room 6A- 32
Bethesda, MD 20892
(301) 496-5248

Supports and conducts research directed toward improving the prevention, diagnosis and treatment of eye disorders. Publications are available upon request, including information on institute-supported research.

**National Heart, Lung, and Blood Institute**
Information Office
9000 Rockville Pike
Building 31
Room 4A-21
Bethesda, MD 20892
(301) 496-4236

Responds to inquiries and conducts research, education and training activities on heart, blood vessel, lung and blood diseases. Develops professional and general information publications.

**National Information Center for Handicapped Children and Youth**
P.O. Box 1492
Washington, DC 20013
(703) 522- 3332
(800) 999-5599

Responds to inquiries from parents of disabled children, disabled adults and professionals regarding available services. Provides publications on handicapping conditions.

**National Institute of Allergy and Infectious Diseases**
9000 Rockville Pike
Building 31
Room 7A-32
Bethesda, MD 20892
(301) 496-5717

Responds to inquiries from consumers and professionals, provides information and publications and conducts and supports research on infectious and allergic disesases.

**National Institute of Arthritis and Musculoskeletal and Skin Diseases**
Office of Scientific and Health Reports
9000 Rockville Pike
Building 31
B2-B15 E

Bethesda, MD 20892
(301) 496-8188

Responds to inquiries from consumers and professionals, provides information and publications and conducts and supports research on arthritis, musculoskeletal disorders and skin diseases.

## National Institute of Child Health and Human Development

Office of Research Reporting
9000 Rockville Pike
Building 31
Room 2A-32
Bethesda, MD 20892
(301) 496- 5133

Responds to inquiries from consumers and professionals. Conducts and supports basic and clinical research and provides publications on topics of maternal and child health and the population sciences.

## National Institute of Dental Research

9000 Rockville Pike
Building 31
Room 2C- 35
Bethesda, MD 20892
(301) 496-8188 (publications)
(301) 496-2883 (audiovisuals)

Responds to inquiries from consumers, educators and health care professionals. Provides information and publications that focus on improving dental health.

## National Institute of Diabetes and Digestive and Kidney Diseases

9000 Rockville Pike
Building 31
Room 9A- 52
Bethesda, MD 20892
(301) 496-5877

Responds to inquiries from consumers and professionals, provides information and publications, and conducts and supports research in diabetes, digestive disorders and kidney diseases.

## National Institute of General Medical Sciences

9000 Rockville Pike
Building 31
Room 4A- 52
Bethesda, MD 20892
(301) 496-7301

Responds to inquiries from consumers and professionals and supports research in the basic biomedical sciences, including genetics and cell biology.

## National Institute of Mental Health

Public Inquiries Section
5600 Fishers Lane
Room 15C-05
Rockville, MD 20857
(301) 443-4513

Responds to inquiries from consumers and professionals, provides information and publications, and conducts and supports research on all areas of mental health and mental illness.

## National Library Service for the Blind and Physically Handicapped

1291 Taylor Street, NW
Washington, DC 20542
(202) 287-5100

Works through local and regional libraries to distribute Braille and recorded materials for persons with visual or physical impairments. Provides information on blindness and physical handicaps for professionals and consumers. A list of participating libraries is available from the National Library Service Reference Section.

## National Maternal and Child Health Clearinghouse

38th and R Streets, NW
Washington, DC 20057
(202) 625-8410

Distributes publications—on adolescent health, adolescent pregnancy, nutritional needs of adolescents, genetics, genetic disorders, genetic counseling, prenatal diagnosis and other maternal and child health topics—produced by the Divison of Maternal and Child Health and Resources Development, the Healthy Mothers/Healthy Babies Coalition, the National Center for Education in Maternal and Child Health, the National Center for Clinical Infant Programs, and others.

## National Maternal and Child Health Resource Center

College of Law Building
University of Iowa
Iowa City, IA 52242
(319) 335-9046 or 335-9067

Collects, analyzes and disseminates information about public health care programs serving mothers and children; conducts research and prepares reports about MCH services; provides consultation and technical assistance to agencies, institutions and organizations; designs education and training materials and programs with respect to children with special health care needs.

### National Resource Institute on Children with Handicaps
University of Washington, Mailstop WJ-10
Seattle, Washington 98195
(206) 543-2213

Develops and provides specialized training in developmental disabilities and the child welfare system; provides a comprehensive information resource; catalyzes team building and training among disciplines and agencies serving children with disabilities.

### National Sudden Infant Death Syndrome Clearinghouse
8201 Greensboro Drive
Suite 600
McLean, VA 22102
(703) 821-8955

Responds to inquiries and provides publications and information on sudden infant death syndrome to health professionals and consumers.

### Office for Substance Abuse Prevention
5600 Fishers Lane
Room 9A54
Rockville, MD 20857
(301) 443-0365

Responds to inquiries from consumers and professionals; develops and collects drug and alcohol abuse prevention literature and materials; sponsors regional and national workshops on the prevention of drug and alcohol abuse and operates a grant program for projects to demonstrate effective models for the prevention, treatment and rehabilitation of drug and alcohol abuse among high risk youth.

### Office of Adolescent Pregnancy Programs
Hubert H. Humphrey Building
200 Independence Avenue, SW
Room 736-E
Washington, DC 20201
(202) 245-7473

Responds to inquiries and funds demonstration programs that deliver comprehensive services to pregnant and parenting adolescents. Publishes the *Office of Adolescent Pregnancy Programs Information Bulletin* which is available to consumers and professionals.

### Office of Maternal and Child Health
5600 Fishers Lane
Room 6-05
Rockville, MD 20857
(301) 443-1080

Provides technical assistance to state MCH programs and service providers. Funds a variety of demonstration, research and training grants. Produces publications that are available from the National Maternal and Child Health Clearinghouse.

### Office of Population Affairs
Hubert H. Humphrey Building
200 Independence Avenue, SW
Room 736-E
Washington, DC 20201
(202) 245-6335

Responds to inquiries from consumers and professionals regarding the Family Planning Program and the Adolescent Family Life Program. Publications are available from Family Life Information Exchange.

### Office on Smoking and Health
Technical Information Center
5600 Fishers Lane
Room 116
Rockville, MD 20857
(301) 443-1690

Responds to inquiries from consumers and professionals, offers bibliographic and reference service to researchers and others and publishes and distributes a number of materials on smoking and health.

### President's Committee on Employment of the Handicapped
1111 29th Street, NW
Room 636
Washington, DC 20036
(202) 653-5044
TTY (202) 653-5050

Responds to inquiries, provides information and a quarterly publication and serves an advocacy and public awareness role in fostering job opportunities for the disabled.

### President's Committee on Mental Retardation
North Building
330 Independence Avenue, SW
Room 4723
Washington, DC 20201
(202) 245-7634

Responds to inquiries and serves as an advocate for mentally retarded persons.

# 4.
# REGIONAL GENETICS SERVICES NETWORKS

## COUNCIL OF REGIONAL NETWORKS FOR GENETICS SERVICES (CORN)

Greater Baltimore Medical Center
Department of Pediatrics
6701 North Charles Street
Baltimore, MD 21204
(301) 828-2780

## *GREAT PLAINS GENETIC SERVICES NETWORK (GPGSN)*

University of Iowa Hospitals and Clinics
Department of Pediatrics
Iowa City, IA 52242
(319) 356-2674

ARKANSAS
IOWA
KANSAS
MISSOURI
NEBRASKA
OKLAHOMA
NORTH DAKOTA
SOUTH DAKOTA

## *MID-ATLANTIC REGIONAL HUMAN GENETICS NETWORK (MARHGN)*

St. Christopher's Hospital for Children
Division of Medical Genetics
Fifth and Lehigh Avenue
Philadelphia, PA 19133
(215) 427-5289

DELAWARE
DISTRICT OF COLUMBIA
MARYLAND
NEW JERSEY
PENNSYLVANIA
VIRGINIA
WEST VIRGINIA

## *GREAT LAKES REGIONAL GENETICS GROUP*

Genetic Diseases Section
Division of Maternal and Child Health
1330 West Michigan Street
Indianapolis
IN 46206-1964
(317) 633-0805

ILLINOIS
INDIANA
MICHIGAN
MINNESOTA
OHIO
WISCONSIN

## *MOUNTAIN STATES REGIONAL GENETICS SERVICES NETWORK*

Colorado Department of Health
Family and Community Health Services Division
4210 East 11th Avenue
Denver, CO 80220
(303) 331-8373

ARIZONA
COLORADO
MONTANA
NEW MEXICO
UTAH
WYOMING

(continued)

## NEW ENGLAND REGIONAL GENETICS GROUP (NERGG)

Children's Hospital
Developmental Evaluation Center
300 Longwood Avenue
Boston, MA 02115
(617) 735-6509

CONNECTICUT
MAINE
MASSACHUSETTS
NEW HAMPSHIRE
RHODE ISLAND
VERMONT

## NEW YORK STATE GENETICS PROGRAM (GENES
### —Genetic Network of the Empire State)

New York State Department of Health
Wadsworth Center for Laboratories and Research
Laboratory of Human Genetics and Birth Defects
   Institute
Albany, NY 12201
(518) 474-6796

NEW YORK

## PACIFIC NORTHWEST REGIONAL GENETICS GROUP (PacNoRGG)

Oregon Health Sciences University
Crippled Children's Division
P.O. Box 574
Portland, OR 97207
(503) 279-8342

ALASKA
IDAHO
OREGON
WASHINGTON

## PACIFIC SOUTHWEST REGIONAL GENETICS NETWORK (PSRGN)

California Department of Health Services
Genetics Disease Branch
2151 Berkeley, Annex 4
Berkeley, CA 94704
(415) 540-2553

CALIFORNIA
HAWAII
NEVADA

## SOUTHEASTERN REGIONAL GENETICS GROUP (SERGG)

Emory University
School of Medicine
2040 Ridgewood Drive Building
Atlanta, GA 30322
(404) 727-5840

ALABAMA
FLORIDA
GEORGIA
KENTUCKY
LOUISIANA
MISSISSIPPI
NORTH CAROLINA
SOUTH CAROLINA
TENNESSEE

# 5.
# REGIONAL AND STATE MCH/CCS SERVICES

Standard federal administrative regions were established to achieve systematic coordination among agencies and federal-state-local governments and to facilitate improvements in management and interagency cooperation. Consultants in the areas of Nursing, Nutrition, Social Work and Maternal and Child Health Programs work with the ten Public Health Service Regional Offices to serve state MCH agencies and service providers. Some regions do not have consultants in all of these categories.

Following the lists of consultants in each region, we have listed the directors of Maternal and Child Health Services and Services for Children with Special Health Care Needs (formerly known as CCS) for each state within that region. Some states combine these functions in one office, or maintain a combined office in addition to separate offices for each program. These agencies administer Title V Block Grant MCH programs and in some cases provide other public health services.

## STANDARD FEDERAL ADMINISTRATIVE REGIONS

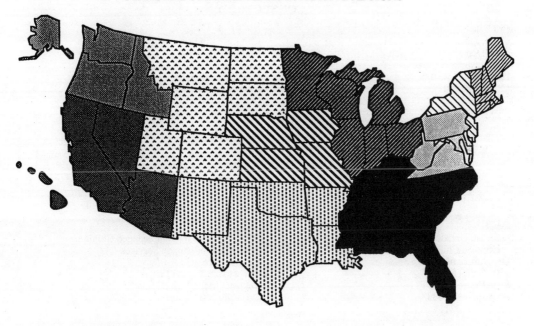

 **REGION I:** Connecticut, Maine, Massachusetts, New Hampshire, Rhode Island, Vermont

 **REGION II:** New Jersey, New York, Puerto Rico, Virgin Islands

 **REGION III:** Delaware, District of Columbia, Maryland, Pennsylvania, Virginia, West Virginia

 **REGION IV:** Alabama, Florida, Georgia, Kentucky, Mississippi, N. Carolina, S. Carolina, Tennessee

 **REGION V:** Illinois, Indiana, Michigan, Minnesota, Ohio, Wisconsin

 **REGION VI:** Arkansas, Louisiana, New Mexico, Oklahoma, Texas

 **REGION VII:** Iowa, Kansas, Missouri, Nebraska

 **REGION VIII:** Colorado, Montana, N. Dakota, S. Dakota, Utah, Wyoming

 **REGION IX:** Arizona, California, Hawaii, Nevada, Pacific Basin∗

 **REGION X:** Alaska, Idaho, Oregon, Washington

∗American Samoa, Commonwealth of the Northern Mariana Islands, Federated States of Micronesia, Guam, Republic of Belau, Republic of the Marshall Islands

# REGION I

(Connecticut, Maine, Massachusetts, New Hampshire, Rhode Island, Vermont)

## *REGIONAL CONSULTANTS*

REGIONAL NURSING CONSULTANT
JFK Federal Building, Room 1401
Boston, MA 02203
(617) 565-1461

REGIONAL NUTRITION CONSULTANT
JFK Federal Building, Room 1401
Boston, MA 02203
(617) 565-1459

REGIONAL PROGRAM CONSULTANT
JFK Federal Building, Room 1401
Boston, MA 02203
(617) 565-1460

## *STATE MCH/CCS DIRECTORS*

### CONNECTICUT

(MCH)
Chief, Maternal and Child Health
State Department of Health
150 Washington Street
Hartford, CT 06106
(203) 566- 5601

(CCS)
Chief, Health Services for Handicapped
Children's Section
State Department of Health
150 Washington Street
Hartford, CT 06106
(203) 566-2057

(MCH, CCS)
Director, Community Health Service
State Department of Health
150 Washington Street
Hartford, CT 06106
(203) 566-4282

### MAINE

(MCH)
Director, Division of Child Health and
   Crippled Children's Services
Department of Human Services
150 Capitol Street
State House-Station 11
Augusta, ME 04333
(207) 289- 3311

(CCS)
Chief, Services for Handicapped Children
Department of Human Services
150 Capitol Street
State House-Station 11
Augusta, ME 04333
(207) 289-3311

### MASSACHUSETTS

(MCH)
Maternal and Child Health Section
Massachusetts Department of Public Health
150 Tremont Street
Boston, MA 02111
(617) 727-0940

(CCS)
Handicapped Children's Section
Massachusetts Department of Public Health
150 Tremont Street
Boston, MA 02111
(617) 727-5812

(MCH, CCS)
Director, Division of Family Health
Massachusetts Department of Public Health
150 Tremont Street
Boston, MA 02111
(617) 727-3372

(continued)

## NEW HAMPSHIRE

(MCH)
Chief, Bureau of Maternal and Child Health
New Hampshire Division of Public Health
   Services
6 Hazen Drive
Concord, NH 03301-6527
(603) 271-4517

(CCS)
Chief, Handicapped Children's Services
New Hampshire Division of Public Health Services
6 Hazen Drive
Concord, NH 03301-6527
(603) 271-4596

(MHC, CCS)
Director, Office of Family and Community Health
New Hampshire Division of Public Health Services
6 Hazen Drive
Concord, NH 03301-6527
(603) 271-4726

## RHODE ISLAND

(MCH)
Chief, Division of Family Health
Department of Health
75 Davis Street, Room 302
Providence, RI 02908
(401) 277-2312

(CCS)
Services for Handicapped Children
Department of Health
75 Davis Street, Room 302
Providence, RI 02908
(401) 277-2312

## VERMONT

(MCH)
Director, Medical Services Division
Vermont Department of Health
1193 North Avenue
P.O. Box 70
Burlington, VT 05402
(802) 863-7347

(CCS)
Services for Handicapped Children
Vermont Department of Health
1193 North Avenue
P.O. Box 70
Burlington, VT 05402
(802) 863-7338

---

# REGION II

(New Jersey, New York, Puerto Rico, Virgin Islands)

## *REGIONAL CONSULTANTS*

REGIONAL NURSING CONSULTANT
Nurse Midwife Advisor
Federal Building, Room 3300
26 Federal Plaza
New York, NY 10278
(212) 264-2544

REGIONAL NUTRITION CONSULTANT
Federal Building, Room 3300
26 Federal Plaza
New York, NY 10278
(212) 264- 2708

REGIONAL PROGRAM CONSULTANT
Federal Building
26 Federal Plaza
New York, NY 10278
(212) 264-4628

REGIONAL SOCIAL WORK CONSULTANT
N.Y. Geographic Rep. for Family Planning
Federal Building
26 Federal Plaza
New York, NY 10278
(212) 264-2538

---

(continued)

## *STATE MCH/CCS DIRECTORS*

### NEW JERSEY

(MCH)
Director, Maternal and Child Health Services
New Jersey Department of Health
CN 364
Trenton, NJ 08625
(609) 292- 5656

(CCS)
Director, Special Child Health Services
120 South Stockton Street
New Jersey Department of Health
CN 364
Trenton, NJ 08625
(609) 292-5676

### NEW YORK

(MCH)
Director, Division of Family Health Services
New York State Department of Health
Tower Building, Empire State Plaza
Room 890
Albany, NY 12237
(518) 473-7922

(CCS)
Director, Bureau of Child Health
New York State Department of Health
Tower Building, Empire State Plaza
Room 878
Albany, NY 12237
(518) 474-3664

(MCH, CCS)
Director, Bureau of Reproductive Health
New York State Department of Health
Tower Building, Empire State Plaza
Room 831
Albany, NY 12237
(518) 474-3368

### PUERTO RICO

(MCH, CCS)
Director, Maternal and Child Health and Crippled Children's Programs
Commonwealth of Puerto Rico
Department of Health
Call Box 70184
San Juan, PR 00936
(809) 763-7104

### VIRGIN ISLANDS

(MCH, CCS)
Assistant Commissioner for Ambulatory Services
P.O. Box 520
Christiansted
St. Croix, VI 00820
(809) 778-6567

# REGION III

(Delaware, District of Columbia, Maryland, Pennsylvania, Virginia, West Virginia)

## *REGIONAL CONSULTANTS*

REGIONAL NURSING CONSULTANT
P.O. Box 13716, Room 4480
Philadelphia, PA 19101
(215) 596- 6686

REGIONAL NUTRITION CONSULTANT
P.O. Box 13716, Room 4479
Philadelphia, PA 19101
(215) 596- 6686

(continued)

REGIONAL PROGRAM CONSULTANT
P.O. Box 13716, Room 4489
Philadelphia, PA 19101
(215) 596-6686

REGIONAL SOCIAL WORK CONSULTANT
P.O. Box 13716, Room 4484
Philadelphia, PA 19101
(215) 596-6686

## STATE MCH/CCS DIRECTORS

### DELAWARE

(MCH)
Director, Maternal and Child Health Services
Division of Public Health
P.O. Box 637
Dover, DE 19903
(302) 736-4785

(CCS)
Director, Handicapped Children's Services
P.O. Box 637
Dover, DE 19903
(302) 736-4786

### DISTRICT OF COLUMBIA

(MCH)
Director, Maternal and Child Health Services
D.C. Office of Maternal and Child Health
1875 Connecticut Avenue, N.W.
Room 804D
Washington, DC 20009
(202) 673-6665

(CCS)
Chief, Crippled Children Unit
D.C. General Hospital
Building 10
19th & Massachusetts Avenue, S.E.
Washington, DC 20003
(202) 675-5214

### MARYLAND

(MCH)
Chief, Division of Infants, Children,
and Adolescents
Preventive Medicine Administration
State Department of Health and Mental Hygiene
201 West Preston Street, 4th Floor
Baltimore, MD 21201
(301) 225-6749

(CCS)
Chief, Children's Medical Services
Mental Retardation and Developmental Disabilities
Administration
State Department of Health and Mental Hygiene
201 West Preston Street, 4th Floor
Baltimore, MD 21201
(301) 225-5880

(MCH, CCS)
Chief, Division of Maternal Health, Family Planning, and Hereditary
Disorders
201 West Preston Street, 3rd Floor
Baltimore, MD 21201
(301) 225-6721

### PENNSYLVANIA

(MCH)
Director, Division of Maternal and Child Health
State Department of Health, Room 725
P.O. Box 90
Harrisburg, PA 17108
(717) 787-7440

(CCS)
Director, Children's Rehabilitative Services
Division of Rehabilitation
State Department of Health, Room 714
P.O. Box 90
Harrisburg, PA 17108
(717) 783-5436

### VIRGINIA

(MCH)
Director, Bureau of Maternal and Child Health
State Department of Health
109 Governor Street
Richmond, VA 23219
(804) 786-7367

(CCS)
Director, Division of Handicapped Children's
Services
State Department of Health
109 Governor Street
Richmond, VA 23219
(804) 786-3691

(continued)

## WEST VIRGINIA

(MCH)
Director, Division of Maternal and Child Health
State Department of Health
1143 Dunbar Avenue
Dunbar, WV 25064
(304) 768-6295

(CCS)
Administrative Director, Division of Handicapped
  Children
West Virginia Department of Human Services
116 Quarrier Street
Charleston, WV 25301
(304) 348-6330

# REGION IV

(Alabama, Florida, Georgia, Kentucky, Mississippi, North Carolina, South Carolina,
Tennessee)

## *REGIONAL CONSULTANTS*

REGIONAL NURSING CONSULTANT
101 Marietta Towers, Suite 1202
Atlanta, GA 30323
(404) 331- 5394

REGIONAL NUTRITION CONSULTANT
101 Marietta Towers, Suite 1202
Atlanta, GA 30323
(404) 331- 5394

ACTING REGIONAL PROGRAM
CONSULTANT
101 Marietta Towers, Suite 1202
Atlanta, GA 30323
(404) 331- 5394

REGIONAL SOCIAL WORK
  CONSULTANT
101 Marietta Towers, Suite 1202
Atlanta, GA 30323
(404) 331- 5394

## *STATE MCH/CCS DIRECTORS*

### ALABAMA

(MCH)
Director, Division of Family Health Services
State Department of Public Health
434 Monroe Street
Montgomery, AL 36130- 1701
(205) 261-5025

(CCS)
Assistant Director, Division of Rehabilitation and
  Crippled Children's Services
2129 East South Boulevard
Montgomery, AL 36111-0586
(205) 281-8780

### FLORIDA

(MCH)
Medical Director, Maternal and Child Health
Department of Health and Rehabilitative Services
1323 Winewood Boulevard
Building 1, Room 204
Tallahassee, FL 32301
(904) 487-1321

(CCS)
Director, Children's Medical Services Program
Department of Health and Rehabilitative Services
1323 Winewood Boulevard
Building 5, Room 127
Tallahassee, FL 32301
(904) 487-2690

### GEORGIA

(MCH)
Director, Family Health Services Section
Division of Public Health
Georgia Department of Human Resources
878 Peachtree Street, N.E.
Suite 217
Atlanta, GA 30309
(404) 894-6622

(CCS)
Manager, Children's Medical Services
Georgia Department of Human Resources
878 Peachtree Street, N.E.
Suite 214
Atlanta, GA 30309
(404) 894-6604

(continued)

## KENTUCKY

(MCH)
Director, Division of Maternal and Child Health
Bureau for Health Services
State Department of Human Resources
275 East Main Street
Frankfort, KY 40621
(502) 564-4830

(CCS)
Executive Director, Commission for Handicapped
   Children
Bureau for Health Services
State Department of Human Resources
1405 East Burnett Avenue
Louisville, KY 40217
(502) 588-4459

## MISSISSIPPI

(MCH)
Chief, Bureau of Personal Health Services
P.O. Box 1700
Jackson, MS 39205
(601) 960-7463

(CCS)
Director, Children's Medical Program
State Department of Health
P.O. Box 1700
Jackson, MS 39205
(601) 960-7613

## NORTH CAROLINA

(MCH)
Chief, Maternal and Child Care Section
Division of Health Services
P.O. Box 2091
1330 St. Mary's Street
Raleigh, NC 27602-2091
(919) 733-3816

(CCS)
Head, Developmental Disabilities Branch
Division of Health Services
P.O. Box 2091
1330 St. Mary's Street
Raleigh, NC 27602-2091
(919) 733-7437

(MCH, CCS)
Maternal and Child Health Branch
Division of Health Services
P.O. Box 2091
1330 St. Mary's Street
Raleigh, NC 27602-2091
(919) 733-7791

## SOUTH CAROLINA

(MCH)
Director, Bureau of Maternal and Child Health
Department of Health and Environmental Control
2600 Bull Street
Columbia, SC 29201
(803) 734-4670

(CCS)
Director, Division of Children's Health and Rehabilitative Services
Department of Health and Environmental Control
2600 Bull Street
Columbia, SC 29201
(803) 734-4739

(MCH, CCS)
Director, Division of Maternal Health and Family Planning
Department of Health and Environmental Control
2600 Bull Street
Columbia, SC 29201

## TENNESSEE

(MCH)
Medical Director, Maternal and
   Child Health Section
Tennessee Department of Health and Environment
100 9th Avenue North
Nashville, TN 37219-5405
(615) 741-7353

(CCS)
Director, Crippled Children's Services
Tennessee Department of Health and Environment
100 9th Avenue North
Nashville, TN 37219- 5405
(615) 741-7353

(continued)

# REGION V

(Illinois, Indiana, Michigan, Minnesota, Ohio, Wisconsin)

## REGIONAL CONSULTANTS

REGIONAL NURSING CONSULTANT
300 South Wacker Drive, 34th Floor
Chicago, IL 60606
(312) 353-1700

REGIONAL NUTRITIONAL CONSULTANT
300 South Wacker Drive, 34th Floor
Chicago, IL 60606
(312) 353-1700

REGIONAL PROGRAM CONSULTANT
300 South Wacker Drive, 34th Floor
Chicago, IL 60606
(312) 353-1700

REGIONAL SOCIAL WORK CONSULTANT
300 South Wacker Drive, 34th Floor
Chicago, IL 60606
(312) 353-1700

## STATE MCH/CCS DIRECTORS

### ILLINOIS

(MCH)
Chief, Division of Family Health
Department of Public Health
535 West Jefferson Street
Springfield, IL 62761
(217) 782-2736

(CCS)
Director, Division of Services for Crippled Children
University of Illinois at Chicago
2040 Hill Meadows Drive, Suite A
Springfield, IL 62702-4698
(217) 793-2340

### INDIANA

(MCH)
Director, Maternal and Child Health
State Board of Health
1330 West Michigan Street, P.O. Box 1964
Indianapolis, IN 46206
(317) 633-0170

(CCS)
Director, Division of Services for Crippled Children
State Department of Public Welfare
141 South Meridian Street
Indianapolis, IN 46225
(317) 232-4283

### MICHIGAN

(MCH)
Chief, State of Michigan Bureau of
    Community Services
Michigan Department of Public Health
3500 North Logan Street
P.O. Box 30035
Lansing, MI 48909
(517) 335-8955

(CCS)
Chief, Division of Services to Crippled Children
Bureau of Community Services
Michigan Department of Public Health
3500 North Logan Street
P.O. Box 30035
Lansing, MI 48909
(517) 335- 8961

### MINNESOTA

(MCH, CCS)
Director, Division of Maternal and Child Health
Department of Health
717 Delaware Street, S.E.
Minneapolis, MN 55440
(612) 623-5166

(continued)

## OHIO

(MCH, CCS)
Chief, Division of Maternal and Child Health
State Department of Health
246 North High Street
Columbus, OH 43266-0118
(614) 466-3263

## WISCONSIN

(MCH)
Supervisor, Maternal and Child Health Unit
Family and Community Health Section
Wisconsin Division of Health
P.O. Box 309
1 West Wilson Street
Madison, WI 53701
(608) 266- 2670

(CCS)
Director, Bureau for Children with Physical Needs
P.O. Box 7841
125 South Webster Street
Madison, WI 53702
(608) 266-3886

# REGION VI

(Arkansas, Louisiana, New Mexico, Oklahoma, Texas)

## *REGIONAL CONSULTANTS*

REGIONAL NURSING CONSULTANT
1200 Main Tower Building, Room 1835
Dallas, TX 75202
(214)767-3903

REGIONAL NUTRITION CONSULTANT
1200 Main Tower Building, Room 1835
Dallas, TX 75202
(214) 767-6538

REGIONAL PROGRAM CONSULTANT
1200 Main Tower Building, Room 1835
Dallas, TX 75202
(214) 767-7337

REGIONAL SOCIAL WORK CONSULTANT
1200 Main Tower Building, Room 1835
Dallas, TX 75202
(214) 767-7337

## *STATE MCH/CCS DIRECTORS*

### ARKANSAS

(MCH)
Director, Division of Maternal and Child Health
State Health Department
4815 West Markham
Little Rock, AR 72201
(501) 661-2762

(CCS)
Medical Director, Crippled Children's Section
  of Social Services
Department of Human Services
P.O. Box 1437
Little Rock, AR 72203
(501) 371-2277

### LOUISIANA

(MCH)
Administrator, Maternal and Child Health Section
Office of Preventive and Public Health Services
P.O. Box 60630
New Orleans, LA 70160
(504) 568-5070

(CCS)
Administrator, Handicapped Children's Services
Office of Preventive and Public Health Services
Department of Health and Human Resources
P.O. Box 60630
New Orleans, LA 70160
(504) 568-5070

(continued)

## NEW MEXICO

(MCH, CCS)
Maternal and Child Health Bureau
Health and Environment Department
1190 St. Francis Drive
Santa Fe, NM 87504
(505) 827-2350

## OKLAHOMA

(MCH)
Medical Director, Maternal and Child Health Services
State Department of Health
1000 N.E. 10th Street, Room 703
Oklahoma City, OK 73152
(405) 271-4476

(CCS)
Assistant Director,
Children's Medical Services
Medical Services Division
Department of Human Services
4001 North Lincoln Boulevard, 4th Floor
Oklahoma City, OK 73105
(405) 521-3902

## TEXAS

(MCH)
Director, Division of Maternal and Child Health
Texas Department of Health
1100 West 49th Street
Austin, TX 78756
(512) 458-7321

(CCS)
Director, Crippled Children's Program
Texas Department of Health
1100 West 49th Street
Austin, TX 78756
(512) 458-2680

---

# REGION VII

(Iowa, Kansas, Missouri, Nebraska)

## *REGIONAL CONSULTANTS*

REGIONAL NURSING CONSULTANT
New Federal Office Building
601 East 12th Street
Kansas City, MO 64106
(816) 374-2924

REGIONAL NUTRITION CONSULTANT
New Federal Office Building
601 East 12th Street, Fifth Floor West
Kansas City, MO 64106
(816) 374-2916

REGIONAL PROGRAM CONSULTANT
New Federal Office Building
601 East 12th Street, Fifth Floor West
Kansas City, MO 64106
(816) 374-2924

REGIONAL SOCIAL WORK CONSULTANT
New Federal Office Building
601 East 12th Street, Fifth Floor West
Kansas City, MO 64106
(816) 758-3915

## *STATE MCH/CCS DIRECTORS*

## IOWA

(MCH)
Deputy Commissioner, Division of Family
   and Community Health
Iowa Department of Health
Lucas State Office Building
Des Moines, IA 50319-0075
(515) 281-4910

(CCS)
Director, Iowa Child Health Specialty Clinics
Hospital School Building, Room 241
Iowa City, IA 52242
(319) 353-4431

---

(continued)

## KANSAS

(MCH)
Director, Bureau of Family Health
Kansas Department of Health and Environment
Landon State Office Building, 10th Floor
900 S.W. Jackson
Topeka, KS 66620-0001
(913) 296-1300

(CCS)
Director, Crippled and Chronically Ill Children's
  Programs
Kansas Department of Health and Environment
Landon State Office Building, 10th Floor
900 S.W. Jackson
Topeka, KS 66620-0001
(913) 296-1310

(MCH, CCS)
Kansas State Department of Health
State Office Building
Topeka, KS 66612
(913) 296-3506

## MISSOURI

(MCH, CCS)
Director, Division of Personal Health Services
Missouri Department of Health
1738 East Elm
P.O. Box 570
Jefferson City, MO 65102
(314) 751-6174

## NEBRASKA

(MCH)
Director, Bureau of Medical Services and Grants
State Department of Health
301 Centennial Mall South, 3rd Floor
P.O. Box 95007
Lincoln, NE 68509
(402) 471-3980

(CCS)
Medical Consultant, Medically Handicapped
  Children's Program
Nebraska Department of Social Services
301 Centennial Mall South, 5th Floor
Lincoln, NE 68509
(402) 471-9283

# REGION VIII

(Colorado, Montana, North Dakota, South Dakota, Utah, Wyoming)

## *REGIONAL CONSULTANTS*

REGIONAL NURSING CONSULTANT
Federal Office Building
1961 Stout Street, Room 11037
Denver, CO 80294
(303) 844-5955

REGIONAL NUTRITION CONSULTANT
Federal Office Building
1961 Stout Street, Room 1194
Denver, CO 80294
(303) 844-5955

REGIONAL PROGRAM CONSULTANT
Federal Office Building
1961 Stout Street, Room 11037
Denver, CO 80294
(303) 844-5955

(continued)

## *STATE MCH/CCS DIRECTORS*

### COLORADO

(MCH)
Director, Family Health Services Division
Colorado Department of Health
4210 East 11th Avenue
Denver, CO 80220
(303) 331-8359

(CCS)
Crippled Children's Program
Colorado Department of Health
4210 East 11th Avenue
Denver, CO 80220
(303) 331- 8404

(MCH, CCS)
Director, Medical Affairs and Special Programs
Colorado Department of Health
4210 East 11th Avenue
Denver, CO 80220
(303) 331-8373

### MONTANA

(MCH)
Perinatal Program
Health Services and Medical Facilities Division
Department of Health and Environmental Sciences
Cogswell Building
Helena, MT 59260
(406) 444-4740

(CCS)
Chief, Clinical Programs Bureau
Health Services and Medical Facilities Division
Department of Health and Environmental Sciences
Cogswell Building
Helena, MT 59620
(406) 444-4740

### NORTH DAKOTA

(MCH)
Director, Division of Maternal and Child Health
State Department of Health
State Capitol Building
Bismarck, ND 58505
(701) 224-2493

(CCS)
Administrator, Crippled Children's Program
Department of Human Services
State Capitol Building
Bismarck, ND 58505
(701) 224-2436

### SOUTH DAKOTA

(MCH, CCS)
Program Director, Maternal and Child Health and Crippled Children's
    Services Program
Division of Health Services
South Dakota State Department of Health
Joe Foss Building, Room 314
523 East Capitol Street
Pierre, SD 57501
(605) 773-3737

### UTAH

(MCH)
Director, Maternal and Infant Health Bureau
Division of Family Health Services
Utah Department of Health
44 Medical Drive
Salt Lake City, UT 84113
(801) 538-4084

(CCS)
Director, Handicapped Children's Services Bureau
Division of Family Health Services
Utah Department of Health
288 North 1460 West
Salt Lake City, UT 84116
(801) 538-6165

(continued)

(MCH, CCS)
Director, Division of Family Health Services
Utah Department of Health
288 North 1460 West
Salt Lake City, UT 84116-0700
(801) 538-6161

## WYOMING

(MCH)
Administrator, Division of Health and
  Medical Services
State Department of Health and Social Services
Hathaway Office Building
Cheyenne, WY 82002
(307) 777-6296

(CCS)
Administrator, Children's Health Services
Division of Health and Medical Services
State Department of Health and Social Services
Hathaway Office Building
Cheyenne, WY 82002
(307) 777-6296

---

# REGION IX

(American Samoa, Arizona, California, Comlth of the Northern Mariana Islands, Federated States of Micronesia, Guam, Hawaii, Nevada, Republic of Belau, Republic of  the Marshall Islands)

## *REGIONAL CONSULTANTS*

REGIONAL NURSING CONSULTANT
Federal Office Building
50 United Nations Plaza
San Francisco, CA 94102
(415) 556-5185

REGIONAL NUTRITION CONSULTANT
Federal Office Building
50 United Nations Plaza, Room 351
San Francisco, CA 94102
(415) 556-1097

REGIONAL PROGRAM CONSULTANT
Federal Office Building
50 United Nations Plaza, Room 306
San Francisco, CA 94102
(415) 556-7370

REGIONAL SOCIAL WORK CONSULTANT
Federal Office Building, Room 347
50 United Nations Plaza
San Francisco, CA 94102
(415) 556-4926

## *STATE MCH/CCS DIRECTORS*

### AMERICAN SAMOA

(MCH, CCS)
Director of Health Services
Department of Health
Pago Pago, American Samoa 96799
(go through overseas operator, [684] 633-5743)

### ARIZONA

(MCH)
Assistant Director, Division of Family
  Health Services
Bureau of Maternal and Child Health
State Department of Health
1740 West Adams
Phoenix, AZ 85007
(602) 255-1223

(CCS)
Manager, Office of Children's Rehabilitative Services
State Department of Health
1740 West Adams, Room 205
Phoenix, AZ 85007
(602) 255-1860

---

(continued)

(MCH, CCS)
Chief, Maternal and Child Health
State Department of Health
1740 West Adams
Phoenix, AZ 85007
(602) 255-1870

## CALIFORNIA

(MCH)
Chief, Maternal and Child Health Branch
State Department of Health
714 P Street, Room 740
Sacramento, CA 95814
(916) 323-3096

(CCS)
California Children's Services
State Department of Health
714 P Street, Room 323
Sacramento, CA 95814
(916) 322-2090

## COMMONWEALTH OF THE NORTHERN MARIANA ISLANDS

(MCH, CCS)
Director, Department of Public Health and Environmental Services
Commonwealth of the Northern Mariana Islands
Saipan, Mariana Islands 96950
(go through overseas operator, [670] 234-8950)

## FEDERATED STATES OF MICRONESIA

(MCH, CCS)
Chief, Bureau of Health Services
Government of the Federated States of Micronesia
Kolonia, Ponape
Eastern Caroline Islands 96941
Telex 729-6807

## GUAM

(MCH, CCS)
Director, Department of Public Health and Social Services
Government of Guam
P.O. Box 2816
Agana, Guam 96910
(go through overseas operator, [671] 734-9910)

## HAWAII

(MCH)
Chief, Maternal and Child Health Branch
State of Hawaii Department of Health
741-A Sunset Avenue
Honolulu, HI 96816
(808) 548-6554

(CCS)
Chief, Crippled Children's Services Branch
State of Hawaii Department of Health
741-A Sunset Avenue
Honolulu, HI 96816
(808) 732-3197

(MCH, CCS)
Director, Family Health Services Division
3652 Kilauea Avenue
Honolulu, HI 96816
(808) 548-6574

## NEVADA

(MCH, CCS)
Administrator, Division of Health
State Department of Human Resources
505 East King Street, Room 205
Carson City, NV 89710
(702) 885-4885

(continued)

## REPUBLIC OF BELAU

(MCH, CCS)
Director, Bureau of Health Services
Republic of Belau
MacDonald Memorial Hospital
Koror, Palau 96940

## REPUBLIC OF THE MARSHALL ISLANDS

(MCH, CCS)
Minister of Health
Republic of the Marshall Islands
Majuro, Marshall Islands 96940

# REGION X

(Alaska, Idaho, Oregon, Washington)

## *REGIONAL CONSULTANTS*

REGIONAL NURSING CONSULTANT
2901 Third Avenue, MS 405
Seattle, WA 98121
(206) 442-1020

REGIONAL NUTRITION CONSULTANT
2901 Third Avenue, MS 405
Seattle, WA 98121
(206) 442-1020

REGIONAL PROGRAM CONSULTANT
2901 Third Avenue, MS 405
Seattle, WA 98121
(206) 442-1020

REGIONAL SOCIAL WORK CONSULTANT
Regional Medical Social Work Consultant
   for Maternal and Child Health
50 United Nations Plaza
Federal Office Building, Room 347
San Francisco, CA 94102
(415) 556-4926

## *STATE MCH/CCS DIRECTORS*

### ALASKA

(MCH, CCS)
Chief, Family Health Section
Department of Health and Social Services
1231 Gamble Street, Room 314
Anchorage, AK 99501-4627
(807) 274-7626

### IDAHO

(MCH, CCS)
Chief, Bureau of Child Health
Idaho Department of Health and Welfare
450 West State Street
Boise, ID 83720
(208) 334-5968

(continued)

# OREGON

(MCH)
Chief, Office of Health Services
Oregon State Health Division
P.O. Box 231
Portland, OR 97207
(503) 229-6380

(CCS)
Director, Crippled Children's Division
Oregon Health Sciences University
P.O. Box 574
Portland, OR 97207
(503) 225-8362

# WASHINGTON

(MCH, CCS)
Director, Bureau of Parent-Child Health Services
Department of Social and Health Services
Airdustrial Park Building 3
Olympia, WA 98504
(206) 753-7021

# 6.
# STATE TREATMENT CENTERS FOR METABOLIC DISORDERS

## ALABAMA

### Birmingham

Sparks Center for Developmental and Learning
  Disorders
University of Alabama–Birmingham
1720 7th Avenue South
Birmingham, AL 35294
(205) 934-5471

### Mobile

University of South Alabama Medical
  College–Mobile
Department of Neurology
Section of Pediatric Neurology
1100 Moorer Building
2451 Fillingim Street
Mobile, AL 36617
(205) 471-2159

## ALASKA

### Juneau

Alaska Department of Health and Special Services
Division of Public Health
Section of Family Health
P.O. Box H-06B
Juneau, AK 99811
(907) 465-3100

## ARIZONA

### Scottsdale

The Genetics Center of the Southwest
  Biomedical Research Institute
6401 Thomas Road
Scottsdale, AZ 85281
(602) 945-4363

### Tucson

Arizona Health Sciences Center
1501 North Campbell
Tucson, AZ 85724
(802) 626-6303

## ARKANSAS

### Little Rock

State Department of Health
Child Health Services

4815 West Markham
Little Rock, AR 72205-3867
(501) 661-2251

Arkansas Children's Hospital and
  University of Arkansas Medical Sciences
4301 West Markham, 512-B
Little Rock, AK 72205
(501) 661-6412

## CALIFORNIA

### Davis

University of California–Davis Medical Center
California Children Services Center for
  Endocrine and Metabolic Disorders
Department of Pediatrics
Davis, CA 95616

Mail Address:    4301 S Street
                 Sacramento, CA 95817 or
Street Address:  2315 Stockton Boulevard
                 Sacramento, CA 95817
                 (916) 453-3112

### Fresno

Valley Children's Hospital
Medical Genetics–PKU Program
3151 North Millbrook Avenue
Fresno, CA 93703
(209) 225-3000, x 234

### Loma Linda

Loma Linda University Medical Center
Metabolic Clinic
Department of Pediatrics/Genetics Division
11234 Anderson Street
Loma Linda, CA 92354
(714) 796-7311, x 2838

### Los Angeles

Children's Hospital of Los Angeles
Medical Genetics Clinic
4650 Sunset Boulevard
Los Angeles, CA 90027
(213) 669-2178

Kaiser Permanente Medical Group
  –Southern California

Regional Metabolic Center
4733 Sunset Boulevard, Room 101
Los Angeles, CA 90027
(213) 667-5316/667- 8868
(714) 829-5425/829-5496

Los Angeles County/University of
  Southern California Medical Center
General Laboratories for Basic and
  Clinical Research,  Room 1G24
1129 North State Street
Los Angeles, CA 90033
(213) 226-3816

University of California–Los Angeles
  Hospitals and Clinics
Newborn Screening Program, Genetics
Department of Pediatrics MDCC 22-499
10833 Le Conte Avenue
Los Angeles, CA 90024
(213) 825-0402/206-6581

*Oakland*

Children's Hospital of the East Bay
Child Development Center
756 52nd Street
Building K
Oakland, CA 94609
(415) 428-3351

Kaiser Permanente Medical Group
  –Northern California
Regional Metabolic Center
280 West MacArthur Boulevard
Oakland, CA 94611
(415) 428-5783

*Orange*

University of California–Irvine Medical Center
Inborn Errors Clinic
Department of Pediatrics/Genetics Division
Route 81, Building 27
101 City Drive, South
Orange, CA 92668
(714) 634-5791/634-6616

*San Diego*

San Diego/Imperial Counties Developmental
  Services, Inc.
4355 Ruffin Road
Suite 205
San Diego, CA 92123- 1648
(619) 576-2932

*San Francisco*

University of California–School of Medicine,
  Department of Pediatrics
PKU & Other Errors of Metabolism Center
HSE 1556
San Francisco, CA 94143
(415) 476-2871/476- 5048

*Stanford*

Stanford Medical Center
Department of Pediatrics, Room F322
300 Pasteur Drive
Stanford, CA 94305
(415) 723- 5791

*Torrance*

Harbor–University of California-Los Angeles
  Medical Center
Medical Genetics-E4
1000 West Carson Street
Torrance, CA 90509
(213) 533-3751

## COLORADO

*Denver*

University of Colorado Health Sciences Center
Inherited Metabolic Diseases Clinic
4200 East Ninth Avenue, Box C233
Denver, CO 80262
(303) 394-7037

## CONNECTICUT

*Farmington*

University of Connecticut
Department of Pediatrics/Genetics Division
Farmington, CT 06032
(203) 674- 2676

*New Haven*

Yale University School of Medicine
Genetic Consultation Service
Department of Human Genetics
333 Cedar Street
New Haven, CT 06510
(203) 785-2660

## DELAWARE

*Wilmington*

Alfred I. DuPont Institute
Department of Developmental Medicine
Box 269
Wilmington, DE 19899
(302) 651-4500

## DISTRICT OF COLUMBIA

### Washington

Children's Hospital National Medical Center
Metabolic Clinic
1111 Michigan Avenue, N.W.
Washington, DC 20010
202) 745-2121

Georgetown University Hospital
Center for Genetic Counseling and
   Birth Defects Evaluation
Department of Pediatrics
3800 Reservoir Road, N.W.
Washington, DC 20007
(202) 625-2348

Howard University Hospital
Department of Pediatrics
2041 Georgia Avenue, N.W.
Washington, DC 20060
(202) 745-1592

## FLORIDA

### Gainesville

Regional Genetics Center
Department of Pediatrics/Genetics Division
Box J-296
J. Hillis Miller Health Center
Gainesville, FL 32610
(904) 392-4104

### Miami

University of Miami
Newborn Screening and Follow-up Program
P.O. Box 016820
Miami, FL 33101

Street Address:   1601 N.W. 12th Avenue
                  Miami, FL 33101
                  (305) 547-6091/547-6006

### Tampa

University of South Florida College of Medicine
Metabolic Disease Section
Regional Metabolic Disease Program
Box 15
Tampa, FL 33612

Street Address:   12901 Bruce B. Downs Blvd.
                  Tampa, FL 33612
                  (813) 974-4214/974-4360

## GEORGIA

### Atlanta

Emory University School of Medicine
Department of Pediatrics/Medical Genetics
   Division
2040 Ridgewood Drive, N.E.
Atlanta, GA 30322
(404) 727-5840

### Augusta

Medical College of Georgia
Genetics and Growth Clinic
Department of Pediatrics
Augusta, GA 30912- 3770
(404) 828-4159/828-2191

## HAWAII

### Honolulu

Medical Genetics Services
1310 Punahou Street
Honolulu, HI 96826
(808) 948-6834/948-6872

## IDAHO

### Boise

State Department of Health and Welfare
Bureau of Child Health
450 West State Street
Boise, ID 83720
(208) 334-5968

## ILLINOIS

### Chicago

University of Illinois at Chicago
Department of Pediatrics
Box 6998
Clinical Sciences Building, Room 1311 N.
Chicago, IL 60680
(312) 996-5305/996-6326

Children's Memorial Hospital
PKU and Metabolic Clinic
2300 Children's Plaza
Chicago, IL 60614
(312) 880- 4012

Rush-Presbyterian-St. Luke's Medical Center
Department of Pediatrics/Genetics Section
1753 West Congress Parkway
Chicago, IL 60612
(312) 942-6299

## INDIANA

### *Indianapolis*

Indiana University Medical Center
James Whitcomb Riley Hospital for Children
Metabolism Clinic, Room A36
702 Barnhill Drive
Indianapolis, IN 46223
(317) 274-3966

## IOWA

### *Iowa City*

University of Iowa Hospitals and Clinics
University Hospital School
Metabolic Management Clinic
Iowa City, IA 52242
(319) 356-2674

## KANSAS

### *Kansas City*

University of Kansas Medical Center
H.C. Miller Building, Room 247
39th and Rainbow
Kansas City, KS 66103
(913) 588-5908

### *Wichita*

University of Kansas School of Medicine–Wichita
Genetic Clinic
1010 North Kansas
Wichita, KS 67214
(316) 261-2622

## KENTUCKY

### *Lexington*

University of Kentucky Medical Center
Department of Pediatrics, MN 480
Endocrine-Metabolic Division
Lexington, KY 40536
(606) 233-5404

### *Louisville*

University of Louisville School of Medicine
Inborn Errors of Metabolism
Department of Pediatrics
Louisville, KY 40292
(502) 562-8825

## LOUISIANA

### *New Orleans*

State Department of Health and Human Resources
Office of Preventive and Public Health Services
Genetic Disease Program
P.O. Box 60630, Room 613
New Orleans, LA 70160

Street Address:  325 Loyola Avenue
New Orleans, LA 70112
(504) 568-5075/568-5070
Tulane Medical Center
Human Genetics Program
1430 Tulane Avenue
New Orleans, LA 70112
(504) 588-5229

## MAINE

### *Bangor*

Eastern Maine Medical Center
Genetics Program
489 State Street
Bangor, ME 04401
(207) 945-7354

### *Scarborough*

Foundation for Blood Research
Metabolic Disease Program/Clinical Genetics
P.O. Box 190
Scarborough, ME 04074
(207) 883-4362

## MARYLAND

### *Baltimore*

Bressler Research Laboratory
655 W. Baltimore St.
Baltimore, MD 21201

Directors:  Miriam Blitzler, Ph.D.
Marcia Schwartz, M.D., Ph.D.
(301) 328-3480
Johns Hopkins Hospital
Pediatric Genetics Clinic
1004 Children's Medical and Surgical Center
Baltimore, MD 21205

Street Address:  600 North Wolfe Street
Baltimore, MD 21205
(301) 955-3071/955-3000

## MASSACHUSETTS

### *Boston*

New England Medical Center Hospital
Amino Acid Disorders Clinic
171 Harrison Avenue
Boston, MA 02111
(617) 956-5531/956-5532

Children's Hospital Medical Center
Inborn Errors of Metabolism/PKU Program
283 Longwood Avenue, Gardiner 6-Room 650
Boston, MA 02115
(617) 735-7945

## MICHIGAN

### Ann Arbor

University of Michigan Medical Center
Pediatric Metabolic Disease Center
Section of Pediatric Neurology
Box 0800, C7123 University Hospital
Ann Arbor, MI 48105
(313) 763-4697

### Detroit

University Health Center
Clinic for Genetic, Metabolic, and
    Developmental Disorders
4701 St. Antoine St.
Detroit, MI 48201
(313) 745-6035

## MINNESOTA

### Minneapolis

University Hospital
Pediatric Clinic-PKU
420 Delaware Street, S.E.
Box 384
Minneapolis, MN 55455
(612) 626-6777

### Rochester

Mayo Clinic
Department of Medical Genetics
Rochester, MN 55905
(507) 284-8397

## MISSISSIPPI

### Jackson

University Medical Center
Department of Preventive Medicine/Medical
    Genetics Division
2500 North State Street
Jackson, MS 39216
(601) 984-1900

## MISSOURI

### Columbia

University of Missouri Health Sciences Center
G-I Metabolism Clinic
Department of Child Health
1 Hospital Drive

Columbia, MO 65212
(314) 882-3996

### Kansas City

Children's Mercy Hospital
Genetic Counseling Center
Section of Genetics
24th at Gillham
Kansas City, MO 64108
(816) 234-3290

### St. Louis

Cardinal Glennon Memorial Hospital for Children
PKU Clinic
1465 South Grand Boulevard
St. Louis, MO 63104
(314) 391-6300

St. Louis Children's Hospital
Washington University School of Medicine
Department of Pediatrics
P.O. Box 1478
St. Louis, MO 63178

Street Address:   400 South Kings Highway
                  St. Louis, MO 63110
                  (314) 454-6093

## MONTANA

### Helena

State Department of Health and Environmental
    Sciences
Maternal and Child Health Bureau
Cogswell Building
Helena, MT 59620
(406) 444-4740

## NEBRASKA

### Omaha

University of Nebraska Medical Center
Pediatric Metabolic Clinic
42nd and Dewey
Omaha, NE 68105
(402) 559- 7350/559-5281

## NEVADA

Contact State Newborn Screening Director for referral.

## NEW HAMPSHIRE

Contact State Newborn Screening Director for referral.

## NEW JERSEY

### Camden

Cooper-Bancroft PKU Program
Cooper Hospital University Medical Center
1 Cooper Plaza
Camden, NJ 08103
(609) 342-2226

Cooper Hospital/University Medical Center
Department of Pediatrics
Division of Pediatric Endocrinology
3 Cooper Plaza
Camden, NJ 08103
(609) 342-2260

### Newark

Children's Hospital of New Jersey
15 South 9th Street
Newark, NJ 07107
(201) 268-8763/279-6273
(201) 268- 8337

University of Medicine and Dentistry of
    New Jersey
Biochemical Genetics Laboratory
100 Bergen Street, Room F545
Medical Science Building
Newark, NJ 07103
(201) 456-5278

### New Brunswick

St. Peter's Medical Center
University Medical and Dental School of
    New Jersey–Rutgers Medical School
Department of Endocrinology
254 Easton Avenue
New Brunswick, NJ 08901
(201) 745-8600, x 8574

## NEW MEXICO

### Albuquerque

New Mexico Scientific Laboratory Division
700 Camino De Salud, N.E.
(505) 982-4564

University of New Mexico Medical Center
Endocrine Clinic
2211 Lomas Boulevard
Albuquerque, NM 87131
(505) 277-4842

## NEW YORK

### Albany

Albany Medical Center Hospital
Inherited Metabolic Disease Treatment Center
47 New Scotland Avenue
Albany, NY 12208
(518) 445-5723

### Buffalo

Robert Warner Rehabilitaiton Center
PKU Clinic
936 Delaware Avenue
Buffalo, NY 14209
(716) 878-7595

Children's Hospital of Buffalo
Metabolic Clinic
219 Bryant Street
Buffalo, NY 14222
(716) 878-7442

### New York

New York University Medical Center
Inherited Metabolic Disease Treatment Center
550 1st Avenue
New York, NY 10016
(212) 340-6266

### Rochester

Strong Memorial Hospital
Inherited Metabolic Disease Treatment Center
Box 777
601 Elmwood Avenue
Rochester, NY 14642
(716) 275-7744

### Stony Brook

State University of New York, Stony Brook–
    School of Medicine
Health Sciences Center
Inherited Metabolic Disease Treatment Center
Department of Pediatrics
Stony Brook, NY 11794-8111
(516) 444-2700

## NORTH CAROLINA

### Chapel Hill

University of North Carolina School of Medicine
Department of Pediatrics
Metabolic/Genetic Division
Chapel Hill, NC 27514
(919) 966-4202

*Charlotte*

Charlotte Memorial Hospital and Medical Center
Clinical Genetics Program
P.O. Box 32861
Charlotte, NC 28232
(704) 338-3156

*Durham*

Duke University Medical Center
Division of Genetics and Metabolism
Box 3028
Durham, NC 27710
(919) 684- 2036/684-3729

*Winston-Salem*

Bowman Gray School of Medicine
Genetic Clinic
Department of Pediatrics/Medical Genetics Section
300 South Hawthorne Road
Winston-Salem, NC 27103
(919) 748-4321

## NORTH DAKOTA

*Fargo*

Fargo Clinic
Pediatric Endocrine and Metabolic Disease Clinic
737 Broadway, Box 2067
Fargo, ND 58123
(701) 237-2431

*Grand Forks*

Medical Center Rehabilitation Hospital
Child Evaluation and Treatment Program
1300 South Columbia Road
Grand Forks, ND 58201
(701) 780-2477

## OHIO

*Akron*

The Children's Hospital Medical Center of Akron
PKU Clinic
281 Locust Street
Akron, OH 44308
(216) 753-0345

*Cincinnati*

Children's Hospital Research Foundation
Institute for Developmental Research
Division of Metabolic Disease
Elland and Bethesda Avenue
Cincinnati, OH 45229
(513) 559-4451

*Cleveland*

Cleveland Clinic Foundation
Pediatrics Desk A- 120
Section on Pediatric and Adolescent Endocrinology
9500 Euclid Avenue
Cleveland, OH 44106
(216) 444-6238

*Columbus*

Children's Hospital
Department of Endocrinology and Metabolism
700 Children's Drive
Columbus, OH 43205
(614) 461-2115

*Dayton*

Children's Medical Center
PKU Clinic
One Children's Plaza
Dayton, OH 45404-1815
(513) 226-8433

*Toledo*

Mercy Hospital
Department of Pediatric Endocrinology
2200 Jefferson Avenue
Toledo, OH 43624
(419) 259-1369

## OKLAHOMA

*Oklahoma City*

Oklahoma Children's Memorial Hospital
Department of Pediatrics
Genetic, Endocrinology, and Metabolic Disease
    Section
The University of Oklahoma Health Sciences Center
940 N.E. 13th Street
Oklahoma City, OK 73190
(405) 271-4401/271- 6764

*Tulsa*

Children's Medical Center
P.O. Box 35648
Tulsa, OK 74153
Street Address:    5300 East Skelly Drive
                   Tulsa, OK 74135
                   (918) 664-6000 Ext. 264 or 240

## OREGON

*Portland*

PKU and Metabolic Birth Defects Center
Child Development and Rehabilitation Center

P.O. Box 574
Portland, OR 97207

Street Address:   707 S.W. Gaines
                  Portland, OR 97207
                  (503) 225-8344

## PENNSYLVANIA

### Hershey

Milton S. Hershey Medical Center
PKU Clinic
Department of Pediatrics
P.O. Box 850
Hershey, PA 17033
(717) 531-8412

### Philadelphia

St. Christopher's Hospital for Children
Handicapped Children's Unit
PKU Program
2603 North 5th Street
Philadelphia, PA 19133
(215) 427-5464

### Pittsburgh

Children's Hospital of Pittsburgh
PKU Clinic
125 DeSoto Street
Pittsburgh, PA 15213
(412) 647-5097/621-2432

## PUERTO RICO

### San Juan

University Pediatric Hospital
Crippled Children's Clinic
GPO Box 5067
San Juan, PR 00936
(809) 763-1093

## RHODE ISLAND

### Providence

Child Development Center
Ambulatory Patient Center Building, 6th Floor
PKU Program
593 Eddy Street
Providence, RI 02902
(401) 277-5071

## SOUTH CAROLINA

### Columbia

State Department of Health and Environmental
   Control
Metabolic Disorders Screening

2600 Bull Street
Columbia, SC 29201
(803) 734-8959

### Greenwood

Greenwood Genetic Center
1 Gregor Mendel Circle
Greenwood, SC 29646
(803) 223-9311

## SOUTH DAKOTA

### Pierre

State Department of Health
Division of Health Services
523 East Capitol
Pierre, SD 57501
(605) 773-3737

## TENNESSEE

### Memphis

University of Tennessee, Memphis
Child Development Center
Inborn Errors of Metabolism Clinic
711 Jefferson
Memphis, TN 38105
(901) 528-6514

## TEXAS

### Dallas

Children's Medical Center
Metabolic Clinic
1935 Motor Street
Dallas, TX 75235
(214) 920-2085/688-3382

### Galveston

University of Texas Medical Branch
PKU Program
Department of Pediatrics
Child Development Division
Galveston, TX 77550
(409) 761-2355

### Houston

Texas Children's Hospital
Birth Defects–Genetics Center
Houston, TX 77030
(713) 791-3261/799-4795

University of Texas Medical School
Department of Pediatrics
P.O. Box 20708
Houston, TX 77225

Street Address:    6431 Fannin Street
Houston, TX 77030
(713) 797-4555/792-5330

## UTAH

### *Salt Lake City*

PKU Clinic
c/o Handicapped Children's Services
P.O. Box 16700
Salt Lake City, UT 84116-0700
(801) 581-3461

## VERMONT

### *Burlington*

Child Development Center
56 Colchester Avenue
Burlington, VT 05401
(802) 863-7315

## VIRGINIA

### *Charlottesville*

University Hospital
Department of Pediatrics/Medical Genetics
  Division
Box 386
Charlottesville, VA 22908
(804) 924-2665

### *Richmond*

Medical College of Virginia
MCV Station
P.O. Box 239
Richmond, VA 23298
(804) 786-9617

## WASHINGTON

### *Seattle*

University of Washington
Child Development and Mental Retardation Center
PKU Program
RD-20
Seattle, WA 98195
(206) 543-3370/545-1364

## WEST VIRGINIA

### *Dunbar*

State Department of Health
Division of Maternal and Child Health
1143 Dunbar Avenue
Dunbar, WV 25064
(304) 768- 6295

### *Morgantown*

West Virginia University Medical Center
Department of Pediatrics
Morgantown, WV 26506
(304) 293-4451

## WISCONSIN

### *Madison*

Waisman Center on Mental Retardation and
  Human Development
Metabolic Clinic
1500 Highland Avenue
Madison, WI 53705-2280
(608) 263-5787/263-5993

### *Marshfield*

Marshfield Clinic
Department of Pediatrics
1000 Oak Avenue
Marshfield, WI 54449
(715) 387-5185

### *Milwaukee*

Children's Hospital of Wisconsin
Child Development Center
PKU Program
P.O. Box 1997
Milwaukee, WI 53201
Street Address:    1700 W. Wisconsin Avenue
Milwaukee, WI 53233
(414) 931-4069

## WYOMING

### *Cheyenne*

State Department of Health and Social Services
Family Health Services
Hathaway Building
Cheyenne, WY 82002
(307) 777-6297

# 7.
# STATE NEWBORN SCREENING DIRECTORS

## STATE NEWBORN SCREENING DIRECTORS

### ALABAMA

MCH Clinical Director
Division of Family Health Services
State Department of Public Health
434 Monroe Street
Montgomery, AL 36130
(205) 261-5661

### ALASKA

Chief, Family Health Section
Department of Health &
  Social Services
Health and Welfare Building
Box H-06B
Juneau, AK 99811
(907) 465-3100

### ARIZONA

Children's Rehabilitative Services
Arizona Department of Health Services
1740 W. Adams, Room 205
Phoenix, AZ 85007
(602) 255-1860

### ARKANSAS

Coordinator
Division of Infant and
  Child Health
Arkansas Department of Health
4815 West Markham
Little Rock, AR 72205-3867
(501) 661-2189

### CALIFORNIA

Chief, Newborn Screening Section
Genetic Disease Branch
State Department of Health Services
2151 Berkeley Way, Annex 4
Berkeley, CA 94704
(415) 540-2534

### COLORADO

Director
Medical Affairs and Special Programs
Colorado Department of Health
4210 East 11th Avenue
Denver, CO 80220
(303) 331-3873

### CONNECTICUT

Chief, Maternal and Child
  Health Section
State Department of Health Services
150 Washington Street
Hartford, CT 06106
(203) 566-5601

### DELAWARE

Director
Maternal and Child Health
Bureau of Personal Health Services
Division of Public Health
802 Silver Lake Boulevard
Robbins Building
Dover, DE 19901
(302) 736-4785

### DISTRICT OF COLUMBIA

Divison of Medical Genetics
Department of Pediatrics and
  Child Health
Howard University College of Medicine
Washington, DC 20059
(202) 636-6380/6340

### FLORIDA

Infant Screening Metabolic Coordinator
Department of Health and
  Rehabilitative Services
Children's Medical Services
1317 Winewood Boulevard
Building 5, Room 127
Tallahassee, FL 32301
(904) 488-6005

### GEORGIA

Genetic Program Manager
Georgia Department of Human Resources
Community Health Section
878 Peachtree Street, N.E., Rm. 102
Atlanta, GA 30309
(404) 894-5307

### HAWAII

Chief
Crippled Children's Services Branch
State of Hawaii Department of Health

741-A Sunset Avenue
Honolulu, HI 96816
(808) 732-3197

## IDAHO

Genetics Program Coordinator
Idaho Department of Health and Welfare
Bureau of Labs
2220 Old Penitentiary Road
Boise, ID 83712
(208) 334-4778

## ILLINOIS

Administrator, Genetic Diseases Program
Division of Family Health
Department of Public Health
535 West Jefferson Street
Springfield, IL 62761
(217) 785-4522

## INDIANA

Chief, Genetic Diseases Section
Division of Maternal and Child Health
State Board of Health
1330 West Michigan Street
P.O. Box 1964
Indianapolis, IN 46206-1964
(317) 633- 0805

## IOWA

Administrator
Birth Defects Institute
Iowa State Department of Health
Lucas Office Building
Des Moines, IA 50319-0075
(515) 281-6646

## KANSAS

Genetic Disease Coordinator
Crippled and Chronically Ill Children's Program
Department of Health and Environment
Forbes Field
Topeka, KS 66620
(913) 862-9360, x 400

## KENTUCKY

Director, Division of Maternal and Child Health
Department of Health Services
Cabinet for Human Resources
275 East Main Street
Frankfort, KY 40621
(502) 564-4430

## LOUISIANA

Genetic Nurse Consultant
Department of Health and Human Resources
Office of Health Services and Environmental
    Quality

P.O. Box 60630
New Orleans, LA 70160
(504) 568-5075

## MAINE

Director, Newborn Screening Program
Division of Maternal and Child Health
Department of Human Services
State House, Station 11
Augusta, ME 04333
(207) 289-3311

## MARYLAND

Chief, Division of Hereditary Disorders
State Department of Health and Mental Hygiene
201 West Preston Street
Baltimore, MD 21201
(301) 225-6730

## MASSACHUSETTS

Director
New England Regional Newborn Screening Program
State Laboratory Institute
State Department of Public Health
305 South Street
Jamaica Plain, MA 02130
(617) 522- 3700, x 160

## MICHIGAN

Genetic Program Coordinator
Bureau of Community Services
Eastern Regional Division
Michigan Department of Public Health
3500 North Logan Street
P.O. Box 30035
Lansing, MI 48909
(517) 378-8892

## MINNESOTA

Administrator
Division of Laboratories
Department of Health
717 Delaware Street, S.E.
P.O. Box 9441
Minneapolis, MN 55440
(612) 623-5640

## MISSISSIPPI

Director
Genetics Project
State Department of Health
P.O. Box 1700
Jackson, MS 39215-1700
(601) 982-6571

## MISSOURI

State Coordinator for Metabolic Screening
Bureau of Maternal and Child Health

Department of Health
1730 East Elm Street
Jefferson City, MO 65101
(314) 751-4667

## MONTANA
Chief
Clinical Programs Bureau
Health Services and Medical Facilities Division
Department of Health and Environmental Sciences
Cogswell Building
Helena, MT 59620
(406) 444-4740

## NEBRASKA
Acting Director
Maternal and Child Health Division
State Department of Health
301 Centennial Mall South, 3rd Floor
P.O. Box 95007
Lincoln, NE 68509
(402) 471-2907

## NEVADA
Chief, Bureau of Community Health Services
505 East King, Room 205
Carson City, NV 89710
(702) 885-4885

## NEW HAMPSHIRE
Chief
Newborn Screening Coordinator
Bureau of Special Medical Services
Health and Human Services Building
6 Hazen Drive
Concord, NH 03301
(603) 271-4518

## NEW JERSEY
Special Child Health Services Program
State Department of Health
CN 364
Trenton, NJ 08625
(609) 984- 0775

## NEW MEXICO
Newborn Genetic Screening Program
Scientific Laboratory Division
700 Camino De Salud, N.E.
Albuquerque, NM 87106
(505) 841-2581

## NEW YORK
Director, Newborn Screening Program
Laboratory of Human Genetics
Wadsworth Center for Laboratories and Research
State Department of Health
Empire State Plaza

Albany, NY 12201
(518) 473-7552

## NORTH CAROLINA
Director, Genetics Program
Division of Health Services
Department of Human Resources
P.O. Box 2091
Raleigh, NC 27602
(919) 733-7437

## NORTH DAKOTA
Director
Division of Maternal and Child Health
State Department of Health
Capitol Building
Bismarck, ND 58505
(701) 224-2493

## OHIO
State Department of Health
P.O. Box 43266- 0118
Columbus, OH 43215
(614) 466-4644

## OKLAHOMA
Director, Pediatric Division
State Department of Health
1000 N.E. 10th Street
P.O. Box 53551
Oklahoma City, OK 73152
(405) 271-4471

## OREGON
Oregon State Health Division
P.O. Box 231
Portland, OR 97207
(503) 229-6390

## PENNSYLVANIA
Director, Neonatal Metabolic Screening Program
State Department of Health
Room 725
P.O. Box 90
Harrisburg, PA 17108
(717) 787-7440

## PUERTO RICO
Dean, School of Medicine
University of Puerto Rico
G.P.O. Box 5067
San Juan, Puerto Rico 00936
(809) 765- 2363

## RHODE ISLAND
Health Laboratory Building
State Department of Health
50 Orms Street

Providence, RI 02904
(401) 274-1011

## SOUTH CAROLINA

Director, Bureau of Maternal and Child Health
Department of Health and Environmental Control
J. Marion Sims Building
2600 Bull Street
Columbia, SC 29201
(803) 734-4670

## SOUTH DAKOTA

Division of Health Services
South Dakota Department of Health
523 East Capitol Street
Pierre, SD 57501
(605) 773-3737

## TENNESSEE

Division of Maternal and Child Health
State Department of Health and Environment
One Hundred 9th Avenue North, 3rd Floor
Nashville, TN 37219-5405
(615) 741-7335

## TEXAS

Coordinator
Newborn Screening Program
Bureau of Maternal and Child Health
Texas Department of Health
1100 West 49th Street
Austin, TX 78756
(512) 458-7700

## UTAH

Genetic Nurse Consultant
Division of Family Health Services
State Department of Health
44 Medical Drive
Salt Lake City, UT 84113
(801) 533-4084

## VERMONT

Director
Medical Services Division
Vermont Department of Health
1193 North Avenue
P.O. Box 70
Burlington, VT 05402
(802) 863-7330

## VIRGINIA

Genetic Metabolic Nurse Coordinator
State Department of Health
Bureau of Maternal and Child Health
109 Governor Street, Room 624
Richmond, VA 23219
(804) 786-7367

## WASHINGTON

Genetic Services Section
Department of Social and Health Services
1704 N.E. 150th Street
Seattle, WA 98155
(206) 545-6783

## WEST VIRGINIA

Division of Maternal and Child Health
State Department of Health
1143 Dunbar Avenue
Dunbar, WV 25064
(304) 768-6295

## WISCONSIN

Director
State Laboratory of Hygiene
465 Henry Mall
Madison, WI 53706
(608) 262-1293

## WYOMING

Director, Family Health Services
State Department of Health and Social Services
Hathaway Office Building, 4th Floor
Cheyenne, WY 82002
(307) 777-6297

# 8.
# THE MATERNAL PKU
# COLLABORATIVE STUDY

The success of the nationwide neonatal phenylketonuria (PKU) screening programs implemented in the early 1960s created an unexpected problem as women with PKU reached childbearing age. Retrospective surveys have revealed that maternal blood phenylalinine (phe) levels ≥ 20 mg/dl during pregnancy are asssociated with a high rate of mental retardation, microcephaly, congenital heart defects and intrauterine growth retardation among offspring of women with untreated maternal PKU.

To study this problem, the National Institute of Child Health and Human Development launched a seven-year collaborative effort involving fifty states, the District of Columbia and all of the provinces of Canada. The Maternal PKU Collaborative Study (MPKUCS) is a prospective, longitudinal, observational investigation designed to evaluate the efficacy of a phe-restricted diet in reducing the morbidity associated with maternal hyperphenylalaninemia (HPA).

The enrollment of HPA subjects commenced on November 1, 1984. Women of childbearing age, whose blood phe concentrations while on unrestricted diets are ≥ 4 mg/dl, are invited to participate in the study. In addition to women planning pregnancy, or at high risk for unplanned pregnancies, all women 18 years of age or older, who are willing to participate in the study, should be enrolled. Early enrollment, independent of plans for pregnancy, is encouraged in order to identify and counsel women about the importance of initiating dietary therapy prior to conception.

The plan of treatment for women desiring pregnancy involves the initiation of diet prior to conception, the provision of adequate nutrition during pregnancy, offering dietary restriction of phe for women with blood phe levels ≥ 10 mg/dl, and dietary supplementation with tyrosine and other micronutrients, as medically indicated.

For purposes of the study's protocol, obstetrical monitoring during pregnancy includes routine prenatal examinations, nutritional evaluations, laboratory tests and ultrasound for the determination of gestational age and intrauterine growth. Offspring will be followed for six years to assess physical, neurological, cognitive and psychosocial development. Data will also be collected on office-matched and familial control subjects and on pregnant mates of HPA males.

Additional information on the MPKUCS may be obtained by contacting the coordinating center in Los Angeles or the contributing center for your region, listed below.

## COORDINATING CENTER

Maternal PKU Collaborative Study
Childrens Hospital of Los Angeles
4650 Sunset Boulevard
Los Angeles, CA 90027
(213) 669-2152

## NICHD

Contracts Management Section
Office of Grants and Contracts
NICHD, NIH
Landow Building, Room 6C-29
7910 Woodmont Avenue
Bethesda, MD 20892
(301) 496-4611

Mental Retardation and Developmental Disabilities Branch
NICHD, NIH
Landow Building, Room 7C-09
7910 Woodmont Avenue
Bethesda, MD 20892
(301) 496-1383

## CONTRIBUTING CENTERS

### NORTHEAST REGION
Connecticut, Delaware, New Hampshire, Maine, Maryland, Massachusetts, New Jersey, New York, Pennsylvania, Rhode Island, Vermont, Virginia, West Virginia, District of Columbia

IEM–PKU Program
Childrens Hospital Medical Center
Gardner 6, Room 650
283 Longwood Avenue
Boston, MA 02115
(617) 735-7945

### SOUTHEAST REGION
Alabama, Arkansas, Florida, Georgia, Louisiana, Mississippi, North Carolina, South Carolina, Tennessee, Texas

Department of Pediatrics
University of Texas Medical Branch
Galveston, TX 77550
(409) 761-2355

## WESTERN REGION
Alaska, Arizona, California, Colorado, Hawaii, Idaho, Montana, Nevada, New Mexico, Oregon, Utah, Washington, Wyoming

PKU Section
Childrens Hospital of Los Angeles
4650 Sunset Boulevard
Los Angeles, CA 90027
(213) 669-2152

### MIDWEST REGION
Illinois, Indiana, Iowa, Kansas, Kentucky, Michigan, Minnesota, Missouri, Nebraska, North Dakota, Ohio, Oklahoma, South Dakota, Wisconsin

Department of Pediatrics
Room 1311-N CSB
840 South Wood Street
Chicago, IL 60612
(312) 996-5305

### CANADA
The Hospital for Sick Children
555 University Avenue
Toronto, Ontario
Canada M5G 1X8
(416) 597-1500

# 9.
# RECREATION RESOURCES

**Accent on Information**
P.O. Box 700
Bloomington, IL 61701
(309) 378-2961

Database information on recreation and disabilities available by phone. All searches charge a small fee.

**American Alliance for Health, Physical Education, Recreation and Dance**
Adapted Physical Activity Council
1900 Association Drive
Reston, VA 22091
(703) 476-3430

Membership organization for recreation teachers and leaders. Publishes *Able-Bodies* newsletter that reports to membership on successful recreation programs, adaptations and methods.

**American Camping Association**
Bradford Woods
5000 State Road 67 North
Martinsville, IN 46151
(317) 342-8456

Accredits camps nationwide and publishes *A Guide to Accredited Camps* ($9.95), which lists over 2,000 approved camps, including listings by disability. Catalog of over 450 titles on camping and nature also available. Orders only, call 1-800-428- 2267.

**American Wheelchair Sailing Association**
Duncan Milne
512 Thirtieth Street
Newport Beach, CA 92663

**Association of Handicapped Artists**
5150 Broadway
Depew, NY 14043
(716) 683-4624

Company that markets cards and calendars of mouth and foot painters. Information on how to join, where to get supplies and adaptive equipment is available by calling or writing.

**Boy Scouts of America, Scouting for the Handicapped**
1325 Walnut Hill Lane
P.O. 152079

Irving, TX 75015
(214) 580-2000

Open to any youth ages 6-20. Boy Scouts will adapt a program to the special needs of the youths involved and work with the parents for support, involvement and leadership. Contact the local Boy Scout Council.

**Canadian Association for Disabled Skiing**
Box 307
Kimberley, British Columbia
Canada V1A 2Y9
(604) 427-7712

Governing body of nine provincial divisions. Specific programs within divisions, no age limits.

**Canadian Recreational Canoeing Association**
P.O. Box 500
Hyde Park, Ontario
Canada N0M 1Z0
(519) 473-2109

More information available in videocassette or manual form.

**Canadian Wheelchair Sports Association**
160 James Naismith Drive
Gloucester, Ontario
Canada K1B 5N4
(613) 748-5685

Governs 10 sports, most with junior divisions. Programs start at age 8. Provincial branches in every province from which 80 juniors participate in competition at one central location.

*Committee on Recreation and Leisure Newsletter*
President's Committee on Employment of People with Disabilities
Washington, DC 20210
(202) 653-5044

Magazine aimed at employers, containing a section devoted to recreation.

**Girl Scouts of the USA**
Martha Jo Dennison
830 Third Ave. & 51st St.
New York, NY 10022
(212) 940-7736

Open to girls ages 5-17, kindergarten-12th grade. National office will help parents coordinate with local Girl Scout Councils.

**Handicapped Scuba Association**
116 W. El Portal, Suite 104
San Clemente, CA 92672
(714) 498-6128

Programs available to young adults. Participation requires another family member or adult to work with the person with a disability in a team.


**HEALTHsports, Inc.**
1455 West Lake Street
Minneapolis, MN 55408
(612) 827-3232

Ski for Light International, an event for blind, physically handicapped and guides. Program also sponsors events at local and regional levels.


**I CAN Network**
University of Virginia
Adapted Physical Education Program
221 Memorial Gymnasium
Charlottesville, VA 22903
PE Helpline: (804) 924-6192

Responds to requests for information regarding physical education and sport opportunities for people with disabilities. Works to facilitate communication between athletes, parents, teachers, professors and students in the field of adapted physical education.


**International Foundation for Wheelchair Tennis**
Peter Burwash Associates
2203 Timberloch Place, Suite 126
The Woodlands, TX 77380
(713) 363-4707

Connects wheelchair tennis players with professional players for lessons.


**International Wheelchair Road Racers Club, Inc.**
Joseph M. Dowling, President
30 Myano Lane
Stamford, CT 06902
(203) 967-2231

Keeps wheelchair road racers up to date on races and other events through newsletters.


*The Itinerary Magazine*
P.O. Box 1084
Bayonne, NJ 07001-1084
(201) 858- 3400

Magazine for travelers with disabilities; also organizes tours.


**National Archery Association**
1750 E. Boulder St.
Colorado Springs, CO 80909
(719) 578-4576

Nationwide program for children under 18. Membership application and more information are available.


**National Foundation for Horsemanship for the Handicapped**
Box 462
Malvern, PA 19355
(215) 644-7414

Advisory center for the evaluation of programs and the exchange of ideas and experience in therapeutic horsemanship. Sponsor of an international conference of riders with disabilities held September 1989.


**National Handicapped Sports and Recreation Association**
1145 19th St. N.W., Suite 717
Washington, DC 20036
(301) 652-7505

Family-oriented programs that focus on involving people with disabilities in various recreational activities. Fifty-seven chapters in 34 states, offering such programs as aerobics, skiing and white-water rafting. Most programs are open to all ages.


*The National Hookup*
Ruth B. Meyette, Editor
32 Margaret Drive
Albany, NY 12211
(518) 459-8563

Newsletter published by Indoor Sports Club for the Physically Disabled. Call or write for information or for a copy of the newsletter.


**National Park Service**
Division of Special Programs and Populations
P.O. 37127
Washington, DC 20013-7127
(202) 343-4747

Provides technical assistance for National Parks to improve accessibility to people with special needs, focuses primarily on correcting architectural barriers.


**National Theater of the Deaf**
P.O. Box 659
Chester, CT 06412
(203) 526-4971

Two touring companies: National Theater of the Deaf and Little Theater of the Deaf, a family oriented program that appears at schools and parks across the country. Tour schedules are available.

**National Therapeutic Recreation Society**
3101 Park Center Drive
Alexandria, VA 22302
(703) 820-4940

Organization serving professionals, associates and
agencies that provide recreational services to people
with disabilities. NTRS also provides information
on local resources and materials.

**National Wheelchair Athletic Association**
1604 E. Pike's Peak Ave.
Colorado Springs, CO 80909
(303) 597-8330

Juniors program for children ages 6-18 offering six
sports: airguns, archery, swimming, table tennis,
track and field and weightlifting.

**National Wheelchair Basketball**
   **Association**
110 Seaton Building
University of Kentucky
Lexington, KY 40506
(606) 257-1623

Juniors Division of NWBA available. Communities
with existing youth teams receive information and
development of the sport. Call or write for an appropriate program in your area.

**National Wheelchair Games**
National Wheelchair Athletic Assoc.
3617 Betty Drive, Suite S
Colorado Springs, CO 80917
(303) 597-8330

Competition limited to athletes 18 years and older.

**National Wheelchair Softball Association**
Jon Speake, Commissioner
P.O. Box 22478
Minneapolis, MN 55422
(612) 437-1792

Governing body for the National Wheelchair Softball tournaments.

**North American Riding for the**
   **Handicapped,   Inc.**
P.O. Box 33150
Denver, CO 80233
(303) 452-1212

Serves more than 18,000 disabled individuals in
over 450 programs in U.S and Canada, including
both youth and adult riders, no age limit.

**Performing Arts Theater of the Handicapped**
   **(PATH)**
P.O. Box 9050
Carlsbad, CA 92208
(619) 438-3498

**Physically Challenged Swimmers of America**
Joan Karpuk
22 William Street, #225
South Glastonbury, CT 06073

**Recreation Information Management**
U.S. Department of Agriculture, Forest Service
South Building
12st St. & Independence Ave., S.W.
Washington, DC 20250
(202) 382-9402

Provides outdoor recreation on national lands. Also
works on projects to improve access for people with
disabilities. Local projects in the works include bro-
chures on the accessibilty of specific regions.

*Slate and Style*
National Federation for the Blind
2704 Beach Drive
Merrick, NY 11566

Quarterly magazine published by the Writers Division of the National Federation of the Blind. Sub-
scriptions are available in cassette, large type
($5/year) or Braille ($10/year) format and include
membership in the Writers Division.

**Special Olympics, Inc.**
1350 New York Ave, N.W.,
Suite 500
Washington, DC 20005
(202) 628-3630

Holds competition in numerous sports for ages 8-
adult. More information on local events is available
through state chapters.

**Special Recreation, Inc.**
International Center on Special Recreation
362 Koser Ave.
Iowa City, IA 52246-3038
(319) 337-7578

Information and referral center with special recreation access library and publications on special recreation, including directories, guides and quarterly
newsletters.

**U.S.A. Toy Library Association**
2719 Broadway Ave.
Evanston, IL 60201
(312) 864- 8240

Individual or organization membership, which includes quarterly newsletter and discounts on publications. Some Lekoteks, toy libraries with

adaptive toys and lists of trained professionals, available.

**United States Cerebral Palsy Athletic
    Association, Inc.**
34518 Warren Road, Suite 264
Westland, MI 48185
(313) 425-8961

Governing body for persons with cerebral palsy involved in sports. Youths ages 8-18 can participate in such events as track and field, swimming and cycling; bocci ball is available for persons with more severe disabilities. Competitions are held on the local, regional, and national level. For more information on local sports clubs and programs, contact the national headquarters.

**United States Association for Blind Athletes**
55 West California Avenue
Beach Haven Park, NJ 08008
(609) 492-1017

Develops sports programs for people with visual impairments and sponsors competitions on regional, national and international level. Trains athletes and provides instructional manuals.

**United States Blind Golfers Association**
c/o Patrick Browne, Jr.
300 Carondelet Street
New Orleans, LA 70130
(504) 522-3203

**United States Organization for Disabled Athletes**
Pan-Am Victory Games for Physically Disabled Youth
1101 E. River Cove Street
Tampa, FL 33604
(813) 978- 0101

Olympic-style national and international competition for youths ages 8-18, open to all disabilities. Write for an application, or to participate call Al Orr at (813) 272-5732. To sponsor a child or for more information call Wanda LaVelle at (813) 978- 0101.

**United States Quad Rugby Association**
2418 W. Fall Creek Court
Grand Forks, ND 58201
(701) 772-1961

Organizes competitive teams of quadriplegics, any age.

**United States Wheelchair Racquet-Sports
    Association**
Chip Parmelly
1941 Viento Verano Drive
Diamond Bar, CA 91765
(714) 861-7312

Purpose of organization is to promote awareness of wheelchair racquetball and provide information on programs and wheelchair racquet sports.

**United States Wheelchair Weightlifting
    Federation**
Bill Hens
39 Michael Place
Levittown, PA 19057
(215) 945-1964

Governing body of wheelchair weightlifting. Junior program for 16-18-year-olds. Call or write for more information on programs, the sport itself, adaptive equipment or what to look for in a weightlifting program.

**Very Special Arts**
1331 Pennsylvania Ave., NW
Suite 1205
Washington, DC 20004
(202) 662-8899

Educational affiliate of the John F. Kennedy Center for the Performing Arts, VSA has programs for all ages in all art forms. Every state has an independent organizational branch.

**Wheelchair Motorcycle Association, Inc.**
101 Torrey St.
Brockton, MA 02401
(508) 583-8614

Requests and information on all-terrain wheelchairs and any off- road transportation either with or without a wheelchair. A newsletter is available and a video is upcoming.

**4-H and Youth Development**
U.S. Department of Agriculture
Extension Service,
Room 3860-S
Washington, DC 20250
(202) 447-5516

Most programs integrate disabled children using the buddy-system approach. Children ages 7-19 years can participate. Contact your local county 4-H extension. Services and programs vary from county to county.

Directory of recreation organizations reprinted with the permission of Exceptional Parent Magazine, 1170 Commonwealth Ave., Boston, MA 02134.

# 10.
# SUPPORT GROUPS IN THE
# UNITED KINGDOM

Alzheimer's Disease Society
Bank Buildings
Fulham, Broadway
London SW6 1EP

Association to Combat Huntington's Chorea
Borough House
34A Station Road
Hinckley
Leics LE10 1AP

Association for Research into Restricted Growth
24 Pinchfield
Maple Cross
Rickmansworth
Herts

Association for Spina Bifida and Hydrocephalus
Tavistock House North
Tavistock Square
London WC1H 9HJ

Association for Tuberous Sclerosis of Great Britain
Little Barnsley Farm
Catshill
Bromsgrove
Worcs B61 0WQ

The British Retinitis Pigmentosa Society
24 Palmer Close
Redhill
Surrey RH 1 4BX

Brittle Bone Society
112 City Road
Dundee DD2 2PW

Cleft Lip and Palate Association
Dental Department
Hospital for Sick Children
Great Ormond Street
London WC1N 3JH

The Coeliac Society of the United Kingdom
PO Box 181
London NW2 2QY

Cornelia De Lange Syndrome Foundation
46 Victoria Street
Staple Hill
Bristol

The Cystic Fibrosis Research Trust
5 Blyth Road
Bromley
Kent BR1 3RS

Disabled Drivers' Association
Registered Office
Ashwell Thorpe
Norwich NOR 89W

Down's Children's Association
4 Oxford Street
London W1

Dystrophic Epidermolysis Bullosa Research
  Association
'Debra'
7 Sandhurst Lodge
Wokingham Road
Crowthorne
Berks RG11 7QD

The Friedreich's Ataxia Group
Burleigh Lodge
Knowle Lane
Cranleigh
Surrey GU6 8RD

The Haemophilia Society
PO Box 9
16 Trinity Street
London SE1 1DE

Infantile Hypercalcaemia Foundation
37 Mulberry Green
Old Harlow CM17 0EY

Muscular Dystrophy Group of Great Britain
26 Borough High Street
London SE1 9QG

National Deaf Children's Society
31 Gloucester Place
London 4EA

National Federation of the Blind of the UK
20 Cannon Close
Raynes Park
London SW20

National Society for Phenylketonuria and Allied
  Disorders
18 Wood Close

Joydens Wood
Bexley
Kent

The Neurofibromatosis Association
Link
1 The Alders
Hanworth
Middlesex TW13 6NU

Research Trust for Metabolic Disease in Children
53 Beam Street
Nantwich
Cheshire
CW5 5NF

Royal National Institute for the Blind
224 Great Portland Street
London W1N 6AA

Royal National Institute for the Deaf
105 Gower Street
London WC1E 6AH

Sickle Cell Society
c/o Brent Community Health Council
16 High Street
Harlesden
London NW10 4XL

UK Thalassaemia Society
107 Nightingale Lane
London N8 7QY

# 11.
# ORGANIZATIONS IN CANADA

## Genetic Counseling Services

### BRITISH COLUMBIA
**Vancouver**
Department of Medical Genetics
Grace Hospital
4490 Oak St.
Vancouver, B.C. V6H 3V5
(604) 875-2157

**Kamloops, Kelowna, Pentington and Vernon Outreach Clinics**
c/o Thomposn-Okanagan Genetic Outreach
   Program
South Okanagan Health Unit
390 Queensway Ave.
Kelowna, B.C. V1Y 6S7
(604) 762-2704

### Alberta
**Calgary**
Medical Genetics Clinic
Alberta Children's Hospital
1820 Richmond
Calgary, Alta. T2T 5C7
(403) 229- 7373 or
229-7376 (collect)

**Edmonton**
Edmonton Genetics Clinic
2C3-44 WC MacKenzie Health Sciences Centre
University of Alberta
Edmonton, Alta.
T6G 2R7
(403) 432-4077 or 432-7006 (collect)

*Hereditary Diseases Program: Outreach Services[a]*

**Fort McMurray**
Fort McMurray & Dist. Health Unit
9921 Main St.
Fort McMurray, Alta.
T9H 4B4
(403) 743-3232

**Lethbridge**
Lethbridge Genetics Clinic
801-1st St. S.

Lethbridge, Alta. T1J 4L5
(403) 327-2166

**Red Deer**
Red Deer Health Unit
4920 51st St.
Red Deer, Alta. T4N 6K8
(403) 346-7741

**Grande Prairie**
South Peace Health Unit
1032 99th St.
Grande Prairie, Alta.
T8Z 6J4
(403) 532-4441

**Medicine Hat**
South East Alberta Health Unit
2948 Dunmore Rd., S.E.
Medicine Hat, Alta.
T1A 8E3
(403) 526-7950

### MANITOBA
**Winnipeg**
Dept. of Genetics
Health Sciences Centre
685 William St.
Winnipeg, Man. R3E 0Z1
(204) 787-4350

### Saskatchewan
*Outreach Services*

**Saskatoon**
Division of Medical Genetics
Dept. of Pediatrics
Room 515, Ellis Hall
University Hospital
Saskatoon, Sask. S7N 0X0
(306) 966-1692

**Regina**
Pediatric Outpatient Dept.
   Regina General Hospital
1440 14th Ave.

[a.] Hereditary Diseases Program Nurse may be contacted at most Health Units in the province.

Regina, Sask.
S4P 0W5
(306) 359- 4289

## ONTARIO

### Hamilton
Human Genetics Program
McMaster University Medical Centre
1200 Main St. W.
Hamilton, Ont. L8N 3Z5
(416) 525- 9140, x 2278

### Kingston
Division of Medical Genetics
Dept. of Pediatrics
Queen's University
20 Barrie St.
Kingston, Ont. K7L 3N6
(613) 545-6310

### London
Regional Medical Genetics Centre
Children's Hospital of Western Ontario
800 Commissionors Rd. E.
London, Ont. N3A 4G5
(519) 685-8140

### Oshawa
Genetic Services
Oshawa General Hospital
24 Alma St.
Oshawa, Ont. L1G 2B9
(416) 686-1888

### Ottawa
Division of Genetics
Children's Hospital of Eastern Ontario
401 Smyth Rd.
Ottawa, Ont. K1H BL1
(613) 737-2275

### Metropolitan Toronto Region
The Credit Valley Hospital
2200 Eglinton Ave. W.
Mississauga, Ont.
L5M 2N1
(416) 820-2696

Clinical Genetics Diagnostic Centre
North York General Hospital and IODE
Children's Centre
4001 Leslie St.
North York, Ont. M2K 1E1
(416) 756-6345

Dept. of Genetics
Hospital for Sick Children
555 University Ave.
Toronto, Ont. M5G 1X8
(416) 598-6390

Toronto General Hospital[a]
200 Elizabeth St.
Toronto, Ont.
M5G 2C4
(416) 595-3019

The Wellesley Hospital[a]
Prenatal Program
160 Wellesley St. E.
Toronto, Ont.
M4Y 1J3
(416) 966-6600

Surrey Place Centre[b]
Dept. of Genetics
2 Surrey Place
Toronto, Ont. M5S 2C2
(416) 925-5141

*Outreach Services*

### North Bay
Genetic Services
North Bay & District Health Unit
P.O. Box 450
200 McIntyre St. E.
North Bay, Ont.
P1B 8V6
(705) 474-1400

### Peterborough
Genetic Services
Peterborough County—City Health Unit
835 Weller St.
Peterborough, Ont.
K9J 4Y1
(705) 743-1160

### Sault Ste. Marie
Genetic Services
Algoma Health Unit
99 Foster Dr.
Sault Ste. Marie P6A 5X6
(705) 759-5289

### Sudbury
Genetic Services
Sudbury & Dist. Health Unit

[a.] Prenatal diagnosis services only.
[b.] Esp. psychiatry and mental retardation.

1300 Paris Ctr.
Sudbury, Ont. P3E 3A3
(705) 522-9200

**Thunder Bay**
Genetic Services
Thunder Bay District Health Unit
999 Balmoral Ave.
P.O. Box 1024
Thunder Bay, Ont. P7C 4Y7
(807) 622-3961

**Timmins**
Genetic Services
Porcupine Health Unit
Postal Bag 2012
Timmins, Ont. P4N 8B7
(705) 267-1181

**Windsor**
Genetic Services
Metro—Windsor—Essex County Health Unit
1005 Quelette Ave.
Windsor, Ont. N9A 4J8
(519) 258-2146

# QUEBEC
**Montreal**
Hôpital Ste.-Justine
Clinique Génétique
3175 Côte- Ste. Catherine
Montréal, Que. H3T 1C5
(514) 345-4727

Montreal Children's Hospital
Division of Medical Genetics
2300 Tupper St.
Montreal, Que.
H3H 1P3
(514) 934-4432

Montreal General Hospital[c]
Division of Medical Genetics
1650 Cedar Ave.
Montreal, Que.
(514) 937-6011

**Quebec City**
Génétique Humain
Centre hospitalier de l'université Laval
2705 Boul. Laurier
Québec (Québec)
G1V 4G2
(418) 656-4141

[c.] Adult service only.

**Sherbrooke**
Centre hospitalier de l'université de Sherbrooke
3001 12$^e$ ave nord
Sherbrooke (Québec)
J1H 5N0
(819) 563-5555

# NOVA SCOTIA
**Halifax**
Atlantic Research Centre for Mental Retardation
Room C-RI, Clinical Research Centre
5849 University Ave.
Halifax, N.S.
B3H 4H7
(902) 494-6491

## Newfoundland
**St. John's**
Genetics Clinic
Janeway Child Health Centre
Newfoundland Dr.
St. John's Nfld. A1A 1R8
(709) 778- 4386

Community Medicine
Health Sciences Centre
St. John's, Nfld.
A1B 3V6
(709) 737-6693

*Note:* Outreach clinics: Fortreau Labrador (for he-mophilia), Gander, and Grand Falls. Referrals for outreach through the Janeway Centre.

**Selection of Voluntary Organizations Involved with Genetic Diseases**

**Achondroplasia and skeletal dysplasias**
Little People of Canada, Inc.
Karen Renner
16585 84th Avenue
Surrey, B.C. V3S 4N7

Little People of Ontario, Inc.
P.O. Box 19
Agincourt, Ont. M1S 2T1

**Amytropic lateral sclerosis**
ALS Society of Canada
234 Eglinton Avenue East
Suite 305
Toronto, Ont. M4P 1K5

**Charcot-Marie Tooth**
Carchot-Marie Tooth International
34-B Bayview Drive
St. Catharines, Ont. L2N 4Y6

**Cleft lip and palate**
Canadian Cleft Lip and Palate Family Association
Suite 649
170 Elizabeth Street
Toronto, Ont. M5G 1E8

**Cystic fibrosis**
Canadian Cystic Fibrosis Foundation
2221 Yonge Street
Suite 601
Toronto, Ont. M4S 2B4

**Down syndrome**
Down Syndrome Association of Metropolitan
   Toronto
307 Lonsdale Road
Toronto, Ont. M4V 1X3

**Dystonia**
Dystonia Medical Research Foundation
777 Hornby Street, #1800
Vancouver, B.C. V6Z 1S4

**Growth**
The Foundation for Growth Problems in Children
Box 4601
London, Ont. N5W 5L7

**Hemophilia**
The Hemophilia Society (Canadian)
100 King Street West #210
Hamilton, Ont. L8P 1A2

**Huntington Disease**
Huntington Society of Canada
13 Water Street North, #3
Box 333
Cambridge, Ont. N1R 5T8

**Kidney disease**

Kidney Foundation of Canada
4060 Ste. Catherine Street W. #555
Montreal, Que. H3Z 2Z3

**Liver diseases**
Canadian Liver Foundation
1320 Yonge St. #301
Toronto, Ont. M4T 1X2

**Lupus**
Lupus Foundation of Canada
Box 3802, Station B
Calgary, Alta. T2M 4LB

Ontario Lupus Association
250 Bloor St. East #401
Toronto, Ont. M4W 3P2

**Malignant hyperthermia**
Malignant Hyperthermia Foundation
2 Bloor Street West
P.O. Box 144
Toronto, Ont. M4W 3E2

**Marfan**
Canadian Marfan Association
RR #2
Luskville, Que. J0X 2G0

**Muscular dystrophy**
Muscular Dystrophy Association of Canada
357 Bay Street
Toronto, Ont. M5H 1T7

**Neurofibromatosis**
Neurofibromatosis Society of Ontario
c/o Division of Neurosurgery
38 Shuter Street
Toronto, Ont. M5B 1A6

**Osteogenesis imperfecta**
Canadian Osteogenesis Imperfecta Society
Box 607, Station U
Toronto, Ont. M8Z 5Y9

**Polyposis**
Polyposis (Familial) Registry
Toronto General Hospital
Eaton Wing, Room 10-315
Toronto, Ont. M5G 1L7

**Prader Willi syndrome**
Prader Willi Association (Ontario)
1788 Stone Path Crescent
Mississauga, Ont. L4X 1X9

**Retinitis pigmentosa**
Retinitis Pigmentosa Foundation of Canada
   (National)
185 Spadina Crescent, #411
Toronto, Ont. M5S 2C6

**Sickle cell disease**
Canadian Sickle Cell Society
1076 Bathurst Street #305
Toronto, Ont. M5R 369

**Spina bifida & hydrocephalus**
Spina Bifida & Hydrocephalus Association of
  Ontario
10 Trinity Square
Toronto, Ont. M5G 1B1

**Thyroid**
Thyroid Foundation of Canada
P.O. Box 1643
Kingston, Ont. K7L 5C8

**Tourette syndrome**
Tourette Syndrome Foundation of Canada
1099 Bay Street #202
Toronto, Ont. M5S 2B3

**Turner syndrome**
Turner Syndrome Society
York University ABS 006
4700 Keele Street
Downsview, Ont. M3T 1P3

**Williams syndrome**
The Canadian Association for Williams Syndrome
1954 West 3rd Avenue, #301
Vancouver, B.C. V6T 1L1

# BIBLIOGRAPHY

Anderson, V.E., W.A. Hauser, J.K. Penny et al. (eds.), *Genetic Basis of the Epilepsies*. New York: Raven Press, 1982.

Atonarakis, S.E., P.G. Waber, S.D. Kittur et al., "Hemophilia A. Detection of Molecular Defects and Carriers by DNA Analysis," *N Eng J Med*, 313(1985): 842.

Applebaum, Eleanor G. and Stephen K. Firestein, *A Genetic Counseling Casebook*. New York: The Free Press (Macmillan, Inc.), 1983.

Arrighi, F.E., E. Stubblefield and P.N. Rao (eds.), *Genes, Chromosomes and Neoplasia*. New York: Raven Press, 1981.

Baird, Patricia A., "Genetic Disorders in Children and Young Adults: A Population Study," *American Journal of Human Genetics*, 42(1988): 677-693.

Bank, A., J.G. Mears and F. Ramirez, "Disorders of Human Hemoglobin," *Science*, 207(1980): 486.

Baraitser, M., *Genetics of Neurological Disorders*. New York: Oxford University Press, 1982.

Beighton, Peter, *Inherited Disorders of the Skeleton*, 2nd ed. New York: Churchill Livingstone Publishers, 1988.

————, *The Man Behind the Syndrome*. New York: Springer-Verlag, 1986.

Bergsma, Daniel, *Birth Defects Compendium*, 2nd edition. New York: Alan Liss, 1979.

Blasi, F. (ed.), *Human Genes and Diseases*. New York: J. Wiley, 1986.

Blau, Sheldon and Dodi Schultz, *The Body Against Itself*. Garden City, N.Y.: Doubleday, 1977.

Blumberg, B., M. Golbus and K. Hanson, "The Psychological Sequelae of Abortion Performed For a Genetic Indication," *Am J Obstet Gynecol*, 122(1975): 799.

Boehm, C.D., S.E. Antonarakis, J.A. Phillips III et al., "Prenatal Diagnosis Using DNA Polymorphisms," *New Eng J Med*, 308(1983): 1054.

Borgaonkar, D.S., *Chromosomal Variation in Man. A Catalog of Chromosomal Variants and Anomalies*. New York: Alan Liss, 1983.

Brock, D.J.H., D. Bedgood, L. Barron et al., "Prospective Prenatal Diagnosis of Cystic Fibrosis," *The Lancet*, 18439 (1985): 1175.

Carter, C.H. (ed.), *Medical Aspects of Mental Retardation*. Springfield: Charles C. Thomas, 1978.

Cavenee, W.K., A.L. Murphree, M.M. Shull et al., "Prediction of Familial Predisposition to Retinoblastoma," *N Eng J Med*, 314(1986): 1201.

Cohen, Felissa L., *Clinical Genetics in Nursing Practice*. Philadelphia: J.B. Lippincott, 1984.

Conneally, P.M., "Huntington's Disease: Genetics and Epidemiology," *Am J Hum Genet*, 36(1984): 506.

Cotlier, E., I.H. Maumenee and E.R. Berman (eds.), *Genetic Eye Disorders: Retinitis Pigmentosa and other Inherited Eye Disorders*. (Birth Defects Original Article Series, vol. 18, no. 6) New York: Alan R. Liss, 1982.

Dalessio, D.J., "Seizure Disorders and Pregnancy," *N Engl J Med*, 3/3(1985): 559.

de Grouchy, J. and C. Turleau, *Clinical Atlas of Human Chromosomes*. New York: John Wiley, 1977.

Der Kaloustian, V.M. and A.K. Kurban, *Genetic Diseases of the Skin*. New York: Springer-Verlag, 1979.

Desnick, R.J. and G.A. Grabowski, "Advances in the Treatment of Inherited Metabolic Diseases," in *Advances in Human Genetics*, vol. 11. New York: Plenum Press, 1981.

Eisenberg, Eileen and Heidi Eisenberg Murkoff, *What to Expect When You're Expecting*. New York: Workman, 1984.

Emery, A.E.H. and D.L. Rimoin (eds.), *Principles and Practice of Medical Genetics*. New York: Churchill Livingstone, 1983.

Eriksson, A.W., H. Forsius, H.R. Nevanlinna, P.L. Workman and P.K. Norio, *Population Structure and Genetic Disorders*. London: Academic Press, 1980.

Federman, D.D., *Abnormal Sexual Development: A Genetic and Endocrine Approach to Differential Diagnosis*. Philadelphia: W.B. Saunders, 1967.

Feigin, R. and J. Cherry, *Textbook of Pediatric Infectious Diseases*. Philadelphia: W.B. Saunders, 1981.

Finnie, Nanci R., I.C.S.P., *Handling the Young Cerebral Palsied Child at Home*. New York: E.P. Dutton, 1975.

Freiherr, G., "Fetal Surgery: Saving the Unborn," *Research Resources Reporter*, 7(1983): 1.

Friedman, T.F., *Gene Therapy: Fact and Fiction in Biology's New Approaches to Disease*. New York: Cold Spring Harbor, 1983.

Fudenberg, H.H., J.R.L. Pink, A.C. Wang and S.D. Douglas, *Basic Immunogenetics*, 2nd ed. New York: Oxford University Press, 1978.

Galjaard, J., *Genetic Metabolic Disease, Early Diagnosis and Prenatal Analysis*. Amsterdam: Elsevier/North Holland, 1980.

Gardner, K.D., Jr. (ed.), *Cystic Diseases of the Kidney*. New York: John Wiley, 1976.

Garver, Kenneth L., *Genetic Counseling for Clinicians*. Chicago: Year Book Medical Publishers, 1986.

*Genetics and Heredity: The Blueprints of Life*. New York: Torstar Books, 1985.

German, J. (ed.), *Chromosomes and Cancer*. New York: John Wiley, 1974.

Glasser, Ronald J., *The Body Is the Hero*. New York: Random House, 1976.

Goldberg, M.F. (ed.), *Genetic and Metabolic Eye Diseases*. Boston: Little, Brown, 1974.

Golbus, M.S., "Antenatal Diagnosis of Hemoglobinopathies, Hemophilia and Hemolytic Anemias," *Clin Obstet Gynecol*, 24(1981): 1055.

Golbus, M.S. and B.D. Hall (eds.), *Diagnostic Approaches to the Malformed Fetus, Abortus, Stillborn and Deceased Newborn*. New York: Alan R. Liss, 1979.

Gomez, M.R. (ed.), *Tuberous Sclerosis*. New York: Raven Press, 1988.

Goodman, Richard M., *Genetic Disorders Among the Jewish People*. Baltimore: Johns Hopkins University Press, 1979.

———, *Planning for a Healthy Baby*. New York: Oxford University Press, 1986.

Goodman, Richard M. and R.J. Gorlin, *Atlas of the Face in Genetic Disorders*, 2nd ed. St. Louis: C.V. Mosby, 1977.

———, *The Malformed Infant and Child*. New York: Oxford University Press, 1983.

Goodman, Richard M. and A.G. Motulsky, *Genetic Diseases Among Ashkenazi Jews*. New York: Raven Press, 1979.

Gorlin, R.J., J.J. Pindborg and M.M. Cohen, *Syndromes of the Head and Neck*, 2nd ed. New York: McGraw-Hill, 1976.

Gottron, H.A. and V.W. Schnyder, *Verebung von Hautkrankheiten*, vol. 7 of "Jadassohn Handbuch." Berlin: Springer-Verlag, 1955.

Graham, John M., *Smith's Recognizable Patterns of Human Deformation*, 2nd ed. Philadelphia: W.B. Saunders, 1988.

Grouse, L.D., "Recognition of Fetal Alcohol Syndrome," *JAMA*, 245(1981): 2436.

Hagerman, R.J. and P.M. McBogg (eds.), *The Fragile X Syndrome*. Dillon, Colorado: Spectra Publishing, 1983.

Harper, P.S., *Practical Genetic Counseling*, 3rd ed. Boston: Wright, 1988.

Harris, H., *The Principles of Human Biochemical Genetics*, 3rd ed. Amsterdam: Elsevier/North-Holland Biomedical Press, 1980.

Hendin, D. and J. Marks, *The Genetics Connection*. New York: Morrow, 1978.

Hobbins, J.C., P.A. Grannum, R.L. Berkowitz et al., "Ultrasound in the Diagnosis of Congenital Anomalies," *Am J. Obstet Gynecol*, 134(1979): 331.

Holbrook, K. (ed.), "Prenatal Diagnosis of Genetic Skin Disease," *Seminars in Dermatology* 3:3(1984).

Holleb, Arthur I. (ed.), *The American Cancer Society Cancer Book*. New York: Doubleday, 1986.

Holm, V.A. and P.L. Pipes, *Prader-Willi Syndrome*. Baltimore: University Park Press, 1981.

Holmes, L.B., H.W. Moser, C.S. Halldorsson, C. Mack, S.S. Paint and B. Matzilevich, *Mental Retardation: An Atlas of Diseases with Associated Physical Abnormalities*. New York: Macmillan, 1972.

Hook, E.B. and P.K. Cross, *Clinical Genetics: Problems in Diagnosis and Counseling*. New York: Academic Press, 1982.

Horrobin, J.M. and J.E. Rynders, *To Give an Edge: A Guide for New Parents of Down's Syndrome (Mongoloid) Children*. Minneapolis: Colwell Press, 1974.

International Commission for Protection Against Environmental Mutagens and Carcinogens, *Perspectives in Mutation Epidemiology*, 6. New York: Elsevier, 1983.

Ionasescu, V. and H. Zellweger, *Genetics of Neurology*. New York: Raven Press, 1983.

Jackson, L.G. and R.N. Schimke (eds.), *Clinical Genetics, A Source Book for Physicians*. New York: John Wiley, 1979.

Jones, Kenneth Lyons, *Smith's Recognizable Patterns of Human Malformation*, 4th ed. Philadelphia: W.B. Saunders, 1988.

Jones, Peter, M.D., *Living With Hemophilia*. Philadelphia: F.A. Davis, 1974, 1984.

Jorgenson, Yoder and Shapiro, *The Pedigree: A Basic Guide*. Grendel Co., 1980.

Kalter, H. and J. Warkany, "Congenital Malformations, Etiologic Factors and Their Role in Prevention," *N Eng J Med*, 308(1983): 425.

Kelly, T.E., *Clinical Genetics and Genetic Counseling*, 2nd ed. Chicago: Year Book Medical Publishers, 1986.

Kessler, S. (ed.), *Genetic Counseling–Psychological Dimensions*. New York: Academic Press, 1979.

Kevles, Daniel J. *In the Name of Eugenics: Genetics and the Uses of Human Heredity*. New York: Knopf, 1985.

Kirkwood, Evelyn and Catriona Lewis, *Understanding Medical Immunology*. New York: John Wiley, 1983.

Kolata, G., "Huntington's Disease Gene Located," *Science*, 222(1983): 913.

Knudson, A.G., "Hereditary Cancer, Oncogenes, and Antioncogens," *Cancer Res*, 45(1985): 1437.

Konigsmark, B.W. and R.J. Gorlin, *Genetic and Metabolic Deafness*. Philadelphia: W.B. Saunders, 1976.

Lammer, E.J., D.T. Chen, R.M. Hoar et al., "Retinoic Acid Embryopathy," *N Eng J Med*, 3/3(1985): 837.

Levitan, Max, *Textbook of Human Genetics*. New York: Oxford University Press, 1977.

Lewontin, Richard C., *Human Diversity*. New York: Scientific American Library, (distributed by) W.H. Freeman, 1982.

Lubs, H.A. and F. De La Cruz (eds.), *Genetic Counseling*. New York: Raven Press, 1977.

Lynch, H.T. (ed.), *Cancer Genetics*. Springfield: C.C. Thomas, 1976.

Lynch, H.T., W.A. Albano, B.S. Danes et al., "Genetic Predisposition to Breast Cancer," *Cancer*, 53(1984): 612.

Macri, J.N., D.A. Baker and R.S. Baim, "Diagnosis of Neural- Tube Defects by Evaluation of Amniotic Fluid," *Clin Obstet Gynecol*, 24(1981): 1089.

Mange, Arthur and Elaine Mange, *Genetics: Human Aspects*. Philadelphia: W.B. Saunders, 1980.

Marimuthu, K.M. and P.M. Gopinath (eds.), *Conference Recent Trends in Medical Genetics* (held in Madras, India, in 1983). New York: Pergamon, 1986.

Maroteaux, P., *Bone Diseases of Children*. Philadelphia: Lippincott, 1979.

McKusick, V.A., *Heritable Disorders of Connective Tissue*, 8th ed. St. Louis: C.V. Mosby, 1988.

———, *Mendelian Inheritance in Man*, new ed. Baltimore: Johns Hopkins University Press, 1986.

Miles, J.H. and M.M. Kaback, "Prenatal Diagnosis of Hereditary Disorders," *Pediatr Clin No Am*, 25(1978): 593.

Milunsky, A. (ed.), *Genetic Disorders and the Fetus: Diagnosis, Prevention, and Treatment*. New York: Plenum Press, 1986.

———, *Know Your Genes*. Boston: Houghton-Mifflin, 1977.

Milunsky, A. and G.J. Annas (eds.), *Genetics and The Law*. New York: Plenum, 1976.

Mulvihill, J.J., R.W. Miller and J.F. Fraumeni (eds.), *Genetics of Human Cancer*. New York: Raven Press, 1977.

Murphy, E.A. and G. Chase, *Principles of Genetic Counseling*. Baltimore: Johns Hopkins University Press, 1975.

National Center for Education in Maternal and Child Health, *State Treatment Centers for Metabolic Disorders*. Washington, D.C.: NCEMCH, 1986.

———, *Social and Psychological Aspects of Genetic Disorders: A Selected Bibliography*. Washington, D.C.: NCEMCH, 1986.

———, *Starting Early: A Guide to Federal Resources in Maternal and Child Health*. Washington, D.C.: NCEMCH, 1988.

National Center for Health Statistics, *Advance Report of Final Mortality Statistics*. Hyattsville, Maryland: NCHS, 1988.

———, *Advance Report of Final Natality Statistics*. Hyattsville, Maryland: NCHS, n.d.

National Clearinghouse for Human Genetic Diseases, *Prenatal Diagnosis and Genetic Counseling*. Washington, D.C.: NCHGD, n.d.

National Institute of Child Care and Human Development, *Diagnostic Ultrasound Imaging in Pregnancy*. Washington, D.C.: NICCHD, 1984.

———, *Mental Retardation and Developmental Disabilities*. Washington, D.C.: NICCHD, 1986.

National Institute of General Medical Sciences, *The New Human Genetics; How Gene Splicing Helps Researchers Fight Inherited Disease*. Washington, D.C.: NIGMS, 1984.

National Organization for Albinism and Hypopigmentation, *What Is Albinism?* Philadelphia: NOAH, n.d.

National Research Council, *Health Risks of Radon and Other Internally Deposited Alpha-Emitters*. Washington, D.C.: NRC, 1988.

Newmark, M.E. and J.K. Penny, *Genetics of Epilepsy: A Review*. New York: Raven Press, 1980.

Newmark, P., "Testing for Cystic Fibrosis," *Nature*, 318(1985): 309.

Nichols, Eve K., *Human Gene Therapy*. Cambridge: Harvard University Press, 1988.

Nora, James J. and F. Clarke Fraser, *Medical Genetics: Principles and Practice*, 3rd ed. Philadelphia: Lea & Febiger, 1989.

Nyhan, William L., *The Heredity Factor: Genes, Chromosomes, and You*. New York: Lea & Febiger, 1989.

O'Brien, R. and M. Chafetz, *The Encyclopedia of Alcoholism*. New York: Facts On File, 1982.

Paluszny, Maria J., *Autism: A Practical Guide for Parents and Professionals*. Syracuse: Syracuse University Press, 1979.

Porter, I.H., N.H. Hatcher and A.M. Willey (eds.), *Prenatal Genetics: Diagnosis and Treatment* (15th New York State Health Department Birth Defects Symposium, Albany, 1984). Orlando: Academic Press, 1986.

Porter, I.H. and E.B. Hook (eds.), *Human Embryonic and Fetal Death*. New York: Academic Press, 1980.

Powledge, T.M. and J. Fletcher, "Ethics of Prenatal Diagnosis," *N Eng J Med*, 300(1979): 168.

President's Commission for the Study of Ethical Problems in Medicine and Behavioral Research, *Screening and Counseling for Genetic Conditions*. Washington, D.C.: U.S. Government Printing Office, 1983.

Pueschel, S.M., *Down Syndrome: Growing and Learning*. Mission, Kansas: Andrews and McNeel, 1978.

Rao, D.C., R.C. Elston, L.H. Fuller et al. (eds.), *Genetic Epidemiology of Coronary Heart Disease: Past, Present, and Future*. New York: Alan R. Liss, 1984.

Reed, S., *Counseling in Medical Genetics*. New York: Alan R. Liss, 1980.

Riccardi, Vincent M., *The Genetic Approach to Human Disease*. New York: Oxford University Press, 1977.

Rimoin, D.L. and R.N. Schimke, *Genetic Disorders of the Endocrine Glands*. St. Louis: C.V. Mosby, 1971.

Rose, N.R., P.E. Bigazzi and N.C. Warner (eds.), *Genetic Control of Autoimmune Disease*. Amsterdam: Elsevier/North Holland, 1978.

Rotter, J.I., "The Modes of Inheritance of Insulin Dependent Diabetes," *Am J Hum Genet*, 34(1981): 835.

Rowley, P.T., "Genetic Screening: Marvel or menace?" *Science*, 225(1984): 138.

Rutter, Michael and Eric Schopler, *Autism: A Practical Guide For Parents and Professionals*. New York: Plenum, 1976.

Schulman, J.D. and J.L. Simpson (eds.), *Genetic Diseases in Pregnancy: Maternal Effects and Fetal Outcome*. New York: Academic Press, 1981.

Schimke, R.N., *Genetics and Cancer in Man*. Edinburgh: Churchill Livingston, 1978.

Scriver, Charles R., Arthur L. Beaudet, William S. Sly and David Valle (eds.), *The Metabolic Basis of Inherited Disease*. New York: McGraw-Hill, 1989.

Scriver, C.R. and L.E. Rosenberg, *Amino Acid Metabolism and Its Disorders*. Philadelphia: W.B. Saunders, 1973.

Shepard, T.H., *Catalog of Teratogenic Agents*, 5th ed. Baltimore: Johns Hopkins University Press, 1986.

Sherlock, P. and S.J. Winawer, "Are There Markers for the Risk of Colorectal Cancer?" *Eng J Med*, 311(1984): 118.

Simoni, G., B. Brambati, C. Danesino et al., "Efficient Direct Chromosome Analyses and Enzyme Determinations From Chorionic Villi Samples in the First Trimester of Pregnancy," *Hum Genet*, 63(1983): 349.

Simpson, J.L., *Disorders of Sexual Differentiation: Etiology and Clinical Delineation*. New York: Academic Press, 1976.

Smithells, R.W., N.C. Nevin, M.J. Seller et al., "Further Experience of Vitamin Supplementation For the Prevention of Neural-Tube Defect Recurrences," *Lancet*, 8332(1983): 1027.

Sorsby, A., *Ophthalmic Genetics*. London: Butterworth, 1970.

Spranger, J.W., L.O. Langer Jr. and J.R. Wiedemann, *Bone Dysplasias. An Atlas of Constitutional Disorders of Skeletal Development*. Stuttgart: Gustav Fischer Verlag, 1974.

Stagnos, S. and R.J. Whitley, "Herpesvirus Infections in Pregnancy," *N Eng J Med*, 313(1985): 1270, 1327.

Stanbury, J.B., J.B. Wyngaarden, D.S. Fredrickson, J.L. Goldstein and M.S. Brown, *The Metabolic Basis of Inherited Disease*, 5th ed. New York: McGraw-Hill, 1983.

Stehm, R. and V. Fulginiti, *Immunologic Disorders in Infants and Children*, 2nd ed. Philadelphia: W.B. Saunders, 1980.

Stewart, R.R. and G.H. Prescott (eds.), *Oral Facial Genetics*. St. Louis: C.V. Mosby, 1976.

Summit, R.L., *Clinical Genetics, A Source Book for Physicians*. New York: John Wiley, 1980.

Taft, L.T., "Mental Retardation Overview," *Pediatr Ann*, 2(1973): 10.

Temtamy, S.A. and V.A. McKusick, *The Genetics of Hand Malformations*. New York: Alan R. Liss, 1978.

Thompson, Charlotte E., *Raising A Handicapped Child*. New York: Ballantine, n.d.

Thompson, J.S. and M.W. Thompson, *Genetics in Medicine*, 4th ed. Philadelphia: W.B. Saunders, 1986.

Tsuang, M.X.T. and R. Vandermey, *Genes and the Mind; Inheritance of Mental Illness*. New York: Oxford University Press, 1980.

United Nations Scientific Committee on the Effects of Atomic Radiation, *1982 Report to the General Assembly: Ionizing Radiation: Sources and Biological Effects*. New York: United Nations, 1982.

U.S. Department of Health and Human Services, *Congenital Malformations Surveillance*. Atlanta: Centers for Disease Control, 1988.

————, *Leading Major Congenital Malformations Among Minority Groups in the United States, 1981–1986*, Morbidity and Mortality Weekly Report. Atlanta: Centers for Disease Control, 1988.

————, *Premature Mortality Due to Congenital Anomalies—United States*, Morbidity and Mortality Weekly Report. Atlanta: Centers for Disease Control, 1988.

U.S. Department of Health, Education and Welfare, *Antenatal Diagnosis*, NIH Publication No. 79. Washington, D.C.: HEW, 1973, 1979.

Vinken, P.J. and G.W. Bruyn (eds.), *Handbook of Clinical Neurology.* Amsterdam: Elsevier/North Holland, 1970 (vol. 10), 1972 (vols. 13, 14), 1982 (vol. 43).

Vogel, F. and A.G. Motulsky, *Human Genetics: Problems and Approaches*, 2nd ed. Berlin: Springer-Verlag, 1986.

Waardenberg, P.J., A. Franceschetti and D. Klein, *Genetics and Ophthalmology.* Springfield, Ill.: C.C. Thomas, 1961 (vol. 1), 1963 (vol. 2).

Warkany, J., *Congenital Malformations.* Chicago: Year Book Medical Publishers, 1971.

Warkany, J., R.J. Lemire and M.M. Cohen, *Mental Retardation and Congenital Malformations of the Central Nervous System.* Chicago: Year Book Publishers, 1981.

Weaver, David D., *Catalog of Prenatally Diagnosed Conditions.* Baltimore: Johns Hopkins University Press, 1989.

Whaley, Lucille, *Understanding Inherited Disorders.* St. Louis: C.B. Mosby, 1974.

Wilson, J.G. and F.C. Fraser (eds.), *Handbook of Teratology*, vols. 1–4. New York: Plenum, 1977.

Wright, E.E. and M.V.Shaw, "Legal Liability in Genetic Screening, Genetic Counseling and Prenatal Diagnosis," *Clinical Obstetrics & Gynecology* (1981).

Wyngaarden, W.B. and L.H. Smith (eds.), *Cecil Textbook of Medicine*, 16th ed. Philadelphia: W.B. Saunders, 1982.

Wynne-Davies, R., *Heritable Disorders in Orthopaedic Practice.* Oxford: Blackwell, 1973.

Yunis, J.J. (ed.), *New Chromosomal Syndromes.* New York: Academic Press, 1979.

# BIOGRAPHICAL SKETCH

James Wynbrandt's writing has been honored by the International Reading Association, the National Society of Professional Engineers, the Fiscal Policy Council, the International Radio Programming Forum and other organizations. In addition to a broad background in scientific subjects, he has authored books on corporate management issues, popular music and sports training. His work frequently appears in magazines and on nationally syndicated radio programs, and he also writes for a variety of corporations and government and international agencies. He lives in New York City.

Mark D. Ludman, M.D., F.R.C.P.C., is a consultant pediatrician and clinical geneticist, with a particular interest in inherited metabolic diseases. Following his undergraduate and medical education at Brown University, he took his postgraduate training in pediatrics and medical genetics at the Mount Sinai Hospital in New York City. After several years on the faculty of the Mount Sinai School of Medicine, he crossed the 49th parallel. He is presently an assistant professor of pediatrics in the Faculty of Medicine of Dalhousie University in Halifax, Nova Scotia, where he is also a senior investigator at the Atlantic Research Centre for Mental Retardation. He is a Fellow of the Royal College of Physicians of Canada and a Diplomate of the American boards of Pediatrics and Medical Genetics. He is married to a child psychologist and has two wonderful sons.

# INDEX

Boldface type indicates main entry.